Medical and Veterinary Entomology

D.S. Kettle
Professor of Entomology
University of Queensland

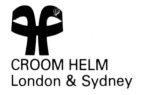

CROOM HELM
London & Sydney

© 1984 D.S. Kettle
Croom Helm Ltd, Provident House, Burrell Row,
Beckenham, Kent BR3 1AT
Croom Helm Australia Pty Ltd, First Floor,
139 King Street, Sydney, NSW 2001, Australia

British Library Cataloguing in Publication Data

Kettle, D.S.
    Medical and veterinary entomology
    1. Entomology
    I. Title
    595.7   QL436
    ISBN 0-85664-839-6

To my Father and Mother whose
unobtrusive sacrifices made my
university training possible

Typeset by Leaper & Gard Ltd, Bristol
Printed and bound in Great Britain by
Mackays of Chatham Ltd

CONTENTS

Part III: Diseases of which the Pathogens are Transmitted by Insects or Acarines

ACKNOWLEDGEMENTS

This book was begun when I was a visiting scholar at Corpus Christi College, University of Cambridge, to which I am indebted for the opportunity to write in a stimulating environment. It was largely completed during a six-months special studies programme free from teaching responsibilities at the University of Queensland.

I am particularly grateful to Dr R. Domrow for his helpful detailed comments on Chapters 20 and 21 (Mites), and to Drs R.L. Doherty and the late R.H. Wharton for their valuable comments on Chapters 24 (Arboviruses) and 30 (Lymphatic Filariasis), respectively. Other colleagues who generously gave of their time and expertise include Drs J.H. Bryan, D. Hoyte, D.E. Moorhouse, R.M. Newson, B.H. Kay, D. Kemp, Mr T. McRae, Drs G. Monteith, D. Murray, M. Ramsamy, M.J. Rice, W.M. Rogoff, J.P. Spradbery, J.B. Walker and T.E. Woodward.

It is a pleasure to acknowledge the exemplary typing of both the draft and final manuscripts by Miss C. Buckley and Mrs R. Crombie, and the invaluable assistance of my wife, Babs Kettle, who carefully and thoughtfully read every chapter, improving the punctuation and drawing attention to obscurities and inconsistencies. I appreciated the helpful co-operation of many librarians, especially those of the Biological Sciences Library at the University of Queensland.

I am indebted to Ms Jane Harthoorn for many excellent detailed original illustrations, not all of which bear her logo, and to Dr Jenny Graaf who, at a critical time, volunteered to do additional illustrations. Figures 2.7, 2.8, 2.10, 2.12, 2.18 and 2.19 are reproduced from Queensland Museum Booklet 13, by permission of the Trustees. Other illustrations are reproduced by permission of: Academic Press (27.1, 28.1); *American Midland Naturalist* (22.1, 22.2); Athlone Press (23.1); Australian Entomological Society (8.6, 8.8); Baillière Tindall (11.1A, 11.1C, 14.6, 16.1B, 18.3, 22.3); *Biological Reviews* (5.1); British Museum (Natural History) (7.6, 7.12); *British Veterinary Journal* (15.7); *Bulletin of Entomological Research* (5.2, 7.11, 16.2); Butterworths (13.4, 14.3, 14.7, 15.4, 15.8); Cambridge University Press (4.4, 4.5, 5.4, 5.5B, 7.5, 7.10 left, 13.5, 19.6, 23.3, 23.4); *Canadian Journal of Zoology* (8.9, 8.10); Freshwater Biological Association (10.4); Gustav Fischer Verlag (4.6); *Journal of Medical Entomology* (8.11, 9.7); *Journal of Parasitology* (21.11, 21.13, 23.2); H.K. Lewis (4.7, 12.1, 12.2, 12.4, 12.5); Liverpool School of Tropical Medicine (8.5, 14.8); Melbourne University Press (2.15, 3.2, 4.2B, 13.1B, 14.1, 17.6); *Microentomology* (7.2); Pacific Coast Entomological Society (19.2, 19.5A); *Physiologia Comparata et Oecologia* (10.5); *Quarterly*

Journal of Microscopical Science (5.5A); Royal Entomological Society of London (8.5, 8.6, 8.7); Royal Highland and Agricultural Society (15.1, 15.5, 15.6, 15.10, 15.11); Royal Society of Edinburgh (11.4, 11.5); Royal Society of London (5.6); Smithsonian Miscellaneous Collection (4.1, 4.9, 4.10); Thacker and Spink (7.7, 7.8, 7.9).

PART 1
GENERAL INTRODUCTION TO MEDICAL AND VETERINARY ENTOMOLOGY

1 INTRODUCTION

The science of Entomology should, strictly speaking, be restricted to the six-legged animals or Insecta, but the applied entomologist is expected to cover a wider field. The agricultural entomologist is often required to advise on soil nematodes and to distinguish between damage done by insects and that due to other pathogens such as viruses. The medical and veterinary entomologist is expected to deal with the Acari, i.e. ticks and mites, and to be reasonably informed on the other terrestrial Arthropoda, e.g. spiders, scorpions etc. In this book I shall use the term 'medical entomologist' in place of the more accurate but cumbersome 'medical and veterinary entomologist,' and references to 'medical entomology' should be taken to include veterinary entomology. Similarly, when used in a general sense the terms 'entomology' and 'insects' should be taken to include the Acari as well as the Insecta.

Medical entomology is concerned with the role of insects in the causation of disease in animals and man. This concern is paramount and hence the centre of interest of the medical entomologist must be disease incidence and disease control, not the insect and insect control. Insect control is one means of disease control and, in a particular setting, may not be the most appropriate method. Where disease incidence is low and the insect widespread, it may be more realistic to treat cases as they arise than to attempt control of the vector. The medical entomologist who forgets this primary involvement with disease and focuses all his attention on the insect does a disservice to his profession. He may be a better entomologist but not necessarily a good medical entomologist.

Animal and human disease arise basically from two causes: the presence of an introduced agent or pathogen upsetting the normal functioning of the organism, or a breakdown of the organism's integrating mechanism leading to the development of organic disease. Medical entomology is obviously only concerned with diseases caused by pathogens. Sometimes the insect itself may be the pathogen as in scabies, a skin disease due to the presence of the mite, *Sarcoptes scabiei*, and pediculosis due to infestation with the human body louse, *Pediculus humanus*, or head louse, *P. capitis*. More commonly the role of the insect is as a vector of the pathogen from one host to another. Insects function as vectors in one of two ways, either mechanically or biologically.

In mechanical transmission the insect acquires the pathogen from one source and deposits it in other locations, where it may infect a new host. The role of houseflies in the transmission of enteric diseases is mechanical. Houseflies are attracted equally to faeces and food on both of which they feed. Consequently organisms picked up in the body of a housefly, when it is feeding on faeces, are carried away and may be deposited on human food, when the fly feeds there. The housefly functions in a similar manner to a pathologist's platinum loop, which is used to lift a sample from faeces and apply it to a suitable agar plate for incubation and isolation of pathogens. The important feature to be recognised is that there are other routes for the spread of enteric diseases, e.g. by faecal contamination of drinking water or by human carriers of the pathogen handling food for human consumption.

In biological transmission the only natural route for the pathogen to take from host to host is through an insect. Thus, while it is possible to transmit malaria by blood transfusion, in nature the only way the malarial organism is passed from man to man is through the bite of the *Anopheles* mosquito. The role of the insect is very important in biological transmission and insect control is a major weapon in the armoury of disease control. There is a fundamental difference in the effect of insect control on disease incidence depending on whether transmission is mechanical or biological. Elimination of the insect vector of a biologically transmitted disease will eliminate the disease whereas eradication of a mechanical vector will only reduce the incidence, but not eliminate the disease. Elimination of *Anopheles* mosquitoes eradicates malaria but removal of houseflies only reduces the incidence of enteric disease; the pathogens will continue to spread through other routes.

Another major difference between biological and mechanical transmission involves the onset and duration of the vector's infectivity. Infectivity of a mechanical vector declines sharply with time and by 24 hours is, to all intents and purposes, nil (see Chapter 11). Biologically transmitted organisms undergo a cycle of development in the vector. Consequently there is a period after ingestion of the pathogen when the infected insect is not infective. When the pathogen's cycle is complete the insect is infective and usually remains so for the rest of its life. Mechanical or biological transmission is a character of the pathogen not of the insect vector. For example, although horseflies (Diptera, Tabanidae) are mechanical vectors of *Trypanosoma evansi*, the causative organism of Surra in horses and camels, they are biological vectors of *Trypanosoma theileri*, a benign parasite of cattle (see Chapter 29).

The greater part of the medical entomologist's work is concerned with diseases in which insects are biological vectors. In the simplest situation there are three different organisms involved: the pathogen, the vertebrate host and the insect vector. Such is the case with malaria involving the malarial parasite *Plasmodium*, man and the *Anopheles* mosquito. The parasite cycles between man and the mosquito. Theoretically there are three ways in which the disease may be controlled: (1) by breaking the man/mosquito contact and preventing transmission; (2) by eradicating the

Anopheles mosquito; and (3) by chemotherapy of the population to eliminate the source of infection of the mosquito. In practice all three approaches are attempted with the emphasis being determined by local circumstances. Eradication of the mosquito is not necessarily required. It is enough to reduce the *Anopheles* population to a level below which no transmission occurs. Transmission is a matter of probability and the epidemiology of malaria is a quantitative relationship between three different organisms — man, *Plasmodium* and *Anopheles*, each with their own ecologies (see Chapter 27).

In medical entomology many disease situations are complicated by the existence of a fourth component, which, from the human point of view, is often referred to as the reservoir host. It is the main population of the pathogen and the source of human infections. In such diseases there are two cycles (1) reservoir host, pathogen, vector and (2) man, pathogen, vector. The pathogen is the same in both cases but the vector is likely to be different. For example, sylvan yellow fever is circulated among primates in the Bwamba Forest, Uganda, through *Aedes africanus* but the virus is transmitted to man by *Aedes simpsoni* which feeds on both man and monkeys and bites the latter when they invade banana plantations. From the pathogen's point of view the significant cycle is that among the reservoir host and human involvement is an accident of little quantitative importance. From the human standpoint the important feature is the relationship between the two cycles.

Certain consequences follow from this dual cycle. Firstly, treatment of human cases may make little or no difference to the incidence of the disease which is maintained by 'spillover' from the reservoir host cycle. This is the case with flea-borne (murine) typhus caused by *Rickettsia mooseri* and transmitted by the tropical rat flea *Xenopsylla cheopis*. Reduction of the disease incidence depends either on dealing with the reservoir cycle or ensuring the separation of the two cycles. In the case of murine typhus, elimination requires reducing the close contact between rats and man. Adequate rat-proofing of human dwellings and storage of food in rat-proof containers will effectively eliminate the risk of murine typhus to man but leave the reservoir cycle in the rat unaffected. Dealing with the reservoir cycle is more often a theoretical than a practical possibility. For example, more than 200 species and subspecies of rodents are capable of harbouring *Yersinia pestis*, the causative organism of human plague. Clearly, in this case, elimination of the reservoir cycle is impractical and ecologically undesirable.

It should be evident now that the role of the medical entomologist is as a member of a team and, if he is to be effective, he must understand the main features of the biology of both pathogen and host. Only then will he be in a position to appreciate those aspects of the ecology and biology of the vector, which are of the greatest importance in the epidemiology of insect-borne disease. Thus to the medical entomologist the study of tsetse flies, *Glossina* spp., is inextricably bound up with the control of trypanosomiasis in man and domestic animals. This approach is not to be interpreted too narrowly and limited solely to those aspects of tsetse biology which are of obvious epidemiological significance but wider investigations must be justified ultimately in their contribution to our understanding of the epidemiology of trypanosomiasis. This is not to deny the value of using medically important insects for the study of fundamental biological problems. The yellow fever mosquito, *Aedes aegypti*, has been colonised for many years and has proved a suitable subject for many biological investigations but it would be simplistic to regard all these investigations as studies in medical entomology. Such studies are clearly of interest to the medical entomologist but so are other biological investigations of fundamental phenomena which are undertaken on organisms of no direct importance to the medical entomologist.

In accordance with this understanding of medical entomology the chapters of this book are arranged in three sections. The first deals with basic introductory entomology, the second with the recognition, biology and bionomics (ecology) of insects of medical importance, and the third with pathogens and diseases, emphasising those aspects which are relevant to an understanding of the insects' role in the epidemiology of disease. The third section will be largely restricted to pathogens of which insects are biological vectors and be highly selective. It will deal cursorily, if at all, with diagnosis, pathology, clinical symptoms and structure and identification of pathogens. Insect-borne pathogens are to be found in a wide range of life forms: Viruses, Rickettsiales, Bacteria, Spirochaetales, Protozoa, Cestoda and Nematoda.

Generalisations and Quantitative Information

It is necessary in a book attempting to deal with a topic as broad as medical and veterinary entomology, to have recourse to generalisations. The reader should appreciate that, when such all-embracing statements are found in the text, they are not infallible. They are considered to have a high probability of being correct but there is also a finite probability of the existence of exceptions. Nevertheless, if this limitation is borne in mind, generalisations can be a valuable aid to learning. The place for the consideration of exceptions is in the advanced text or monograph. Every teacher will have learned to his dismay that however briefly in the course of a lecture an exception is mentioned, there is a perverse streak in the learning processes of students whereby the exception will be the one firm fact that will be retained.

For example, it would not be unreasonable to make the general statement that all species of *Anopheles* mosquitoes are biologically capable of transmitting malaria. There are exceptions to this generalisation. In the laboratory, some species of *Anopheles* are difficult to infect with certain strains of plasmodia to which they are not exposed in nature. However, the generalisation that all species of *Anopheles* are biologically competent to transmit malaria has value but it must not be extrapolated and misinterpreted as indicating that all species of *Anopheles* are of equal importance in a field situation. This is quite untrue. The significant difference between species of *Anopheles*, which are major vectors of malaria in the field, compared with those which are unimportant, does not lie in their susceptibility to infection but in their behaviour, in particular the frequency with which they feed on man.

The medical and veterinary entomologist is concerned with the epidemiology of human and animal disease. The qualitative aspects of disease transmission form the framwork within which epidemiology seeks to quantify the relationships between the various components (pathogen, vector, host) of the system. For this reason a certain amount of numerical information will be included in the text. As with generalisations, such numerical data should not be regarded as having the precision of physical constants but as indicators of the order of magnitude of the factor concerned. This information should provide the reader with a numerical framework within which he can begin to quantify a problem. It is important, for example, to know the approximate fecundity of a vector, the frequency with which it oviposits and the length of its life cycle. Many of these quantities are variable being dependent on environmental conditions, particularly temperature, and therefore the figures quoted will refer to optimal conditions. The numerical data presented in the text can prove useful, providing they are regarded as approximations, indicating an order of magnitude.

Nomenclature

The classification of living organisms is built on the concept of a species. Species are the building blocks out of which the edifice displaying relationships within the animal kingdom is constructed. A precise definition of a species is difficult, if not impossible. Definitions range from the valuable, but largely theoretical, 'a species is a population of animals which interbreed, producing fertile offspring', to the more practical, but decidedly vague, definition that, 'a good species is one recognised by a good taxonomist'. Notwithstanding this difficulty the species remains the basic unit of classification.

Each species has a name based on the binomal system devised by the Swedish naturalist, Linnaeus, in the eighteenth century. The name consists

Binomal system

of two components, the generic and specific names. The specific name, once published, in inviolable but the genus to which the species is referred may change with increased knowledge of the group. The full name of a species includes the author and the year in which the description was first published, e.g. *Musca domestica* Linnaeus, 1785, the common housefly. When, at a later date, a species is placed in a different genus from that to which it was referred by the author, then the author's name is placed in parentheses, e.g. *Aedes aegypti* (Linnaeus, 1762). When Linnaeus described *aegypti* he placed it in the genus *Culex* which he had created in 1758. The genus *Aedes* was not established by Meigen until 1818. The reader should note that the generic name always begins with an upper case letter while the specific name starts with a lower case letter, although botanical taxonomists use an upper case letter when a species has been named after a particular person.

Two sources of error can arise within this system. A species may be described more than once or several species may be confused and regarded as a single species. The first error is, in theory, the easier to deal with. Two or more names for the same species are synonyms and the earliest description has priority. For example the yellow fever mosquito was named *Culex aegypti* by Linnaeus in 1762, *Culex argenteus* by Poiret in 1787, and *Culex fasciatus* by Fabricius in 1805. These three names are synonyms and the earliest description, that of Linnaeus, has priority and the specific name of the mosquito is *aegypti*. Synonyms confound the reader but do not invalidate observations on the several 'species' since the observations are equally applicable to the single species.

In a large genus it is convenient to establish subgenera and the subgenus is then shown in parentheses after the generic name, e.g. *Aedes (Stegomyia) aegypti* (Linnaeus, 1762). *Stegomyia* was established by Theobald in 1901 as a genus distinct from *Aedes* but later workers include it as a subgenus of *Aedes*. The decision as to whether a group of species is best regarded as constituting a genus or included as a subgenus within an existing genus, is largely a matter of judgement by the individual taxonomist, to which he will need to bring a wide range of knowledge of the whole group.

The second error is more important. It involves homonyms in which two or more species have been confused and referred to by the same name. This often invalidates all previous biological data because it is uncertain as to which of the two or more entities the observations apply. For example, the common European malarial mosquito *Anopheles maculipennis* Meigen, 1818, has proved to be a complex of at least six species (see Chapter 6), including a revised description of *An maculipennis* Meigen, 1818; *An sacharovi* Favre, 1903; *An labranchiae* Falleroni, 1926; and *An melanoon* Hackett, 1934. It is usual for the full name of the species to be given only in taxonomic papers. Most journals require the author's name, but not the year, to be given when a species is first cited in a scientific paper. After this the author's name is omitted and the generic name abbreviated to a single capital letter. Where such abbreviation might cause confusion, as for example when *A.* could refer to *Aedes* or *Anopheles*, mosquito taxonomists use two-letter abbreviations for the genera of mosquitoes and *Aedes* and *Anopheles* are abbreviated to *Ae* and *An*, respectively.[3]

Sometimes a trinomial system is used with the third name denoting a subspecies, e.g. *Anopheles melanoon melanoon* Hackett, 1934, and *Anopheles melanoon subalpinus* Hackett and Lewis, 1935. *An m. melanoon* is widely distributed in Southern Europe extending from Spain in the west to Iran in the east while *An m. subalpinus* has been recorded only from Albania and Turkey. It is desirable to keep the use of subspecific names to a minimum and to avoid the naming of numerous 'varieties'. Species complexes, such as that of *An maculipennis*, appear now to be common in widespread species and considerably complicate the work of the medical entomologist. This topic will be considered in greater detail in Chapter 6.

Species are placed in a genus (plural genera), genera are associated into tribes, tribes into subfamilies and so on into increasingly large aggregations designated families, superfamilies and orders. Since in many cases the words for these different levels may use the same stem it is important to appreciate the significance of the endings which, fortunately, are standardised.

Grade	*Ending*	*Example*
Order	-ptera (commonest ending)	Diptera
Superfamily	-oidea	Muscoidea
Family	-idae	Muscidae, Culicidae
Subfamily	-inae	Muscinae, Culicinae
Tribe	-ini	Culicini

Zoogeographical Regions

As a result of the past history of the continents, especially their degree of isolation from other land masses, and the geographical origin of the various animal groups, the faunas of different parts of the world are distinctive. It is useful to be able to describe the distribution of an insect or a disease by reference to zoogeographical regions rather than to constantly changing national boundaries. For this purpose six main regions are recognised. They are:

Palaearctic — Europe, Africa north of the Tropic of Cancer but including the Sahara; China north of 30°N; Asiatic USSR; Korea and Japan

Nearctic	—	USA, Canada, Greenland, Alaska and North Mexico
Afrotropical	—	the whole of Africa south of the Tropic of Cancer but excluding the Sahara
Oriental	—	India, Pakistan, south-east Asia, China south of 30°N, Malaysia and Indonesia
Australian	—	Australia, New Guinea, New Zealand and the Pacific Islands
Neotropical	—	Southern Mexico, Central America and South America

There are common elements in the faunas of the Nearctic and Palaearctic regions and they are referred to collectively as the Holarctic region. The Afrotropical region is more commonly designated the Ethiopian region, but since Ethiopia forms only a very small part of the region, Crosskey and White[2] proposed the more appropriate term, Afrotropical region.

Introduction to the Literature

The intention of this book is to provide the reader with sufficient background to be able to delve into the literature with some confidence. The text attempts to provide an outline sketch of the vectors, their biologies and the diseases they transmit.

In the text references are indicated by superior numbers and listed in numerical and alphabetical order at the end of each chapter. They do not represent an exhaustive coverage of the literature nor are the references cited necessarily the most important papers published. Very often they have been selected because they illustrate a particular point which has been made in the chapter. Their role is to provide the student with an entry into the literature. Each paper cited will, in turn, give references to earlier work and enable the reader to explore the subject as fully as he/she needs.

Through the references cited at the end of each chapter the reader will become acquainted with the earlier literature. The problem will be to keep abreast of new developments. The medical and veterinary entomologist is favourably placed for keeping up to date through the Review of Applied Entomology, Series B, Medical and Veterinary[4], which appears monthly. Some idea of the expansion of medical entomology during the 1970s can be obtained from the growth in the number of articles abstracted in the Review. In the late 1960s the Review was about 250 pages long and included about 900 abstracts. Between 1969 and 1976 it expanded linearly, abstracting another 400 articles and adding 106 pages to its length each year, until by 1976 the Review was abstracting more than 3,000 papers per annum and covering more than 1,000 pages. (There was a change of format between 1972 and 1973 and the pages for the earlier years have been standardised for size and number of printed lines.) In part the increase may represent a change in editorial policy but it would be unreasonable to attribute this growth solely to a change in policy. It would imply that in the 1960s less than 30 per cent of the papers published in medical and veterinary entomology were being included in the Review (Figure 1.1). This is not credible.

Several factors may explain increased research into medical and veterinary entomology during the 1970s. The greatest contribution that medical and veterinary entomology can make to human development is in the tropics and subtropics where arthropod-borne diseases are most abundant. The tropics is also the region where the greatest number of 'under-

Figure 1.1: Growth of Medical and Veterinary Entomology in the Decade 1967-77, as shown by number of reviews (Y_1) and number of pages (standardised) (Y_2) in the Review of Applied Entomology, Series B, Medical and Veterinary

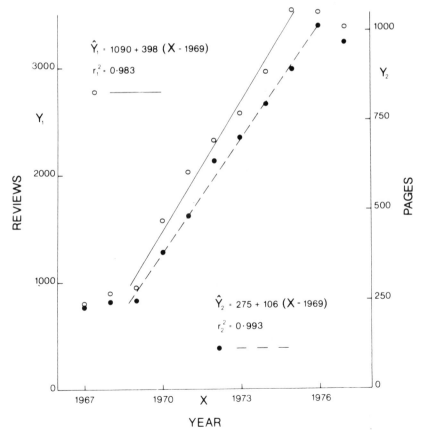

$\hat{Y}_1 = 1090 + 398 \, (X - 1969)$

$r_1^2 = 0.983$

$\hat{Y}_2 = 275 + 106 \, (X - 1969)$

$r_2^2 = 0.993$

developed' countries are to be found. Many of these have only relatively recently obtained independence and there has been a drive by the United Nations, and independent foundations and grant-giving bodies to improve human welfare in the newly independent countries by eliminating or reducing substantially diseases of man and his animals.

The United Nations Development Programme with the World Bank and the World Health Organization has formulated a 'Special Programme for Research and Training in Tropical Disease'. This programme, which commenced in 1975, listed seven major human diseases, of which five: malaria, filariasis, African trypanosomiasis, Chagas' disease and leishmaniasis, involved medical entomology. It has been estimated[5] that in 1981, 1,800 million people in 107 countries were exposed to malaria (see Chapter 27) and 150 million new cases occurred each year. Several hundred million people were affected by onchocerciasis and lymphatic filariasis (see Chapters 30, 31). African trypanosomiasis threatened 45 million people in 38 countries, and Chagas' disease 65 million people in Latin America with 24 million persons chronically infected (see Chapter 29). Leishmaniasis (see Chapter 29) claimed 400,000 new cases a year.

Another abstracting journal of interest to the medical entomologist is The Tropical Diseases Bulletin.[6] This publication deals with the whole range of tropical diseases, whether or not they involve arthropods and deals with aspects of the disease, e.g. pathology and medication, which are remote from medical entomology. Nevertheless the Bulletin has a section devoted to medical entomology and is a useful source especially when a wider understanding of a particular disease is required. The Annual Review of Entomology[1] is another publication in which articles of interest to the medical and veterinary entomologist appear. However, medical and veterinary entomology is only one aspect of entomology covered by the Annual Review.

References

1. Annual Review of Entomology, Annual Reviews Inc., Palo Alto, California, USA
2. Crosskey, R.W. and White, G.B. (1977). The Afrotropical Region a recommended term in zoogeography. *Journal of Natural History 11*: 541-4
3. Reinert, J.F. (1975). Mosquito generic and subgeneric abbreviations (Diptera: Culicidae). *Mosquito Systematics 7*: 105-10.
4. Review of Applied Entomology, Series B, Medical and Veterinary, Commonwealth Agricultural Bureaux, Slough, England
5. Special Programme for Research and Training in Tropical Diseases, *Newsletter 18*: 6-8. May 1982
6. Tropical Diseases Bulletin, Bureau of Hygiene and Tropical Diseases, London, England

2 CLASSIFICATION OF ARTHROPODA AND THE MEDICAL IMPORTANCE OF GROUPS OF MINOR SIGNIFICANCE

The largest phylum in the animal kingdom is the Arthropoda, which contains about 80 per cent of the known species of animals. They are bilaterally symmetrical, segmented animals with jointed legs. Each segment consists of a dorsal sclerotised plate, the tergum, and a similar ventral plate, the sternum, the two being jointed together laterally by membranous pleura (singular pleuron). The terga and sterna of successive segments are separated by intersegmental membranes which, together with the pleura, provide flexibility. The primitive arthropod was probably a worm-like creature with some cephalisation at the anterior end, and metameric segmentation, i.e. each segment being similar to the one before and behind. Each segment bore a pair of appendages, and those on segments incorporated into the head formed the mouthparts. The exoskeleton provides a limit to growth and periodically arthropods have to develop a new skin under the existing one and then cast the old skin. The process is known as ecdysis or moulting and, in the Insecta, the interval between ecdyses is an instar. Internally arthropods have the typical invertebrate arrangement of ventral nerve cord and dorsal heart, the reverse of the vertebrate arrangement.

Arthropod Venoms

Before considering the classification of the Arthropoda in more detail it will be useful to examine the part played by arthropods in causing disease. Their main economic importance is as vectors of pathogens to man and domestic animals. The vectors are species of insects and acarines, but a larger range of arthropods can cause severe reactions and even death by their stings or bites. The subject of arthropod venoms has been reviewed recently under the editorship of Bettini.[3] This substantial work includes six chapters on the venoms of spiders; six on Hymenoptera (ants, bees and wasps); four on scorpions; one each on centipedes, millipedes and ticks; one on other arachnids; and four on different insect orders, but not including the Diptera. It was originally planned to include a chapter on the Diptera but this was abandoned as the information available was 'so scanty'.

Classification of Arthropoda

The Arthropoda may be divided into those with antennae, the Antennata, and those lacking antennae but possessing chelicerae, the Chelicerata. The chelicerae are mouthparts (see Chapter 20). Two classes of Arthropoda are especially important to the medical entomologist — the Insecta in the Antennata and the Arachnida in the Chelicerata. Three other classes are of minor significance.

Class Crustacea

Strictly speaking the Crustacea are outside the scope of this book, but they are common and of minor medical importance. With few exceptions the

Figure 2.1: Dorsal View of a Chilopod, *Lithobius erythrocephalus*

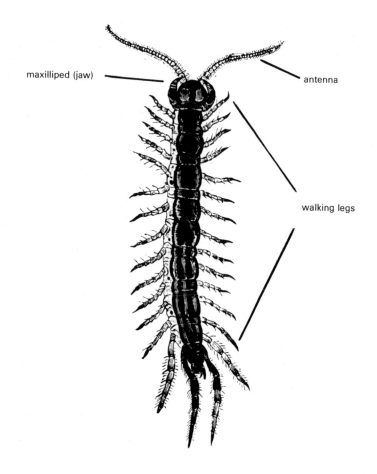

maxilliped (jaw)

antenna

walking legs

Crustacea are aquatic, and the majority are marine. Their bodies are organised into a cephalothorax and a posterior abdomen. They possess two pairs of antennae, which may be reduced, and at least five pairs of legs. This class includes the crabs, lobsters, shrimps and water fleas. They are medically important as intermediate hosts of helminths, e.g. the river crab (*Eriocheir japonicus*) is an intermediate host of the lung fluke *Paragonimus ringeri*, and copepods of the genus *Cyclops* are intermediate hosts of the guinea worm *Dracunculus mediensis*. Human beings become infected by eating inadequately cooked river crabs or by drinking water containing infected *Cyclops*.

Class Chilopoda (Centipedes) (see Figure 2.1)

Chilopods are long, snake-like, terrestrial arthropods, which are dorsoventrally flattened. They have one pair of antennae on the head and three pairs of appendages associated with the mouth. Behind the head the body is metamerically segmented and composed of at least 17 segments, each of which, with the exception of the last segment, bears a pair of legs. The first pair of legs act as powerful jaws which can inflict a painful bite on a man. The jaws of a chilopod are pierced by a duct through which the secretion of the venom glands is injected into the victim. The venom of centipedes is used to kill prey and in defence. It probably also has a digestive function. Large centipedes may cause pain but rarely death in man. Chilopods seek dark, humid shelters and can cause considerable irritation, when, in search of such refuges, they enter the natural openings of the body of a vertebrate.

Figure 2.2: Lateral View of a Diplopod, *Iulus terrestrias*

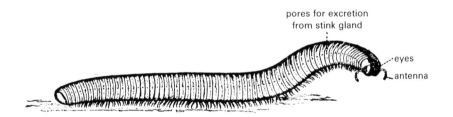

pores for excretion
from stink gland

eyes

antenna

Class Diplopoda (Millipedes) (see Figure 2.2)

Millipedes are obviously metamerically segmented, terrestrial arthropods with cylindrical, worm-like bodies made up of many segments. They have one pair of antennae and two pairs of appendages associated with the mouth. Each apparent segment bears two pairs of legs and two pairs of spiracles, i.e. respiratory openings. Millipedes do not possess biting jaws of the centipede type but produce a defensive secretion from segmental glands. Benzoquinones and phenolic derivatives have been identified in these secretions. In *Apheloria corrugata* the secretion contains hydrogen cyanide.[11] They are reputed to be one of the few creatures which predacious safari (doryline) or army ants are said to leave untouched.

Class Arachnida[7, 16]

The Arachnida are carnivorous, terrestrial, chelicerate arthropods which have no antennae. They have one pair of chelicerae used in feeding, a pair of pedipalps whose function varies from order to order and four pairs of walking legs. The Arachnida is a large class containing nine orders of which three are of medical importance.

Order Scorpiones (Scorpions) (see Figure 2.3)

About 600 species of scorpions have been described throughout the world. They are large Arachnids with powerful, chelate pedipalps and whose abdomens end in a globular sting terminating in a large curved spine. Scor-

Figure 2.3: Ventral View
of a Scorpion

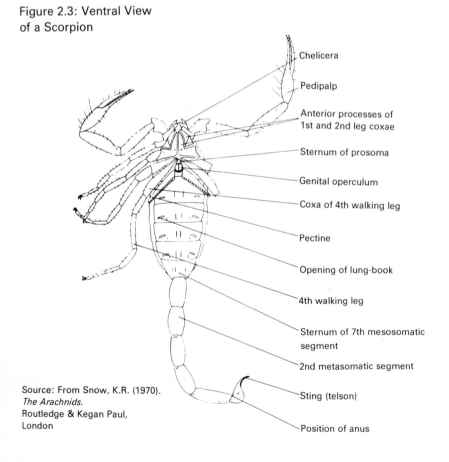

Chelicera

Pedipalp

Anterior processes of
1st and 2nd leg coxae

Sternum of prosoma

Genital operculum

Coxa of 4th walking leg

Pectine

Opening of lung-book

4th walking leg

Sternum of 7th mesosomatic
segment

2nd metasomatic segment

Sting (telson)

Position of anus

Source: From Snow, K.R. (1970).
The Arachnids.
Routledge & Kegan Paul,
London

pions are nocturnal creatures which hide away by day under stones, bark and other objects. Desert species frequently burrow to depths of up to 2.4 m.[11] Scorpions lie in ambush for their prey, the approach of which is detected with the pectines. The pectines are large plate-like structures on the ventral surface of the body, immediately posterior to the fourth pair of legs. They are sensitive to vibrations, and, when held in contact with the ground, provide sensory information on the approach of potential prey. When the prey is seized in the pedipalps the sting is brought rapidly over the top of the body and thrust into the victim. Through the sting a toxin is forcibly injected into the prey by muscular action. When, in the laboratory, ejection is artificially stimulated the toxin may be propelled tens of centimetres.

The effect of the toxin on mammals depends on the species of scorpion and is independent of size. The large *Hadrurus arizonensis* is comparatively harmless while the small *Centruroides sculpturatus* is deadly. There is variation within a genus. Thus *C. sculpturatus* and *C. limpidus* are dangerous while *C. pantherinus* and *C. vittatus* are not.[11] Most of the dangerous species are in the family Buthidae, which contains about half the described species of scorpions. Death is due to cardiac failure or to paralysis of the respiratory muscles and occurs within a few hours. Treatment may be provided by specially prepared sera.

Scorpion venom has been likened to Cobra venom because of the similarity of the victim's response but the two venoms are distinct. Scorpion venoms are homologous for amino acid sequences as are the venoms of elapid snakes but the sequences in the two groups are quite different. They also act differently on the nervous system. Elapid toxins produce an anti-depolarising block of the end plate, while scorpion venoms depolarise different target cells.[22] The result may be the same but the method of bringing it about is distinct.

Scorpions will not attack but will defend themselves when apparently threatened. Most stings occur because scorpions have taken shelter in shoes or clothing or because inquisitive humans too casually explore under stones or into holes in the ground. About 30 of the world's most dangerous species of scorpions have been recently reviewed by Keegan.[9]

Order Araneae (Spiders) (see Figure 2.4)

More than 20,000 species of spiders have been described. They are characterised by having a uniform prosoma (anterior portion of the body) joined by a narrow pedicel to an unsegmented opisthosoma (hind portion). The pedipalps are tactile, leg-like structures, shorter than the ambulatory legs. In the male they are modified as intromittent organs and male spiders are readily recognised by the terminal swelling on the pedipalp. The chelicerae are two-segmented but not chelate. The distal segment is sharply pointed and bears at its tip the opening of the poison duct. The poison gland may

Figure 2.4: Dorsal (left) and Ventral (right) Views of a Mygalomorph Spider

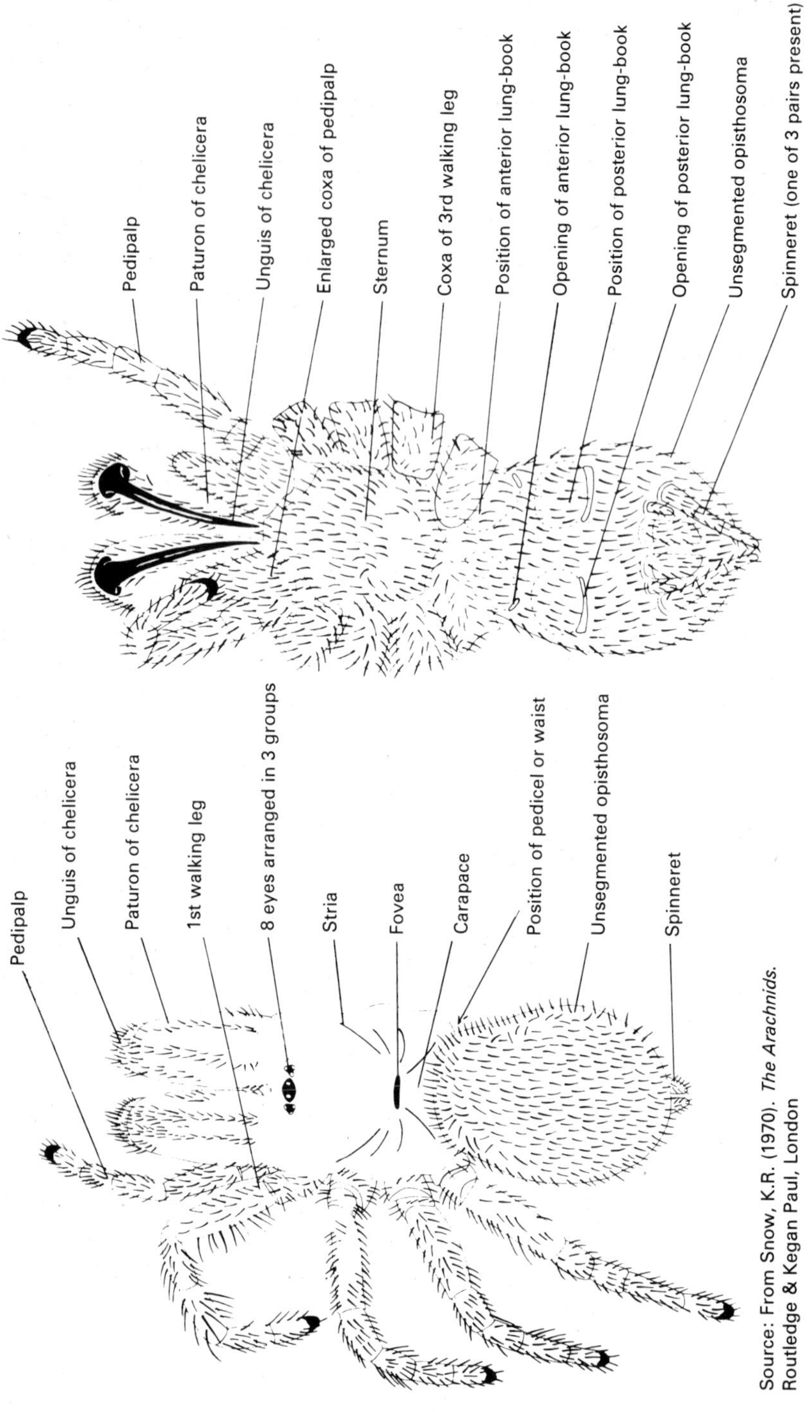

Pedipalp

Paturon of chelicera

Unguis of chelicera

Enlarged coxa of pedipalp

Sternum

Coxa of 3rd walking leg

Position of anterior lung-book

Opening of anterior lung-book

Position of posterior lung-book

Opening of posterior lung-book

Unsegmented opisthosoma

Spinneret (one of 3 pairs present)

Pedipalp

Unguis of chelicera

Paturon of chelicera

1st walking leg

8 eyes arranged in 3 groups

Stria

Fovea

Carapace

Position of pedicel or waist

Unsegmented opisthosoma

Spinneret

Source: From Snow, K.R. (1970). *The Arachnids.*
Routledge & Kegan Paul, London

be contained in the basal segment of the chelicera or, more usually, occupies the anterior part of the prosoma. In the majority of spiders (suborder Araneamorphae) the chelicerae are fixed vertically with the terminal segment, the fang (unguis), being concealed in a groove in the larger basal segment. In action the fangs converge towards the midline horizontally. In the Mygalomorphae the chelicerae are directed forwards horizontally and in action the parallel fangs strike vertically downwards. Spider venom is adapted to the prey species on which the spider feeds, mostly invertebrates, but the mygalomorph spider, *Selonocosmia javanensis*, attacks and kills birds.

Most spiders are harmless being either unable to penetrate the human skin or having ineffective venom. Some of the larger species may cause a temporary local reaction and a few may produce a severe, or even a fatal, response. The Australian funnel web spider, *Atrax robustus*, a mygalomorph, has caused the deaths of adult humans,[19] and all species of the genus should be regarded as dangerous. Species of *Latrodectus*, an araneomorph genus, produce a neurotropic venom and cause a severe human reaction but rarely death in adults of good health. The *L. mactans* complex is a group of black spiders with red or yellow patches on the opisthosoma. They are widely distributed throughout the warmer parts of the world with several different subspecies being recognised. *L.m. mactans* is the black widow spider of the USA; *L.m. tridecimguttatus* is in southern Europe; and *L.m. hasselti* is the Australian red-backed spider. An effective antivenom has been available to combat bites of *L.m. hasselti* since 1956 and in 1980 an effective antivenom was produced against *A. robustus.*[21]

Araneomorph spiders of the genera *Loxosceles* and *Lycosa* produce a necrotic venom, which causes tissue destruction. The initial bite may be painless and pass unnoticed, but locally extensive, necrotic patches develop around the location of the bite. *Lycosa raptoria* has caused 200 cases a year in Brasil and an antivenom serum has been produced for their treatment. Over a 20-year period in Chile *Loxosceles laeta* caused five deaths among 133 cases.[17] The brown recluse spider, *Loxosceles reclusa*, causes necrotic damage to man in the USA.

Order Acari (Mites and Ticks) (see Figure 2.5)

The Acari are sometimes treated as a subclass of the Arachnida. They are small arthropods 0.3–0.5 mm long varying widely in form but in which the prosoma and opisthosoma are broadly fused and abdominal segmentation is inconspicuous or absent. The pedipalps are short sensory structures associated with the chelicerae in a discrete gnathosoma. Acarines are extremely important agents of disease and vectors of pathogens, and will be considered in detail in Chapters 20-23.

Figure 2.5: Dorsal View
of an Acarine, *Zercoseius
ometes*, Acari

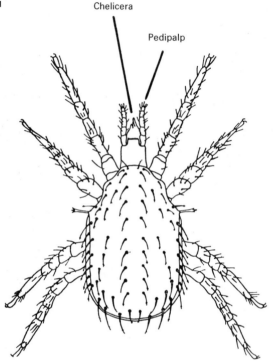

Orders of Minor Interest (see Figure 2.6)

The solifugids (sun or camel spiders) are an ancient order of Arachnida, being known as fossils from the Carboniferous period. They are large, hairy, nocturnal, carnivorous arachnids of desert areas in the tropics and subtropics. About 800 species have been described. Solifugids are easily recognised by their possession of large, powerful, chelate chelicerae with which they seize their prey (Figure 2.6D). They will attack any suitable prey including small vertebrates and each other. However, they have no poison glands and rely solely on the crushing power of the chelicerae.

The Uropygi (whip-scorpions) and Amblypygi (whip-spiders) are flat-bodied, mainly tropical arachnids, which are nocturnal predators with powerful pedipalps, but lacking poison glands. In both orders only the posterior three pairs of legs are used for walking and those of the first pair are tactile and, in action, are stretched out in front of the animal. In the

Figure 2.6: A, a Uropygid, *Thelyphonus insularis*; B, an Amblypygid, *Stegophrynus dammermani*; C. a Pseudoscorpion, *Chelifer cancroides*; D, a Solifugid, *Galeodes arabs*

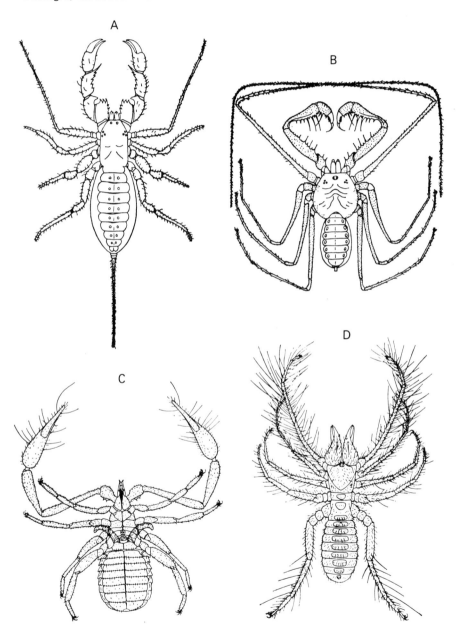

amblypygids the first pair of legs is excessively long, more than twice the length of the walking legs (Figure 2.6B). In the uropygids the abdomen terminates in a segmented flagellum, as long as the rest of the abdomen (Figure 2.6A).

The pseudoscorpions are a widely distributed order of small arachnids (<8 mm) with large chelate pedipalps, superficially resembling small scorpions but they lack a sting (Figure 2.6C). They are common in soil and decaying vegetation, and a few species are to be found in food stores and among books, presumably feeding on book-lice (psocids).

Figure 2.7: Lateral View of a Collembolan

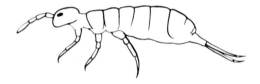

Superclass Hexapoda[5, 6, 13]

The Hexapoda are characterised, as the name implies, by having three pairs of walking legs. They also have three pairs of mouthparts, and the genital area placed posteriorly. This superclass contains the Insecta and three other groups of small hexapods. The latter are entognathous and prognathous, that is, the mouthparts and preoral cavity are enclosed and forwardly directed. Of the three groups only the Collembola (Springtails; Figure 2.7) are common, and are likely to be encountered when examining soil samples and material from humid habitats.

Class Insecta (Insects) (see Figure 2.8)

Insects are ectognathous and usually hypognathous, i.e. the mouthparts are exposed and directed ventrally. The body of an insect is organised into three regions — head, thorax and abdomen. The head bears a pair of sensory antennae, large compound eyes and three pairs of mouthparts (mandibles, 1st maxillae and labium or fused 2nd maxillae).

Figure 2.8: Lateral View of a Generalised Insect

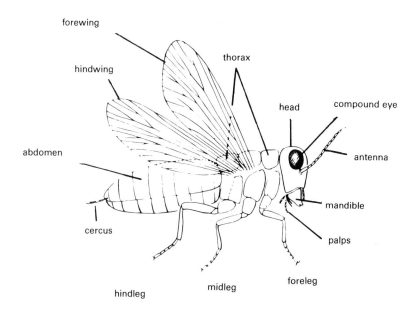

Structure of Insects

Head (see Figure 2.9). The insect head is a rigid capsule formed from a series of sclerotised plates. The anterior wall of the capsule is formed by the frons, which articulates dorsally with the vertex and ventrally with the clypeus. The dorsal and lateral walls are formed by the vertex and genae (singular gena) respectively. The incomplete posterior wall is the occiput, which articulates with the neck and surrounds the occipital foramen through which the nerve cord, gut and dorsal aorta pass.

The antennae are inserted between the eyes and, in action, are directed forwards. Their structure is very variable, ranging from being many-segmented, long and slender in cockroaches (Figure 2.13) to being three-segmented, short and stout in fleas (Figure 2.20). The compound eyes are placed dorsolaterally and an insect is said to be dichoptic when the eyes are separated and holoptic when they are contiguous in the middorsal line. Many insects have ocelli (singular ocellus) on the head. They are dark, hemispherical structures projecting above the general level of the head surface. Typically there are three ocelli forming an inverted triangle antero-dorsally, but in Diptera they are placed more dorsally and are located on the vertex.

The labrum or anterior lip, which is broadly joined to the clypeus, forms the anterior wall of the preoral cavity, exterior to the mouth. The other

Figure 2.9: Anterior (left) and Lateral (right) Views of a Generalised Insect Head

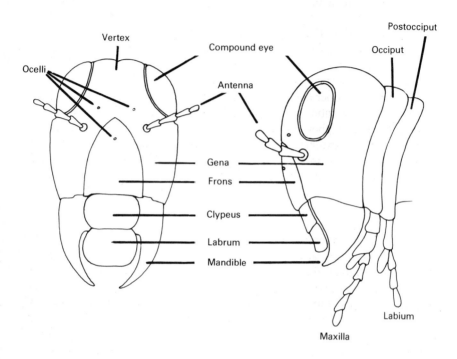

limits to the cavity are formed by the mouthparts, the mandibles and maxillae laterally and the labium posteriorly. The maxillae and labium may carry sensory palps. The mouthparts of medically important insects are described in more detail in Chapter 4.

Thorax (see Figure 2.8). The thorax is composed of three segments, named anteroposteriorly, prothorax, mesothorax and metathorax. In a typical adult insect each segment bears a pair of legs and, in the Pterygota, the mesothorax and metathorax a pair of wings. When both pairs of wings are fully developed the meso- and metathoraces are fused to form the pterothorax, which is very much larger than the prothorax. In the Diptera, there is only one pair of functional wings, the mesothoracic, consequently the mesothorax is highly developed and the prothorax and metathorax correspondingly reduced (see Chapter 3). The lateral walls of the thorax are pierced by the mesothoracic and metathoracic spiracles, openings of the respiratory system.

The legs are made up of a number of segments which provide flexibility. There are two small segments at the base, the coxa which articulates with the thorax and the trochanter (Figure 2.10). They are followed successively by two longer segments, the femur and tibia. The leg terminates in the tarsus, composed of one to five short segments or tarsomeres. The basal segment may be referred to as the metatarsus or basitarsus. The terminal tarsal segment bears the pretarsus, which in Diptera consists typically of a pair of claws and pad-like pulvilli (singular pulvillus) and a median empodium which may be setaceous (hair-like) or pulvilliform (Figure 2.11).

The typical insect wing is a thin, transparent membrane, composed of closely adherent upper and lower layers which enclose a series of longitudinal strengthening tubes, the veins. These are connected by cross-veins which are few in higher insects such as the Diptera. Each vein contains a trachea and an extension of the blood-containing haemocoele. The arrangement of veins in the wing is characteristic of the insect and referred to as its wing venation. It affords a very useful character for identification and it is often possible to decide the family or genus of an insect solely on its wing venation.

Abdomen. The abdomen is primitively 11-segmented, and only in the Apterygota are there appendages on the pregenital segments. In primitive insects the terminal abdominal segment may bear a pair of long, lateral cerci (singular cercus) and, less frequently, a median caudal filament or appendix dorsalis. Laterally the abdomen may bear up to eight pairs of spiracles. The gonopore opens on segment 9 in the male and behind segment 8 in the female. In the Pterygota highly modified appendages are associated with the gonopore and are involved in copulation and insemination. These terminalia, particularly those of males, provide useful characters for species identification, but their treatment is highly specialised and outside the scope of this book.

Figure 2.10: Segments of a Typical Insect Leg, a Mosquito

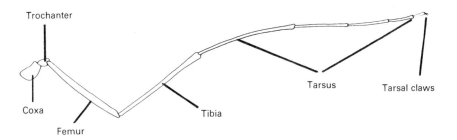

Figure 2.11: Tarsal Claws and Associated Structures: A, *Lucilia cuprina* with large seta which overlies the empodium, omitted; B, a Tabanoid

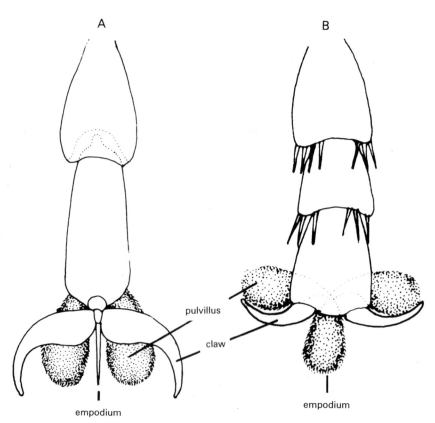

In the Diptera the first abdominal segment becomes progressively reduced and the 10th and 11th are fused to form the protiger which bears the reduced cerci and the anal opening. In the higher Diptera the abdominal segments are telescoped so that only a small number are normally visible externally.

Subclass Apterygota (see Figure 2.12)

These primitive, wingless insects possess an appendix dorsalis. They continue to moult throughout their lives. Some of the Thysanura are minor household pests and include the silverfish, *Lepisma saccharina*, and the firebrat, *Lepismodes inquilinus*.

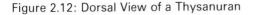

Figure 2.12: Dorsal View of a Thysanuran

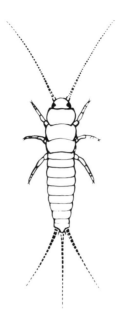

Subclass Pterygota

The Pterygota are winged or secondarily wingless insects in which an appendix dorsalis is rare and moulting ceases at sexual maturity. There are two distinct forms of development. In exopterygote (hemimetabolic) development the wing rudiments are present externally in the nymphal stages and increase in size at each moult, becoming functional only in the adult and in the winged preimaginal stage of the Ephemeroptera (mayflies). Except in aquatic forms the nymphs are similar to the adults both in appearance and mode of life. In endopterygote (holometabolic) insects wings develop internally, and the larval stages are quite unlike the adult in appearance and lead an entirely different mode of life. Transition from larva to adult requires extensive reorganisation and is effected in a non-feeding and usually non-motile stage, the pupa. This strategy allows the separate adaptation of larva and adult to their respective habitats and has been most successful as 86 per cent of all insects are endopterygotes.

The type of life cycle has practical implications. There is usually only one control strategy possible against exopterygotes but there is a choice of two against endopterygotes when actions may be directed against the adult or the immature stages. Thus any action taken against exopterygote pests such as lice or cockroaches will operate equally on the immature stages (nymphs) and adults which share the same habitat, whereas with houseflies and mosquitoes there is a choice of actions. Control measures can be directed against the adults as, for example, when deposits of residual insecticides are applied to the inner surfaces of houses or animal shelters or, on the other hand, measures can be directed against the immature stages by eliminating breeding sites or by rendering them unsuitable. The strategy adopted will depend upon circumstances with the general rule being to attack the pest where it is more concentrated and accessible. Where breeding sites are abundant the only practical method may be to attack the adults. When breeding sites are limited it will be preferable to direct control measures against the immature stages. In general, when the adult insect is the pest, it is preferable to control the immature stages and cut the pest off at its source.

Two main divisions are recognised within the Pterygota. Two ancient orders are included in the Palaeoptera while the bulk of insect species are in the Neoptera. Members of the Palaeoptera are characterised by an inability to fold the wings against the body when the insect is at rest. The wings are either held vertically above the body or horizontally laterally. The two palaeopteran orders are the Odonata (dragonflies, damselflies) and the Ephemeroptera (mayflies). Neither order is of medical importance but their immature stages are often abundant in aquatic habitats and will be found when searching for the larvae of mosquitoes or blackflies. The Odonata are predacious in all stages and both adults and nymphs may play a minor role as predators of mosquitoes.

The Neoptera include the Endopterygota and two exopterygote groups, the Blattoid-Orthopteroid and the Hemipteroid. The Blattoid-Orthopteroid group includes many well-known and easily recognised insects such as locusts, crickets, stick insects, earwigs, preying mantids and termites. It includes only one order of medical importance the Blattodea (cockroaches). Members of the Blattoid-Orthopteroid group have generalised mandibulate (chewing) mouthparts and the forewings are usually thickened to provide protection to the folded hind wings. The Hemipteroid group is characterised by having specialised mouthparts which are often suctorial. Two of the four orders in the Hemipteroid group, the Phthiraptera (lice) and the Hemiptera (bugs) include families of medical and veterinary importance. The other two orders in this group are the plant-feeding thrips (Thysanoptera) and the scavenging psocids (Psocoptera). The two orders of major medical importance in the Endopterygota are the Siphonaptera (fleas) and the Diptera (mosquitoes, flies). The Endopterygota also includes three of the best-known orders of insects, the Coleoptera (beetles), the Lepidoptera (butterflies and moths) and the Hymenoptera (ants, bees and wasps). A very small number of these three orders have some medical and veterinary importance.

Order Blattodea (Cockroaches) (see Figure 2.13)

Cockroaches are dorsoventrally flattened, exopterygote, terrestrial insects with long antennae and wings, when present, folded flat over the body. The mouthparts are mandibulate and the legs cursorial, i.e. adapted for running, at which cockroaches are very adept. The hardened forewings, called tegmina (singular tegmen), overlap and cover much of the dorsal surface of the body, protecting the more delicate hind wings, which are the effective flying organs. The abdomen ends in paired, jointed cerci. The eggs are enclosed in a hardened, purse-like case, the ootheca. Internally the nervous system has discrete segmental ganglia and there are numerous malpighian tubes. More than 3,500 species have been described of which a small number have become domestic pests. As synanthropic insects, i.e. adapted to living closely with man, they have been carried around the world by him in his baggage. The main pest species are the large *Periplaneta americana* and *P. australasiae* and the smaller *Blatella germanica* and *Blatta orientalis*.

Figure 2.13: Dorsal View of a Cockroach, *Periplaneta americana*

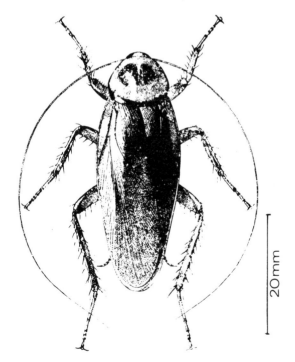

20mm

Source: From Patton, W.S. (1931). *Insects, Ticks, Mites and Venomous Animals, Part II: Public Health.* H.R. Grubb, Croydon

Cockroaches are active, nocturnal insects, whose main period of activity is after 'lights out'. The full extent of an infestation is only appreciated when the householder returns to the kitchen some time after all the lights have been put out. The sight can be most displeasing. Apart from their presence being aesthetically unacceptable they produce a characteristic offensive odour. They are scavengers which are attracted to any organic material which may serve as food. They are equally at home in the sewers and in the kitchen. The sewers of tropical cities often support unbelievable populations of cockroaches which on warm nights emerge and are attracted to lights around and inside houses.

Cockroaches will feed on human food, excreta, sputa and, when food is scarce, the bindings of books and even paper. This wide-ranging feeding habit makes cockroaches potential mechanical vectors of pathogens but their precise role in any particular situation has to be assessed individually. The relationship of cockroaches with pathogenic organisms and other life forms has been comprehensively reviewed by Roth and Willis in two publications.[14, 15] Cockroaches can carry infected material on their bodies when their legs and mouthparts become contaminated while feeding on it. In addition, while feeding they defaecate, and pathogens can remain fully viable after passage through the cockroach gut. In some situations cockroaches may be more important than houseflies as mechanical vectors of human disease.

Order Phthiraptera (Lice)

Lice are small, dorsoventrally flattened, exopterygote, wingless, obligatory ectoparasites of birds and mammals. Two different forms of lice have evolved — the Mallophaga retain the primitive insectan mandibulate mouthparts and feed on epidermal structures of birds and mammals, while the Anoplura have evolved specialised mouthparts for blood-feeding and are found only on mammals.

Suborder Anoplura (= Siphunculata) *(Suckling lice)* (see Figure 2.14). Sucking lice have relatively long, narrow heads on which the mouthparts are not discernible externally. They are retracted into the head (see Chapter 4). The three thoracic segments are fused to form a single structure. The most important siphunculate louse is *Pediculus humanus*, a parasite of man. The human louse has had a major impact on human history and social development by being the biological vector of epidemic typhus and epidemic relapsing fever (see Chapters 25 and 26).

Suborder Mallophaga (Chewing Lice) (see Figure 2.15). The heads of chewing lice are broad to accommodate mandibulate mouthparts and their associated muscles. These mouthparts are obvious externally. The prothorax is free from the mesothorax, which may be fused to, or separate from, the metathorax. The chewing lice are mainly ectoparasites of birds but some species occur on mammals.

The Phthiraptera are considered in more detail in Chapter 19.

Order Hemiptera (Bugs) (see Figure 2.16)

The Hemiptera are exopterygote insects with highly specialised mouthparts produced into a ventrally reflected proboscis. Most Hemiptera feed on the fluid contents of plants either by tapping the phloem or by piercing the cells of the mesophyll. This habit of piercing plants makes them ideal vectors of plant pathogens and they are vectors of viruses which cause disease among crops and are therefore of considerable importance to agriculturalists and horticulturalists. Some Hemiptera are predacious and a few feed on blood, including the Cimicidae (bedbugs) and some Reduviidae (assassin bugs). The latter are vectors of Chagas' disease caused by *Trypanosoma cruzi* (Chapter 29).

Figure 2.14: Dorsal View of *Linognathus vituli*, the Long-nosed Cattle Louse (Phthiraptera, Anoplura)

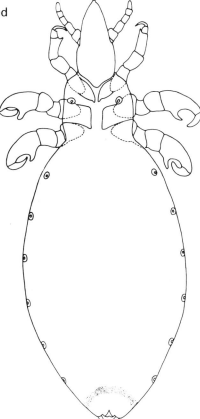

Figure 2.15: Dorsal View of
Paraheterodoxus insignis
(Phthiraptera, Mallophaga,
Boopidae)

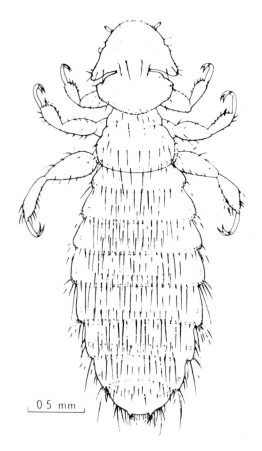

0·5 mm

Order Coleoptera (Beetles) (see Figure 2.17)

Beetles are endopterygote, mandibulate insects with thickened forewings
known as elytra (singular elytron), which meet edge to edge in the middorsal line. The Coleoptera is the largest order containing 40 per cent of
the known species of insects, but it is only of very minor importance in
medical entomology. When some beetles are disturbed they produce a vesicating fluid. Members of the Meloidae are known as blister-beetles, of
which the best-known member is the southern European species *Lytta
vesicatoria* popularly known as Spanish-fly (Figure 2.17A). The active
agent in the vesicating secretions is cantharadin, a highly toxic material,
which at one time was used medicinally as a counter irritant[1] and illegally
as an aphrodisiac.

Rove beetles (Staphylinidae) of the genus *Paederus* (Figure 2.17B)
secrete a vesicating fluid when crushed or irritated. This phenomonen has
been recorded in the southern hemisphere and the Oriental region. In
Australia the species usually involved is *Paederus cruenticollis*,[10] and in

Figure 2.16: Ventral View of a
Hemipteran, a Cicada

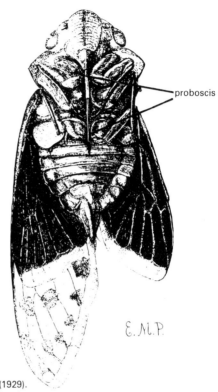

proboscis

E. M. P.

Source: From Patton, W.S. and Evans, A.M. (1929).
Insects, Ticks, Mites and Venomous Animals, Part I:
Medical. H.R. Grubb, Croydon

East Africa it is the Nairobi eye-fly (*Paederus cribripunctatus*). The fluid is usually secreted when the insect lands on bare skin and is injudiciously brushed off or when it becomes trapped between clothing and skin. There is no immediate response to the fluid but in a day or two's time an angry red weal will appear and be followed by the formation of blisters.

Order Hymenoptera (Ants, Bees, Wasps) (see Figure 2.18)

The Hymenoptera are endopterygote, mandibulate insects in which the forewings are larger than the hind wings and both fore and hind wings are coupled mechanically to function as a single entity. Many Hymenoptera have a complex social organisation. The female ovipositor is often modified into a sting which is used to immobilise prey, as in the hunting wasps, or in defence of the colony, as in ants and bees. Although a wasp or bee sting is painful the main danger lies in an allergic response, which may lead to anaphylactic shock and rapid collapse of the person stung. In this way wasp and bee stings caused 61 deaths in England and Wales during the period 1959 to 1971.[18]

Figure 2.17: Coleoptera — Dorsal Views of *Lytta versicatoria* (A) and *Paederus sabeus* (B)

A   B

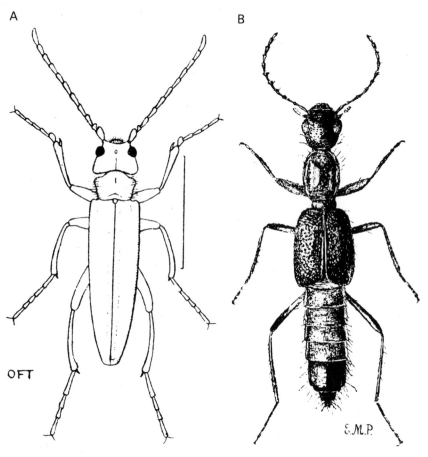

OFT

E.M.P.

Source: From Patton, W.S. (1931). *Insects, Ticks and Venomous Animals, Part II: Public Health.* H.R. Grubb, Croydon

Order Lepidoptera (Butterflies, Moths) (see Figure 2.19)

Lepidoptera are endopterygote insects whose body, legs and wings are covered with detachable scales, which are morphologically flattened hairs. The scales produce colourful patterns which make members of this order so attractive and the object of collectors. The larval stage is a caterpillar with chewing mandibulate mouthparts, while the adult has a coiled proboscis for feeding on nectar. In West Africa a very few moths, mainly species of *Acyophora* (Noctuidae), have been found to feed on secretions of the eyes of cattle.[4, 12] In south-east Asia one Noctuid *Calpe eustrigata* actually

Figure 2.18: Dorsal View of a Hymenopteran

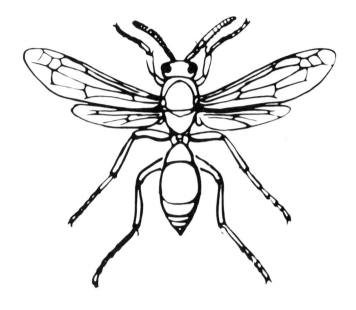

Figure 2.19: Dorsal View of a Lepidopteran

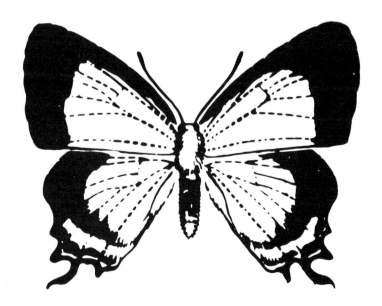

pierces the skin of mammals and feeds on blood.[2] This species is nocturnal, feeding between 20.00 and 02.00 hours with the actual feeding process taking 12 to 30 minutes. *C. eustrigata* has been observed feeding on a range of large mammals including elephant, rhino, tapir and Artiodactyla.

Many caterpillars are covered with long hair, e.g. processionary caterpillars (Notodontidae) and the Australian white cedar moth *Leptocneria reducta*.[20] Such larvae should be handled with care as the hairs are often urticating. In addition allergic responses can be induced among sensitive individuals by exposure to the scales and hairs of Lepidoptera. A few caterpillars secrete noxious fluids, e.g. formic acid by *Dicranura vinula*[13] and *Heterocampa mantea*.[8]

Order Siphonaptera (Fleas) (see Figure 2.20)

Fleas are laterally flattened, wingless, endopterygote, blood-sucking ectoparasites of birds and mammals. The larva is apodous (legless) while in the adult the hind legs are saltatorial, i.e. adapted for leaping, and the source of the familiar escape response of adult fleas. Fleas are important vectors of disease, of which the major one is plague (Chapter 26) and are dealt with in Chapter 17.

Order Diptera (Two-winged Flies) (see Figure 2.21)

Diptera are endopterygote insects with only one pair of functional wings, the mesothoracic pair, the metathoracic pair being modified into halteres, which play an important role in flight. Halteres are stalked, knobbed struc-

Figure 2.20: Lateral View of
a Flea (Siphonapteran)

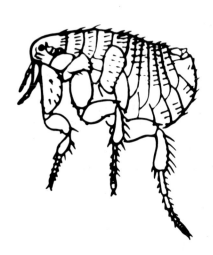

tures which function as alternating gyroscopes providing, in most Diptera, essential sensory information for the stabilisation of flight. Some Diptera, e.g. horseflies (Tabanidae), can still fly properly when the halteres have been surgically removed, but most Diptera, e.g. the blowfly, *Calliphora*, cannot.[23] Dipterous larvae are apodous; those of the higher Diptera have very reduced heads and some are known as maggots. From a medical point of view the Diptera is the most important order of insects and its classification will be considered in detail in the next chapter.

Figure 2.21: Dorsal View of a Dipteran

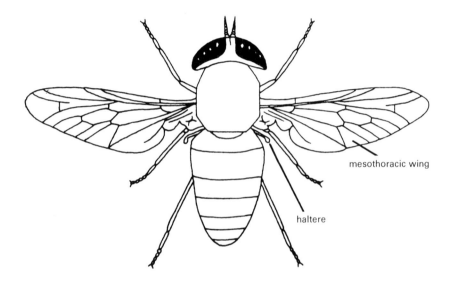

mesothoracic wing

haltere

References

1. Ainley Wade (ed.) (1977). *Martindale: The Extra Pharmacopoeia.* Pharmaceutical Press, London
2. Banziger, H. (1975). Skin-piercing blood-sucking moths. I. Ecological and ethological studies on *Calpe eustrigata* (Lepidoptera; Noctuidae). *Acta Tropica 32*: 125-44
3. Bettini, S. (ed.) (1978). *Arthropod Venoms.* Springer-Verlag, Berlin
4. Buttiker, W. and Nicolet, J. (1975). Observations complémentaires sur les lépidoptères ophthalmotropes en Afrique occidentale. *Revue d'Elevage et de Médecine Vétérinaire des Pays Tropicaux 28*: 319-29
5. Chapman, R.F. (1971). *The Insects: Structure and Function.* Hodder and Stoughton, London
6. CSIRO (1970). *The Insects of Australia.* Sponsored by the Division of Entomology, CSIRO, Canberra
7. Grassé, Pierre-P. (1949). *Traité de Zoologie, Anatomie, Systématique, Biologie. VI. Oncychophores, Tardigrades, Arthropodes — Trilobitomorphes Chélicérates.* Masson et Cie, Paris

8. Kearby, W.H. (1975). Variable oakleaf caterpillar larvae secrete formic acid that causes skin lesions (Lepidoptera: Notodontidae). *Journal of the Kansas Entomological Society* 48: 280-2
9. Keegan, H.L. (1980). *Scorpions of Medical Importance.* University Press of Mississippi, Jackson, Mississippi
10. McKeown, K.C. (1951). Dermatitis apparently caused by a staphylinid beetle in Australia. *Medical Journal of Australia* 2: 772-3
11. Minton, S.A. (1974). *Venom Diseases.* Charles C. Thomas, Springfield, Illinois
12. Nicolet, J. and Buttiker, W. (1975). Observations sur la kératoconjonctivitis infectieuse du bovin en Côte d'Ivoire. 2. Etude sur la rôle vecteur des lépidoptères ophthalmotropes. *Revue d'Elevage et de Médecine Vétérinaire des Pays Tropicaux* 28: 125-32
13. Richards, O.W. and Davies, R.G. (1977). *Imms' General Textbook of Entomology.* Chapman and Hall, London
14. Roth, L.M. and Willis, E.R. (1957). The medical and veterinary importance of cockroaches. *Smithsonian Miscellaneous Collections 134* (10): 1-147
15. _____ and Willis, E.R. (1960). The biotic associations of cockroaches. *Smithsonian Miscellaneous Collections 141*: 1-470
16. Savory, T.H. (1977). *Arachnida.* Academic Press, London
17. Schenone, H., Rubio, S., Villarroel, F. and Rojas, A. (1975). Epidemiologia y curso clinico del loxoscelismo. Estudio de 133 casos causados por la mordedura de la araña de los rincones (*Loxosceles laeta*). *Boletin Chileno de Parasitologia 30*: 6-17
18. Somerville, R., Till, D., Leclercq, M and Lecomte, J. (1975). Les morts par piqûre d'hymenoptères Aculéates en Angleterre et au Pays de Galles (Statistiques pour la periode 1959-1971). *Revue Médicale de Liège 30*: 76-8
19. Southcott, R.V. (1978). *Harmful Arachnids.* Mimeographed by author, 2 Taylors Road, Mitcham, South Australia 5052
20. _____ (1978). Lepidopterism in the Australian Region. *Records of the Adelaide Children's Hospital 2*: 87-173
21. Sutherland, S.K. (1980). The biochemistry and actions of some Australian venoms with notes on first aid. *Chemistry in Australia 47*: 351-6
22. Watt, D.D., Babin, D.R. and Mlejnek, R.V. (1974). The protein neurotoxins in scorpion and Elapid snake venoms. *Journal of Agricultural and Food Chemistry 22*: 43-51
23. Wigglesworth, V.B. (1972). *The Principles of Insect Physiology.* Chapman and Hall, London

3 CLASSIFICATION AND STRUCTURE OF THE DIPTERA

Before considering the classification of the Diptera it will be necessary to examine briefly some features of their structure. The antennae are typically many-segmented, long and slender in the Nematocera and three-segmented and short in the Cyclorrhapha. In the latter the characteristic antenna has two, short, basal segments, and a long, third segment bearing a dorsal arista (Figure 3.1). In most Cyclorrhapha the antennae are surrounded dorsally and laterally by an inverted U-shaped frontal or ptilinal suture.

Figure 3.1: Heads of A, an Aschizan, and B, a Schizophoran

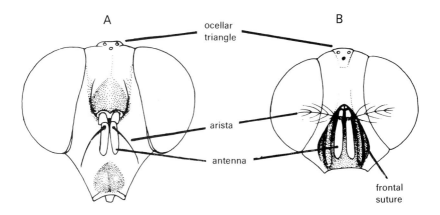

Structure of the Diptera

Thoracic Sclerites and Chaetotaxy[2, 5]

The greater part of the dorsal surface of the thorax is formed by the mesonotum, which is usually subdivided into three areas: an anterior prescutum (sc_a; Figure 3.2), separated by the transverse suture (ss) from the scutum (sc_b), and a small, posterior scutellum (s). Posterior to the mesonotum and between the scutellum and the postnotum (mdt) in the Tachinidae, there is a prominent, convex, transverse ridge, the subscutellum (ssc) or postscutellum. The chaetotaxy, i.e. the arrangement of bristles and setae, on the mesonotum includes the acrostichals (ac), a row of bristles either side of the middorsal line on the prescutum and scutum; and a more-or-less parallel row of dorsocentral (dc) bristles between the acrostichals and more laterally placed bristles. The scutellum carries a row of bristles along its free margin.

Figure 3.2: Thoracic Structure and Chaetotaxy of a Cyclorrhaphan (Tachinidae).

an, mesopleuron (anepisternum); *cx₁, cx₂, cx₃,* coxae of pro-, meso- and metathoraces respectively; *h,* haltere; *mdt,* postnotum (mediotergite); *mp,* meropleuron (hypopleuron); *mtp,* metapleuron; *np,* notopleuron; *pac,* postalar callus; *plt,* pleurotergite of postnotum; *ppl,* propleuron; *ppn,* pronotum; *ps,* pleural suture; *ptp,* pteropleuron; *s,* scutellum; *scₐ,* prescutum; *scᵦ,* scutum; *sp₂, sp₃,* meso- and metathoracic spiracles respectively; *ss,* transverse suture; *ssc,* subscutellum (postscutellum); *stp,* sternopleuron (katepisternum). Bristles in A: *ac,* acrostichal; *dc,* dorsocentral; *hm,* humeral; *in,* intraalar; *ph,* posthumeral; *pr,* presutural; *sa,* supraalar

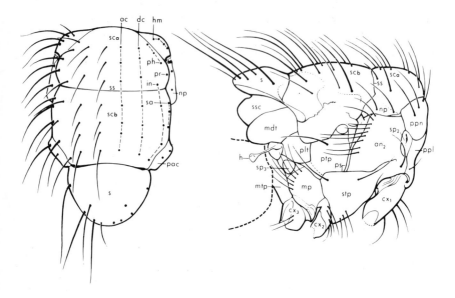

Source: From Colless and McAlpine in CSIRO[2]

The lateral walls of the thorax are formed from sclerites and their chaetotaxy provides useful characters for identification, particularly in the Cyclorrhapha. The notopleuron (*np*) is a triangular sclerite dorsolaterally placed, adjoining the transverse suture. The mesopleuron (*an*) or anepisternum lies below the notopleuron and posterior to the mesothoracic spiracle (*sp2*). It abuts on the ventral sternopleuron (*stp*) or katepisternum. Posterior to these two sclerites there is an upper pteropleuron (*ptp*) and a lower meropleuron (*mp*) or hypopleuron. The pteropleuron lies below the insertion of the wing. The upper posterior corner of the meropleuron adjoins the metathoracic spiracle (*sp3*).

Wing Structure and Venation[2, 5, 7]

The wing may have up to three basal lobes posteriorly — the alula and two squamae (singular squama). The alula has the same appearance as the wing membrane but is separated from it by a deep incision. The squamae or calypters are thicker and more opaque than the wing membrane. One is attached to the base of the wing and the other to the thorax, and when the latter is well developed it overlies the haltere, which is not visible from above.

Two systems of classifying wing veins are in general use. The Comstock-Needham system is widely used by entomologists, but many dipterists use a numerical system. The two systems will be compared using the wing venations of a calliphorid and a mosquito (Figures 3.3 and 3.4). In both systems the vein supporting the anterior margin of the wing is the costa, and it usually ends towards the apex of the wing. Posterior to the costa there is a shorter, longitudinal vein, the subcosta, which is unbranched, but may be two-branched in other Diptera.

Figure 3.3: Wing of *Musca domestica* (Cyclorrhapha, Muscidae). cv = cross-vein

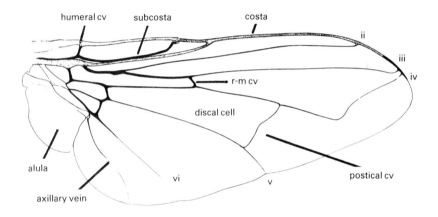

Figure 3.4: Wing of an *Anopheles* Mosquito

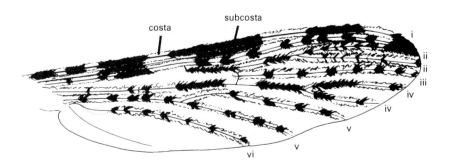

Proceeding posteriorly the longitudinal veins are successively the radius, media, cubitus and anal. The radius forks near the base of the wing, giving rise to an unbranched vein (R_1 or vein i) and the radial sector (Rs), which may have four branches (R_2 to R_5). Branches of veins are referred to by an initial followed by a number with the veins being numbered anteroposteriorly. In the calliphorid, vein ii ($R_2 + R_3$) is unbranched, but in the mosquito vein ii is branched, i.e. R_2 and R_3 are separate, and are referred to, in the numerical system, as the anterior and posterior branches of vein ii. This applies to other branched numbered veins. Vein iii (R_4 and $R_5 = R_{4+5}$) is unbranched in both the mosquito and calliphorid. The media vein may be four-branched (M_1 to M_4). In the calliphorid vein iv (M_{1+2}) is unbranched, but in the mosquito there is an anterior branch to vein iv (M_1) and a posterior branch (M_2). Vein v (M_{3+4}) is unbranched in calliphorids, and with anterior and posterior branches in the mosquito. Vein vi is formed from the cubitus and anal, and there may be an axillary vein.

In the Diptera there are relatively few cross-veins, but the following are usually present: a humeral cross-vein, running between the costa and subcosta at the base of the wing; an r-m cross-vein between veins iii and iv in the middle of the wing; and a postical or posterior cross-vein between veins iv and v. Areas of the wing separated by veins are referred to as cells, and named after the vein forming the anterior border of the cell. Cells do not have to be bound on all borders by veins, and are often open at the wing margin.

Classification of the Diptera[2]

The Diptera are divided into two suborders, the Nematocera and Brachycera.[2] The Nematocera are usually small, delicate, gnat-like flies, with long filamentous antennae composed of many similar, freely articulated segments (more than six). The single pair of palps are three- to five-jointed and usually pendulous but are porrect, i.e. stiff and forwardly directed, in mosquitoes. The larval stage has a well-developed head. The Brachycera are small to large, stout-bodied flies with short antennae, often composed of three segments and never more than six, freely articulated segments. The palps are one- or two-jointed and porrect. The larval stage has a reduced head.

Suborder Nematocera

Four of the 18 families in the Nematocera are of medical and veterinary importance. They are the Culicidae (mosquitoes), the Psychodidae (true sandflies), the Ceratopogonidae (biting midges) and the Simuliidae (blackflies). The characters by which the adults of these families may be recognised and the diseases and pathogens with which they are associated are given briefly below.

Family Culicidae (Mosquitoes) (see Chapter 7)

Adult culicids have scales on their wings and body and a characteristic wing venation, in which the longitudinal veins (i to iv) run more or less parallel to the long axis of the wing and end at the wing tip. Veins ii and iv are forked while veins i and iii are unbranched (Figure 3.4). There is a long, forwardly directed proboscis, which is longer than the head and thorax combined and the palps are porrect. Mosquitoes are vectors of pathogenic protozoans, viruses and nematodes which cause such diseases as malaria., yellow fever and lymphatic filariasis to man and related diseases in domestic animals.

Family Ceratopogonidae (Biting Midges) (see Chapter 8)

Ceratopogonids are small, compact flies with short legs, a short vertical proboscis and pendulous palps (Figure 8.1). The wing venation is reduced with only two veins (iv and v) in the posterior half of the wing (Figure 8.2). They are both two-branched. Members of this family are important pests of man and vectors of pathogens to livestock, including bluetongue virus to sheep and nodule-forming nematodes to cattle.

Family Psychodidae (Sandflies, Mothflies) (see Chapter 9)

These small flies have their bodies and wings covered with hairs but no scales. The wing venation is characterised by having veins ii and v branched, and iii and iv unbranched (Figure 9.2). The proboscis is short and directed vertically downwards and the palps are pendulous (Figure 9.1). The true sandflies (Phlebotominae) are vectors of several diseases of which the most important is leishmaniasis, caused by infection with the protozoan *Leishmania.* The mothflies are of no medical or veterinary importance.

Family Simuliidae (Blackflies) (see Chapter 10)

Simuliids are small, hump-backed flies with a short vertical proboscis and pendulous palps. The antennae have eleven segments but appear shorter due to the individual segments being globular. The wing has strongly developed anterior veins and weakly developed posterior veins (iv, v and vi) (Figure 10.3). They are important vectors of filarial nematode worms, including *Onchocerca volvulus,* the cause of river blindness in man.

Suborder Brachycera

The classification used here is taken from *Insects of Australia* and recognises two divisions within the Brachycera, the Orthorrhapha and the Cyclorrhapha[2]. Another classification in common use recognises three suborders within the Diptera — Nematocera, Brachycera and Cyclorrhapha.[5, 7] The relationship between the two classifications is that in the second system the divisions of the first are raised to the status of suborders and the term Orthorrhapha replaced with Brachycera. The category Brachycera, as defined in the first system, disappears.

Division Orthorrhapha

The Orthorrhapha are large, stout-bodied flies, the adults and larvae of which are largely predacious. The structure of the antennae is variable, the palps are one- or two-segmented and the abdomen has seven visible segments. The head of the larva is retractable into the thorax and the pupa is free of the larval exuviae, i.e. it is obtect. Only one of the 15 families in this division, the Tabanidae, is of medical importance.

Family Tabanidae (Horseflies, Marchflies) (see Chapter 11)

Tabanids are stout-bodied flies with antennae, which are stiff and forwardly directed, and eyes, which are often coloured. The wing venation of a tabanid is characteristic but is not exclusive to the family. All the wing veins are well developed and there is an enclosed discal cell in the distal half of the wing (Figure 11.2). The squamae are large, obscuring the halteres from dorsal view. The empodium is padlike and hence the last tarsal segment of the leg carries three pads and two claws (Figure 2.11). They are vectors of loiasis to man and surra to livestock.

Division Cyclorrhapha

These flies have three-segmented antennae with the third segment bearing an arista on its dorsal surface (Figure 3.1). The abdomen rarely has as many as seven segments visible. The larvae are acephalic, i.e. the head is vestigial, and they live in organic matter. The pupa is enclosed in the last larval skin or puparium, i.e. coarctate. The Cyclorrhapha is composed of two series, the Aschiza and the Schizophora. The Aschiza contains six families of medically unimportant Diptera, which do not have a ptilinum (see below) and therefore lack a frontal suture on the head (Figure 3.1).

The Schizophora contains a large number of families which have both a ptilinum and a frontal suture. When the fly emerges from the pupa the suture is open. This allows the flap, carrying the antennae, to hinge on its lower edge, permitting eversion of a balloon-like structure, the ptilinum, from the head. The larvae of Schizophora often burrow into the soil before pupariation to reduce predation and parasitisation of the immobile puparium. The newly-emerged fly is able to force its way to the surface of the soil by alternately inflating and retracting the ptilinum. While it is being retracted the fly climbs up into the space vacated. Using this structure

Figure 3.5: A, Head of a Chloropid; B, Wing of a Chloropid

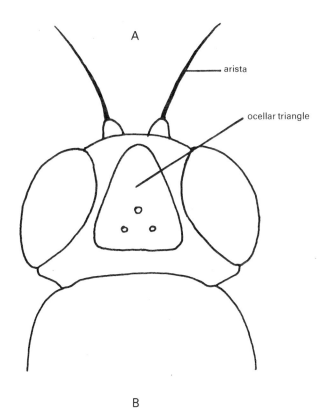

houseflies can reach the surface from considerable depths. Once the fly reaches the surface the ptilinum is withdrawn and the suture closed.

The Schizophora is a large assemblage of nearly 50 families of Diptera which are grouped into superfamilies of which one, the Muscoidea, is of considerable medical and veterinary importance. In addition the Chloropidae, a family of the Drosophiloidea, is of medical importance.

Family Chloropidae (Eyeflies)

Eyeflies are small, very shiny flies about 2 mm long. Their antennae are short, with the third segment being nearly globular and the arista either bare or with very short branches. The ocellar triangle is very large (Figure 3.5). The thorax has no distinct transverse suture and the squamae are small, not obscuring the halteres from dorsal view. The wings have no markings, the subcosta is rudimentary and vein vi is absent.

The adults of some species are attracted to body secretions and feed on sweat, at sores, and are particularly attracted to eyes, especially eyes which have a copious discharge. They scrape the conjunctival surface of the eye with the spiny tips of the pseudotracheal rings on the labella (see Chapter 4). This irritation increases the flow of secretion, attracting more eyeflies. By moving from one individual to another eyeflies can act as mechanical vectors of yaws[4] and conjunctivitis. In the Oriental region *Siphunculina funicola* is the main species associated with man; and in the southern states of the USA, *Hippelates pusio* in the east and *H. collusor* in the west.[6] *H. pusio* oviposits in freshly cultivated or otherwise disturbed soil,[1, 3] where the larvae are widely dispersed in the soil and under favourable conditions peak emergence of adults will occur three weeks after oviposition. Other species breed in plant or vegetable debris.

Superfamily Muscoidea

These are moderately large flies in which the thorax has a distinct transverse suture and the squamae are usually well developed. The commonest form of mouthparts in the Muscoidea is the lapping type, adapted for feeding on surface films and secretions. A small number of species have evolved piercing mouthparts adapted for feeding on blood, and a small number have vestigal, i.e. non-functional, mouthparts.

Family Glossinidae (Tsetse Flies) (see Chapter 12)

Tsetse flies are medium to large, brown, blood-sucking flies, which at the present day are confined to Africa south of the Sahara. They have a long, forwardly directed, piercing proboscis. The wing venation is unique being characterised by a 'hatchet-shaped' cell, more or less in the centre of the wing (Figure 12.3). The cell is limited by veins iv and v anteriorly and posteriorly, respectively, and cross-veins proximally and distally. Tsetse flies are viviparous, depositing fully-developed, non-feeding larvae, which burrow into the substrate and pupariate. Tsetse flies are biological vectors of pathogenic trypanosomes, which cause sleeping sickness in man and trypanosomiasis in animals.

Family Muscidae (Houseflies, Stableflies) (see Chapter 13)

Houseflies are medium sized, rather dull coloured flies usually without bristles on the pteropleura and meropleura. Their mouthparts are either lapping or piercing. Vein iv is either parallel to vein iii or gently curved towards it in the distal half of the wing, and vein vi does not reach the wing margin (Figure 13.2). Muscids breed commonly in material of vegetable origin, grass cuttings, straw, and the dung of herbivores. Houseflies are important mechanical vectors of intestinal pathogens, such as those which cause typhoid, and amoebic and bacillary dysenteries. Blood-sucking stableflies can act as mechanical vectors of surra in camels and horses.

Family Calliphoridae (Blowflies) (see Chapter 14)

Calliphorids are medium to large flies often metallic in colour, dark green or blue. Their mouthparts are of the lapping type. The arista is plumose to beyond halfway. Vein iv is quite sharply bent towards vein iii and the two veins are very close together when they meet the wing margin (Figure 3.3). Both the meropleura and pteropleura bear bristles, and there are two stout bristles on the notopleura. Calliphorid larvae feed on organic material of animal origin and serve a useful purpose in breaking down carrion, but some feed on living animal flesh causing a condition known as myiasis.

Family Sarcophagidae (Grey Fleshflies) (see Chapter 14)

Sarcophagids are similar in appearance to calliphorids but their bodies are grey with black longitudinal stripes on the thorax. In addition they have three or more bristles on the notopleura and usually only the basal half of the arista is plumose. A few species of sarcophagids are associated with myiasis, but most breed in carrion.

Families Oestridae, Hypodermatidae, Cuterebridae and Gasterophilidae (see Chapter 15)

These families were, at one time, included in a single family, an enlarged 'Oestridae', on the grounds that they were all large bee-like flies with vestigal mouthparts and usually densely clothed with bushy hair. The adults do not feed and therefore are relatively shortlived and uncommon. The larvae are endoparasites of vertebrates, causing myiasis in livestock.

Families Hippoboscidae (Keds), Streblidae and Nycteribiidae
(see Chapter 16)

Members of the these families are leathery, dorsoventrally flattened, blood-sucking ectoparasites of birds and animals. In adaptation to this mode of life the legs bear well-developed claws, and all nycteribiids and many other species are wingless. The females are viviparous with the larva being retained in the body of the female until it is fully developed. The larva is immobile and pupariates where it has been deposited. At one time it was considered that the female deposited a puparium and these three families were grouped together as the Pupipara. The main species of economic importance is the sheep ked, *Melophagus ovinus.*

References

1. Burgess, R.W. (1951). The life history and breeding habits of the eye-gnat *Hippelates pusio* Loew in the Coachella Valley, Riverside County, California. *American Journal of Hygiene* 53: 164-77
2. CSIRO (1970). *The Insects of Australia.* Sponsored by the Division of Entomology, CSIRO, Canberra
3. Dow, R.P. and Hutson, G.A. (1958). The measurement of adult populations of the eye gnat, *Hippelates pusio. Annals of the Entomological Society of America* 5: 351-60
4. Nicholls, L. (1936). Framboesia tropica — a short review of a colonial report concerning statistics and *Hippelates flavipes. Annals of Tropical Medicine and Parasitology 30*: 331-5
5. Richards, O.W. and Davies, R.G. (1977). *Imms' General Textbook of Entomology.* Chapman and Hall, London
6. Rogoff, W.M. (1978). *Methods for collecting eye gnats (Diptera: Chloropidae).* United States Department of Agriculture, Science and Education Administration, ARM-W2
7. Smith, K.G.V. (ed.) (1973). *Insects and Other Arthropods of Medical Importance.* British Museum (Natural History), London

4 MOUTHPARTS OF INSECTS OF MEDICAL AND VETERINARY IMPORTANCE

The mouthparts of medically important insects deserve special consideration because they are the main, but not the only, route whereby pathogens are transmitted from host to host. Even when no pathogen is involved, the mouthparts are the structures which pierce the skin and cause irritation. It is preferable to deal with the mouthparts on a comparative basis rather than to describe them separately for each group of insects.

Basic Chewing Mouthparts — Mallophaga (see Figure 4.1)

The mouthparts of a primitive insect are chewing structures capable of dealing with a wide range of potential food material. Three pairs of appendages are associated with the mouth. They are the mandibles, first maxillae, and the labium, which is formed from the fused second maxillae. Both the maxillae and the labium may bear sensory palps. The mouthparts have evolved from appendages, and are therefore external to the mouth and border the preoral cavity. In hypognathous insects, the preoral cavity is bordered anteriorly by the labrum-epipharynx (referred to hereafter as the labrum), composed of an inner sensory surface, the epipharynx, and an external strongly-sclerotised labrum or upper lip. The lateral walls of the preoral cavity are formed by the mandibles and maxillae, and the posterior wall by the labium. The hypopharynx is an unpaired, median, tongue-like structure, located internally to the labium, and associated with the opening of the salivary duct.

At the start of feeding, potential food is palpated by the palps which have sensilla concentrated at their free ends. If the appropriate sensory information is received the food is crushed by the mandibles and the exuding fluid passes over the sensory areas of the labium and maxillae. If the fluid contains the appropriate stimulating substances the maxillae and labium participate in feeding. Both structures have cutting blades which finely divide the food and during this process saliva is poured out and mixes with the food.

Chewing mouthparts of this type are found in cockroaches, beetles and locusts. They are modified in the Mallophaga with the labium being reduced to a simple broad plate to which the maxillae are attached laterally. There are no palps in the suborder Ischnocera, and only a pair of maxillary palps in the other suborder the Amblycera.

Figure 4.1: Mouthparts of an Amblyceran (Mallophaga). A, ventral view of head; B, mandibles; C, maxilla; D. labium and maxillae

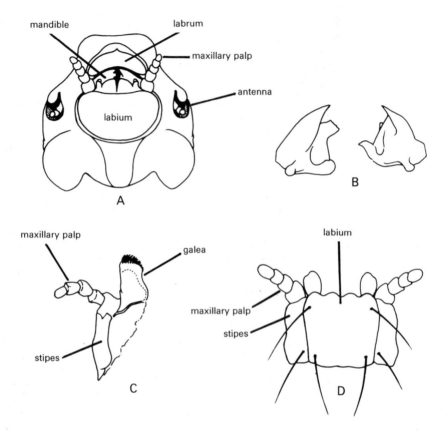

Source: Redrawn from Snodgrass, R.E. (1943). *Smithsonian Miscellaneous Collections 104* (7). By permission of the Smithsonian Institution Press, Smithsonian Institution, Washington D.C.

Blood-sucking Mouthparts — Nematocera (see Figure 4.2)

In blood-sucking Nematocera the mouthparts have to perform two functions, to pierce the skin and imbibe blood. The mouthparts are essentially the same in all four families of blood-sucking Nematocera (Culicidae, Ceratopogonidae, Simuliidae and Phlebotominae), although they are greatly elongated in the Culicidae. They contain the same elements as in the Mallophaga. Only the maxillary palps are present. However, the primitive mouthparts have been greatly modified for feeding on blood. The labium forms a protective sheath for the effective structures and it ends in

Figure 4.2: A, Mouthparts of a Female Mosquito (antennae incomplete); B, Transverse Section of Proboscis of *Aedes aegypti* towards Apex

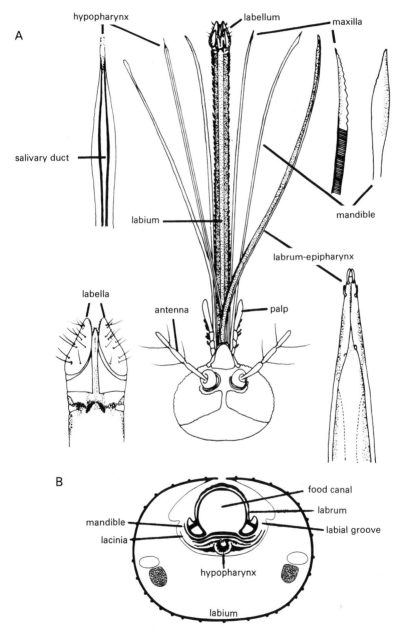

Source: A, redrawn from Patton, W.S. and Evans, A.M. (1929). *Insects, Ticks, Mites and Venomous Animals, Part I: Medical.* H.R. Grubb, Croydon; B (1970), from *Insects of Australia.* Melbourne University Press

two sensory lobes, the labella (singular, labellum). The main cutting function is undertaken by the mandibles and maxillae which are slender structures, finely toothed at the distal ends. The labrum is curled inwards at the edges to form an almost complete tube, and the gap is closed by the mandibles to form the food canal. Blood is sucked up by two muscular pumps, which are separated from each other and the midgut by sphincter muscles. The cibarial pump operates at the base of the food channel and the pharyngeal pump between the cibarium and the midgut.

When a mosquito feeds the labella test the surface of the skin and select a suitable location. The labrum, mandibles and maxillae (lacinia in Figure 4.2B) are closely associated to form the fascicle, which operates as a single structure. The tips of the labrum and the hypopharynx are also toothed. The fascicle moves up and down, supported by the labella, and penetrates the skin. The fascicle is then inserted and the flexible labium, which remains outside the host, becomes bowed posteriorly. The fascicle is either inserted into a capillary or it is moved about to lacerate capillaries and to facilitate the formation of a pool of blood.[7] Saliva is poured into the wound through a duct which runs the entire length of the hypopharynx, opening at its tip. The function of the saliva is to bring about the release of histamine and the consequent dilation of the capillaries, thus ensuring a good flow of blood. The saliva may or may not contain an anticoagulant. The saliva of *Anopheles maculipennis* does, and that of *An claviger* does not.[12] An anticoagulant is not essential for blood-feeding.

Most Nematocera are pool feeders but the long proboscis of mosquitoes enables them to use either pool feeding or capillary feeding. In the blood-sucking Nematocera only the female takes blood. The mandibles and maxillae are reduced or absent in the male, which feeds only on nectar. This implies that only the female can be a vector of disease. Some pathogens, such as viruses and the sporozoites of the malaria parasite, pass down the salivary duct and into the host with the saliva. Infective larvae of filarial worms are too large to use that route. They enter the blood space in the labium and escape by rupturing it near the labella while the insect is feeding. The filarial larvae then enter the host through the feeding site.

Species of blood-sucking Nematocera differ in the degree to which they scrape away the surface of the skin or pierce it more cleanly. This has an effect on their vectorial status. The microfilariae of *Onchocera volvulus* are in the skin and are acquired by *Simulium damnosum* as it scrapes through the skin. *Culicoides austeni* picks up microfilariae of *Dipetalonema perstans* from circulating human blood, but not those of *D. streptocerca*, which are in the skin. On the other hand, *Culicoides grahamii* more easily acquires *D. streptocerca* than *D. perstans*.

Blood-sucking and Lapping Mouthparts of Tabanids (see Figure 4.3)

The mouthparts of tabanids combine the blood-sucking mouthparts of the Nematocera with the lapping mouthparts of the Cyclorrhapha. The fascicle lacks the delicacy which this structure shows in the Nematocera. The mandibles are flat, broad, saw-like blades, the maxillae are narrow, toothed files and the food canal is formed from a stout labrum and a narrow hypopharynx. The fascicle is accommodated in the labial gutter, a groove in the anterior side of the labium. The short, but stout-bodied labium bears terminally a pair of large, fleshy, inflatable labella. The detailed structure of the labella will be given when considering the lapping mouthparts of the Cyclorrhapha.

As in the Nematocera, only the female tabanid is haematophagous, i.e. blood-feeding, while the male feeds only on nectar. When the female tabanid feeds, the labella are retracted to expose the fascicle which pierces the skin and lacerates the tissues for pool-feeding. During this process the mandibles move with a scissor-like action and the maxillae move forwards and backwards.[3] Insertion of the large fascicle is usually painfully obvious. When feeding ceases the fascicle is withdrawn and as the labella come together they trap a film of blood. This is of great importance in the mechanical transmission of diseases because the enclosed film is protected

Figure 4.3: Mouthparts of a Female *Tabanus striatus*. Mandible on left omitted

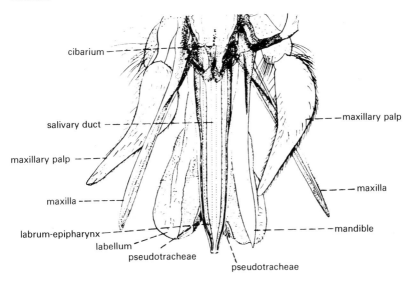

Source: From Patton, W.S. and Evans A.M. (1929). *Insects, Ticks, Mites and Venomous Animals, Part I: Medical.* H.R. Grubb, Croydon

from drying and pathogens such as *Trypanosoma evansi* may survive for an hour or more.

Tabanids are vectors of the filaroid worm *Loa loa* and the infective stage of the nematode enters the labium and escapes from it while the tabanid is feeding.

Lapping Mouthparts of Cyclorrhapha (see Figures 4.4 and 4.5)

Most cyclorrhaphous flies have lapping mouthparts, designed for feeding on liquids, particularly when present in thin films. Under such conditions a food canal, which functions like a drinking straw, is ineffective as it cannot be immersed in a thin film. What is required is an absorbent structure and this has been developed from the labella, which have been greatly enlarged and modified for this function. At rest the inner surfaces of the labella are in close contact and kept moist by secretions from the labial salivary gland.

Figure 4.4: Left, Anterior and Right, Lateral Views of Head and Mouthparts of *Calliphora erythrocephala*

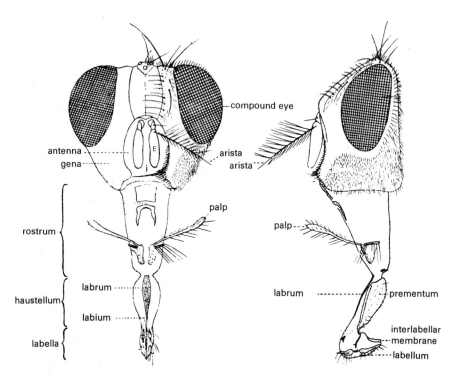

Source: From Graham-Smith, G.S. (1930). *Parasitology*. Cambridge University Press

Figure 4.5: Positions Assumed by Labella of *Calliphora* (A,B,C) and *Musca* (D,E). A, resting position; B, filtering position; C, direct feeding position; D, surface view of labella in filtering position; E, single straightened pseudotracheal ring and flattened portion of pseudotrachea

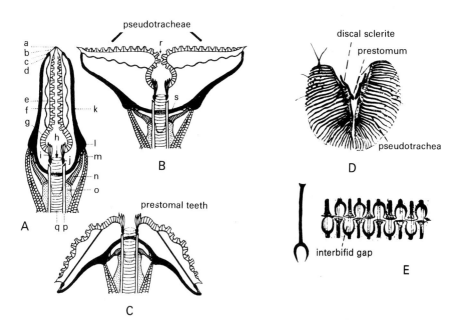

Source: A, B, C from Graham-Smith, G.S. (1930). *Parasitology*, Cambridge University Press; D, E from Patton and Evans, *op. cit.*

These inner surfaces are covered with, more or less, parallel rows of pseudotracheae, which converge on the prestomum or opening of the food canal.

Pseudotracheae are incomplete tubes, the side walls of which are closely opposed, effectively completing the tube. The tubes are supported by numerous interrupted rings of chitin. It is the presence of these rings which cause the tubes to be named pseudotracheae by analogy with the tubular vertebrate trachea which is supported by cartilaginous rings. Each chitin ring has one end simple, and the other end bifurcate, and they are arranged on the pseudotracheae so that simple and bifurcate ends alternate. The membrane supported by the rings is complete everywhere except in the interbifid space, the gap between the arms of each bifurcation. Fluid flows through the interbifid gap by capillary action and is drawn to the prestomum by the sucking action of the cibarial pump acting via the food canal.

The interbifid space acts as a filter, limiting the size of particle which may enter. In *Musca domestica* the diameter of a pseudotrachea ranges from 8-16 μm and the interbifid space from 3-4 μm.[9] This clearly influences the size of pathogen which may be ingested. However, the labella can be retracted and particles enter the food canal directly. The labella are broadly joined to the body of the labium, known as the haustellum, which bears the labial gutter anteriorly. The mandibles and maxillae have been lost, and only the labrum and the hypopharynx are housed in the labial gutter. The haustellum is a rather fleshy structure, supported posteriorly by the prementum, a chitinised plate, and anteriorly by the sclerotised floor of the labial gutter. The cuticle joining these two strengthening structures is thin and flexible.

Plate 4.1: Scanning Electron Micrograph of Everted Labellum (position shown diagrammatically in Figure 4.5C) of Female *Lucilia cuprina*. Note parallel rows of pseudotracheae, and prestomal teeth directed upwards

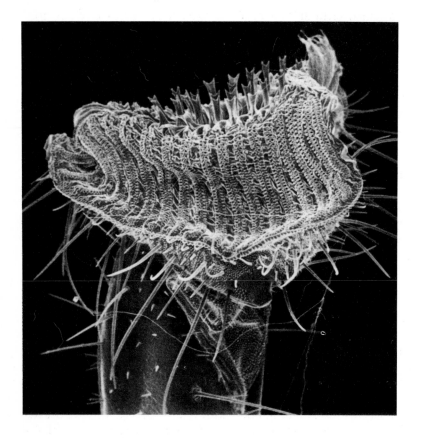

Courtesy of J.V. Hardy, M.J. Rice and S.M. Waladde

The labium is joined proximally to a specialised part of the head capsule, the rostrum, which can be lowered or retracted by inflating or deflating air sacs in the head. When the rostrum is retracted and the haustellum raised to a horizontal position the mouthparts cannot be seen from dorsal view and are inconspicuous in profile. In action the rostrum is lowered by inflation of air sacs and the haustellum directed downwards by muscular action. The labella are expanded by blood pressure and rotated to expose their inner surfaces which form a more or less flat, horizontal surface with the pseudotracheae on the underside. When the pseudotracheal surface is placed on films or liquids, fluid will flow into the pseudotracheae and on to the prestomum, where it will be sucked up the food canal by the cibarial pump and onwards to the gut. At rest the labella collapse as the blood escapes into the circulation, the rostrum is retracted and the haustellum raised to a vertical position.

There are minute teeth around the prestomum, which are used to scrape at material for direct ingestion into the food canal. In some muscid flies these prestomal teeth are enlarged and used to scrape away scabs from wounds and clots from milk, exposing the underlying fluid on which the muscid feeds. Patton and Cragg[9] have described a series of Indian muscids of the genus *Philaematomyia* (now included in different subgenera of *Musca*), in which the teeth get larger and the scraping gets deeper until some can bore through unbroken skin by rapidly applying and withdrawing prestomal teeth. However, the evolution of the mouthparts of truly blood-sucking muscoidea, e.g. *Glossina*, has followed a somewhat different route.

The Mouthparts of Blood-sucking Muscoidea (see Figures 4.6 and 4.7)

The ancestors of the blood-sucking Cyclorrhapha probably had lapping mouthparts and they had certainly lost the mandibles and maxillae. These are the skin-piercing tools of the blood-sucking Nematocera and a substitute has to be developed. The labella have been adapted for this purpose by being reduced in size and the pseudotracheae, if they were present originally, have been replaced by sharp teeth.

In action the labella are pressed on the skin, pulled apart by muscular action and, when the muscles relax, they recoil from the pressure of displaced blood. To function effectively the labella need to be rigidly supported in order to maintain adequate pressure on the host's skin. Rigidity is produced by reducing the zone of thin cuticle between prementum and labial gutter, thus strengthening the haustellum. However, a rigid haustellum cannot bend, as the labium does in the blood-sucking Nematocera when the fascicle is inserted into the host. It is necessary now for both the labium and the enclosed food canal to be inserted. This has been achieved by lengthening the haustellum and concentrating the labellar muscles at its

Figure 4.6: Above, Mouthparts of *Stomoxys*; Below, Transverse Section of Proboscis. *A*, apodeme; *F*, fulcrum; *H*, hypopharynx; *J*, endoskeleton; *L*, labium; *Lp*, labrum-epipharynx; *M*, muscles; *O*, oesophagus; *S*, tendon to labella; *SP*, salivary gland; *T*, trachea; *Ts*, palp

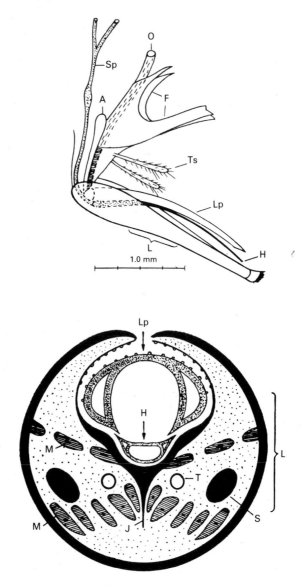

Source: From Zumpt, F. (1973). *Stomoxyine Biting Flies of the World*. Gustav Fischer Verlag, Stuttgart

Figure 4.7: Mouthparts of *Glossina* in Lateral View. *cbp*, cibarial pump; *clp*, clypeus; *csd*, common salivary duct; *ful*, fulcrum; *h*, hypopharynx; *hu*, haustellum; *l*, labrum; *lab*, labellum; *o*, oesophagus; *p*, palp; *th*, theca

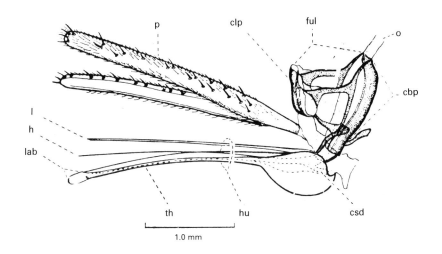

Source: From Buxton, P.A. (1955). *A Natural History of Tsetse Flies.* H.K. Lewis, London

base. The muscles are connected to the labella by long tendons which run throughout the space within the haustellum. To accommodate the concentrated muscles a noticeable swelling or bulb is developed at the base of the haustellum. The rostrum is reduced and the long, rigid haustellum cannot be concealed, being always visible from dorsal and/or lateral views. Mouthparts of this type are found in the Stomoxinae, *Glossina* and the Hippoboscidae.

In feeding, the haustellum is turned vertically downwards and the sensory receptors of the labella are used to select the site for penetration. When the labella are pulled apart and recoiled, the teeth on the labella rasp away the skin. This action is repeated in rapid sequence and the haustellum pierces the skin. Saliva passes down the duct in the hypopharynx and blood is sucked up the food canal by the cibarial pump.

In the Stomoxinae the mouthparts form a stout, robust structure (Figure 4.6). In *Glossina* they have been refined and form a slender, relatively delicate, but highly efficient structure (Figure 4.7). At rest the forwardly directed haustellum is protected by the palps, which flank it on either side. The main support of the haustellum is provided by the sclerotised labial gutter. The prementum is much reduced. The labrum is a delicate structure, held in the labial gutter by teeth on its outer surface. It forms almost a complete tube and the hypopharynx is little more than a sclerotised salivary duct. The labella are narrow structures, each bearing three finely toothed rasps, additional larger teeth and sensilla.[8]

The haustellum is so long that, in feeding, the tsetse fly has to rear up on its hindlegs in order to get the haustellum vertical. It should be noted that there is no connection between the salivary duct and the food canal except at the tip of the haustellum where they both open. This is important in the development of trypanosomes. The proboscis of *Glossina* has relatively few chemoreceptors and these are of two types only. They are so distributed that one type (LR7) is exposed before piercing and the other type (LR5) after penetration (10). Another class of chemo-receptors is present in the labrocibarial region and monitors incoming material before swallowing (11). Feeding of *Glossina austeni* is stimu-lated by the presence of ATP (adenosine triphosphate) and less by ADP and AMP.[6] *Aedes aegypti* shows a similar feeding response to adenosine nucleotides,[5] while the rat flea, *Xenopsylla cheopis*, responds only to ATP.[4]

In the hipposcids the bulb of the haustellum is concealed in a recess in the head, and the thin proboscis is protected by the palps. The labrum,

Figure 4.8: Head and Prothorax of a Flea

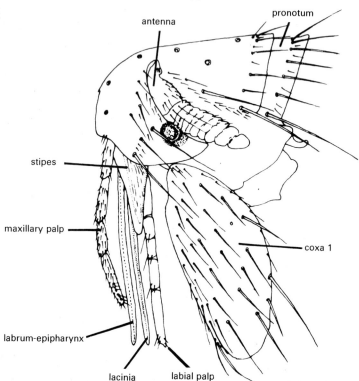

labial gutter and prementum are all sclerotised structures, but the hypopharynx is delicate.

Mouthparts of Fleas (see Figure 4.8)

There have been different views regarding the homologies of the structures composing the mouthparts of fleas. The present view is that fleas have lost the mandibles but retained both labial and maxillary palps. The maxillae are represented by two elements, the lacinia and stipes. The labrum is well

Figure 4.9: Mouthparts of *Cimex lectularius.* A, lateral view of head; B, ventral view of head; C, transverse section of proboscis (rostrum)

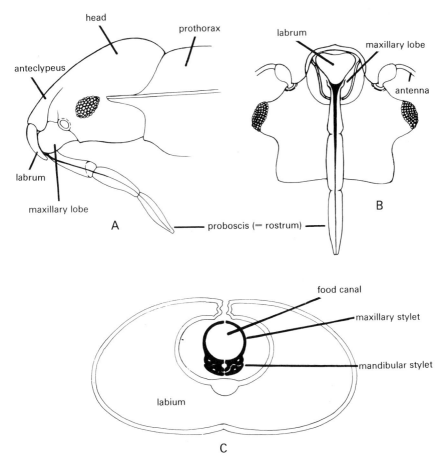

Source: Redrawn from Snodgrass, R.E. (1943). *Smithsonian Miscellaneous Collections 104* (7). By permission of the Smithsonian Institution Press, Smithsonian Institution, Washington, D.C.

Figure 4.10: Longitudinal Section Through Head of an Anopluran Louse (above) and Transverse Section Through Head and Stylet Sac (below)

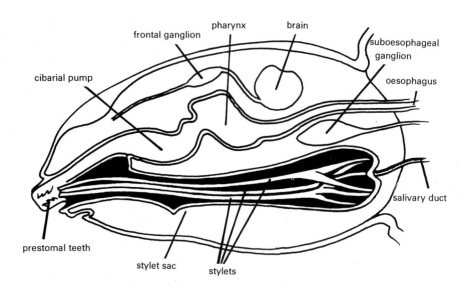

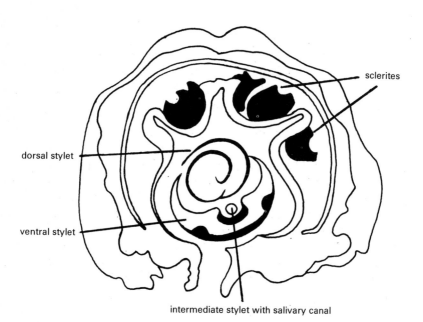

Source: Redrawn from Snodgrass, R.E. (1943). *Smithsonian Miscellaneous Collections 104* (7). By permission of the Smithsonian Institution Press, Smithsonian Institution, Washington, D.C.

developed and forms the food canal. The hypopharynx is very short, and an alternative route has to be found to convey the saliva to the distal end of the mouthparts. This is provided by the laciniae, which are grooved along their length, and the two grooves are closely opposed to form a tube. The labial palps form a protective sheath around the fascicle of laciniae and labrum. When the flea feeds the mouthparts are steadied by the broad, triangular stipites (plural of stipes), which are directed laterally. The toothed laciniae pierce the skin, and as the fascicle is inserted the labial palps separate. Saliva is poured in and blood sucked up the food canal. Fleas infected with plague bacilli become blocked and blood cannot be forced into the midgut by the cibarial pump. When the muscles of the pump relax, blood and part of the bacillary clot flow back into the host and infect it with plague bacilli.

Mouthparts of Blood-sucking Hemiptera (see Figure 4.9)

The proboscis of an hemipteran consists of a jointed labium (rostrum) which encloses a fascicle formed from the closely opposed maxillae and mandibles. There are no palps, the hypopharynx is greatly reduced, and the labrum is short and entirely external to the labium and functional mouthparts. The mandibles, which form the inner core of the fascicle, bear two longitudinal grooves, which are closely opposed. One of these forms the food canal, and the other conveys saliva. When the hemipteran is feeding the fascicle penetrates the skin, and the jointed, labial sheath is bowed posteriorly in a similar manner to the labium of mosquitoes, except that in mosquitoes the labium is unjointed. In *Cimex* and *Rhodnius* the fascicle enters a blood vessel of suitable calibre, and they are capillary feeders.[2]

Mouthparts of Anoplura (see Figure 4.10)

The mouthparts of blood-sucking lice are aberrant and impossible to homologise with those of other insects. They consist of three stylets, housed in the stylet sac, a diverticulum from the floor of the cibarium. The anterior opening of the foregut, the prestomum, is located at the anterior extremity of the head. It is sometimes referred to as the haustellum. Lined internally with small teeth the prestomum is inverted in feeding, and the teeth firmly secure the louse to the skin of its host. The opening of the stylet sac is then brought up to the prestomum and the stylets pierce the skin. Blood is sucked up by the cibarial pump.[1]

References

1. Buxton, P.A. (1950). *The Louse.* Edward Arnold, London
2. Dickerson, G. and Lavoipierrre, M.M.J. (1959). Studies on the methods of feeding of blood-sucking arthropods. II. The method of feeding adopted by the bed-bug (*Cimex lectularius*) when obtaining a blood-meal from the mammalian host. *Annals of Tropical Medicine and Parasitology 53*: 347-57
3. _____ and Lavoipierre, M.M.J. (1959) Studies on the methods of feeding of blood-sucking arthropods. III. The method by which *Haematopota pluvialis* (Diptera, Tabanidae) obtains its blood-meal from the mammalian host. *Annals of Tropical Medicine and Parasitology 53*: 465-72
4. Galun, R. (1966). Feeding stimulants of the rat flea *Xenopsylla cheopis. Life Sciences 5*: 1335-42
5. _____ Avi-Dor, Y. and Bar-Zeev, M. (1963). Feeding response in *Aedes aegypti*: stimulation by adenosine triphosphate. *Science 142*: 1674-5
6. _____ and Margalit, J. (1969). Adenosine nucleotides as feeding stimulants of the tsetse fly *Glossina austeni* Newstead. *Nature, London 222*: 583-4
7. Gordon, R.M. and Lumsden, W.H.R. (1939). A study of the behaviour of the mouthparts of mosquitoes when taking up blood from living tissue; together with some observations on the ingestion of microfilariae. *Annals of Tropical Medicine and Parasitology 33*: 259-78
8. Jobling, B. (1933). A revision of the structure of the head, mouthparts and salivary glands of *Glossina palpalis* Rob. Desv. *Parasitology 24*: 449-90
9. Patton, W.S. and Cragg, F.W. (1913). *A Textbook of Medical Entomology.* Christian Literature Society for India, London
10. Rice, M.J., Galun, R. and Margalit, J. (1973). Mouthpart sensilla of the tsetse fly and their function. II. Labial sensilla. *Annals of Tropical Medicine and Parasitology 67*: 101-7
11. _____ Galun, R. and Margalit, J. (1973). Mouthpart sensilla of the tsetse fly and their function. III. Labrocibarial sensilla. *Annals of Tropical Medicine and Parasitology 67*: 109-16
12. Yorke, W. and Macfie, J.W.S. (1924). The action of the salivary secretion of mosquitoes and of *Glossina tachinoides* on human blood. *Annals of Tropical Medicine and Parasitology 18*: 103-8

5 INTERNAL STRUCTURE AND FUNCTION OF INSECTS[10]

This chapter presents a general account of the internal structure and physiological organisation of insects, emphasising those features in which insects differ markedly from vertebrates, and which are relevant to medical entomology.

Cuticle (see Figure 5.1)

Many of the features peculiar to insects have their origin in the cuticle, which acts as both a limiting membrane or skin, and as a skeleton for the attachment of muscles. The cuticle is composed of a single layer of cells, the epidermis, which rests upon a basement membrane, and three outer non-living layers, the endocuticle, exocuticle and epicuticle.

Figure 5.1: A, Section of Typical Insect Cuticle; B, Detail of Epicuticle

a, laminated endocuticle; *b*, exocuticle; *c*, epicuticle; *d*, bristle; *e*, pore canals; *f*, duct of dermal gland; *g*, basement membrane; *h*, epidermal cell; *i*, trichogen cell; *k*, tomogen cell; *l*, oenocyte; *m*, haemocyte adherent to basement membrane; *n*, dermal gland; *o*, cement layer of epicuticle; *p*, wax layer; *q*, polyphenol layer; *r*, cuticulin; *s*, pore canal

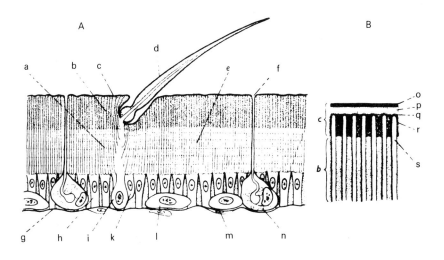

Source: From Wigglesworth, V.B. (1948). *Biological Reviews 23*: 409

Epicuticle

The epicuticle is about 1 μm in thickness and composed of several layers. Its innermost layer is a refractile, inelastic, amber coloured membrane, the cuticulin layer, largely composed of lipoprotein. To allow for growth and stretching this layer is often wrinkled. Outside the epicuticle is a very thin, wax layer (0.25 μm), which is covered by a cement layer of uncertain chemical composition. The function of the cement is to protect the vital wax layer, which provides essential waterproofing to enable insects to survive desiccation in unsaturated atmospheres. Waterproofing is independent of the thickness of the cuticle, being solely dependent upon the existence of the wax layer, of which the most important component is an orientated monolayer closely adherent to the cuticulin layer.[1]

The arrangement has applied implications. Firstly, the wax has a particular melting point, and there exists a critical temperature, about 5 to 10°C below the melting point, at which the monolayer becomes disorganised and water is rapidly lost from the organism. This temperature may be higher than the insect's thermal death point. Secondly, the wax layer can be removed by abrasive materials greatly increasing the rate of water loss. Abrasive dusts have been applied to clothing for the control of sucking lice. Thirdly, the wax layer is a barrier to the inward passage of foreign materials. Water-soluble materials are excluded, but lipid-soluble materials may dissolve in the wax and enter the insect. It is notable that the synthetic contact insecticides, e.g. DDT, are lipid-soluble and owe their activity on contact to this property.

Exocuticle

The exocuticle is a thick, rigid, amber coloured layer which forms the main skeletal component. It is composed of chitin and protein. Chitin is a nitrogenous polysaccharide, composed of long chains of acetylated glucosamine residues. The rigidity is provided by the tanned protein, sclerotin. The exocuticle is absent from areas such as the integmental membranes, where the body is flexible.

Endocuticle

The endocuticle is a thick, elastic layer composed of chitin and protein, which has not been tanned. It provides flexible support. In some areas requiring great elasticity, as in the cibarial pump of Diptera,[9] the rubber-like protein, resilin, occurs in the endocuticle.

Pore Canals

The endocuticle and exocuticle are penetrated by pore canals, protoplasmic extensions of the epidermal cells. There may be 200 pore canals per epidermal cell and it is likely that they penetrate the cuticulin layer and are involved in secreting the wax layer. The endocuticle and exocuticle are deposited by the pore canals while the cement layer is secreted by dermal glands which penetrate the cuticle.

Water Absorption

The structure of the cuticle makes it more permeable to the passage of water into the body than out.[1] The pupating larva of the oriental rat flea, *Xenopsylla cheopis,* can take up moisture from air at a relative humidity of 45 per cent and may increase its weight by as much as 29 per cent before pupation.[6] Ixodid ticks have a similar ability to absorb water from unsaturated air. This ability is important to the survival of starving or non-feeding stages.

Growth

Since parts of the cuticle are rigid, e.g. the head capsule, there arises a stage in the growth of an individual when a new cuticle is required. The epidermis separates itself from the existing cuticle, a process known as apolysis, and lays down the cuticulin layer of the epicuticle, followed by the exocuticle, which, at this stage, is as flexible as endocuticle, as it is not sclerotised until after the moult. The endocuticle is not secreted until after ecdysis. The cuticulin layer is, of course, wrinkled to provide room for expansion when the old cuticle is cast. The moulting fluid, containing appropriate enzymes, is secreted into the space between the old and new cuticles and completely

Figure 5.2: Changes in the Abdominal Air Sacs of *Lucilia* at Various Stages of Adult Development

A, fly just emerged; B, after five minutes — gut filled with air, abdomen distended; C, after ten hours — gut collapsed, air sacs distended; D, fully fed for six days — ovaries and fat body fill abdomen, air sacs collapsed again. *a,* air sacs; *b,* gut; *c,* ovaries; *d,* fat body

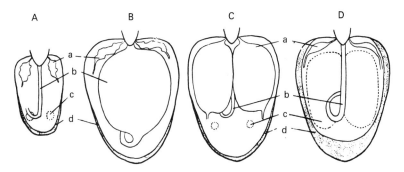

Source: From Evans, A.C. (1935). *Bulletin of Entomological Research 26:* 115

digests the old endocuticle, the products of which are absorbed. This has the effect of reducing the ecdysial suture to the epicuticle as no exocuticle is present under the suture. Shortly before ecdysis the wax layer is secreted and the cement layer shortly after the moult is completed. When an insect completes virtually all the moult except for the final discarding of the old cuticle the hidden new stage is referred to as pharate. Thus the mature flea pupa contains a pharate adult awaiting the stimulus of a host's arrival to cast its pupal cuticle and become a free adult.

The newly moulted insect is usually very pale because sclerotisation has not begun. It immediately expands to a new size by increasing its volume by swallowing air or water. The newly emerged adult blowfly *Calliphora* increases its volume by 128 per cent by swallowing air (Figure 5.2). Formation of exocuticle and the laying down of the new endocuticle proceed rapidly. Newly emerged adults, which remain soft and pliable, are referred to as teneral.

Mosquito larvae have four instars in which only the head capsule is sclerotised. The abdomen and thorax continue to grow steadily throughout larval life but the head increases dramatically at each moult. The following change was observed in *An sergenti* within a minute of the old skin being cast.[7]

	Head		Thorax	
	Breadth	Length	Breadth	Length
Before ecdysis	128 μm	116 μm	184 μm	265 μm
After ecdysis	230 μm	219 μm	196 μm	276 μm
% increase	80	89	4	6

The increase in volume was achieved by swallowing water and pumping blood anteriorly to expand the head capsule, which increased in volume six-fold. This step-wise increase of larval head size has a useful application. Most keys to the identification of *Anopheles* larvae apply to the 4th or final instar larvae. The 4th instar can be recognised by the size of the head capsule (Figure 7.9).

The cuticle cast at ecdysis is called an exuviae (unchanged in the plural). Exuviae are taxonomically important because they retain the external features of the stage. It is therefore possible to associate a particular adult insect with its own larval and pupal exuviae.

Digestive Tract and Digestion (see Figure 5.3)

The gut of an insect is composed of three main regions — foregut, midgut and hindgut. It is unusual in that the foregut and hindgut develop from

Figure 5.3: Diagrammatic Longitudinal Section of a Generalised Insect

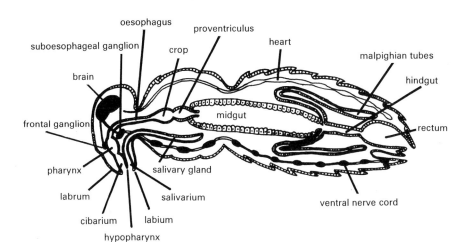

ectodermal invaginations, and consequently are lined with a thin layer of cuticle. At ecdysis these cuticular linings are shed with the exuviae. In vertebrates the proctodeal and stomodeal invaginations are very short. Only the midgut of an insect is comparable to the vertebrate digestive tract.

The mouth leads into the buccal cavity and thence to the pharynx, which may be developed as a muscular pump moving food down the narrow oesophagus to the storage organ or crop. In Diptera the crop is a blind diverticulum from the oesophagus. In the Cyclorrhapha the crop functions as a store passing food to the midgut as required. In mosquitoes, and probably in other blood-sucking Nematocera, blood is stored in the midgut and sugar solutions in the crop. In the tabanid *Haematopota*, blood passes to the stomach and the overflow to the crop. The crop is purely storage and secretes no enzymes. Any digestion that occurs in the crop is due to the action of enzymes contained in the saliva.

The foregut ends in the proventriculus, which, in most medically important insects, has become a valve preventing regurgitation of food from the midgut. It is a very prominent structure in fleas being lined with backwardly directed spines said to be involved in rupturing red blood cells. Other blood-feeding insects manage without these spines. The spines are very important medically because it is in the interstices of the proventricular spines that plague bacilli multiply.

The midgut of many insects is lined with a non-adherent, thin, transparent tube, the peritrophic membrane. Its function is to protect the midgut from abrasion by food particles. It is therefore not always well developed in blood-sucking insects. The peritrophic membrane is secreted at the anterior end of the midgut and moulded by an invagination of the oesophagus. The peritrophic membrane is present in *Glossina*, where it influences the development of trypanosomes. It is present in the larvae of mosquitoes, simuliids, tabanids and fleas but absent in adult tabanids and fleas, and adult and nymphal Siphunculata. In adult mosquitoes, phlebotomine sandflies[5] and simuliids[8] a short-lived peritrophic membrane is secreted around the blood meal by the midgut epithelium.

Figure 5.4: Alimentary Canal of *Glossina*, Showing the Structure of the Different Parts of the Midgut

1, oesophagus; 2, proventriculus; 3, duct of crop; 4, 'mycetome'; 5, junction of anterior and middle segments of midgut; 6, malpighian tubes; 7, hindgut; 8, rectum. A,A', transverse sections of anterior segment of midgut; B,B', same of middle segment; C,C', same of posterior segment; D, detail of 'mycetome'; E,F,F', transverse sections through 'mycetome' showing intracellular rod-like organisms

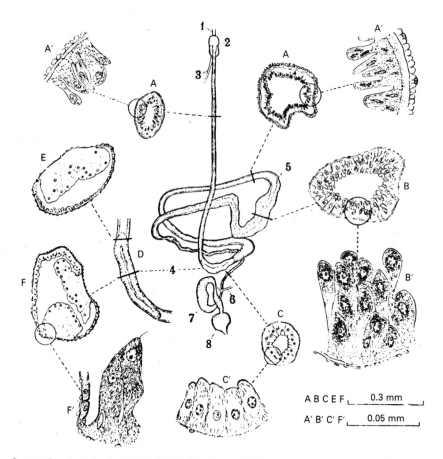

The midgut is the main digestive organ. In fleas and mosquitoes it forms a capacious stomach for the reception and digestion of blood. The oocysts of the malaria parasite develop on the outer side of the midgut in *Anopheles* mosquitoes. In blood-sucking bugs the anterior part of the midgut is storage and is separated from the posterior digestive part by a sphincter. In the Cyclorrhapha food is stored in the crop and the midgut is a relatively narrow tube with functional divisions. The anterior division is concentrative, removing excess water, the middle division digestive and the hind division absorptive. These divisions are apparent in adult *Glossina* (Figure 5.4) and in *Lucilia* larvae. In most nematocerous larvae the midgut bears caeca anteriorly which are considered to be absorptive and secretory. The midgut is separated by the pyloric sphincter from the hindgut. The midgut enzymes are adapted to the diet of the insect. Thus the midgut of blood-feeding *Glossina* secretes a very active protease but little carbohydrase and that of *Calliphora* which feeds on sweet substances produces little protease and abundant carbohydrases. *Chrysops*, which feeds on both nectar and blood secretes an active protease and an active carbohydrase.

The main function of the hindgut is the absorption of water from the faeces and urine. Urine passes into the hindgut from the malpighian tubules, which open just behind the midgut. When water is freely available as in aquatic insects and liquid-feeding adults, faeces and urine are watery, but most insects need to conserve water. Desiccation is an ever present threat. Water is absorbed from the hindgut especially by the rectal glands, and faeces are excreted as dry pellets and nitrogenous waste as uric acid. Water economy is practised in the excretion of nitrogenous waste, which passes, in solution, into the lumen of the malpighian tubes as the relatively soluble potassium acid urate, where it is converted in the presence of carbon dioxide to potassium bicarbonate and relatively insoluble uric acid. This enables a small amount of water to circulate repeatedly from hindgut to malpighian tubes via the body cavity, and bring about the elimination of large amounts of nitrogenous waste (Figure 5.5).

Bursell[2] recognises in Diptera three substances as being capable of oxidation at a rate adequate to support flight. In species in which only the female is haematophagous, e.g. *Tabanus*, or in which neither sex is blood-sucking, e.g. *Musca*, energy for flight is provided by pyruvate oxidation. In facultative blood-sucking species, such as those in the Stomoxinae, pyruvate and proline are the substrates. In obligatory haematophagous Diptera, e.g. *Glossina*, energy is derived from the oxidation of proline.

Symbiotic Organisms in Blood-sucking Insects

Insects have different vitamin requirements from those of vertebrates. They do not require ascorbic acid (vitamin C) but do require a source of sterols and some specifically need cholesterol. All insects require certain fractions of the B group of vitamins and these are often provided by micro-organisms living in the food source or in the gut of the insect. Blood is an incomplete food for insect growth and sexual maturity, and insects that

Figure 5.5: Above, Diagram of Water-circulation in Alimentary and Excretory Systems of an Insect. Below, Diagram Showing Possible Mechanism by Which Free Uric Acid is Precipitated in the Lower Segment of the Malpighian Tubes in *Rhodnius*. Shaded part represents upper segment of tube

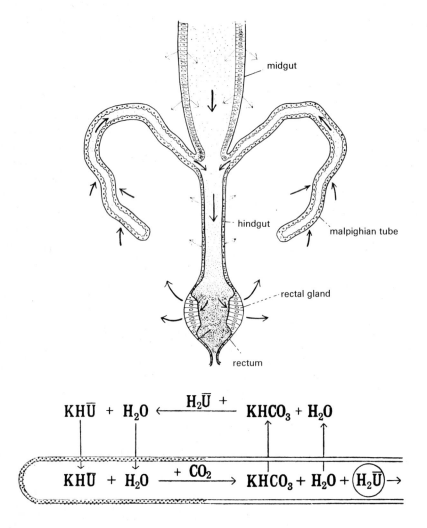

feed in all stages of their life only on blood, have special arrangements for the cultivation of symbiotic micro-organisms. In the blood-sucking reduviid bugs the organisms are free in the lumen of the midgut diverticula; in the Hippoboscidae the organisms inhabit cells in the wall of the midgut diverticula. In the Siphunculata and *Glossina* a special zone of the midgut, the 'mycetome', is composed of cells laden with micro-organisms (Figure 5.4D). In the bedbug *Cimex*, the mycetome is remote from the gut, being located elsewhere in the body cavity.

Holometabous insects whose larval stage is free-living, e.g. mosquitoes, fleas, tabanids, *Stomoxys*, do not have mycetomes. Presumably enough essential materials are acquired by their larvae to meet the needs of the adults. If the symbionts are removed from nymphs of *Pediculus* they die in a few days and female *Pediculus*, deprived of symbionts, are sterile.

Respiration (see Figure 5.6)

In insects air is carried direct to the tissues by special tubes, the tracheae. These are ectodermal invaginations and are consequently lined with thin cuticle which is thrown into folds which follow a spiral course round the trachea. These spiral thickenings resist compression and enable the tracheae to recoil quickly from deformation. The tracheae open to the

Figure 5.6: Tracheal System of *Xenopsylla* (Left Side Only). *Th.I, Th.II,* thoracic spiracles; Abd. i-viii, abdominal spiracles

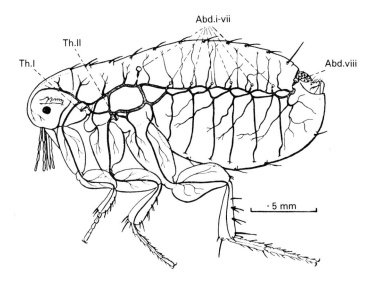

Source: From Wigglesworth, V.B. (1935). *Proceedings of the Royal Society B118*: 398

exterior at the spiracles, of which there are typically two pairs on the thorax and eight pairs on the abdomen. The tracheae anastomose, usually forming paired longitudinal trunks which run the length of the body and extend into the head. The tracheae branch among the tissues with the branches becoming narrower in diameter. The finest branches, the tracheoles, lack obvious spiral thickenings and are closely applied to the tissues and may even penetrate individual cells.

The fine endings of the tracheoles commonly contain fluid. When the tissue is active, as for example muscle following contraction, the liquid is withdrawn, presumably as a result of increasing osmotic pressure caused by metabolites in the tissue, and air temporarily extends to the termination of the tracheole. Oxygen reaches the tissues by diffusion along the tracheae, and in larger and/or very active insects diffusion is supplemented by active ventilation of the tracheae. Carbon dioxide, the final product of metabolism, may diffuse into the atmosphere along the tracheae but it is quite likely to diffuse through the general body cuticle rather as it does through the skin of a frog.

Open spiracles represent a major source of water loss and elaborate arrangements are made to restrict this. The spiracles of most terrestrial insects have a closing mechanism, which limits water loss. It operates in response to the accumulation of carbon dioxide and not to a deficiency of oxygen. When the flea, *Xenopsylla cheopis*, is placed in an atmosphere of 5 per cent carbon dioxide the spiracles remain open, and it loses water at twice the rate it does in air. It is of interest to note that in vertebrates respiratory movements are also controlled by the concentration of carbon dioxide in the circulating blood and not by a lack of oxygen.

In many insects the tracheal system has large thin-walled dilations, the air sacs. These aid in ventilating the tracheal system and are common in active insects but they also have the function of keeping the external shape of an insect constant in spite of extensive internal changes, e.g. egg maturation. The newly emerged adult *Lucilia* inflates itself to its full size by swallowing air. Initially this air is taken into the gut but ten hours later the gut has returned to its normal size and the air sacs are inflated (Figure 5.2). The volume of the air sacs is adjusted to keep the fly's total volume constant when food is imbibed or eggs matured. In the gravid female the ovaries almost fill the abdomen and the air sacs are insignificant (Figure 5.2). Possession of a constant external shape must simplify flight by eliminating one variable, aerodynamic shape.

The respiration of aquatic larvae will be considered when dealing with individual families.

Insects are less dependent on a continuous supply of oxygen than vertebrates. Certain important cells in the vertebrate central nervous system are irreversibly damaged by being deprived of oxygen. Insects lack these cells and readily survive periods of oxygen deprivation. Insect tissues are able to build up an oxygen debt by respiring anaerobically. This debt is discharged when oxygen becomes available later. When the cockroach, *Blatta orientalis*, is deprived of oxygen for half an hour it sustains an oxygen debt which requires one and a half to two hours to be repaid and the extra oxygen consumed is equivalent to that expected to be used in half an hour.[4]

Circulatory System (see Figure 5.7)

Insect blood or haemolymph is clear and contains no respiratory pigment. The carriage of oxygen to the tissues is the function of the tracheal system. The function of the circulatory system is to transport food to the tissues, to remove the products of metabolism, and to convey hormones around the body. The haemolymph is circulated by a dorsal heart, which is a longitudinal contractile tube, which impels the blood anteriorly. Haemolymph enters the heart via openings, the ostia, of which there is one pair in each abdominal segment. There are no veins obviously recognisable as such. The coelom which forms the body cavity in vertebrates is greatly reduced and its place has been taken by the haemocoele, which can be regarded as a

Figure 5.7: Diagram of Fully Developed Circulatory System

A, lateral view; B, transverse section of thorax; C, transverse section of abdomen. Arrows show course of circulation. *a*, aorta; *apo*, accessory pulsatile organ; *d*, dorsal diaphragm with aliform muscles; *h*, heart; *n*, nerve cord; *o*, ostia; *pc*, pericardial sinus; *pn*, perineural sinus; *po*, mesothoracic and metathoracic pulsatile organs; *s*, septa dividing appendages; *v*, ventral diaphragm; *vs*, visceral sinus

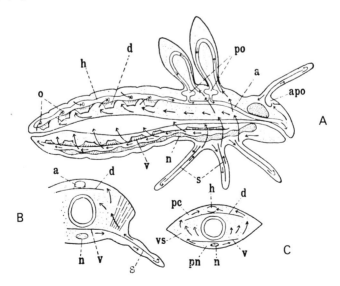

Source: From Wigglesworth, V.B. (1972). *Principles of Insect Physiology*. Chapman & Hall, London

greatly enlarged venous system. Haemolymph passes from the arteries to the haemocoele and from there by various routes to the dorsal pericardial sinus where it enters the heart through the ostia. In the heart the haemolymph is propelled forward by a steady contractile wave, which passes along the heart from the posterior end. In most insects there are supplementary pulsating organs which drive the haemolymph through the appendages. In mosquitoes there are pulsating organs which drive haemolymph into the antennae.[3]

Nervous System (see Figures 5.3 and 5.8)

Primitively the nervous system of an insect consists of a ring of nervous tissue around the oesophagus in the head, and paired ganglia in each thoracic and abdominal segment, connected to each other in the midline, and anteriorly and posteriorly by connectives. The oesophageal ring includes concentrations of nervous tissue into supraoesophageal and suboesophageal ganglia. The supraoesophageal ganglion or brain receives sensory information from the eyes and antennae. It has an overriding excitatory or

Figure 5.8: Successive Stages in the Coalescence of Thoracic and of Abdominal Ganglia in Diptera. A, *Chironomus* (Nematocera); B, *Empis* (Orthorrhapha); C, *Tabanus* (Orthorrhapha); D, *Sarcophaga* (Cyclorrhapha)

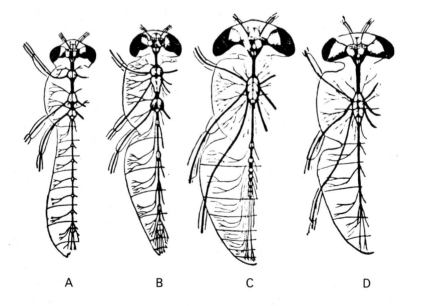

A   B   C   D

inhibiting effect on other centres of activity. The suboesophageal ganglion innervates the mouthparts and has a general excitatory effect on the thoracic ganglia. In higher insects there is a tendency to concentrate the paired segmental ganglia and in Cyclorrhapha they are fused into a single ganglionic mass in the thorax. There is considerable segmental autonomy, and decapitation does not lead to the immediate death of the insect. Providing the loss of haemolymph is prevented, a headless insect is able to walk and oviposit and, providing the critical stage has been passed before decapitation, it will moult.

Various endocrine glands are associated with the nervous system. Secretions of neurosecretory cells in the brain pass along axons to the corpus cardiacum and the corpora allata. The corpora allata secrete neotenin (the juvenile hormone) which controls the expression of immature characters during development, ensures the deposition of yolk in developing eggs, and influences reproductive behaviour. Under stimulation by neurosecretions the thoracic glands secrete ecdyson, the moulting hormone.

Sensory receptors play a major role in insect behaviour but their treatment is outside the scope of this book. Reference will be made to particular receptors when describing the biology of a taxonomic group.

Reproduction

In insects the sexes are separate, and the sex of an individual is determined by its complement of chromosomes. The genes for sex determination act directly on the cells in which they are located, and not via released chemicals (hormones) operating at a distance from the site of secretion. Consequently loss of sex chromosomes during development produces gynandromorphs with a mosaic of female and male characters, and not intersexes with intermediate characters.

The female reproductive organs (Figure 5.9) consist of paired ovaries and oviducts, a common oviduct which opens into the vagina and spermathecae. Each ovary consists of a variable number of ovarioles, two in *Glossina*, and 2,000 in certain termites. Each ovariole is a tube containing a string of oocytes, of which the one nearest the oviduct is the first to mature. When the mature ovum is shed, the empty sac contracts, but often remains as a discrete body. The persistence of these relict bodies has been used to determine the physiological age of individual insects and construct life tables of frequences of different age classes. This technique has been particularly applied to populations of *Anopheles* and *Glossina*.

At oviposition the egg moves down the oviduct and passes the opening to the spermatheca. As it does so sperm are extruded on the micropyle, an area where the chorion (shell) of the egg is very thin and penetration is easy.

Figure 5.9: Female Reproductive System

AcGl, accessory gland; *Clx*, calyx; *ET*, egg tube; *Fol*, follicle; *GC*, vagina; *Gpr*, gonopore; *Grm*, germarium; *Lg*, ligament; *Odc*, common oviduct; *Odl*, lateral oviduct; *Ov*, ovary; *Ovl*, ovariole; *Pdcl*, pedicel; *Spt*, spermatheca; *SptGl*, spermathecal gland; *TF*, terminal filament; *Vtl*, Vitellarium

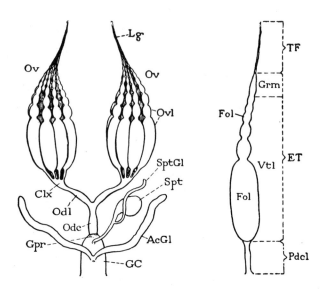

Source: From Snodgrass, R.F. (1935). *Principles of Insect Morphology*. McGraw-Hill, New York (reproduced with permission)

The male reproductive system (Figure 5.10) consists of paired testes, paired vesicula seminales in which the spermatozoa are stored, accessory glands and an ejaculatory duct through which the spermatozoa are deposited in the female. In many insects the spermatozoa are transferred, enclosed in a spermatophore, a proteinaceous membrane formed from secretions of the accessory glands. After deposition the spermatozoa are finally stored in the spermathecae where they may remain viable for years. Queen bees are inseminated during their sole nuptial flight. Fertilised eggs give rise to females, workers or queens, while unfertilised eggs develop into males (drones). A queen may fertilise eggs for many years before producing only drones and causing the death of the colony. Single mating is common in insects.

Most insects are oviparous, laying eggs which undergo embryonic development before hatching. In *Oestrus ovis* and *Sarcophaga* the eggs are retained until embryonic development is complete. The larva emerges as soon as the egg is deposited. This is ovoviviparity. Viviparity involves retention of the egg until hatching and subsequent growth of the larva within the body of the female. *Musca bezzii* and *M. planiceps* retain larvae for one or two ecdyses and deposit them in the 2nd and 3rd instars respectively. These larvae are not full grown and have an active, free-living, feeding period. In *Glossina* the larva completes its development in the female and has only a very brief free-living period, during which it does not feed, but crawls away and buries itself. In the Pupipara, e.g. *Melophagus ovinus*, the larva is deposited fully grown. It is immobile and pupariates where it has been deposited.

Figure 5.10: Male Reproductive System

AcGls, accessory glands; *Dej*, ejaculatory duct; *E.sh*, epithelial sheath; *Gpr*, gonopore; *Pen*, penis; *SpT*, spermatic tube; *Tes*, testis; *Vd*, vas deferens; *Ve*, vas efferens; *Vsm*, vesicula seminalis

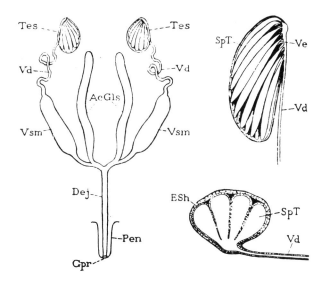

Source: From Snodgrass, R.F. (1935). *Principles of Insect Morphology*. McGraw-Hill, New York (reproduced with permission)

References

1. Beament, J.W.L. (1945). The cuticular lipoids of insects. *Journal of Experimental Biology 21*: 115-31
2. Bursell, E. (1975). Substrates of oxidative metabolism in dipteran flight muscle. *Comparative Biochemistry and Physiology B 52*: 235-8
3. Clements, A.N. (1963). *The Physiology of Mosquitoes*. Pergamon Press, Oxford
4. Davis, J.G. and Slater, W.K. (1926). The aerobic and anaerobic metabolism of the common cockroach (*Periplaneta orientalis*). Part I. *Biochemical Journal 20*: 1167-72
5. Dolmatova, A.V. (1942). The life cycle of *Phlebotomus papatasii* (Scopoli). *Meditsinskaya Parazitologiya 11*: 52-70

6. Edney, E.B. (1947). Laboratory studies on the bionomics of the rat fleas, *Xenopsylla brasiliensis*, Baker, and *X. cheopis*, Roths. II. Water relations during the cocoon period. *Bulletin of Entomological Research 38*: 263-80

7. Kettle, D.S. (1948). The growth of *Anopheles sergenti* Theobald (Diptera, Culicidae), with special reference to the growth of the anal papillae in varying salinities. *Annals of Tropical Medicine and Parasitology 42*: 5-29

8. Lewis, D.J. (1953). *Simulium damnosum* and its relation to onchocerciasis in the Anglo-Egyptian Sudan. *Bulletin of Entomological Research 43*: 597-644

9. Rice, M.J. (1970). Function of resilin in tsetse fly feeding mechanism. *Nature, London 228*: 1337-8

10. Wigglesworth, V.B. (1972). *The Principles of Insect Physiology*. Chapman and Hall, London

6 SPECIES COMPLEXES, AND VARIATION IN *AEDES AEGYPTI*

In 1898 when Ronald Ross was investigating the transmission of malaria in India, knowledge of the systematics of mosquitoes was very rudimentary. Ross recognised only grey and dapple winged mosquitoes and showed that *Plasmodium relictum*, a bird malaria, developed in the grey but not in the dapple winged mosquitoes. In the following year Grassi in Italy extended this observation to human malaria and showed that it developed in *Anopheles* mosquitoes. It was later shown that there were two tribes of mosquitoes of which the Anophelini were vectors of human malaria and the Culicini of bird malaria. Therefore control of malaria became equated with control of *Anopheles* mosquitoes. This led to intensive study of the Anophelini and it was quickly appreciated that not all species of *Anopheles* were equally important. Some, such as *An minimus* and *An fluviatilis*, were dangerous vectors, and others, like *An subpictus*, were unimportant; the main difference being a simple feature of their behaviour: whether or not they bit man, i.e. anthropophilic, or animals, i.e. zoophilic. This recognition gave rise to the concept of 'species sanitation', in which control was concentrated on the important species, after which it was often found that the minor species could be disregarded. Species sanitation gave excellent results in the tropics and subtropics but by 1920 there was some disquiet in Europe.

The European problem will be considered in some depth, because it was the first detailed study of a species complex in medical entomology and is the most complete, and not because it is necessarily the most important. Species complexes abound in medical entomology and some understanding of them is essential to the medical entomologist.

Anopheles maculipennis and Malaria in Europe[9]

The malaria problem in Europe appeared to be relatively simple being very largely concerned with *Anopheles maculipennis*. This species is widely distributed in the Palearctic region from Japan to the Atlantic. In the Nearctic there is the very similar *An quadrimaculatus* but this account will be restricted to Europe. The problem that European malariologists encountered was that the distribution of malaria and the distribution of *An maculipennis* were not closely correlated. Malaria was largely coastal while *An maculipennis* was widely distributed both at the coast and in inland areas. This discrepancy undermined confidence in species sanitation. To resolve this problem the Rockefeller Foundation founded a Malaria Institute in Rome and a field station in Albania across the Adriatic sea. Even in coastal areas of Italy malaria was not uniformly present. In the coastal marshes of Salerno and Volturno, south and north of Naples respectively, and in the Pontine marshes south of Rome *An maculipennis* was abundant. Thousands of them could be collected from animal shelters, the human population was obviously unhealthy, and malaria was rife. Yet further north around Pisa and Florence there were also thousands of *An maculipennis* present in stables, but the human population was vibrantly healthy, and there was no malaria. Hence the phrase 'Anophelism without malaria' was coined. What was the explanation of this quite striking difference?

Theories

In the absence of reliable data hypotheses and guesses abounded. There were the healthy-living propagandists, like Cirio, who argued that good food and drink would make people resistant to disease and the solution was to improve living standards. Cirio was prepared to test his hypothesis and he set up a community in the Pontine marshes which ended in disaster with the well-fed people becoming victims of malaria. Improved living standards will only be successful if they incidentally interfere with the habitat of the mosquito or reduce the *Anopheles*/man contact.

Grassi suggested that mosquitos bred in salt water were larger and stronger. These super mosquitoes fed more avidly and lived longer. Greater longevity would permit longer survival after becoming infected and therefore would enhance malaria transmission. The view of Alessandrini was the direct opposite. He reasoned that mosquitoes reared in fresh water were larger and, being stronger, were resistant to malaria. He did not attempt the simple test of feeding mosquitoes reared from fresh water on persons suffering from malaria. Had he done so he would have found that fresh water *An maculipennis* were equally susceptible to infection by *Plasmodium*.

The French malariologist, Roubaud, came nearer to the truth, when in 1921 he proposed the existence of two races, differing in the number of teeth on their mandibles and maxillae. The multidentate race with more teeth fed on cattle, while the paucidentate race with fewer teeth was unable to pierce the skin of cattle and fed on man. As an elaboration of this hypothesis the natural decline of malaria, which had been observed in some areas, was attributed to competition between the two races with the multidentate race replacing the paucidentate. This mechanical hypothesis gave rise to a great deal of work in which mouthparts were dissected and the numbers of teeth counted. This activity has extended to other blood-feeding Nematocera, but the rewards have been slight. There appears to be little correlation between the hosts of a species and the number of teeth on its mandibles and maxillae.

Malaria in Holland

The strain of malaria present in Holland was unusual in that the incubation period in man was many months compared with the usual ten to twelve days. One leading malariologist, Swellengrebel, deliberately allowed himself to be bitten by an infected *An maculipennis* on 30 October but the primary attack of malaria did not occur until nine months later in July of the next year.

Normally in mosquitoes there is gonotrophic concordancy in which each blood meal is followed by the maturation of a batch of eggs, except that in the autumn mosquitoes, preparing for hibernation, feed on blood, develop fat body not eggs, and then seek a cool sheltered location in which to remain until the next spring. In Holland some *An maculipennis* hibernate in this fashion but others come indoors, stay in the warm and have disso-ciated blood-feeding and ovarian development. These individuals feed at intervals during the winter but develop no eggs until the spring. Malaria infections acquired in the winter do not produce clinical disease until the next summer. If there are both a carrier of malaria and feeding *Anopheles* present in a house, there is a high chance of the mosquitoes becoming infective and transmitting the disease to other members of the household during their winter feeding. This association of carrier and *Anopheles* gave rise to the so-called 'malaria houses', which occured in Holland and also in Norfolk in England. The existence of two behavioural patterns in adult *An maculipennis* recalls Roubaud's two races. Van Thiel made attempts to characterise them and by 1924 he was able to discriminate between a long-winged, hibernating form and a short-winged, non-hibernating form. The latter he named *atroparvus* (little, black), but size and colour are particu-larly variable characters being influenced by food and temperature. Wing length enabled populations to be separated but was less useful in categoris-ing individual mosquitoes.

Recognition of Forms of An maculipennis

The precipitin test was developed in the 1920s enabling the source of a blood meal to be determined from the stomach contents of individual mosquitoes. It was applied to the malaria problem in Europe and by 1930 the precipitin test had confirmed that in malaria-free areas *An maculipen-nis* was zoophilic and in malarious areas it was anthropophilic. But there was still no means of differentiating the two forms.

In the meantime in Italy, Falleroni, a retired sanitary inspector, had collected female *Anopheles* as a hobby and allowed them to lay eggs. He found that the eggs of *An maculipennis* were patterned dark grey and silvery white and he described these in a paper in 1926.[8] He figured five patterns but grouped them into two types — grey and dark eggs which he named *labranchiae* and *messeae*, respectively, after two former colleagues

Figure 6.1: Eggs of Species of the *Anopheles maculipennis* Complex. Top row, from left to right — *An sacharovi, An labranchiae, An atroparvus;* bottom row — *An maculipennis, An messeae, An melanoon, An melanoon subalpinus*

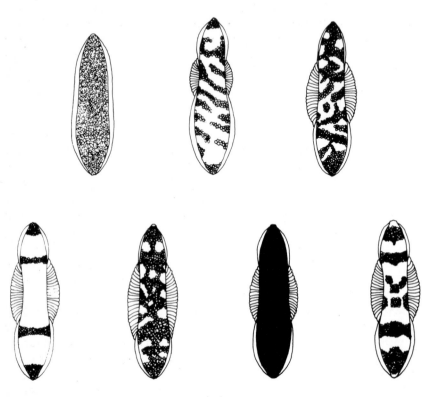

Redrawn from various sources

(Figure 6.1). Falleroni's observations lay dormant for five years and were rediscovered in 1931. Could egg pattern be the vital character required to discriminate between the two forms of *An maculipennis*? To be a useful character all the eggs of a female must conform to the same pattern and the patterns must be consistent throughout the range of *An maculipennis*. Surveys quickly revealed that malaria was associated with females that laid grey eggs and absent where females laid only dark eggs.

The actual situation proved to be much more complicated than originally envisaged. There were not merely two different egg patterns but seven, all of which were consistent. Three types of grey eggs were named *labranchiae, atroparvus* and *sacharovi* and the four types of dark eggs were designated *typicus* (now *maculipennis*), *messeae, melanoon* and *subalpinus*. *Messeae* proved to be Van Thiel's long-winged hibernating species in

Holland and his name *atroparvus* was retained for the egg pattern of the short-winged non-hibernating form. *Sacharovi* had long been recognised as a separate form of *An maculipennis* by its possession of a uniformly red-brown scutum compared with the longitudinal pale, broad, scutal band in *An maculipennis*. The ability to identify forms at the egg stage enabled accurately identified larvae and adults to be reared for critical examination. Such studies have revealed very minor differences between the forms which can only appreciated by an expert in the group. For practical purposes only *sacharovi* can be readily distinguished in the adult and none in the larval stage.

Status of Forms of An maculipennis

There remains the problem as to the taxonomic status to be accorded these seven forms. Are they true species, subspecies or what? Earlier (p. 7) a species was defined as a population of similar individuals, which breeds together and produces fertile offspring. It is usually difficult to effect mating, let alone cross-mating, in Nematocera but in *An maculipennis* one form, *atroparvus*, proved very easy to colonise in the laboratory and it is now a standard laboratory animal. *Labranchiae* and *sacharovi* can be colonised with difficulty but the other forms are refractory. *Atroparvus* mates in small cages without swarming first and its males were crossed with females of the other forms. The results of hybridisation indicated a wide range of degrees of compatibility.

The most successful cross was of *atroparvus* and *labranchiae* in which all the females were normal but only some of the males. The *atroparvus melanoon* cross gave females of which half were sterile as were all the males. Healthy but completely sterile adults resulted from the *atroparvus maculipennis* cross. When *atroparvus* was crossed with *sacharovi* and *messeae* no adults were produced, death occurring in the larval and egg stages, respectively.

On the basis of these results six species and one subspecies were recognised within the *An maculipennis* complex.[11] They were: *An atroparvus* Van Thiel; *An labranchiae* Falleroni; *An maculipennis* Meigen; *An melanoon melanoon* Hackett; *An melanoon subalpinus* Hackett and Lewis; *An messeae* Falleroni and *An sacharovi* Favre. More recently (1976) Russian workers on cytological evidence (see below), have added another species *An beklemischevi* Stegnii and Kabanova to the *An maculipennis* complex.[19]

In passing it is worthwhile drawing attention to the difficulty of breeding many mosquitoes. To achieve success with *An messeae* and *An maculipennis* a large cage was built in Tirana, Albania, to accommodate a stable, donkey, pond and vegetation. Thousands of both species were released in the cage but only a few eggs of *An maculipennis* were laid and none of *An messeae*. *An messeae* is particularly refractory in mating in confinement.

Although *An messeae* females mated with *An atroparvus* males and *An messeae* males mated with *An atroparvus* females they did not mate with each other. Some essential factor was lacking. These observations emphasise how complex the conditions for successful mating may be. If a species mates readily there is no problem; if it does not, a long, arduous study is likely to be required to give success.

Distrubution of Species of the An maculipennis Complex

The species of the *An maculipennis* complex have different geographical distributions with only three species occurring north of the Alps. *An sacharovi* occurs in the eastern Mediterranean, Iraq, Iran, southern Greece, southern Italy and Turkey. *An labranchiae* is found south of 45°N in Sicily, Sardinia, southern Italy and in North Africa, where it is the only species of the complex present. The closely allied *An atroparvus* has very little overlap with *An labranchiae* being mainly found north of 45°, occurring in northern Europe, UK, Holland, northern Italy and Spain. *An messeae* occurs in northern and central Europe, in USSR and UK, and *An maculipennis* in continental Europe, Spain and Iran. *An melanoon melanoon* has been recorded from Italy, Corsica, Sicily and Albania and *An m.subalpinus* from Albania, Turkey and Iran.

Although the breeding places may be characterised as brackish or fresh water there is considerable selection of microhabitats within the larger setting. Thus the freshwater species differ in their oviposition sites, ovipositing in narrow drainage channels, at the lake edge and in vegetation remote from the edge. Although in Italy *An labranchiae* and *An sacharovi* are strictly coastal in distribution, when they are the only members of the complex present they extend into freshwater habitats as *An labranchiae* does in N. Africa and *An sacharovi* in Israel. This expansion is considered to reflect lack of competition.

Status of Vectors of Malaria

An labranchiae and *An sacharovi* are important vectors of malaria throughout their ranges. *An atroparvus* is a vector of malaria but its importance depends on local conditions, as in Holland, or by being present in large numbers. *An messeae* is usually of no importance but can, when present in large numbers, be a vector of malaria. It was the most important vector of malaria in the USSR.

Anopheles gambiae[6,26]

Anopheles gambiae is one of the most efficient vectors of malaria and filariasis in the world, and is widely distributed throughout the Afrotropical region. Although in most of the region it breeds in small, sunlit, freshwater pools, which are often temporary and devoid of vegetation, larvae are also found at the coast in intertidal, salt water swamps. Morphological variation was noted in the banding of the palps, i.e. three or four pale bands, with larvae from salt water giving rise to a higher proportion of adults with four-banded palps, and eggs laid by adults from salt water were longer and broader than those laid by adults from fresh water. On the basis of these differences salt water *An gambiae* were assigned to two new species, *An melas* in West Africa and *An merus* in East Africa.

There was still doubt about the homogeneity of freshwater *An gambiae*. In the absence of morphological differences two lines of investigation, one biological and the other cytological, were possible. The biological method involves the cross-mating of established laboratory strains, and the cytological method the study of giant chromosomes in the population.

Laboratory colonies of *An gambiae* were established from individual, mated females, obtained from the wild. (The wild population may be mixed, and hence the need to found the colony from single females.) In the laboratory, mated blood-fed females readily deposit fertile eggs, which can be reared to the adult. There is then the problem of mating. If this does not occur naturally, a form of artificial insemination can be achieved by lightly anaesthetising a female and bringing a male to her in such a way that the terminalia make contact. This is usually sufficient to achieve coupling and subsequent insemination. Should there be any reluctance of males to mate or females to deposit eggs, inhibition can be removed by decapitation.

Having established colonies from single females from two or more localities their compatibility can be tested by crossing males of one colony with females from another and vice versa. Progeny of these matings have to be reared to adult and mated to determine the fertility of the F_1 generation. It will be apparent that this method requires meticulous attention to maintaining colony integrity. Any mixing would be disastrous. By this laborious method Davidson *et al.*[6] and Davidson and Hunt[5] have shown that freshwater *An gambiae* is a complex of four species, which were designated provisionally A, B, C and D. The validity of this separation has been confirmed by study of their giant chromosomes by Coluzzi and Sabatini[2, 3] and Davidson and Hunt[5] (Figure 6.2). Coluzzi and Sabatini[4] have also shown that the patterns on the giant chromosomes of *An melas* and *An merus* are equally distinctive. The technique will be outlined below when considering the *Simulium damnosum* complex.

Crosses between the four species gave rise to adults of which the females were reproductively normal, but the males were sterile. Both sexes showed the increased vigour associated with hybrids. Species A and B are both vectors of malaria and bancroftian filariasis but not necessarily of equal status. They are widely distributed in the Afrotropical region and may be present in the same locality, i.e. they may be sympatric. In one survey of 57 breeding sites species A and B were present together in 24 (42 per cent) of

Figure 6.2: Polytene Chromosomes of Species in the *Anopheles gambiae* Complex. Above, salivary gland chromosomes of *An arabiensis*; below, ovarian chromosomes of species D

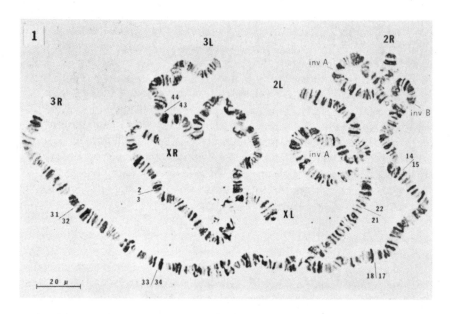

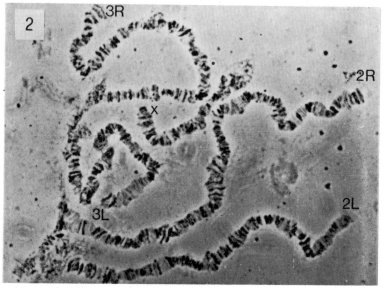

Source: Reproduced with permission from *Parassitologia*. A, from Coluzzi, M. and Sabatini, A. (1967), *9*: 78; and B, from Davidson, G. and Hunt, R.H. (1973), *15*: 129

them. Both species are endophilic, although this is more strongly developed in species A, and in the absence of cattle are 100 per cent anthropophilic. When cattle are present species A is more anthropophilic (88 per cent) than B (39 per cent), and B is more exophilic.[28] Species C is zoophilic and not a vector of malaria or filariasis. It is restricted to eastern Africa, Ethiopia, Zanzibar, Zimbabwe and Swaziland. Species D has a restricted distribution in the Bwamba Forest in Uganda. It breeds in mineralised water rather than fresh water. It is anthropophilic and, if huts are available, endophilic. It is a vector of malaria and probably of bancroftian filariasis.[25]

As a result of these investigations it has been established that *An gambiae* is a complex of six species, two saltwater and four freshwater. The two saltwater species are *An melas* and *An merus*. The name *An gambiae* Giles has been retained for species A; species B has been named *An arabiensis* Patton, and species C, *An quadriannulatus* Theobald by redefining earlier synonyms of *An gambiae*.[27] When *An gambiae* refers to species A it is followed by the abbreviation s.s. (*sensu stricto*), and when it refers to the complex the abbreviation s.l. (*sensu lato*) is appended.

Simulium damnosum

Simulium damnosum is widely distributed in the Afrotropical region, where in certain areas it is the vector of a filarial worm, *Onchocerca volvulus*, which may produce blindness in infected individuals. Like other simuliids, *S. damnosum* breeds in running water and the condition is known as river blindness. There is great variation throughout the range of *S. damnosum* in the incidence of onchocerciasis and blindness. The question therefore arose as to whether *S. damnosum* was a single species or a complex, and it has been subjected to a rigorous study of its giant chromosomes.

In many Diptera giant or polytene chromosomes occur in large cells of the salivary glands, malpighian tubes and rectum. It is considered that the nuclei of these large cells are polyploid, possible 1,024 times: that is to say that the chromosomes have divided nine times ($2^{10} = 1,024$) without cell division occurring. The homologous chromosomes align themselves with the same orientation, and when appropriately fixed and stained these giant chromosomes show transverse banding, which is consistent from tissue to tissue of the same individual. The banding can be mapped and the maps made from different individuals compared. The pattern of banding is unique to each species.

Detailed study of the polytene chromosomes of *S. damnosum* has revealed a bewildering array of different patterns, sibling species, of which Dunbar and Vajime[7] recognise 26 (Figure 6.3). Sixteen of these forms occur in eastern Africa, eight in West Africa and two species are present in both East and West Africa. The forms have been arranged in three species

Figure 6.3: Phylogenetic Relationships of Members of the *Simulium damnosum* Complex. Twenty-four species are included. Formal names for eight West African cytospecies are shown in italics and provisional names for 16 East African siblings are capitalised

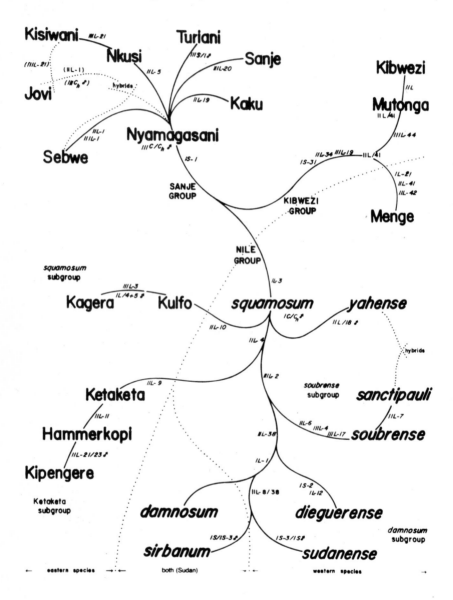

Source: Reproduced with permission from Dunbar, R.W. and Vajime, C.G. (1981), in *Blackflies*, Academic Press, London

groups — Sanje, Kibwezi and Nile. The eight species of the Sanje group are found in East Africa, where they are not associated with onchocerciasis. The three species of the Kibwezi group occur in East Africa and one of them has also been found in Cameroon, West Africa. Fourteen species are included in the Nile group, of which five occur in eastern Africa, eight in West Africa and one extends from West Africa into Uganda, East Africa. The Nile group includes the vectors of onchocerciasis in West Africa, and Vajime and Dunbar[23] have published formal specific names for seven of these species and redefined *S. damnosum.* One species from Ethiopia has not been assigned to a group. *S. damnosum* s.s. refers to the species and *S. damnosum* s.l. to the complex.

The Implications of Species Complexes for the Medical Entomologist

Species complexes are not uncommon and have been described in *Anopheles,* e.g. *An punctulatus*[1]; in culicines, e.g. *Cx pipiens*[12]; in simuliids, e.g. *S. neavei*[17]; and analyses of four species complexes of holarctic simuliids have been presented by Rothfels.[18] The possibility that an abundant, widely distributed species may, on closer examination, prove to be a complex of species, should always be borne in mind. The existence of a complex is only likely to be recognised when a species has been subjected to detailed study, and therefore species complexes appear to be commoner in economically important species.

The medical entomologist should appreciate the implications of species complexes. Firstly, identification of the members of a complex is highly specialised requiring the services of an expert. This means that individuals are unlikely to be able to do their own identifications. Secondly, previous work done on the species may be inapplicable to the worker's current situation. It gives a new twist to the aphorism 'Every malaria problem is a local one', which was coined originally to emphasise that control must be based on intimate knowledge of the local situation. Now it implies that the local vector population may be different and results obtained elsewhere be inapplicable. Thirdly, differences in observations made in different areas may not be artifacts due to techniques or competence of the operator but reflect genuine differences in the vector population. Fourthly, ecological studies must be interpreted cautiously if the adults of the species in a complex are virtually indistinguishable. Ecological results may give a hybrid picture in which specific differences are masked.

Aedes aegypti (see Figure 6.4)

The yellow fever mosquito, *Aedes aegypti,* is widely but sporadically distributed throughout the tropical and subtropical areas of the world. Its distribution appears to be related to the 20°C isotherm which roughly correlates with latitudes 40°N and 40°S. It is a highly domesticated mosquito which can complete its entire life cycle within the confines of a single human dwelling. The female lays its eggs in small containers, such as flower vases, water storage jars and other containers holding water in houses. It will also lay eggs in small amounts of peridomestic water which collects in tyres, plastic containers and other debris associated with human settlement. When the embryo inside the egg of *Ae aegypti* has developed to a certain stage the egg becomes resistant to desiccation. It may then enter diapause in which it can remain for about a year. When the eggs are flooded they hatch and the larvae commence their development immediately. This ability of *Ae aegypti* to produce diapausing eggs enables the species to survive in areas with prolonged dry seasons while the rapid hatching of the eggs on flooding and the speedy development of the immature stages are adaptations to breeding in temporary collections of water.

Adult *Ae aegypti* emerging from breeding sites indoors can complete their cycle without going outside. Swarming is not an essential component of mating. Males orientate to females by responding to the female's wing beat and specific identification is achieved by a contact pheromone on the female. Although in domestic female *Ae aegypti* autogeny is low,[21] blood-feeding presents no problem because the female is strongly anthropophilic and feeds readily on the human inhabitants of the dwelling. The blood-fed

Figure 6.4: Female *Aedes aegypti*

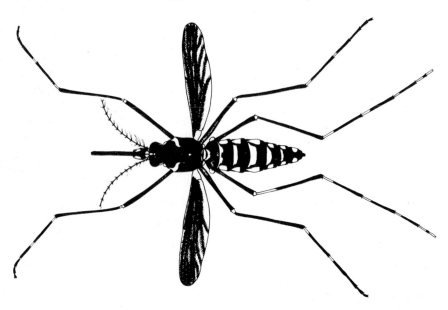

female rests in the house while maturing her ovaries and then deposits her eggs in domestic water containers. The cycle is then complete. It is not surprising that a species with such modest requirements had readily adapted to laboratory colonisation. The fact that *Ae aegypti* produces diapausing eggs made it easy to disseminate material widely throughout the world, even before the days of air transport, and colonies of *Ae aegypti* have been maintained for many years at centres in the northern hemisphere without the introduction of new genetic material. Such colonies form valuable material for studying biological processes but caution must be used in applying the results obtained on such material to 'natural populations'.

Taxonomic Status of Aedes aegypti

The origin of *Ae aegypti* is uncertain but in the post-glacial period it was endemic to Africa from which man has distributed it around the world. Not perhaps unexpectedly, considerable variation in form has been reported in this well-marked, abundant and widely distributed species. Mattingly[13] reviewed the information then available, and postulated three forms of *Ae aegypti* on the basis of colour and associated behavioural characters. The type form *Aedes aegypti aegypti* is a brown or blackish form widely distributed throughout the range of the species, but absent from inland areas of the Afrotropical region. *Ae a.queenslandensis* is a pale form with a similar distribution to that of the type. *Ae a. formosus* is a black form confined to the Afrotropical region, where it is the only form which occurs, except in coastal areas and a few areas of limited inland penetration.

The type form and *queenslandensis* are comparatively recent introductions from the coastal regions of Africa into other parts of the world, where their distribution is sporadic and mainly coastal. These two forms feed and oviposit in and around human habitations in all parts of their range. In addition the type form possesses some ability to breed and feed in natural habitats and in some parts of its range may become semi-wild but not fully wild. In contrast, *Ae a.formosus* commonly exists as a fully wild species, which may become largely domesticated under rural or urban conditions, when human settlement moves into its habitat. *Ae mascarensis* is either another form of *Ae aegypti* or a closely related species. It is a feral, zoophilic taxon, restricted to the high lands above 300 m in Mauritius. Hybridisation of *Ae mascarensis* and *Ae aegypti* was freely accomplished without obvious sterility.[15] *Ae mascarensis* is of no medical importance.

Subsequent authors have recognised three different associations between *Ae aegypti* and man. These have been designated domestic, peridomestic and feral, i.e. wild. The criteria used to differentiate these three associations have varied with the author. Hervy[10] used as criteria the kind and location of larval breeding sites which were either within human dwellings (domestic) or outdoors in artificial containers (peridomestic) or in naturally occurring sites (feral), e.g. tree holes, rock holes. VandeHey *et al.*[24] used the same criteria for classifying breeding sites with the restriction that feral breeding sites must be at least 3 km from human dwellings. In addition VandeHey *et al.*[24] classified adult *Ae aegypti* as domestic or peridomestic on the basis as to whether they bit man indoors or outside houses.

McClelland[14] interprets the relationship between *Ae aegypti* and man in evolutionary terms. He considers that the primitive condition occurs where the human population is either sparse or where there are no sociocultural patterns of water storage. In such areas only the dark form (*Ae a. formosus*) is present and breeds mostly outside but occasionally invades houses. Where the pale and dark forms are sympatric and where the sociocultural patterns favour water storage in houses the pale form is synanthropic, breeding in houses, while the dark form breeds outside. Where the pale form is geographically isolated it breeds mainly inside or around houses but often breeds in rain-filled containers some distance from houses. In McCelland's view, when water and man are continually present the pale form will exclude the dark form from close association with man and the reverse will occur where breeding sites are rain-filled.

McClelland[14] proposes that *Ae aegypti* is in reality two species, *Ae formosus* and *Ae aegypti*. It is commonly accepted that there are two forms of *Ae aegypti* and that there is little justification for recognising both a type form and *queenslandensis*. However, there is less consensus on recognising two separate species. Indeed there is debate as to whether *Ae aegypti* is polytypic or polymorphic, that is, whether there is more than one type (form) of *Ae aegypti* or whether *Ae aegypti* is a single, very variable species. In a polymorphic species there would be free gene flow throughout the population whereas in a polytypic species there would be limited, if any, gene flow between the forms.

Available evidence is conflicting. From a study in East Africa Tabachnick and Powell[20] concluded that significant genetic differences existed between populations in villages, which were less than 2 km apart. These findings implied that the surrounding field-breeding outdoor *Ae aegypti* did not act as a genetic bridge between adjacent populations of indoor breeding *Ae aegypti*. This conclusion is supported by VandeHey *et al.*,[24] who studied 25 different populations of *Ae aegypti* and concluded that, although it was not possible always to identify individual mosquitoes to subspecies, it was possible to attribute populations to either *Ae a. formosus* or *Ae a. aegypti*. They considered that hybridisation and gene flow between the subspecies were rare. Working in the same area Moore[16] found that in the laboratory random mating occurred between domestic and sylvan (feral) *Ae aegypti*, and that there was no evidence of hybrid breakdown. He concluded that *Ae aegypti* was a single species but did not exclude the possibility in nature of other barriers limiting cross-mating between the two forms.

Working in West Africa, Hervy[10] concluded that *Ae aegypti* was a poly-morphic species and he did not accept the concept of subspecies. He considered that, although there was a feral strain which was morphologi-cally distinct, gene flow did occur from the feral to the domestic and peri-domestic population in the rainy season in areas where the feral popula-tion was in close proximity to the domestic-peridomestic population. He also provided evidence of differences in behaviour between the two strains. He reared adults from domestic, peridomestic and feral breeding sites, and, after the newly emerged adults had been marked and released, collections were made in a number of localities. He found that no feral female was recaptured indoors, but that the recapture rate of domestic and peridomes-tic females was the same both indoors and outdoors. This was clear evidence of a behavioural difference between the feral and the domestic+ peridomestic strains and evidence for combining the last two.

A similar experiment in East Africa in which equal numbers of marked domestic, peridomestic and feral *Ae aegypti* were released in a peridomes-tic habitat gave different results.[22] Both experiments resulted in a few or no feral *Ae aegypti* being taken indoors, but in East Africa many more domes-tic than peridomestic *Ae aegypti* (338:63) were taken feeding on humans inside houses.

In summary, *Ae aegypti* is best regarded as being composed of two distinct subspecies, *Ae a.aegypti* and *Ae a.formosus*.[11] *Ae a.aegypti* is pri-marily a coastal subspecies, widely but erratically distributed throughout the tropics and subtropics. It is closely associated with man and, on a global basis, a most important vector of arboviruses to man. *Ae a.formosus* is a dark, feral form which may have little connection with man but can, under certain conditions, form urban populations which are anthropophilic, as in Dar es Salaam.[14]

References

1. Bryan, J.H. (1974). Morphological studies on the *Anopheles punctulatus* Donitz complex. *Transactions of the Royal Entomological Society of London 125*: 413-35
2. Coluzzi, M. and Sabatini, A. (1967). Cytogenetic studies on species A and B of the *Anopheles gambiae* complex. *Parassitologia 9*: 73-88
3. _____ and Sabatini, A. (1968). Cytogenetic observations on species C of the *Anopheles gambiae* complex. *Parassitologia 10*: 155-65
4. _____ and Sabatini, A. (1969). Cytogenetic observations on the salt water species, *Anopheles merus* and *Anopheles melas*, of the *gambiae* complex. *Parassitologia 11*: 177-87
5. Davidson, G. and Hunt, R.H. (1973). The crossing and chromosome characteristics of a new, sixth species in the *Anopheles gambiae* complex. *Parassitologia 15*: 121-8
6. _____ and Paterson, H.E., Coluzzi, M., Mason, G.F. and Micks, D.W. (1967). The *Anopheles gambiae* complex. pp. 211-50 in *Genetics of Insect Vectors of Disease*, J.W. Wright and R. Pal (eds.), Elsevier, Amsterdam
7. Dunbar, R.W. and Vajime, C.G. (1981). Cytotaxonomy of the *Simulium damnosum* complex. pp. 31-43 in *Blackflies*, Marshall Laird (ed.), Academic Press, London

8. Falleroni, D. (1926). Fauna anofelica italiana e suo habitat' (paludi, risaie, canali). Metodi di lotta contro la malaria. *Rivista di Malariologia* 5: 553-93
9. Hackett, L.W. (1937). *Malaria in Europe*, Oxford University Press, London
10. Hervy, J.P. (1977). Expérience de marquage-lâcher-recapture, portant sur *Aedes aegypti* Linné en zone de savane, soudanienne ouest africaine. II. Relations entre habitat, morphologie et comportement. *Cahiers ORSTOM Entomologie Médicale et Parasitologie 15*: 365-72
11. Knight, K.L. and Stone, A. (1977). A catalog of the mosquitoes of the world. *The Thomas Say Foundation 6*: 1-611
12. Laven, H. (1967). Speciation and evolution in *Culex pipiens*. pp. 251-75 in *Genetics of Insect Vectors of Disease*, J.W. Wright and R. Pal (eds.), Elsevier, Amsterdam
13. Mattingly, P.F. (1957). Genetical aspects of the *Aedes aegypti* problem. I. Taxonomy and bionomics. *Annals of Tropical Medicine and Parasitology 51*: 392-408
14. McClelland, G.A.H. (1974). A worldwide survey of variation in scale pattern of the abdominal tergum of *Aedes aegypti* (L.) (Diptera: Culicidae). *Transactions of the Royal Entomological Society of London 126*: 239-59
15. _____ (1967). Speciation and evolution in *Aedes*. pp. 277-311 in *Genetics of Insect Vectors of Disease*, J.W. Wright and R. Pal (eds.), Elsevier, Amsterdam
16. Moore, D.F. (1979). Hybridisation and mating behaviour in *Aedes aegypti* (Diptera: Culicidae). *Journal of Medical Entomology 16*: 223-6
17. Pal, R. (1978). Species complexes in the Simuliidae. *Bulletin of the World Health Organisation 56*: 53-61
18. Rothfels, K. (1981). Cytotaxonomy: principles and their application to some northern species-complexes in *Simulium*. pp. 19-29 in *Blackflies*, Marshall Laird (ed.), Academic Press, London
19. Stegnii, V.N. and Kabanova, V.M. (1976). Cytoecological study of natural populations of *Anopheles* in the territory of the USSR. Report I. Isolation of a new species of *Anopheles* in the *maculipennis* complex by the cytodiagnostic method. *Meditsinskaya Parazitologiya i Parazitarnye Bolezni 45*: 192-8
20. Tabachnick, W.J. and Powell, J.R. (1978). Genetic structure of the East African domestic populations of *Aedes aegypti*. *Nature, London 272*: 535-7
21. Trpis, M. (1977). Autogeny in diverse populations of *Aedes aegypti* from East Africa. *Tropenmedizin und Parasitologie 28*: 77-82
22. _____ and Hausermann, W. (1975). Demonstration of differential domesticity of *Aedes aegypti* (L.) (Diptera, Culicidae) in Africa by mark-release-recapture. *Bulletin of Entomological Research 65*: 199-208
23. Vajime, C.G. and Dunbar, R.W. (1975). Chromosomal identification of eight species of the subgenus *Edwardsellum* near and including *Simulium* (*Edwardsellum*) *damnosum* Theobald (Diptera: Simuliidae). *Tropenmedizin und Parasitologie 26*: 111-38
24. VandeHey, R.C., Leahy, M.G. and Booth, K.S. (1978). Analysis of colour variations in feral, peridomestic and domestic populations of *Aedes aegypti* (L.) (Diptera: Culicidae). *Bulletin of Entomological Research 68*: 443-53
25. White, G.B. (1973). Comparative studies on sibling species of the *Anopheles gambiae* Giles complex (Dipt., Culicidae). III. The distribution, ecology, behaviour and vectorial importance of species D in Bwamba County, Uganda, with an analysis of biological, ecological, morphological and cytogenetic relationships of Uganda species D. *Bulletin of Entomological Research 63*: 65-97
26. _____ (1974). *Anopheles gambiae* complex and disease transmission in Africa. *Transactions of the Royal Society of Tropical Medicine and Hygiene 68*: 278-98
27. _____ (1975). Notes on a catalogue of Culicidae of the Ethiopian region. *Mosquito Systematics 7*: 303-44
28. _____ and Rosen, P. (1973). Comparative studies on sibling species of the *Anopheles gambiae* Giles complex (Dipt., Culicidae). II. Ecology of species A and B in savanna around Kaduna, Nigeria, during the transition from wet to dry season. *Bulletin of Entomological Research 62*: 613-25

PART II
INSECTS AND ACARINES OF MEDICAL AND VETERINARY IMPORTANCE

7 CULICIDAE (MOSQUITOES)

There are two families of Nematocera, the Chaoboridae and the Dixidae, which are closely related to the Culicidae. They have been regarded as subfamilies of an enlarged Culicidae but are now treated as separate families. The blood-sucking habit is found only in the Culicidae, and it is adequate for our purpose to recognise that there are these two other families which may be confused with mosquitoes.

Dixidae: Adult dixids have short mouthparts; no scales on the wings and a wing venation, which is a distorted version of that of the culicidae, with the second vein strongly arched (Figure 7.1). Dixid larvae occur at the edges of streams and may be mistaken for *Anopheles* larvae, but in the dixid the three thoracic segments are not fused; there are pseudopods on abdominal segments 1 and 2, and ambulacral combs on segments 5, 6 and 7,[53] with which it can climb out of water (Figure 7.2). Larvae of *An wellcomei* are unusual in that they can climb out of water,[20] but they lack pseudopods and ambulacral combs.

Figure 7.1: Above, Wing of a Chaborid; Below, Wing of a Dixid

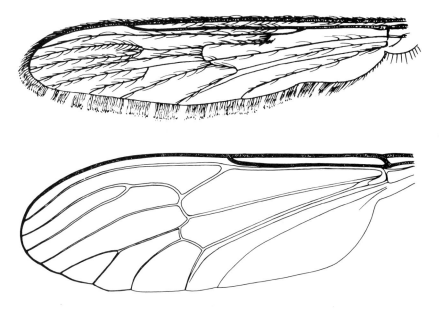

Figure 7.2: Larva of *Dixa brevis*. Dorsal view (left) and ventral view (right)

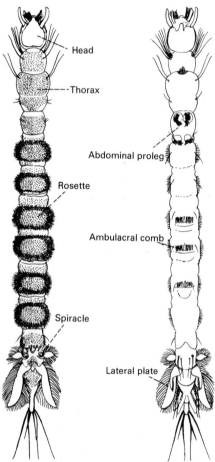

Source: From Nowell[53]

Chaoboridae (phantom midges): Adult chaoborids have short mouth-parts; scales on the wings forming a fringe on the posterior margin and a few on the veins; wing venation inseparable from that of the Culicidae with the second vein running parallel to the first and third veins (Figure 7.1). Chaoborid larvae are aquatic predators.

Culicidae (mosquitoes): Culicid adults have a long forwardly directed proboscis, equal in length to the head and thorax combined (Figure 7.3); wings with scales along the veins and forming a fringe; second vein not arched but running parallel to veins i and iii (Figure 3.4). Culicid larvae are aquatic but in only a relatively small number of species are they predatory.

Figure 7.3: Female *Anopheles annulipes*

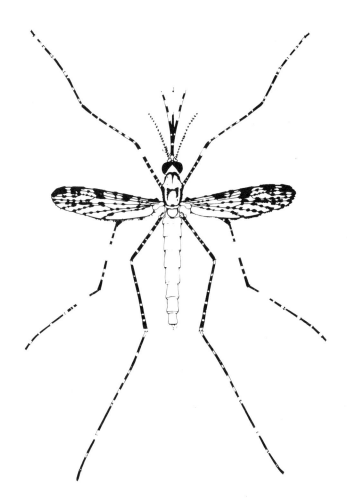

Culicidae

Three subfamilies are recognised among the Culicidae: the Toxorhynchitinae, Anophelinae and Culicinae.

Toxorhynchitinae

This subfamily includes only one genus *Toxorhynchites* which occurs mainly in the tropics and subtropics of the Oriental, Neotropical and Afrotropical regions (Table 7.1). Steffan and Evenhuis[66] have recently reviewed the biology of *Toxorhynchites* and they recognise 69 species, five more than in Table 7.1. *Toxorhynchites* are very large, metallic coloured

Table 7.1: Zoogeographical Distribution of Culicidae

	No. of species	Number of species of each genus in each region					
		Australian	Nearctic	Neotropical	Oriental	Palaearctic	Afrotropical
Anophelinae	389						
Anopheles	377	24	16	76	118	39	118
Bironella	8	8					
Chagasia	4			4			
Culicinae	2,612						
Aedeomyini	7						
Aedeomyia	7	2		1	1		3
Aedini	1,115						
Aedes	914	215	73	118	288	79	189
Armigeres	46	6			41	1	
Eretmapodites	44						44
Haemagogus	28			28			
Heizmannia	29				29		
Opifex	1	1					
Psorophora	47		14	41			
Udaya	2				2		
Zeugnomyia	4	1			4		
Culicini	763						
Culex	744	121	32	313	173	40	137
Deinocerites	18		4	16			
Galindomyia	1			1			
Culisetini	36						
Culiseta	36	14	8	1	4	15	2
Ficalbiini	40						
Ficalbia	7	1			3		4
Mimomyia	33	7			9		19

Table 7.1 continued

	No. of species	Number of species of each genus in each region					
		Australian	Nearctic	Neotropical	Oriental	Palaearctic	Afrotropical
Hodgesiini	11						
Hodgesia	11				4		4
Mansoniini	79						
Coquillettidia	55	14	1	13	8	2	21
Mansonia	24	7	2	13	5		2
Orthopodomyiini	24						
Orthopodomyia	24	1	3	7	10	1	5
Sabethini	355						
Limatus	8			8			
Malaya	12	3			5		6
Maorigoeldia	1	1					
Phoniomyia	22			22			
Sabethes	29			29			
Topomyia	32	1			31		
Trichoprosopon	33			33			
Tripteroides	111	62			52	1	
Wyeomyia	107		4	105			
Uranotaeniini	182						
Uranotaenia	182	31	2	28	76	2	47
Toxorhynchitinae	64						
Toxorhynchites	64	4	1	17	30	3	12
TOTAL	3,065	528	160	874	893	183	613

Note: Sum of regional totals (3,251) exceeds number of species (3,065) because some species occur in more than one region.

Source: Extracted from Knight and Stone[42] and Knight[41]).

mosquitoes, which do not suck blood and in which the proboscis is markedly bent (Figure 7.4). Morphologically they resemble culicine mosquitoes in the structure of the larva and the adult. They breed in small collections of water, e.g. tree holes, where their larvae are predacious on other mosquito larvae. They have been introduced into French Polynesia and Samoa to control *Aedes* (*Stegomyia*) *aegypti* and *Ae* (*Stg*) *Polynesiensis.*[12,60] Throughout this chapter and elsewhere the generic and subgeneric abbreviations proposed by Reinert[59] will be used.

Anophelinae

Three genera of mosquitoes are included in the Anophelinae but only one, *Anopheles,* of which there are nearly 400 species, is widely distributed (Table 7.1). *Bironella* is confined to New Guinea and tropical Australia and *Chagasia* to the Neotropical region. *Anopheles* are medically important, being the sole vectors of malaria, and they play a substantial role in transmitting lymphatic filariasis due to *Wuchereria bancrofti.* *Bironella* and *Chagasia* are medically unimportant. The morphological characters distinguishing Anophelinae and Culicinae will be given later when their life cycles have been considered.

Culicinae

There are more than 2,500 species of Culicinae of which the main genera are *Aedes* with over 900 species, *Culex* with nearly 750 species and the medically unimportant *Uranotaenia* with more than 180 species. Culicine genera are usually widespread, although *Eretmapodites* occurs only in the Afrotropical region, *Haemagogus* in the Neotropical region, *Psorophora* in

Figure 7.4: Heads of *Toxorhynchites speciosus* — male on left and female on the right

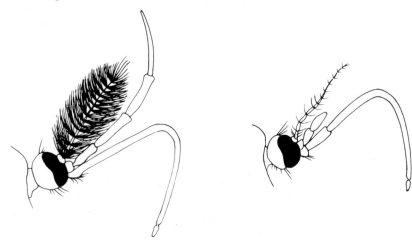

the Nearctic and Neotropical regions and *Heizmannia*, with one exception, in the Oriental region.

The Sabethini are predominantly Neotropical in distribution with four of the eight genera being restricted to that region (Table 7.1). *Wyeomyia* has four species in the adjoining Nearctic region; *Topomyia* is virtually confined to the Oriental region, and *Tripteroides* to the Oriental region and tropical and subtropical parts of the Australian region. The small genus *Malaya* has a wide distribution in the Old World tropics but is of no importance because its adults are not haematophagous. Female *Malaya* have an unusual method of feeding. The female stops foraging ants of the genus *Cremastogaster*, inserts its proboscis into the ant's mouth and sucks up honey-dew which the ant has collected from plant-sucking bugs.[13] Sabethines breed in small collections of water associated with plants, e.g. leaf axils of epiphytic bromeliads, pitcher plants, tree holes and bamboo. *Sabethes chloropterus* is an inefficient vector of yellow fever but it is long-lived and could be involved in the survival of the virus over the dry season.[14,61]

Mattingly[45] classifies the Culicinae ecologically into four groups, which are more or less self-contained. The aedine genera *Aedes* and *Psorophora* have drought-resistant eggs, enabling them to breed in temporary ground pools and small containers. The quasi-sabethines exhibit both aedine and sabethine characters, breed in containers such as bamboo, tree holes and leaf axils, and include such genera as *Eretmapodites*, *Haemagogus* and *Armigeres*. A third group is associated with dense aquatic vegetation and includes *Ficalbia*, *Coquillettidia* and *Mansonia*. The fourth group is an assemblage of miscellaneous genera of which the largest is *Culex* and one, *Deinocerites*, is associated with crab holes in the Nearctic and Neotropical regions.[3,36]

Culicines are important vectors of human disease and are the major vectors of arboviruses and filarias, e.g. *Ae aegypti* of yellow fever and dengue; *Cx tarsalis* of western equine encephalitis; *Cx quinquefasciatus* of *Wuchereria bancrofti*; and *Mansonia uniformis* of *Brugia malayi* (see Chapters 24 and 30).

Life Cycle of *Anopheles*

Egg

The female *Anopheles* mosquito lays a batch of 100-150 eggs usually at night on the surface of the water. They are cigar-shaped objects about 1 mm long and bearing paired lateral air-filled floats, which are characteristic of anopheline eggs (Figure 7.5). In the spring *An sacharovi* lays eggs with small floats but in the summer its eggs lack floats.[50] The fine structure of *Anopheles* eggs has been studied by Hinton,[32] and he suggests that the fine network of the outer layer of the chorion acts as a plastron facilitating respiration when the egg is submerged. The surface structure of the egg is such that eggs will attach end to end or side to side but never end to side. They become attached by surface forces to objects projecting from the water and this property prevents eggs drifting into open stretches of water. The eggs of *An multicolor* are laid side by side in a row resembling cartridges in a bandolier.[36] Anopheline egs develop directly into larvae and only rarely undergo diapause. Ho *et al.*[34] have reported that *An lesteri* overwinters in the egg stage. Under optimal conditions anopheline eggs hatch in 1-2 days.

Larva

The larva emerges from the egg by using a small egg tooth, placed postero-dorsally on its head. Three regions can be differentiated in the body of the larva: a well developed sclerotised head; a broad thorax in which the three segments are fused; and a segmented abdomen (Figure 7.6). The larva is apterous and apodous, having neither wings nor legs. When anopheline larvae come to the water surface they swim backwards by lateral movements of the abdomen until the caudal setae on the anal segment of the abdomen are in contact with a solid object, e.g. vegetation or stone. The larvae are postively thigmotactic.

The larva lies parallel to the water surface supported by the paired prothoracic notched organ, the posterior spiracular apparatus and paired palmate hairs (Figure 7.7B).[58] Palmate hairs are present on most

Figure 7.5: Lateral (left) and Dorsal (right) Views of an Anopheline Egg

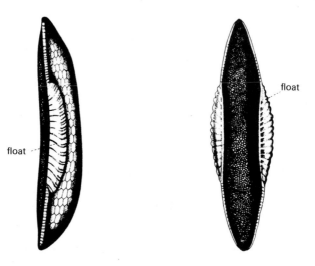

Source: From Nuttall, G.H.F. and Shipley, A.E. (1901) *Journal of Hygiene 1*

Figure 7.6: Larva of *Anopheles maculipennis* Viewed From Above. The anal segment is twisted round to display the ventral brush and caudal hairs

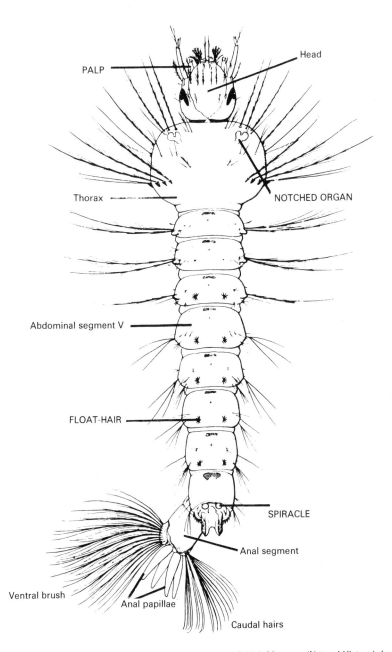

Source: From Marshall (1938). *The British Mosquitoes*. British Museum (Natural History), London

abdominal segments and occasionally on the thorax. They have short, stout bases from which radiate 10-20 leaflets and are unique to anopheline larvae (Figure 7.8). When the palmate hair is in contact with the water surface the leaflets spread out and support the larva. When the larva comes to the water surface its dorsal side is uppermost and the mouthparts are directed downwards. The larva possesses a pair of mouth brushes in addition to the usual complement of mouthparts. Two methods of feeding, film-feeding and free-feeding, have been described.[58] The larva rotates its

Figure 7.7: A, Lateral View of Culicine Larva Showing Feeding Currents (dotted lines). B, Lateral View of an Anopheline Larva Feeding at the Water Surface. Dotted lines indicate depth and direction of current set up by larva. C, Dorsal View of Currents Set Up by Feeding Anopheline Larva

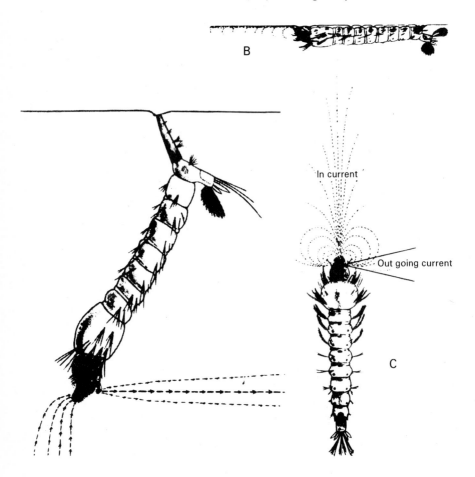

Source: Reproduced with permission from Puri[58]

head through 180° and either feeds directly on the surface bacterial film using slow movements of the mouth brushes or they are moved rapidly backwards and forwards drawing a subsurface current of water towards the head (Figure 7.7C), where it impinges on the labium and is deflected laterally through the maxillae, which act as strainers, filtering out small particles, and transferring them to the mouth.[58]

Like most small-particle feeders, size of particle is an important factor in determining its acceptability. Small particles are ingested and larger ones rejected although, on occasions, the mandibles may be used to nibble at larger particles. Advantage can be taken of this method of feeding to control *Anopheles* by the application of finely powdered Paris green, a complex of copper metarsenite and copper acetate, to the surface. At a dosage of 1.14 kg/ha Paris green, applied as a dust, settles on the surface film, and the feeding larva filters out the poison, ingests it and is killed. The

Figure 7.8: Part of Dorsal Surface of Abdominal Segment V of *Anopheles culicifacies* (above) With a Few Leaflets of a Palmate Hair From Abdominal Segment IV (below)

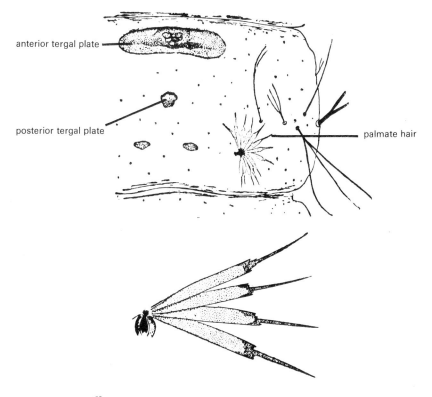

dosage selectively kills *Anopheles* larvae and leaves other organisms unharmed. The efficiency of Paris green as a larvicide against *Anopheles* is thoroughly attested by it being the only larvicide used by Soper and Wilson[65] in their eradication of *An gambiae* from Brazil in the 1930s.

Anopheline larvae breathe atmospheric air through a pair of spiracles at the posterior end of the abdomen, i.e. the larva is metapneustic. The opening of the spiracles is in the floor of the spiracular apparatus, which pierces the surface. To prevent water entering the spiracles a film of oil is secreted by the perispiracular glands.[37] The oil secretion repels water but allows oil to enter and this is the rationale for the use of oil as a mosquito larvicide. To be effective the oil has to have a low viscosity so that it readily enters the spiracles and penetrates the tracheae, and it has to be toxic. Toxicity is provided by including small amounts of organic insecticides, such as DDT or temephos, an organophosphorus insecticide. In passing it might be noted that larvae of the ephydrid fly, *Psilopa petrolei*, live in oil pools in southern California and Thorpe[68] considers that they prevent oil entering their tracheae by the perispiracular glands secreting water.

The larva grows steadily and under optimal conditions will pupate in 7-10 days but the duration of the larval stage is temperature dependent, and in the cool season in subtropical areas the larval stage may last several months, e.g. *An pharoensis* in Egypt. At intervals, the larva moults and, as

Figure 7.9: Growth of Head Capsule of *Anopheles maculatus* var. *willmori* Larva. Note that the collar increases in width during instars 1 to 3 but not in instar 4

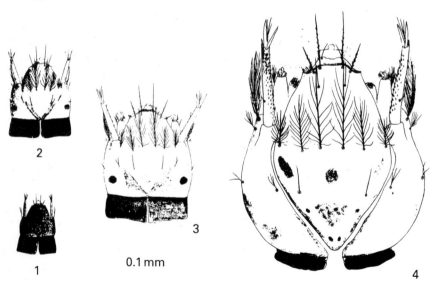

Source: From Puri[58]

described earlier (p. 68), the head capsule is rapidly inflated to the size characteristic of the next instar. Head size increases geometrically from instar to instar and follows Dyar's law (Figure 7.9). In *An sergenti* the head breadth increased by about 50 per cent at each moult and the mean measurements in the four instars were 170,260, 395 and 600 μm.[38] A linear increase of × 1.524 in head size at each moult implies an increase in volume of × 3.5. During the first three instars the head capsule increases in length by the addition of a collar but in the fourth instar the collar remains a narrow band. The only efficient criteria for identifying fourth instar larvae are head size and the extent of the collar. Other body dimensions, such as length, increase steadily throughout larval life and there is an overlap between instars. The fully grown fourth instar larva moults into the pupa.

Pupa

The head and thorax of the pupa are combined into a single division, the cephalothorax, which is joined posteriorly to a segmented abdomen (Figure 7.10). At rest the pupa floats at the water surface with the abdomen reflected under the cephalothorax. The pupa does not feed and is therefore unaffected by Paris green but it breathes through a pair of broad trumpets dorsally placed on the cephalothorax, i.e. it is propneustic, and is susceptible to oil treatment. The ninth segment of the abdomen carries a pair of broad, flat plates, the paddles. The pupa remains quiescent unless disturbed, when the abdomen is straightened out, the paddles spread widely, and then the abdomen is rapidly flexed. Depending upon the orientation of the cephalothorax this movement of the abdomen serves to drive the pupa forward or to dive below the surface where it may merely float to the surface again or stay down without any apparent further effort.[20] Pupae can complete their development out of water; presumably either the pupa itself or the enclosed pharate adult has a complete waterproofing wax layer. On a dry surface pupae can jump about, which is possibly a defence mechanism against predators.[20]

It has been shown recently that *Anopheles* pupae can be killed by applying a monolayer of a water-insoluble surfactant, e.g. lecithin, to their breeding sites.[48,49] The pupae are unable to pierce the monolayer to make contact with the air, and die of lack of oxygen. Other aquatic creatures, dependent for respiration on oxygen dissolved in the water, are unaffected.

Adult Emergence

The pupal skin splits dorsally and the adult emerges. Careful movements are required to ensure that the adult mosquito does not fall sideways and be trapped in the surface film. (Adult *Opifex fuscus* are able to tumble around, on and in water, without becoming trapped.[44]) This danger is particularly acute when the adult is largely out of the pupal exuviae but the terminal segments of the appendages are still not free. At that stage the

Figure 7.10: A, Pupa of *Anopheles maculipennis*; B, Dorsal View of Terminal Segments of Abdomen of Pupa of *Anopheles hilli*

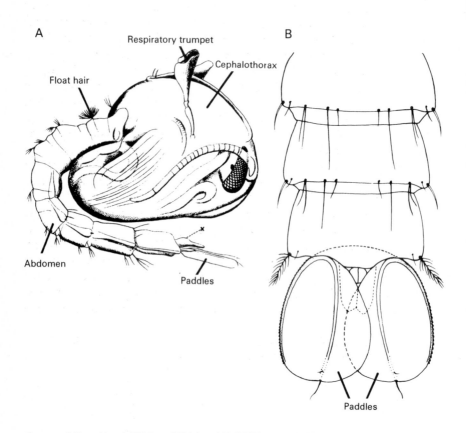

Source: A From Nuttal, G.H.F. and Shipley, A.E. (1901). *Journal of Hygiene 1*

exuviae is largely full of air and the centre of gravity is well above the water surface making for instability. Finally the legs come free and spread on the water surface giving stability. The newly emerged adult inflates its wings, and separates and grooms its head appendages before flying away. Behaviour of the adult mosquito will be given in the section on bionomics below.

Life Cycle of Culicinae

This account will emphasise those features in which culicines differ from anophelines.

Egg

The eggs of *Aedes* are laid in a batch but are not attached to each other. They differ from those of *Anopheles* by the absence of floats. Eggs of *Aedes* are laid on the moist surface at the water's edge and not on the water itself. When the eggs are first laid they are susceptible to desiccation, and collapse and die if dried. When the embryo is fully developed, eggs can withstand desiccation and remain viable in the dried state for many months, depending on the species. The production of eggs resistant to desiccation makes *Aedes* species ideal colonisers of temporary collections of water, e.g. salt marshes, tree holes, etc. When the eggs are flooded, most of them hatch immediately, but some will remain dormant and hatch at the second or third flooding. The early emergence of larvae is essential if the life cycle is to be completed before the habitat dries up. Similar dormant eggs are produced by other aedine genera including *Haemagogus* and *Psorophora*.

Gillett[20] points out that the egg raft, commonly regarded as typical of the Culicinae, is produced in only four genera: *Culex, Culiseta, Coquillettidia* and *Uranotaenia*. Rafts commonly measure 3-4 mm long and 2-3 mm wide, but the precise form is a specific attribute, and Gillett[19] has shown that the shape of the egg raft is a specific character in six species of *Coquillettidia* in the Afrotropical region (Figure 7.11). The lower side of the raft on the water is convex and the other side concave. The eggs are orientated

Figure 7.11: Egg-rafts of Five Species of *Coquillettidia*. A, *C. metallica*; B, *C. maculipennis*; C, *C. fraseri*; D, *C.fuscopennata*; E; *C. aurites*

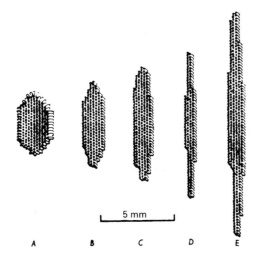

5 mm

A B C D E

at right angles to the water surface, but arranged so that the larva is head down in the egg and emerges from the underside of the raft. The eggs cannot withstand desiccation and, if dried, the eggs collapse and the embryos die.

The eggs of *Mansonia* are laid in clusters on the undersurface of floating leaves of aquatic plants such as *Salvinia*. The eggs are tapered at the free end and the cluster of eggs has the appearance of a miniature pin-cushion.[20,73] The eggs of *Sabethes chloropterus* are unusual in being rhomboidal in shape.[14]

Larva

Culicine larvae differ from those of *Anopheles* by their possessing a siphon on the penultimate segment of the abdomen (Figure 7.12). The tracheae are continued into the siphon and the spiracles open at its tip. Within the subfamily there is great variety in the shape and size of siphons. In *Aedes* the siphon is typically short; in *Mansonia* it is short and highly specialised; and in *Culex* the siphon is long and slender. Possession of the siphon enables culicine larvae to hang head down from the surface film, and simultaneously respire and feed below the surface (Figure 7.7A).

Eretmapodites larvae, inhabiting shallow collections of water in leaf axils, have short siphons but elongated abdomens enabling them to breathe at the surface and feed upon the bottom at the same time. *Aedes* larvae may feed at the surface while respiring by twisting the abdomen to bring the mouthparts into contact with the surface film. They also feed on the bottom out of contact with the surface. Larger larvae of *Eretmapodites* are commonly facultative predators upon smaller larvae within their restricted habitat.[27] The larvae of *Psorophora* (*Psorophora*), *Aedes* (*Mucidus*) and *Culex* (*Lutzia*) are obligatory predators on larvae of their own or other species.[45]

When non-predatory culicine larvae are feeding, the current created by the mouth brushes passes from in front of the larva, through the mouth-parts and out behind. Consequently, as the larva is freely suspended from the water surface, it moves slowly forward while feeding (Figure 7.7A).[58] As the culicine larva hangs head down from the surface it does not possess palmate hairs or prothoracic notched organs and, as they feed below the surface, they are not vulnerable to Paris green applied as a dust to the surface. If Paris green is applied as a water-based suspension it becomes distributed throughout the water body and is available to culicine larvae, which filter out and ingest the poison and are killed. This treatment is only feasible where the breeding site is very shallow and the water volume small. Culicine larvae breathe at the water surface and are therefore susceptible to control by oil.

The larvae of *Mansonia* and *Coquillettidia* have short conical siphons with enlarged, heavily sclerotised valves (Figure 7.13), which are used to

Figure 7.12: Main Features of a Culicine Larva

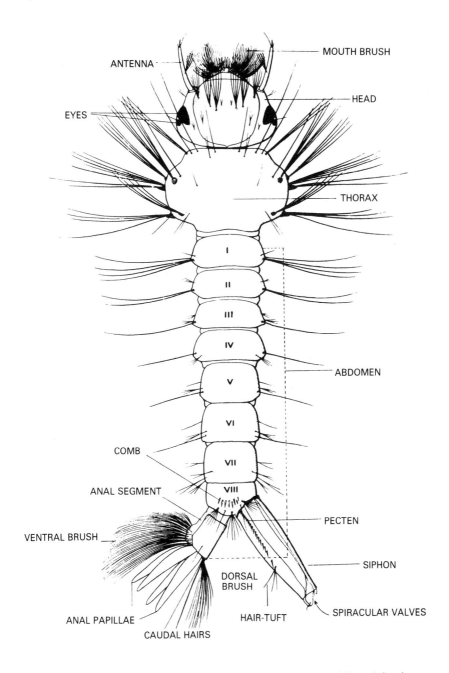

Source: From Marshall (1935). *British Mosquitoes*. British Museum (Natural History). London

pierce aquatic plants and acquire air via the air canals of the plant. This behaviour renders the larva dependent upon emergent aquatic vegetation, but more or less immune to larvicides applied to the surface. Larvae of *Ma uniformis* and *Ma africana* show no selection for any particular plant species and will attach to brown paper in the laboratory.[43] These larvae can respire at the surface but are unable to moult, for which they need to be attached to an object when the exuviae is left *in situ* and the newly moulted larva reattaches. In other culicine larvae the valves of the siphon close the opening and prevent the entry of water, when submerged.

Pupa

The culicine pupa is very similar to that of the Anophelinae, apart from the differences in the shape of the respiratory horn which is tubular, compared with the distally expanded horn in the Anophelinae. In *Mansonia* and *Coquillettidia* the respiratory horns of the pupa are modified for penetrating plant tissue (Figure 7.13) and, on pupation, the larval exuviae is not shed until the pupa has firmly attached itself to the plant. When this is achieved the pupa gives a quick flick and the larval exuviae is both shed and detached from the plant. In these genera, at eclosion, the pupa frees

Figure 7.13: Left, Terminal Segments of the Abdomen of Larva of *Mansonia uniformis*; Right, Respiratory Trumpet of Pupa of *M. uniformis*

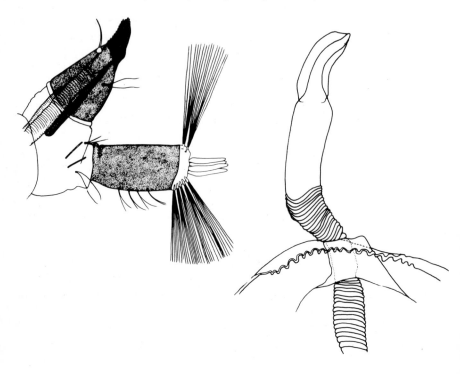

itself from the plant, leaving behind the tips of the respiratory horns, and rises to the surface where it respires in the same manner as other culicine pupae.[20]

In general the development times for culicines are as short or shorter than those of *Anopheles*, but the life cycles of *Mansonia* and *Coquillettidia* are particularly protracted. At 23°C *Cq aurites* takes 40-50 days to develop from egg to adult while *Ae aegypti* completes development in 10 days at the same temperature, and at 26-30°C *Ma uniformis* and *Ma africana* develop in 25-40 days.[20,43]

Morphological Differences Between Adult Anophelinae and Culicinae

Alive

Living adults can be readily recognised by the stance they adopt when resting on a flat surface. Adult *Anopheles* rest with the proboscis, head, thorax and abdomen in one straight line making an acute angle with the surface (Figure 7.14A). In some species, e.g. *An balabacensis*, the adult appears to stand almost on its head while other species, such as *An culicifacies*, as the specific name implies, have a more culicine-like stance. The culicine adult rests with its body angled and the abdomen directed back towards the surface on which it is resting (Figure 7.14). The proboscis, head and anterior part of the thorax form one line and the posterior part of the thorax and the abdomen another. This difference enables selective hand collections to be made of living material, but this character does not apply to dead mosquitoes.

Dead Adults

Dead adults can be classified after examination of the antennae and palps. Most male mosquitoes of all three subfamilies have plumose antennae, and females have pilose antennae with fewer, shorter hairs. This difference is a functional one, the antennae being sound receptors enabling the male to locate the female by the sound of her wing beat. In the female anopheline the palps are as long and straight as the proboscis, while the palps of the female culicine are considerably shorter, usually about one quarter of the length of the proboscis (Figure 7.15). The palps are often closely applied to the proboscis so that the culicine proboscis appears to have a thickened base and the anopheline proboscis to be trifid at the tip.

In the anopheline male the palps are as long as the proboscis and clubbed at the distal end where the last two segments are swollen (Figure 7.16). In the typical culicine male the palps are as long as the proboscis and taper distally, but the tapering is sometimes obscured by the development of tufts of hair on the distal segments (Figure 7.16). In a number of culicine genera, including *Sabethes*, *Uranotaenia* and *Wyeomyia*, the palps of the male are short and similar to those of the female.[46] When the palps of the male are long they are often upturned in Culicinae and laterally directed in the Anophelinae. In the Toxorhynchitinae the palps are of the culicine type, being short in the female and long and tapering in the male (Figure 7.4).

Figure 7.14: Resting Stances of Living Mosquitoes — *Anopheles* (above) and Culicine (below)

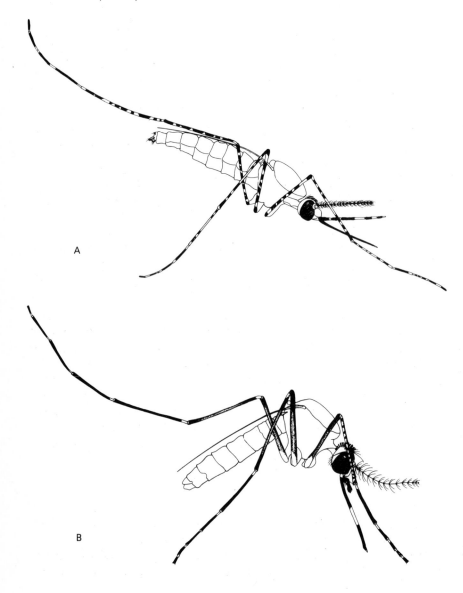

Figure 7.15: Heads of Female Mosquitoes — *Anopheles annulipes* (left) and *Culex annulirostris* (right)

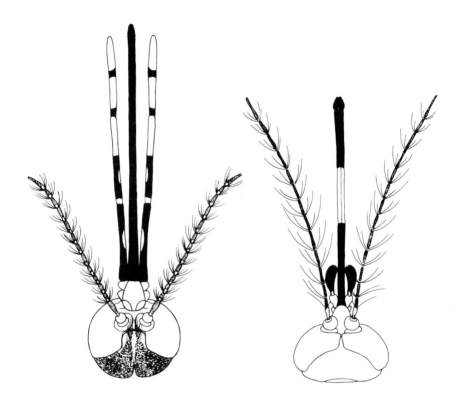

There are also differences between the subfamilies in the distribution of scales on the body, the shape of the scutellum and the number of spermathecae. In the Anophelinae the abdominal sterna and usually also the terga, are completely or largely devoid of scales, but in the Culicinae the abdomen is covered with a uniform layer of scales.[46] The scutellum is evenly curved in the Anophelinae and there is a regular row of setae on the posterior border (Figure 7.17). In the Culicinae the scutellum is trilobed and the setae are grouped on the lateral and median lobes. There are three spermathecae in most Culicinae, two in *Mansonia* and only a single one in the Anophelinae and *Uranotaenia* and *Aedeomyia*.[20]

General Culicid Bionomics

In this section a generalised account of the bionomics of mosquitoes will be given. Most of the features are common to all mosquitoes.

When the progeny of any one egg batch emerge as adults the males emerge first. This is not uncommon in insects, and in mosquitoes there is a

Figure 7.16: Heads of Male Mosquitoes — *Anopheles annulipes* (left) and *Culex annulirostris* (right)

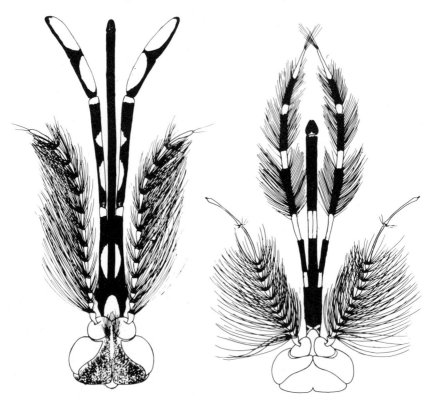

special reason. The male terminalia have to rotate through 180° before the male is ready for mating. This process takes about 24 h so that by the time the females emerge the males are competent for mating. The males obtain additional energy for flight by taking nectar from plants, as do the females. In the Arctic tundra both sexes of mosquitoes may be collected from flowers and be found with orchid pollinia on their heads, indicating that they have probed deeply into orchids.[70] Both sexes of the saltmarsh mosquito, *Ae taeniorhynchus*, show a marked circadian pattern of nectar feeding with peaks in the early morning and from late afternoon until nearly midnight. During the brief periods before sunrise and after sunset, when the males were swarming, no nectar feeding occurred.[29]

Female mosquitoes are referred to as endophilic or exophilic depending on whether they rest indoors or outdoors, and as endophagic or exophagic on whether they feed indoors or outdoors. *An balabacensis* is both exophilic and exophagic; *An maculatus* is exophilic and endophagic, while *An minimus* is both endophilic and endophagic.

Figure 7.17: Scutella of an *Anopheles* (left) and a Culicine (right)

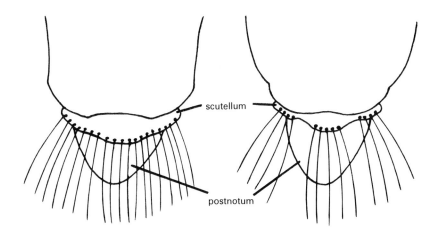

Mating

Mating is often preceded or accompanied by swarming in which the males associate over a marker and fly in a particular manner. Markers are visually prominent objects such as the tops of tall trees or ground objects which contrast with the background.[11] The males face into the wind and fly forward until they are vertically over the front edge of the marker, when they cease flying and are carried backwards. As they pass over the hind edge of the marker active flight is stimulated and the males fly forward again over the marker.[11] Such oscillatory flight is characteristic of males in swarms. The long slender hairs or fibrillae on the plumose antennae of the male are erected from the shaft and increase the receptivity of the antenna to sound waves. In some species, e.g. *Ae aegypti*, the fibrillae remain erected permanently and in other species, e.g. *An gambiae*, the fibrillae undergo a circadian rhythm of being erect or recumbent.[6,8] Sound waves impinging on the fibrillae cause the shaft of the antenna to vibrate and stimulate sensory cells in Johnston's organ in the pedicel, the swollen second segment of the antenna.[8]

In *An melas* it is considered that the adults first orientate to an 'arena', an open flat area and then to markers within the arena. Male swarms form over the markers and virgin females orientating to markers will encounter swarming males. Males recognise a female from a short distance and fly directly towards her and attempt to couple and, if successful, the pair leave the swarm *in copulo* with insemination being completed elsewhere. Charlwood and Jones[7] point out that a female spends less than 30 s in the swarm and at any one time the proportion of males to females would be of the order of 600:1 and hence copulating pairs are seen infrequently.

During mating spermatozoa are deposited in the bursa copulatrix of the female, from which they move to the spermathecae. Wharton[72] described the arenas used by anophelines in Malaya as 'relatively open, flat areas free from overhead obstructions and surrounded by trees or other objects', and the arena of *An melas* was similar.

In *An claviger* insemination occurs in flight, the couples separating when they reach the ground. This behaviour frustrated attempts to colonise this species until it was appreciated that the solution was to have a cage of sufficient height that the coupled pair did not reach the ground until insemination had occurred.[1]

Swarming requires sufficient illumination for the males to be able to see the marker, and a low enough wind speed so that the males can orientate to it. Downes[11] gives the range of wind speed for *Ae hexodontus* to swarm, as 0.2-3.5 m/s. Swarming occurs commonly at sunset when the wind tends to die away, and the rapidly fading light has a stimulating effect on mosquito activity. Wharton[72] observed swarming in five species of *Anopheles* in the same area. They varied in the height at which the swarm formed, with swarms of *An indiensis* occurring 0.3-0.6 m above the ground and swarms of *An maculatus* at 4.5-6.0 m. Most observations were made on *An philippinensis* which began to swarm about 5 min after sunset and continued for about 20 min. Copulating pairs were seen flying in the vicinity of swarms with the period of copulation lasting from 10-25 s. Similar observations were made by Russell and Rao[62] on *An culicifacies* with the difference that most (19/23) of the copulating females had already taken a blood meal whereas copulating female *An philippinensis* were newly emerged.

Some mosquitoes, such as *Ae aegypti*, mate without swarming; with the male responding to the sound of the female's wing beat, which in 3-4 day-old females ranges from 450-600 c/s with an average of 500 c/s.[75] Males show a strong response to sounds within the range of 400-600 c/s and particularly to sounds of 500-550 c/s, and are therefore adapted to respond to the flying female. Male *Ae aegypti* can detect females up to a distance of 25 cm and respond to a sound of approximately 20 decibels.[75] Male *Ae aegypti* have higher wing-beat frequencies than females, but as both sexes have lower frequencies early in adult life the wing beat of young males and old females are similar.[8]

Although only female *Ae aegypti* are blood feeders, both sexes have similar bimodal, diurnal landing rates on man with coinciding peaks before sunset between 17.00-18.00 h. In the morning the peak landing rate for females occur just after sunrise, 06.00-07.00 h, while the male peak is about 2 h later.[10] This suggests that in nature mating occurs in the vicinity of the host. Discrimination between species and inseminated females is achieved by the presence of a contact pheromone on virgin female *Ae aegypti*.[52] When mating and blood-feeding are separated both in space and in time a contact pheromone is not necessary and is not present in *An gambiae*.[6] It was pointed out earlier (Chapter 6) that male *An atroparvus* would mate with females of other species in the *An maculipennis* complex and, in that case, either there is no contact pheromone or the pheromones are so similar that males fail to discriminate between virgin females in the complex.

In some species the male antennae are pilose, like the female's, and sexual recognition is based on other than auditory stimuli. Males of *Deinocerites cancer* search the surface of breeding sites for female pupae and mate with the female when she emerges. Female pupae are recognised through a contact pheromone which the male detects with its antennae.[31] Males of *Opifex fuscus* are capable of mating within an hour of emergence and will copulate with females, while they are still within the pupal exuviae. *Op fuscus* males do not distinguish between male and female pupae but do not attempt to copulate with males.[39,44] In *Sabethes chloropterus* the male hovers over the resting female and tests her receptivity by tapping the hind legs of the female with his mid-tarsi.[14]

During mating, secretions from the accessory glads of the male produce a mating plug in the female. In *Ae aegypti* it has been shown that the plug contains matrone, a substance which stimulates oviposition and inhibits mating. Matrone consists of two fractions, one of which stimulates oviposition while the other has no obvious effect on its own, but both fractions are required to inhibit further mating.[33]

Host Finding

In some species, e.g. *Cx molestus*, the first egg batch may be matured autogenously, i.e. without a blood meal, but most mosquitoes require a blood meal for ovarian development. The source of the blood meal is a major factor in determining the potential of a species to be a vector of disease. Tempelis[67] recognises nine basic feeding patterns among mosquitoes, including species that feed: almost entirely on mammals, e.g. *An gambiae, Culiseta inornata*; almost entirely on birds, e.g. *Culiseta melanura*; readily on both birds and mammals, e.g. *Cx quinquefasciatus*; almost exclusively on amphibians, e.g. *Cx territans*; predominantly on reptiles, e.g. *Deinocerites dyari*; and a remarkable species, *Uranotaenia lateralis*, which feeds on the mudskipper, a fish, which lies out of the water on mud banks with its tail in the water.

Within the mammal-feeding mosquitoes further subdivisions can be made into those which are anthropophilic, feeding on man, e.g. *An gambiae* s.s., and those which are zoophilic, such as *An maculatus* in Nepal.[17] Garrett-Jones *et al*.[17] have reviewed the feeding habits of *Anopheles* species.

There are several stages in the feeding behaviour of mosquitoes, which are designated activation, orientation, landing and probing. Most mosquitoes have a crepuscular or nocturnal circadian cycle of activity, which is stimulated by rapidly fading illumination. Orientation is both visual and chemical. The maximum distance at which orientation occurs is less than 20 m. Bidlingmayer and Hem[4] found that most adult mosquitoes were attracted to large, unpainted plywood suction traps from 15-19 m. The anthropophilic *Ae vexans* was most responsive; the ornithophilic *Cs melanura* showed an average response for the ten species tested; but *Cx quinquefasciatus* was relatively unresponsive and its visual range was less than 7.5 m.

Gillies and Wilkes[25] found that mosquitoes orientated to a single bait from similar distances. *An melas* and other *Anopheles* species responded from a distance of 13.5-18 m; *Cx tritaeniorhynchus* from 9-18 m, and members of the *Cx decens* group from only 5 m. For those species for which information was available orientation to carbon dioxide was from less than 15 m. Carbon dioxide acts as an attractant to mosquitoes which fly upwind in response. To be fully effective the carbon dioxide must be pulsed or accompanied by other host odours. In still air carbon dioxide activates the mosquitoes but there is no orientation to the source.[24] In its upwind movement a mosquito uses visual clues, but many mosquitoes are active on the darkest nights when visibility would be minimal and Gillett[21] has proposed that mosquitoes orientate themselves upwind by adopting an undulating flight pattern.

Gillies and Wilkes, working in West Africa, found that a significant number of *Mansonia* (*Mansonioides*) spp. reached their host by flying downwind at a low level.[26]

Convection currents given off by a warm body enable mosquitoes to orientate to a host very effectively over short distances,[8] and Brown[5] has shown that in the field *Aedes* mosquitoes were attracted to a warm body when the air temperature was less than 15°C.

Biting Cycle

Blood-feeding follows a circadian rhythm with most species of mosquitoes being nocturnal or crepuscular and a smaller number diurnal. Most species of *Anopheles* are nocturnal and many, including major disease vectors such as *An gambiae*, *An minimus* and *An farauti*, have their peak biting rate in the early hours of the morning after midnight.[51] *Ae africanus* is crepuscular with its biting activity being largely concentrated into a 20-minute period following sunset, but there is no similar period of activity at sunrise.[20] Species of *Aedes* (*Stegomyia*), including the disease vectors *Ae aegypti*, *Ae polynesiensis* and *Ae scutellaris*, are diurnal. *Ae aegypti* has two peaks of activity, one just after dawn 06.00-07.00 h and before sunset 17.00-18.00 h. Similar proportions of nulliparous and parous females were present at both times indicating that the bimodality was a general property of the species and was not due to females of different ages feeding at different times.

Most mosquitoes show gonotrophic concordancy in which there is strict alternation of blood-feeding and oviposition, with each blood meal being followed by the maturation and oviposition of a batch of eggs. Gillies[23] has shown that *An gambiae* and *An funestus* require two blood meals to mature the first batch of eggs but only 2 per cent and 4 per cent, respectively, feed twice in subsequent ovarian cycles. *Ae aegypti* also feeds twice during the maturation of its first batch of eggs,[10] and a proportion of the population may take a second blood meal during later ovarian cycles.[47,64] In the calculations of Conway *et al.*[9] this proportion was variously estimated as 6 per cent and 49 per cent. In *Ae aegypti* most nullipars (58 per cent) were inseminated before the first meal, some (17 per cent) were mated between feeds and 25 per cent were inseminated between the second feed and the first oviposition.[10] In *An gambiae* and *An funestus* 26 per cent and 65 per cent, respectively, were inseminated before the first blood meal and the rest between meals.[23] In *An freeborni* blood feeding during development of the ovaries is inhibited by the hormone ecdysone which is produced by the ovaries during oogenesis.[2]

The biting cycle has practical implications in that mosquito nets are effective against nocturnal species, especially those which feed after midnight, whereas they give little protection against crepuscular species, which require house screening or the use of repellents and protective clothing.

Mosquitoes are not limited in their activity to ground level where man spends his time. In forests, potential hosts are to be found from ground level up to the canopy, the domain of birds and primates. In Zika Forest, a tropical rainforest in Uganda, the ground level is heavily shaded and covered with shrubs and small trees; the canopy lies between 12 m and 18 m; the zone between at 6 m is void of vegetation, being above the shrubs and below the canopy; emergent trees rise above the canopy with the tallest reaching to 36 m. A tower was built to provide catching stations from ground level to 36 m at 6 m intervals. Collections were made on human bait at all levels over the full 24 h period. Haddow and Ssenkubuge[28] gave some of the results obtained. *An implexus* was rarely taken above ground level where 98.7 per cent (387/392) of this species were collected; *Cq aurites* was taken at all levels with a maximum at 36 m; and 66 per cent (7,550/11,410) were taken above the canopy at 24-36 m. *Ae africanus* was also collected at all levels but with a maximum (63 per cent) in the canopy.

Although circadian rhythms are characteristic of species they can be modified by environmental conditions. *Mansonia uniformis* and *Ma africana* showed marked peaks of activity immediately after sunset and before sunrise at the catching stations above the canopy (24-36 m). At 6-18 m the bimodality was less marked with increased activity occurring throughout the night, and at ground level bimodality was lost and a high level of activity occurred from sunset to sunrise. *Ae ingrami* showed even greater changes in rhythm with height. It was not taken above 24 m and at that height it was crepuscular with greatest activity at sunset and none between sunrise and sunset; at ground level activity was almost reversed, being virtually confined to sunrise to sunset and with very little activity after sunset. When the catches of *Ae ingrami* during specified periods of the diel are plotted against height, maximum activity shifts from ground level at 09.00-15.00 h to 18 m between 19.00-06.00 h and back again. It recalls the vertical movement of plankton over the diel but in this case there is no evidence of movement of *Ae ingrami* from one level to another. The same result could be produced by insects at the various levels showing differing biting rhythms. Nevertheless, the important conclusion to be drawn is that circadian rhythms can be modified by local conditions and that, particularly in forests, ground level observations give little indication as to what is occurring at higher levels.

Blood-feeding and Ovarian Development

Blood-feeding takes only a few minutes. When pool feeding the female waits until sufficient blood has collected before it is ingested rapidly and the stomach becomes visibly distended. Some species, e.g. *Ae aegypti*, pass drops of clear fluid from the anus while they are feeding, and others, e.g. *An stephensi*, pass apparently unchanged blood from the anus. *Ae aegypti* ingests 4.2 mm^3 of blood, of which 1.5 mm^3 of clear fluid is passed within 15 minutes of feeding. The larger *Cx quinquefasciatus* ingests 10.2 mm^3 of blood when feeding on a chicken.[8]

In the tropics the gonotrophic cycle of blood ingestion and ovarian development takes about 48 h. Following nocturnal activity four categories of resting females can be recognised in the early morning: those which had fed the previous night and are full of blood; those which had fed the night before and contained some dark blood and developing eggs; fully gravid females, which will oviposit during the succeeding night, and empty females either nulliparous or parous females, which have oviposited but not yet fed again. The feeding and oviposition cycles have a minimum duration of 2-3 days.

In *Ae aegypti* ovarian development is triggered by the midgut being stretched, as happens when a blood meal is ingested. The oocytes immediately begin developing, presumably in response to a nervous impulse, but the second phase of yolk deposition is under hormonal control. Distension of the midgut for a prolonged period stimulates the release of a vittellogenic hormone from the corpora allata, leading to yolk deposition in the developing oocytes.[8,18,20]

In each ovarian cycle only one egg is developed in each ovariole and therefore the number of eggs matured in an egg batch cannot exceed the number of ovarioles. The number of eggs matured will depend upon the species and on the source of the blood meal. *An melanoon* laid up to 500 eggs in its first gonotrophic cycle[8] and *Cx pipiens pipiens* developed an average of 121 eggs on 3.0 mg of human blood and 255 eggs from 3.1 mg of canary blood.[76]

Oviposition

Oviposition follows a circadian rhythm in *Ae aegypti* and probably does so in other mosquitoes. In the laboratory peak oviposition of *Ae aegypti* occurs just before sunset and remains so even when the period of daylight is varied substantially. The factor which controls oviposition is the onset of darkness and not the length of daylight. Oviposition occurs 21-23 h after the onset of darkness the previous day. If the species is reared in continuous light, oviposition becomes arrhythmic and eggs are deposited when they are mature. If arrhythmic *Ae aegypti* are then plunged into continuous darkness oviposition becomes rhythmic and the first egg batches are laid 22 h later and thereafter at approximately 24 h intervals for the next five days, i.e. the cycle is said to be 'free running'. Similarly, adults maintained in continuous darkness become rhythmic after exposure to light, which may be as brief as 5 s and become free running.[20,22]

Selection of Breeding Site

Gravid females seek a suitable site for oviposition. General descriptions of the breeding sites of any particular species can readily be given but exceptions will be encountered. The experienced entomologist will know which breeding sites to examine for a particular species. The criteria used by the entomologist, while effective, are almost certainly quite different from those used by the gravid female in search of an oviposition site, as Muirhead-Thomson[51] elegantly showed for *An minimus* in Assam.

Larvae of *An minimus* are to be found in the grassy margins of lightly shaded, flowing streams. These sites are readily recognisable during the daytime on the criteria of shade, and air and water temperatures in the breeding site and outside, but these differences do not apply when gravid *An minimus* are searching for an oviposition site after midnight on moonless nights. There was no difference in illumination under the light shade of the breeding site and in the open, and differences in air and water temperatures, which had been so marked in the afternoon, were no longer present. *An minimus* only oviposited in these sites and only in these sites in the field could its larvae survive.

Larvae of *An minimus* have a relatively low thermal death point and would be killed, if they were exposed in shallow, sunlit pools, and hence they occur in cooler running water. However, they are weak swimmers and can only maintain their position in running water if there is grass to provide shelter and reduce the current. In heavily shaded sections of hill streams there is inadequate illumination to maintain grass and the banks are bare and larvae of *An minimus* are absent. These requirements restrict the immatures of *An minimus* to lightly-shaded portions of flowing water.

The larval habitat is selected by the ovipositing female, and since conditions in the breeding site are likely to change after oviposition it would be anticipated that the female will select a narrower range of conditions than those which can be tolerated by the larvae. Thus larvae, which are normally found in strongly saline waters, are able in the laboratory to complete their development in tap water, e.g. *An multicolor*, and the larvae of *An sergenti*, which occur in nature in fresh water, actually develop more quickly in the laboratory in water with a salinity equivalent to 0.5-0.75 per cent Nac1.

It seems that there will be some species of mosquito which will breed in virtually every naturally occurring collection of water, with the exception of excessively hot springs and large bodies of water with clean edges. Mosquito larvae cannot withstand wave action, and this was used to eliminate *Anopheles* breeding from the river Jordan, by daily fluctuations in the water level by varying the discharge through the hydroelectric turbines. Daily fluctuations in water level eliminated the marginal vegetation and mosquito breeding. Modification of breeding sites is a powerful weapon in mosquito control but it requires knowledge about all species in the area. For example, malaria was reduced in parts of Malaya by exposing hill streams to sunlight and eliminating the vector, *An umbrosus*. In other areas this technique failed because the sunlit streams provided suitable breeding sites for *An maculatus*, another vector of malaria.[51] In the last situation the attempt at control had merely changed one vector for another with little effect on malaria transmission.

Larvae of *An culicifacies* occur in rice fields when the plants are small, but they disappear as the rice develops into tall plants. The water is still suitable for larval development because larvae introduced into the water among tall rice plants develop normally. Their absence, as the crop matures, is the result of the behaviour of the ovipositing female which drops its eggs while hovering 5-10 cm above the water surface. As plants grow taller the female is forced to hover at higher and higher levels and, when this reaches 40-50 cm, the female does not oviposit.[62,63]

Gravid *Cx tarsalis* are attracted to oviposit in water containing egg rafts of the same species or to water in which egg rafts have been laid previously. The attractant is an ether-soluble pheromone which was not attractive to *Ae aegypti* or *Cx pipiens pipiens*.[55]

Although it is possible to describe the typical breeding site characteristic of a species, there is a good deal of variation from the norm and one is always being surprised at finding species in unusual habitats. Breeding sites can be classified in a number of ways. Mattingly[45] recognises two basic types, running and still water habitats. The latter he subdivided into ground water, subterranean and container habitats. In turn most of these can be further classified as fresh or salt water, and as polluted or unpolluted.

In considering different habitats species will be cited as examples of mosquitoes which breed in such habitats, but each species has a limited geographical distribution. Running water habitats are important sources of *Anopheles* mosquitoes. The grassy edges of sunlit, flowing water breed species such as *An maculatus* and *An fluviatilis*. *An minimus* and *An umbrosus* are found in the grassy edges of shaded streams. Larvae of *An superpictus* hide among pebbles at the edges of shallow, bare, hill streams.

Permanent ground habitats, such as large swamps and vegetated lakes, are the breeding sites of species of *Mansonia, Coquillettidia, An funestus* and *An hyrcanus*. Rice fields are semi-permanent man-made swamps and are suitable for *An pharoensis* and *Cx tritaeniorhynchus*. *An funestus* occurs only where the water is clear and unpolluted but *Mansonia* and *Cx tritaeniorhynchus* thrive in moderately polluted water. *Cs melanura* breeds in oligotrophic waters of swamps and *Ae communis* in pools made by melting snow on the tundra.

In Indonesia *An sundaicus*, a vector of malaria, breeds in permanent salt-water fish ponds. The ponds carry a luxuriant growth of floating green algae, which form the food of the herbivorous fish and the breeding site for *An sundaicus*. The local economy is dependent on its fish culture and removal of the green algae for malaria control is unacceptable. An ingenious solution involved the digging of a deep trench at the edges of the ponds. When the main body of water was drained out of the ponds the fish survived in the water-filled trench but most of the green algal mat was stranded on the pond floor. Exposure to the sun killed the green algae. The ponds were then flooded to a depth adequate to support the growth of blue-green algae at the bottom of the pond. The fish feed on the blue-green algae and there was no floating algae to support *An sundiacus*.[71]

Temporary freshwater ground pools are the main breeding sites of *An gambiae* and *Cx annulirostris*, although both breed in more permanent waters particularly during the dry season. Temporary ground pools of salt water are formed in coastal salt marshes and are a prolific source of anthropophilic *Aedes* mosquitoes in almost all parts of the world. In the

Caribbean and the eastern coast of the USA salt marshes breed *Ae taeniorhynchus* and *Ae sollicitans*; in the Palaearctic region they breed species such as *Ae caspius* and *Ae detritus* and in the Australian region *Ae vigilax*. Species that breed in temporary pools show marked fluctuations in the density of adults. There are periods of the year when the *Aedes* population in a coastal locality may consist only of dormant eggs. Following flooding of the breeding sites there is mass hatching of the eggs and ten days later there is a massive emergence of blood seeking females, which invade adjoining residential areas.

Underground water habitats are mostly artefacts, such as storage tanks and wells. In the Mediterranean area *An claviger* breeds in wells and cisterns, and its counterpart in the Oriental region is *An stephensi*. Both species are anthropophilic and, living in close association with man, they are locally important vectors of malaria. Neither species is restricted to underground water and *An claviger* breeds in cool waters in other habitats and *An stephensi* occurs in irrigation ditches in Basra. *Cx p. pipiens* breeds in storage tanks of clean water and *Cx quinquefasciatus* in highly polluted water, such as that found in soakage pits, flooded latrines and the settling ponds of sewage works. Crab holes are natural underground water habitats and in the Neotropical region breed *Deinocerites cancer*.

Container habitats are prolific sources of mosquitoes. All the Sabethini and Toxorhynchitinae breed in them and many Culicini but few Anophelinae. Adaptations to these specialised habitats involve morphological changes in larva and adult, and modifications of oviposition behaviour. Larval modifications include reduced head setae, enlarged maxillary spines and numerous large stellate hairs on the thorax and abdomen. *Armigeres dolichocephalus* has a long narrow thorax, which enables the adult female to enter small holes in bamboo for oviposition.[20] Ovipositing *Sabethes chloropterus* hover in front of vertical holes in bamboo and flick eggs through the hole, one at a time.[14]

Container habitats include tree holes, a source of *An plumbeus, Ae aegypti formosus* and *Ae africanus*; collections of water in bamboo internodes breed *Sa chloropterus*; leaf axils are a source of *Ae simpsoni*; pitchers of plants breed species of *Tripteroides* (*Rachisoura*); epiphytic bromeliads are a source of *Anopheles* (*Kerteszia*), including *An bellator*; fruits and husks breed *Ae albopictus* and *Eretmapodites* species; artificial containers, such as vases, water jars, tyres, etc., breed *Ae aegypti*; and snail shells, *Eretmapodites*.

Dispersal

In the laboratory in still air adult *Ae aegypti* are randomly orientated and have an average ground speed of 17 cm/s. In moving air the substrate appears to move forwards and the mosquito responds by facing into the wind and increasing its flight speed, so that in a wind of 33 cm/s *Ae aegypti* still maintained a ground air speed of 16 cm/s indicating that its average air speed was 49 cm/s. *Ae aegypti* is able to maintain forward movement, but at a steadily reducing rate up to wind speeds of 150 cm/s (= 5.45 km/h).[8] Above this limit mosquitoes either settle or are carried downwind.

In the field species vary greatly in the extent to which they disperse widely from their breeding sites. This can be an important factor in mosquito control because it indicates the distance larval control measures need to be extended in order to protect a community. Assuming, unrealistically, that breeding sites are uniformly distributed, then doubling the distance over which larval control must be carried out, quadruples the area to be treated and the cost.

The flight range of a species can be considered in terms of probability. It is not a limit beyond which a species will not fly but an indication of the distance beyond which the species will be present only in insignificant numbers. Such an estimate is obviously subjective and it would be preferable to give the probability of an individual dispersing more than a fixed distance from the breeding site. This approach emphasises the fact that the greater the population emerging from the site, the larger the number of mosquitoes that will reach a fixed distance, and the greater the maximum distance reached by some members of the population. Dispersal is influenced by the prevailing wind, by longevity of the species and by the presence of suitable hosts.

Mattingly[45] comments that forest mosquitoes appear to have a more restricted flight range than those that breed in open situations. Where suitable domestic breeding sites are available *Ae aegypti* is unlikely to disperse in significant numbers more than 0.5 km. Sheppard *et al.*[64] estimated that the average distance covered by *Ae aegypti* in 24 h was 37 m but Conway *et al.*,[9] working in a different continent, considered that this might be an overestimate and that their 1 ha site might have contained several, relatively distinct, small populations of *Ae aegypti*.

In the tropics larval control against *Anopheles* mosquitoes is usually effective if extended for 3 km. Many species occur abundantly 1 km from their breeding site but rarely reach 5 km, e.g. only 20 per cent of a population of *An funestus* was considered to disperse further than 0.8 km from the breeding site with a practical limit of dispersal of 7 km[36]; and few female *An gambiae* s.s. dispersed further than 3 km with the average being 1.0 to 1.6 km.[74]

An pharoensis is a large mosquito which breeds abundantly in the Delta of Egypt and regularly disperses 6 km from its breeding site and, on occasions, disperses with the wind for distances of 100 km. In 1942 in the Western desert, when the opposing armies were lined up at El Alamein, remote from any water, there were two occasions when troops of both armies were attacked by large numbers of *An pharoensis* which, it is considered, had flown on a south-easterly wind, an unusual direction, from Wadi el Natrun and the Nile Delta.[15] Garrett-Jones[16] presents evidence for this species dispersing 280 km with the prevailing wind.

Salt marsh mosquitoes seem to be particularly addicted to long-distance dispersal flights. The New World species *Ae taeniorhynchus* and *Ae sollicitans* emerge in vast numbers after their breeding sites have been inundated and disperse tens of kilometres. Hocking[35] studied the intrinsic range of flight of four species of *Aedes* and found that three of them were capable of flying nearly 50 km in still air after one feed of nectar and the other species exceeded 20 km. This represents a potential for flight and other aspects of behaviour will decide whether this maximum is ever realised.

Female *Aedes taeniorhynchus* begin to migrate when they are 6-14 h old and their ovaries are immature.[30] They may continue to disperse during the period of normal activity for four consecutive days,[56] carrying large numbers of mosquitoes into urban areas to the dismay of the inhabitants. Female *Ae taeniorhynchus* have been recovered up to 40 km from their site of origin.[57] At low wind velocities (0.25 m/s) they disperse upwind and at high velocities (1.5-2.0 m/s) downwind.[30] In eastern Australia *Ae vigilax* behaves in a comparable manner. In the Middle East *An sacharovi* has a prehibernation flight from Lake Huleh to Rosh Pinah, 14 km away,[40] and during this flight it feeds and lays down fat body for hibernation, requiring three or four blood meals to develop the fat body to its maximum.[50]

In *Ae taeniorhynchus* mating occurs either at the breeding site or in the early stages of migration, because males rarely disperse more than 5 km. This illustrates a general feature of mosquito biology that males do not disperse as far as females. Indeed, if males are found, it is an indication that the breeding site is close at hand, often within 200 m.

Hibernation, Aestivation and Seasonal Cycles

In tropical regions breeding of most species continues throughout the year and seasonal fluctuations in numbers are related to the rainy and dry seasons. In the severe dry season breeding either continues in relation to reduced bodies of permanent water or the population survives this hostile period as dormant eggs or aestivating adults. Aestivation is either a rare phenomenon or has been poorly studied. In the valley of the White Nile in Sudan, *An arabiensis* (*An gambiae* auct.) maintains itself through the dry season by low-level breeding, but in the more arid areas, 20 km from the Nile valley, there is evidence that the females aestivate.[54,74] There is much more information available on the effect of low temperature on mosquito biology. In the subtropics and adjoining areas of the warmer temperate regions the main response to lower temperature in the cool season is to slow down the rate of biological processes. Ovarian development may take 10-14 days, compared with 2-3 days under optimum conditions and development from egg to adult takes 2-3 months. This response is shown by *An pharoensis* in Egypt and by *Cx tritaeniorhynchus* in parts of its range. Further north the latter species enters hibernation. There is gonotrophic dissociation and females develop fat-body after a blood meal. They then seek a cool shelter to pass the approaching winter. Hibernation is induced in a developing generation by exposure to decreasing hours of daylight, reinforced by lower temperatures. Hibernation of inseminated females is probably the commonest way of surviving winter in species which do not produce dormant eggs. Other species pass the winter as larvae in waters that are protected from freezing, e.g. *An claviger* in wells, *Cs melanura* in bogs and *Ae triseriatus* in tree holes.

In the humid tropics breeding may be continuous throughout the year with little variation in the size of the adult populations. In Bangkok Sheppard *et al.*[64] found that differences in the monthly population of *Ae aegypti* were non-significant until movement was taken into account, when the differences were significant but only at the 5 per cent level. It was not possible to attribute these fluctuations to either rainfall or temperature. Females survived better than males with a daily survival of 81-84 per cent compared with 70-72 per cent for the males. In the subtropics with hot dry summers mosquito populations are commonly bimodal with peaks in the spring and autumn and lower populations during the summer. Mer[50] found that there was some decline in fecundity of *An sacharovi* in the late spring. In addition lower survival during the hot dry summer months would lead to fewer egg batches being laid and lower populations. In more temperate regions one or two generations may occur during the warmer months of each year.

References

1. Bates, M. (1949). *The Natural History of Mosquitoes.* Macmillan, New York
2. Beach, R. (1979). Mosquitoes: biting behavior inhibited by ecdysone. *Science 205*: 829-31
3. Belkin, J.N. and Hogue, C.L. (1959). A review of the crabhole mosquitoes of the genus *Deinocerites* (Diptera, Culicidae). *University of California Publications in Entomology 14*: 411-58
4. Bidlingmayer, W.L. and Hem, D.G. (1980). The range of visual attraction and the effect of competitive visual attractants upon mosquito (Diptera: Culicidae) flight. *Bulletin of Entomological Research 70*: 321-42
5. Brown, A.W.A. (1951). Studies of the responses of the female *Aedes* mosquito. Part IV. *Bulletin of Entomological Research 42*: 575-82
6. Charlwood, J.D. and Jones, M.D.R. (1979). Mating behaviour in the mosquito

Anopheles gambiae s.1. I. Close range and contact behaviour. *Physiological Entomology 4*: 111-20

7. _____ and Jones, M.D.R. (1980). Mating in the mosquito, *Anopheles gambiae* s.1. II. Swarming behaviour. *Physiological Entomology 5*: 315-20

8. Clements, A.N. (1963). *The Physiology of Mosquitoes.* Pergamon Press, Oxford

9. Conway, G.R., Trpis, M. and McClelland, G.A.H. (1974). Population parameters of the mosquito *Aedes aegypti* (L.) estimated by mark-release-recapture in a suburban habitat in Tanzania. *Journal of Animal Ecology 43*: 289-304

10. Corbet, P.S. and Smith, S.M. (1974). Diel periodicities of landing of nulliparous and parous *Aedes aegypti* (L.) at Dar es Salaam, Tanzania (Diptera, Culicidae). *Bulletin of Entomological Research 64*: 111-21

11. Downes, J.A. (1969). The swarming and mating flight of Diptera. *Annual Review of Entomology 14*: 271-98

12. Engber, B., Stone, P.F. and Pillai, J.S. (1978). The occurrence of *Toxorhynchites amboinensis* in Western Samoa. *Mosquito News 38*: 295-6

13. Farquharson, C.O. (1918). *Harpagomyia* and other Diptera fed by *Cremastogaster* ants in sourthern Nigeria. *Proceedings of the Entomological Society of London* 29-39

14. Galindo, P. (1958). Bionomics of *Sabethes chloropterus* Humboldt, a vector of sylvan yellow fever in middle America. *American Journal of Tropical Medicine and Hygiene 7*: 429-40

15. Garrett-Jones, C. (1950). A dispersion of mosquitoes by wind. *Nature, London 165*: 285

16. _____ (1962). The possibility of active long-distance migrations by *Anopheles pharoensis* Theobald. *Bulletin of the World Health Organization 27*: 299-302

17. _____ Boreham, P.F.L. and Pant, C.P. (1980). Feeding habits of anophelines (Diptera: Culicidae) in 1971-78, with reference to the human blood index: a review. *Bulletin of Entomological Research 70*: 165-85

18. Gillett, J.D. (1956). Initiation and promotion of ovarian development in the mosquito *Aedes* (*Stegomyia*) *aegypti* (Linnaeus). *Annals of Tropical Medicine and Parasitology 50*: 375-80

19. _____ (1961). Laboratory observations on the life-history and ethology of *Mansonia* mosquitos. *Bulletin of Entomological Research 52*: 23-30

20. _____ (1971). *Mosquitos.* Weidenfeld and Nicolson, London

21. _____ (1979). Out for blood; flight orientation up-wind in the absence of visual clues. *Mosquito News 39*: 222-9

22. _____ Corbet, P.S. and Haddow, A.J. (1961). Observations on the oviposition cycle of *Aedes* (*Stegomyia*) *aegypti* (Linnaeus). VI. *Annals of Tropical Medicine and Parasitology 55*: 427-31

23. Gillies, M.T. (1955). The pre-gravid phase of ovarian development in *Anopheles funestus. Annals of Tropical Medicine and Parasitology 49*: 320-5

24. _____ (1980). The role of carbon dioxide in host-finding by mosquitoes (Diptera: Culicidae): a review. *Bulletin of Entomological Research 70*: 525-32

25. _____ and Wilkes, T.J. (1970). The range of attraction of single baits for some West African mosquitoes. *Bulletin of Entomological Research 60*: 225-35

26. _____ and Wilkes T.J. (1974). Evidence for downwind flight by host seeking mosquitoes. *Nature, London 252*: 388-9

27. Haddow, A.J. (1946). The mosquitoes of Bwamba County, Uganda. IV. Studies on the genus *Eretmapodites* Theobald. *Bulletin of Entomological Research 37*: 57-82

28. _____ and Ssenkubuge, Y. (1965). Entomological studies from a high steel tower in Zika Forest, Uganda. Part I. The biting activity of mosquitoes and tabanids as shown by twenty-four-hour catches. *Transactions of the Royal Entomological Society of London 117*: 215-43

29. Haeger, J.S. (1955). The non-blood feeding habits of *Aedes taeniorhynchus* (Diptera, Culicidae) on Sanibel Island, Florida. *Mosquito News 15*: 21-6

30. _____ (1960). Behavior preceding migration in the salt-marsh mosquito, *Aedes taeniorhynchus* (Wiedemann). *Mosquito News 20*: 136-47

31. _____ and Phinizee, J. (1959). The biology of the crab hole mosquito *Deinocerites cancer* Theobald. *Report of the Florida Antimosquito Association 30*; 34-7

32. Hinton, H.E. (1968). Observations on the biology and taxonomy of the eggs of *Anopheles* mosquitoes. *Bulletin of Entomological Research* 57:495-508
33. _____ (1981). *Biology of Insect Eggs. 1*: 43-7 Pergamon Press, Oxford
34. Ho Ch'i, Chou Tsu-chieh, Ch'en Teng'hung and Hsüch Ai-tseng (1962). The *Anopheles hyrcanus* group and its relation to malaria in east China. *Chinese Medical Journal 81*: 71-8
35. Hocking, B. (1953). The intrinsic range and speed of flight in insects. *Transactions of the Royal Entomological Society of London 104*: 223-345
36. Horsfall, W.R. (1955). *Mosquitoes: their Bionomics and Relation to Disease*. Constable, London
37. Keilin, D., Tate, P. and Vincent, M. (1935). The perispiracular glands of mosquito larvae. *Parasitology 27*: 257-62
38. Kettle, D.S. (1948). The growth of *Anopheles sergenti* Theobald (Diptera, Culicidae) with special reference to the growth of the anal papillae in varying salinities. *Annals of Tropical Medicine and Parasitology 42*: 5-29
39. Kirk, H.B. (1923). Notes on the mating-habits and early life-history of the culicid *Opifex fuscus* Hutton. *Transactions and Proceedings of the New Zealand Institute 54*: 400-6
40. Kligler, J. and Mer, G. (1930). Studies on malaria: VI. long-range dispersion of *Anopheles* during the prehibernating period. *Rivista di Malariologia 9*: 363-74
41. Knight, K.L. (1978). Supplement to a catalog of the mosquitoes of the world. *Thomas Say Foundation Supplement* to vol. 6: 1-107
42. _____ and Stone, A. (1977). A catalog of the mosquitoes of the world (Diptera: Culicidae). *Thomas Say Foundation 6*: 1-611
43. Laurence, B.R. (1960). The biology of two species of mosquito, *Mansonia africana* (Theobald) and *Mansonia uniformis* (Theobald) belonging to the subgenus *Mansonioides* (Diptera, Culicidae). *Bulletin of Entomological Research 51*: 491-517
44. Marks, E.N. (1958). Notes on *Opifex fuscus* Hutton (Diptera: Culicidae) and the scope for further research on it. *New Zealand Entomologist 2*: 20-5
45. Mattingly, P.F. (1969). *The Biology of Mosquito-Borne Disease*. Allen and Unwin, London
46. _____ (1973). Culicidae (Mosquitoes). pp. 37-107 in *Insects and Other Arthropods of Medical Importance*, K.G.V. Smith (ed), British Museum (Natural History), London
47. McClelland, G.A.H. and Conway, G.R. (1971). Frequency of blood feeding in the mosquito *Aedes aegypti*. *Nature, London 232*: 485-6
48. McMullen, A.I. and Hill, M.N. (1971). Anoxia in mosquito pupae under insoluble monolayers. *Nature, London 234*: 51-2
49. _____ Reiter, P. and Phillips, M.C. (1977). Mode of action of insoluble monolayers on mosquito pupal respiration. *Nature, London 267*: 244-5
50. Mer, G. (1931). Notes on the bionomics of *Anopheles elutus*, Edw. (Diptera, Culicidae). *Bulletin of Entomological Research 22*: 137-45
51. Muirhead-Thomson, R.C. (1951). *Mosquito Behaviour in Relation to Malaria Transmission and Control in the Tropics*. Edward Arnold, London
52. Nijhout, H.F. and Craig, G.B. (1971). Reproductive isolation in *Stegomyia* mosquitoes III. Evidence for a sexual pheromone. *Entomologia Experimentalis et Applicata 14*: 399-412
53. Nowell, W.R. (1951). The dipterous family Dixidae in western North America (Insecta: Diptera). *Microentomology 16*: 187-270
54. Omer, S.M. and Cloudsley-Thompson, J.L. (1970). Survival of female *Anopheles gambiae* Giles through a 9-month dry season in Sudan. *Bulletin of the World Health Organization 42*: 319-30
55. Osgood, C.E. (1971). An oviposition pheromone associated with the egg rafts of *Culex tarsalis*. *Journal of Economic Entomology 64*: 1038-41
56. Provost, M.W. (1952). The dispersal of *Aedes taeniorhynchus*. I. Preliminary studies. *Mosquito News 12*: 174-90
57. _____ (1957). The dispersal of *Aedes taeniorhynchus*. II. The second experiment. *Mosquito News 17*: 233-47
58. Puri, I.M. (1931). Larvae of anopheline mosquitoes, with full descriptions of those of

the Indian species. *Indian Medical Research Memoirs 21*: 1-225

59. Reinert, J.F. (1975). Mosquito generic and subgeneric abbreviations (Diptera: Culicidae). *Mosquito Systematics 7*: 105-10

60. Rivière, F., Pichon, G., Duval, J., Thirel, R. and Toudic, A. (1979). Introduction de *Toxorhynchites (Toxorhynchites) amboinesis* (Doleschall, 1857)(Diptera, Culicidae) en Polynésie Française. *Cahiers ORSTOM Entomologie médicale et Parasitologie 17*: 225-34

61. Rodaniche, E. de, Galindo, P. and Johnson, C.M. (1959). Further studies on the experimental transmission of yellow fever by *Sabethes chloropterus. American Journal of Tropical Medicine and Hygiene 8*: 190-4

62. Russell, P.F. and Rao, T.R. (1942). On the swarming, mating and oviposition behaviour of *Anopheles culicifacies. American Journal of Tropical Medicine 22*: 417-27

63. _____ and Rao, T.R. (1942). On relation of mechanical obstruction and shade to ovipositing of *Anopheles culicifacies. Journal of Experimental Zoology 91*: 303-29

64. Sheppard, P.M., Macdonald, W.W., Tonn, R.J. and Grab, B. (1969). The dynamics of · an adult population of *Aedes aegypti* in relation to dengue haemorrhagic fever in Bangkok. *Journal of Animal Ecology 38*: 661-702

65. Soper, F.L. and Wilson, D.B. (1943). *Anopheles gambiae in Brazil 1930 to 1940.* The Rockefeller Foundation, New York

66. Steffan, W.A. and Evenhuis, N.L. (1981). Biology of *Toxorhynchites. Annual Review of Entomology 26*: 159-81

67. Tempelis, C.H. (1975). Host feeding patterns of mosquitoes, with a review of advances in analysis of blood meals by serology. *Journal of Medical Entomology 11*: 635-53

68. Thorpe, W.H. (1930). The biology of the petroleum fly (*Psilopa petrolei* Coq.). *Transactions of the Entomological Society of London 78*: 331-43

69. Reference deleted.

70. Walch, E.W. and Schuurman, C.J. (1929). Saltwater fishponds and malaria. *Mededelingen van den Dienst der volksgezondheid in Nederlandsch-Indie 18*: 341-66

71. Wharton, R.H. (1953). The habits of adult mosquitoes in Malaya. IV. Swarming of anophelines in nature. *Annals of Tropical Medicine and Parasitology 47*: 285-90

72. _____ (1962). The biology of *Mansonia* mosquitoes in relation to the transmission of filariasis in Malaya. *Institute for Medical Research, Federation of Malaya, Bulletin 11*: 1-114

73. White, G.B. (1974). *Anopheles gambiae* complex and disease transmission in Africa. *Transactions of the Royal Society of Tropical Medicine and Hygiene 68*: 278-98

74. Wishart, G. and Riordan, D.F. (1959). Flight responses to various sounds by adult males of *Aedes aegypti* (L.) (Diptera: Culicidae). *Canadian Entomologist 91*: 181-91

75. Woke, P.A. (1937). Comparative effects of the blood of man and of canary on egg-production of *Culex pipiens* Linn. *Journal of Parasitology 23*: 311-13

8 CERATOPOGONIDAE (BITING MIDGES)

Ceratopogonids are popularly referred to as biting midges in Scotland and sandflies in the Caribbean and Australia. They are distinguished from the closely-related, dancing midges or Chironomidae by the following characters. Ceratopogonids are generally smaller with blood-sucking species rarely having a wing length greater than 2 mm (many tropical species have wing lengths less than 1 mm); at rest they fold their wings scissor-like over the abdomen (Figure 8.1); and their swarms are small and inconspicuous. Chironomids are larger; at rest they hold their wings roof-like over the abdomen; and often form large obvious swarms near water. Morphologically ceratopogonids have a forked media vein (M_1, M_2) (Figure 8.2); piercing mouthparts; front pair of legs not lengthened; and postnotum gently rounded and without longitudinal groove. Chironomids have an unbranched media; reduced mouthparts; front pair of legs lengthened; and postnotum more prominent and usually with a median longitudinal groove.[19]

The Ceratopogonidae is a large family, which includes more than 60 genera and nearly 4,000 species.[64] The females are mostly predatory on other insects; ectoparasitic on insects or blood-sucking on vertebrates. Both males and females feed on nectar, and females of several species of *Forcipomyia* are pollinators of the cocoa tree (*Theobroma cocao*).[63] Most females require a protein meal for maturation of the ovaries and female *Atrichopogon* obtain theirs by feeding on pollen. In only four genera is the protein meal obtained by feeding on warm-blooded animals and therefore relevant to medical entomology. The largest of these is the genus *Culicoides*, of which nearly 1,000 species have been described, and the smallest genus is *Austroconops* with only one species. About 80 species are included in the genus *Leptoconops*, of which several subgenera are recognised and reference will be made to *Holoconops*, *Styloconops* and *Leptoconops*. In the genus *Forcipomyia* blood-sucking is restricted to the subgenus *Lasiohelea* which is represented by about 50 species.

The Ceratopogonidae is divided into four subfamilies: Leptoconopinae, Forcipomyiinae, Dasyheleinae and Ceratopogoninae. The Leptoconopinae includes only one genus, *Leptoconops*, which is distinguished by possession of milky-white wings, which contrast sharply with the black head and thorax; there are no macrotrichia (obvious hairs) on the wings; no r-m cross-vein (Figure 8.3); and in the female the antenna has 12-14 segments. In other ceratopogonids the r-m cross-vein is present and the antennae are composed of 15 segments. The Forcipomyiinae contains the subgenus *Forcipomyia* (*Lasiohelea*) which has densely hairy wings, a well-

137

developed empodium on the last tarsal segment, and a long second radial cell (Figure 8.3). No member of the Dasyheleinae is of medical or veterinary importance. They have hairy wings, short second radial cell, vestigial empodium, and sculptured antennal segments. There is considerable variation within the Ceratopogoninae but they have vestigal empodia and

Figure 8.1: Female *Culicoides* at Rest With Wings Folded Scissor-like (above) and With Wings Spread Laterally (below) (×50)

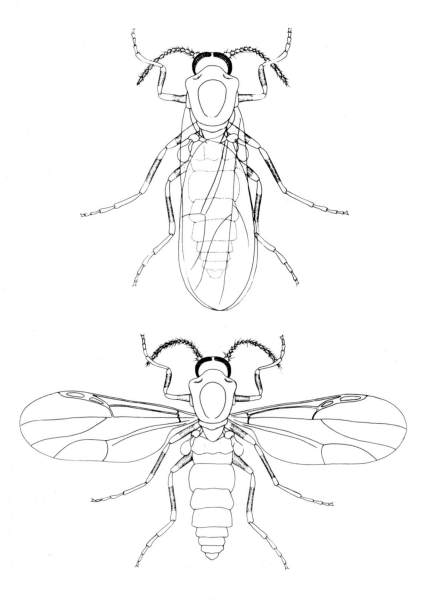

Figure 8.2: Wing of Female *Culicoides marmoratus* ($\times$ 85)

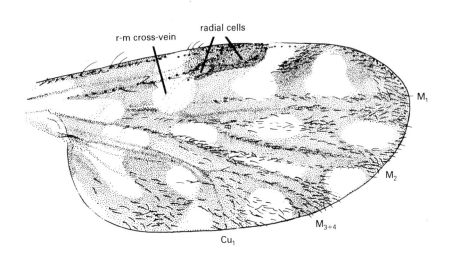

their antennal segments are not sculptured. This subfamily contains the important genus *Culicoides* and also *Austroconops*.

Most species of *Culicoides* have dark and light patterned wings (Figure 8.2). The pattern is due to pigmentation in the wing membrane and therefore it cannot be rubbed off, as can the coloured scales, which form the wing pattern in the Culicidae. However, the pigment fades in specimens stored in alcohol and exposed to light. *Culicoides* have a petiolate media, i.e. vein M forks distally of the r-m cross-vein; the costa extends more than half way and less than two thirds along the front margin of the wing; the radius forms two, small, more-or-less equal cells (the radial cells), one or both of which may be obliterated; distinct humeral pits are located antero-laterally on the scutum; and the claws of both sexes are small, equal and simple (Figure 8.4).

The genus *Culicoides* is widely distributed in the world from the tropics to the tundra, and from sea level to 4,200 m in Tibet, where members of the first Everest expedition of 1921 complained of being bitten persistently.[25] *Austroconops* has only been recorded from near Perth in Western Australia. *Lasiohelea* is associated with tropical and subtropical rainforests, although *F. (L.) sibirica* is a pest at Krasnoyarsk in Siberia.[23] *Leptoconops* species are largely restricted to the warmer areas of the world with the subgenera *Holoconops* and *Styloconops* being associated with sandy coasts, e.g. *L. (H.) becquaerti* in the Caribbean,[49] *L. (S.) spinosifrons* in the Indian Ocean,[16,43] while the subgenus *Leptoconops* is more prevalent in inland locations, e.g. *L. (L.) torrens* in Utah, USA.[59]

Figure 8.3: Above, Wing of Female *Leptoconops (Styloconops) australiensis,* (× 70); Below, Wing of Female *Forcipomyia (Lasiohelea) townsvillensis* (× 115)

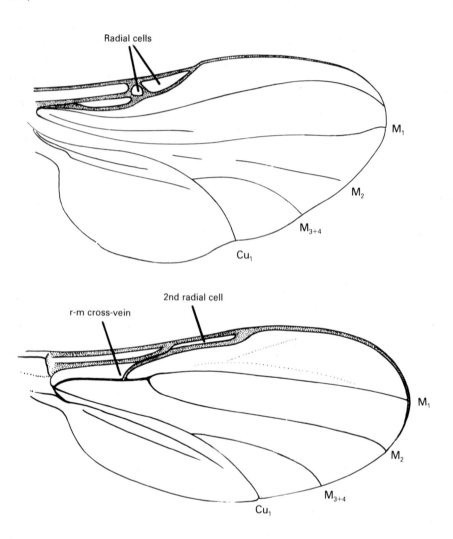

Life Cycle

The life cycle of *Culicoides* will be considered first and then differences shown by *Leptoconops* and *Lasiohelea* will be indicated. Eggs of *Culicoides* are laid in batches, which vary from 30-40 in *C. brevitarsis*[7] and up to 450 with a mean of 250 in *C. circumscriptus.*[3] The eggs are small, dark in colour, and slender, measuring between 350-500 μm in length and

65-80 µm in breadth.[24] They are covered with small projections (ansulae), which are particularly evident on the concave side and probably function as a plastron by retaining a film of air in contact with the egg, facilitating diffusion of oxygen for respiration when the egg is covered by water. In most species the eggs hatch in a few days at favourable temperatures, but those of the northern species, *C. grisescens*, do not hatch for 7-8 months in the laboratory and this species probably overwinters in the egg stage.[56] Another Palaearctic species, *C. vexans*, breeds in temporary, open pools and has a single generation in the spring. Its eggs lie dormant over the summer and hatch in the autumn, when the breeding site is unlikely to dry up.[28] This behaviour is comparable to that of *Aedes* eggs (p. 113).

The larva, which emerges from the egg, is a typical nematoceran larva, with a well sclerotised head, 11 body segments, and no appendages (Figure 8.5). The three thoracic segments are similar to the eight abdominal segments, being not fused together and no broader than the abdominal seg-

Figure 8.4: Lateral View of Female *Culicoides brevitarsis* (×50)

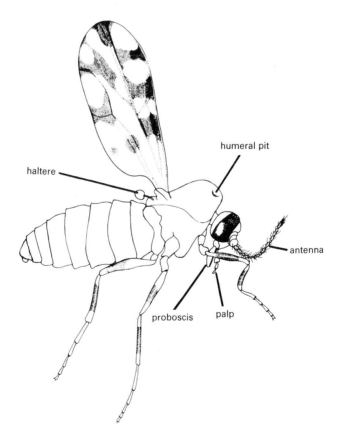

Figure 8.5: Left, Larva of *Culicoides impunctatus* (length 5.0 mm); Right, Lateral and Dorsal Views of Pupa of *Culicoides nubeculosus*. ant. d, ant. m., d.m. and dors. indicate various setae on pupa; halt., haltere

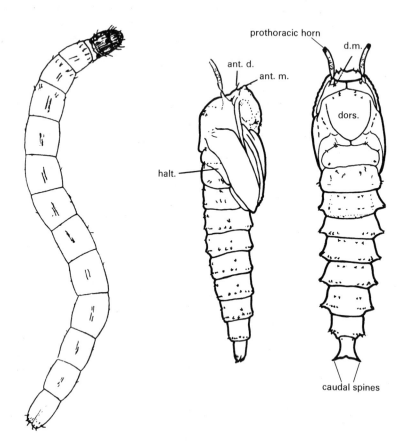

Sources: Larva from Hill,[24] and pupa from Lawson[44]

ments. In late fourth instar larvae the abdomen becomes full of opaque white fat body, which is absent from the thorax, where the imaginal wing and limb buds are developing.

The larva swims by an oscillatory motion, involving flexure about anterior and posterior nodes in the region of the metathorax and seventh abdominal segment.[44] In water, progress appeared not to be commensurate with the energy expended, but this motion is more effective in the wet, semi-solid media in which most species of *Culicoides* occur. There are paired tracheae but the spiracles are closed, and respiration is cutaneous. Two pairs of narrow, bifid anal papillae can be extruded from the anus or retracted into the rectum (Figure 8.6C).

Presumably, as in the Culicidae, the papillae are concerned with the absorption of salts from the surrounding medium. Unlike culicid larvae with their highly developed chaetotaxy, *Culicoides* larvae have only scanty, inconspicuous, unbranched setae. A few species, notably those that breed in tree holes, e.g. the Australian *C. angularis*[34] and the Neotropical *C. hoffmani*[51] have four pairs of long perianal setae (Figure 8.6A). Tree hole species probably spend more time free in water than do the larvae of other species and the long perianal setae may serve to amplify the body oscillations and increase the larva's speed of movement in water, enabling it to catch prey or to avoid predators.

Figure 8.6: Terminations of Anal Segments. A, *Culicoides angularis*; B, *Culicoides marmoratus*; C, extruded bifid anal papillae of *C. nubeculosus*

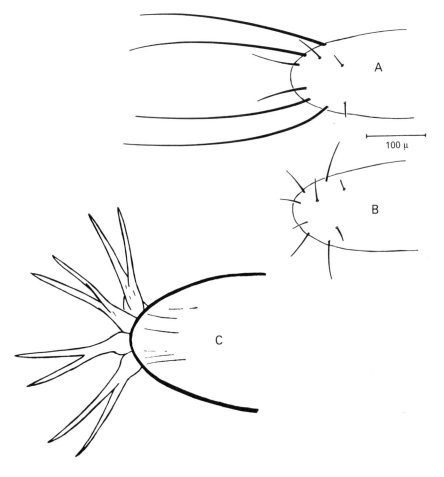

100 μ

A

B

C

Sources: A and B from Kettle and Elson,[34] C from Lawson[44]

The most prominent, internal structures in the head are the epi-pharynges, of which two main forms, heavy or light, occur (Figures 8.7, 8.8). In heavy epipharynges the lateral arms, body and combs are strongly sclerotised. Together with the hypopharynx, they act as a crushing structure, functioning like a pestle and mortar moving in one plane. Heavy epipharynges have, so far, only been reported in a small number of species belonging to the subgenus *Monoculicoides,* including the Palaearctic *C. nubeculosus,*[44] the closely-related Nearctic *C. variipennis,*[27] and the Afro-tropical *C. cornutus.*[40] Larvae of these species occur in muddy substrates and Megahed[53] has described how larvae of *C. nubeculosus* browse upon the surface bacterial film, and on algal and fungal growth. *C. variipennis* has been mass colonised for many years with the larvae being fed on micro-organisms.[29]

In light epipharynges the arms and medium body are only moderately sclerotised, and the combs, of which there are usually two to four, are finely and delicately toothed (Figure 8.8). In spite of the fact that the mandibles are not opposable, larvae with light pharynges are predators. Several species, e.g. *C. austropalpalis,*[39] have been reared from egg to adult on free-living nematodes; and several other species, e.g. *C. furens,*[45] feed

Figure 8.7: Hypopharynx (hypo.); Mandible (mnd.); and 'Heavy' Epipha-rynges (epi.) of Larva of *Culicoides nubeculosus.* l. a. epi. = lateral arms of epipharynx

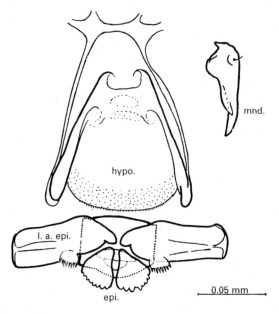

Figure 8.8: 'Light' Epipharynges of Some Australian *Culicoides* Larvae. A, *C. brevitarsis*; B, *C. subimmaculatus*; C, *C. marmoratus*

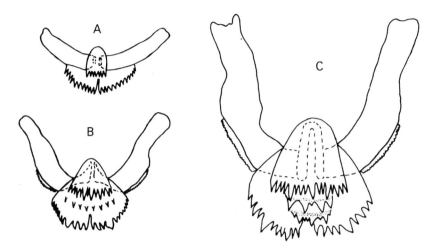

Source: from Kettle and Elson[34]

readily on nematodes in the laboratory. In the field *Culicoides* larvae probably feed on a range of organisms, which they encounter during their movement through the surface layers of the substrate.

There are four larval instars, and the fourth ecdysis gives rise to the pupa, which is culicid in appearance (Figure 8.5). The head and thorax are fused and bear a pair of moderately long, tubular prothoracic horns for respiration. These open to the atmosphere through a number of terminal and a smaller number of lateral openings, i.e. the pupa is propneustic with open spiracles. The segmented abdomen ends in a pair of caudal spines by which the pupa moves over the substrate. The pupa is a short-lived, non-feeding stage which gives rise to the winged adult. Before emergence the pupa, which is usually buried in the substrate with only the prothoracic horns reaching the surface, moves upwards to facilitate eclosion.

The development of *Culicoides* is generally much slower than in the Culicidae under comparable conditions. The egg stage and pupa are, with few exceptions, of short duration, and there is no record of hibernation or aestivation in adult *Culicoides*. The greater part of the life of an individual *Culicoides* is spent in the larval stage. This may be as short as two to three weeks in dung breeding *C. brevitarsis*,[8] two to three months in the sub-tropical, salt marsh *C. subimmaculatus*,[20] nearly a year in the temperate region, bogland species, *C. impunctatus*, and nearly two years in some arctic species.[14] In temperate regions species are commonly univoltine with one generation a year, and even in the tropics there may be only three or four generations in a year.

Other Ceratopogonid Larvae

Two forms of larvae occur in the Ceratopogonidae, the vermiform, apodous, prognathous larva described above for *Culicoides* and the crawling larva of the Forcipomyiinae. The latter has anterior and posterior pseudopods or prolegs (Figure 8.9), comparable to those found in larvae of the Chironomidae; hypognathous head with its long axis at right angles to that of the body and the mouth directed ventrally; and prominent pectinate setae on the head and body.[58] Larvae of *Lasiohelea* occur in drier habitats than the vermiform larvae of other ceratopogonids, and Saunders[58] has found them associated with mosses. In the Dasyheleinae the anterior pseudopod has been lost and the posterior pseudopod has been reduced to a circlet of hooks, which can be extruded from and withdrawn into the rectum. Remnants of an anterior pseudopod are found in first instar larvae of some, but not all, *Culicoides*, e.g. *C. nubeculosus*,[44] *C. vexans*,[28] and vestiges of a posterior proleg have recently been found in first instar larvae of *C. cordiger*.

In *Leptoconops* the larval head (Figure 8.11) has only localised sclerotised thickenings and there is a system of internal, sclerotised rods which extend into the prothorax.[59] This may be an adaptation to life in a sandy habitat because sclerotisation of the head capsule is much reduced in the

Figure 8.9: Larva of *Forcipomyia (Lasiohelea) cornuta*. A, lateral view; B, head; C, posterior pseudopod; D, prothoracic pseudopod

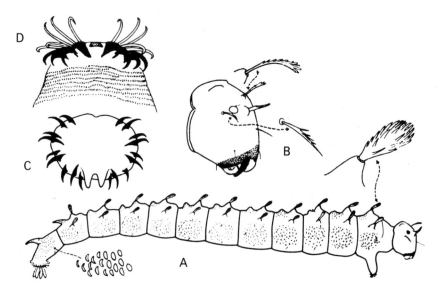

Source: from Saunders[58]

sand-dwelling larvae of the Nearctic *C. melleus,* and the Australian *C. molestus* and *C. subimmaculatus.*[34] Larvae of *Leptoconops* appear to have more than the expected number of body segments due to the inclusion of intercalary segments, giving the appearance of 21 or 23 body segments.[59] The pupae of *Lasiohelea* (Figure 8.10) and *Leptoconops* (Figure 8.11) are very similar to that of *Culicoides* (Figure 8.5), but with a marked tendency for their prothoracic horns to be shorter.

Figure 8.10: Right, Dorsal View of Pupa of *Forcipomyia (Lasiohelea) cornuta*; Left, Two Variations on Its Prothoracic Horn

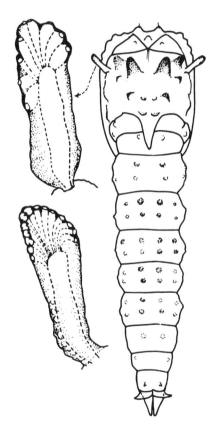

Source: from Saunders[58]

Bionomics

Atchley *et al.*[1] have compiled a useful bibliography on biting midges up to 1978. The bionomics of the blood-sucking genera have been reviewed by

Kettle[33] and form the basis for the account given here. In their bionomics blood-sucking midges have many features in common with mosquitoes. The males commonly emerge before the females but there is no permanent rotation of the terminalia, although during mating they are inverted through 180°.[15] Male *C. melleus* are competent to mate within minutes of emergence and male potency reaches a peak 4-8 h after emergence.[47] Some species mate without swarming, e.g. *C. melleus*,[47] but probably in most

Figure 8.11: Left, Lateral View of Larva of *Leptoconops spinosifrons*; Centre, Lateral View of Larval Head; Right, Lateral View of Pupa of *L. spinosifrons*. A, antenna; C_1, C_2, epipharynges; D, S sclerites; E, eye; Ls, labial sclerite; Mx, maxilla; P, pigment; V, ventral rod

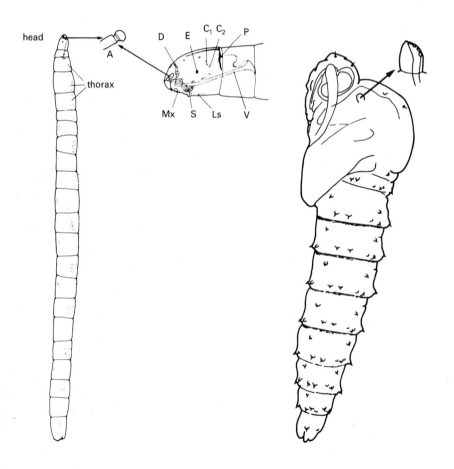

Source: from Saunders[58]

species the males swarm, and in *C. nubeculosus* mating can occur with or without swarming.[13]

Autogeny has been shown to occur commonly among *Culicoides* species, including anthropophilic species such as *C. furens, C. subim-maculatus,*[20,50] but all require a blood meal to mature second and subsequent egg batches and many species, e.g. *C. brevitarsis* and *C. puncticollis,* require a blood meal to mature the first egg batch.[7,33] In *L. (H.) becquaerti* there exist two forms, a short-winged, autogenous form, and a long-winged, anautogenous form.[46] The latter is responsible for most of the nuisance caused by this species to man.

Species feed on a range of hosts: some are anthropophilic, others, such as *C. brevitarsis,* feed mainly on cattle; and yet others are ornithophilic, including the chicken-biting species *C. arakawae* and *C. odibilis.*[41] *C. anophelis* is said to feed on mosquitoes, but this may be a case of phoresy, with the midge being transported by the mosquito rather than the midge being ectoparasitic, feeding either on the mosquito's haemolymph or blood meal.[10]

Blood-sucking midges are exophilic and exophagic, although in areas of high density biting midges will enter houses but in much smaller numbers than are present outside. Feeding preferences may be so strongly marked as to make subjective impressions of non-anthropophilic species very misleading. At Onderstepoort in South Africa human beings were quite untroubled by biting midges, but light traps revealed very large populations of *C. imicola* (= *C. pallidipennis* auct.), which were feeding on horses kept on the pasture at night. Such was the exophagy of this species that the risk of African horse sickness (see Chapter 24) could be greatly reduced, simply by stabling horses at night.

The biting cycle follows a circadian rhythm. Species of *Leptoconops* and *Lasiohelea* are diurnal, as are a small number of *Culicoides,* e.g. *C. nubeculosus* and *C. heliophilus,* but most *Culicoides* are crepuscular and/ or nocturnal. Diurnal species commonly show two peaks of activity, in the morning and in the afternoon. The morning peak occurs two to three hours after sunrise and is commonly the larger of the two peaks, e.g. *L. bec-quaerti* and *C. phlebotomus.*[55] The afternoon peak occurs close to sunset, and in the case of *L. sibirica* may occur as late as 21.00 h in the long summer days of high latitudes.[23]

In Jamaica the pest species, *C. furens* and *C. barbosai,* showed peaks of activity at sunrise and sunset, presumably being initiated by rapidly changing light intensity. Between these peaks biting continued at a reduced rate throughout the night with a smaller peak around midnight.[32] Both species continued to bite during the morning until such activity was terminated by adverse meteorological conditions, especially increasing wind speed and temperature. Environmental conditions may modify basic activity patterns and Reuben[57] caught *C. impunctatus,* mainly a crepuscular and nocturnal species, throughout the 24 hours. Even at times when females were not actively seeking a host, the arrival of a host induced activity in nearby resting, hungry females.

C. *imicola* and C. *schultzei* are two nocturnal species in East Africa, and Walker[61] found that while the numbers of C. *imicola* biting were fairly constant throughout the night, those of C. *schultzei* rose to a peak just after midnight.

Ovarian development and digestion of the blood meal follows the usual pattern of gonotrophic concordancy. Oviposition has not been observed in the field and only the eggs of *L. (S.) spinosifrons* have been found in nature, where they were mostly found at a depth of 30-60 mm in the sand of the breeding site.[16] Female *Leptoconops* burrow into the substrate in the laboratory and presumably do so in the field to rest and oviposit.

Gravid female C. *nubeculosus* oviposit more readily when in groups, than when held singly in tubes, and this may indicate the release of a pheromone at this time. Ismail and Kremer[26] have described the secretion of a pheromone by virgin females, when they are unfed and again when they are gravid. This pheromone attracts males and stimulates mating, but its effect on female behaviour has not been studied.[42] Linley and Carlson[48] have found a contact mating pheromone in C. *melleus*.

Breeding Sites

The breeding sites of blood-sucking ceratopogonids are commonly in wet soil in the ecotone between aquatic and terrestrial habitats, or in moist decaying vegetable material. *Culicoides* larvae burrow into the surface of the substrate and only rarely swim freely in the overlying water. Larvae of *Holoconops* and *Styloconops* occur in coastal areas in almost pure sand at the high spring tide level or even above it in sites inundated by exceptionally high tides.[16,43,59] Larvae of the subgenus *Leptoconops* occur inland in clay-silt soils where they may occur at considerable depths, e.g. *L. (L.) torrens* in the Sacramento Valley in California. When the soil cracks during the dry season the larvae of *L. torrens* pupate, and the adults emerge to feed and oviposit deep within the soil.[59] This has led to control by treating the soil so that cracking no longer occurs and adult emergence is therefore prevented.

Several coastal species of *Culicoides* breed in sand, e.g. C. *melleus,* C. *hollensis* and C. *molestus*. As the mud content in the substrate increases there is a range of habitats, culminating in mangrove swamps in the tropics and mud flats in the temperate regions. In the more sandy habitats of coastal eastern Australia C. *subimmaculatus* breeds in association with a surface-tunnelling soldier crab, *Mictyris livingstonei*.[52] In more muddy habitats in the Caribbean C. *furens* and C. *barbosai* breed in association with mangroves but only C. *barbosai* is dependent on the mangroves, and disappears when the mangroves are felled. C. *furens* continues to breed in high density in the absence of mangroves.[11]

The point is worth making that although there is an association between mangroves and many tropical anthropophilic *Culicoides* the breeding sites of the midge form only a minor part of the mangrove forest. Felling mangroves to control *Culicoides* is economically wasteful and ecologically damaging. The use of selective measures against the restricted larval habitat is more efficient and less costly. In Europe salt mud flats breed *C. halophilus* and *C. circumscriptus*, and *C. maritimus* breeds in vegetated salt marshes.[35] There is an even greater range of freshwater breeding sites. Open, muddy sites, often contaminated with animal excreta are the breeding grounds of *Monoculicoides*, as described earlier, and temporary pools in pasture in Europe produce *C. vexans*.

Vegetated swamps where the water table is above the soil surface, are the breeding grounds of *C. pulicaris* and *C. odibilis* in Europe,[35] while in Japan the latter species occurs in both the same type of habitat and also in rice fields, along with *C. arakawae*, which appears to be restricted to that habitat.[41] Marshland areas, where the water in winter is below the soil level, breed *C. pallidicornis* in Europe and *C. marksi* in Australia. Edges of lakes breed *C. austropalpalis* in Australia and *C. fascipennis*, *C. achrayi* and *C. duddingstoni* in Europe.

In Australia larvae of *C. bundyensis*, *C. bunroensis* occur in sandy creek beds. In Canada *C. denningi* breeds in the Saskatchewan River, and hibernates as a larva under ice in winter.[22] In oligotropic peaty areas characterised by *Sphagnum*, the bog moss, and *Polytrichum*, the *Culicoides* fauna is endemic and includes in Europe *C. impunctatus*, *C. truncorum* and *C. albicans*, and in North America *C. sphagnumensis*.

The faunas of saltwater, eutrophic freshwater, and oligotrophic bogland habitats are largely exclusive. This was demonstrated in north-west Scotland, where an outcrop of limestone supported a typical eutrophic flora and *Culicoides* fauna, sharply differentiated from the surrounding flora and fauna, in spite of its being isolated from other eutrophic areas by a vast sea of acid bogland.

The immature stages of many species of *Culicoides* are found only in small, specialised habitats, usually of vegetable origin. These include tree holes, producing *C. fagineus*, *C. angularis*, *C. hoffmani* and *C. guttipennis*. A comparable habitat to tree holes is water collecting in dugout canoes, from which in West Africa Carter *et al.*[9] bred two species of *Culicoides*. Species of the subgenus *Avaritia*, such as *C. brevitarsis*, *C. pallidipennis*, *C. dewulfi* and *C. chiopterus*, breed in dung, especially that of cattle. The New World *C. copiosus* group of species breed in rotting cacti, and *C. loughnani* has been introduced into Australia with the moth *Cactoblastis cactorum*, when it was introduced to control prickly pear.[17]

In West Africa *Culicoides* have been reared from the rotting stems of bananas; in Trinidad Williams[62] has recorded ten species, including the anthropophilic *C. paraensis* breeding in decaying cocoa pods; and Buxton[6] bred *C. scoticus* from large fungi of the Agaricaceae, Polyporaceae and Boletaceae. *C. heliconiae* breeds in the axils of the epiphytic bromeliad, *Heliconia*.[21] Woodland leaf litter, which in other countries has proved an unrewarding habitat to examine for *Culicoides*, in the eastern USA breeds the anthropophilic *C. sanguisuga*.[27]

From the foregoing, it is clear that species of *Culicoides* are able to exploit a wide range of moist habitats, but individual species utilise only a very limited range of breeding sites. This is of great practical importance because, where it is necessary to carry out larval contol, measures can be restricted to the breeding sites of the target species, minimising costs and environmental damage.

The same necessity to know the range of species in a locality before attempting control by habitat modification, applies to ceratopogonids as it did to culicids. In Jamaica an enterprising hotelier cut down the mangroves in the adjoining swamp, burnt the trash, and filled the swamp with sand dredged from offshore. It had the desired effect of eliminating *C. furens*, the original pest species, but the sand-filled swamp created ideal conditions for the breeding of *L. (H.) becquaerti*, which had previously been a rarity in the area. *L. becquaerti* was a far greater threat to the hotel's trade because its biting activity coincided with the periods of maximum tourist relaxation on the beach. The new situation was worse than the original. Effective control required the swamp to be filled to a depth greater than that which subsoil water can ascend by capillarity (750-1,100 mm) and/or covering the surface with marl and establishing and binding the surface with grass.[49]

Flight Range

In general, most species disperse only short distances from their breeding sites, and control of all breeding sites within 500 m is enough to reduce substantially the nuisance caused by species such as *C. molestus* and *C. subimmaculatus*. There is a difference between dispersal by active flight and passive wind carriage. In woodland *C. impunctatus* disperses only a short distance from its breeding site, the density decreasing rapidly to a tenth of the initial value 70 m from the breeding site.[30] This observation appeared to offer the prospect of protecting midge-infested areas by limited larval control. Unfortunately in the open *C. impunctatus* disperses downwind over 1,000 m without any noticeable reduction in density. Indeed the population density was more a function of the availability of suitable hosts than distance from the breeding site.[31]

Culicoides are mainly troublesome under calm conditions and numbers decline rapidly with increasing wind speed until few are encountered at wind speed exceeding 2.5 m/s. Female *F. (L.) sibirica* cease to bite at wind speeds in excess of 1.3 m/s,[23] while those of *C. phlebotomus*, another day biting species, remain active at wind speeds of 3.3 m/s,[55] and female *L. (H.) becquaerti* continue biting in wind speeds up to 5.0 m/s and have been collected in wind traps at greater wind speeds. Such small creatures are unlikely to be able to orientate to a host in other than winds of low speed. There is some evidence of a dispersal flight by *C. furens*, when large numbers were trapped in a truck trap, but only negligible numbers were biting.[4]

Specific Behaviour in Biting

Even when several species feed on the same host at the same time their behaviour is likely to be specific and different. In Jamaica three species, *C. furens*, *C. barbosai* and *L. becquaerti*, were anthropophilic and all actively biting at the same time in the one locality.[36,37,38] They differed in their relative densities on the limb exposed (leg or arm), although the 'bait' was seated on the ground and only offering an arm or a leg. In the morning, the arm:leg ratio for catches of *C. barbosai* was 3:2 and for *C. furens* 2:3 and for *L. becquaerti* 1:4. There was therefore a six-fold difference in the distribution of *C. barbosai* and *L. becquaerti*. Although *C. furens* and *L. becquaerti* were commoner on the leg, *L. becquaerti* fed on the sunlit upper surface while *C. furens* fed on the shady underside.

Four 'baits' were used, of whom two were Caucasian (K, L) and two were dark skinned West Indians (C, S). S caught fewest of all these species but the relative catches made by C, K and L differed according to the species. They all caught equal numbers of *C. barbosai*; K and L caught significantly more *L. becquaerti* than C but the catches of *C. furens* made by each 'bait' were significantly different with C catching the most, K less and L the least. The three species were responding differently to the three baits under exactly the same conditions. This emphasises the specific nature of the biting response and the inadequacy of any simple explanation implying attraction to pale or dark skins. Actually *C. impunctatus* and other species are attracted to dark cloth and this has been used as a sampling technique for estimating population size.[24] Other evidence showed that an individual's 'attractiveness' was not constant, but changed with conditions.

Survival and Frequency of Feeding

Study of the age-structure of populations of *Culicoides* has benefited greatly from Dyce[18] recognising that a burgundy-red pigment is laid down in the surface layers of the abdomen during the first ovarian cycle. This has now been confirmed for many species of *Culicoides*. The duration of the ovarian cycle is dependent on temperature and is two to three days in *C. phlebotomus*, a tropical species, and four days in members of the *C. obsoletus* group in the summer in southern England.[5,55]

The ability of a species to be a vector of blood-dwelling pathogens will be a function of the frequency with which blood meals are taken and the daily survival rate. In *C. phlebotomus* Nathan[54] found that the daily survival rate was about 0.90 in the first three days of life, declining to 0.69 at six days; but these observations were made on midges infected with *Mansonella ozzardi*, which may have affected their survival.

Birley and Boorman[5] developed a general method for determining survival and feeding frequency, which they applied to females of the *C. obsoletus* group. They obtained a daily survival rate of 0.74, and a four-day interval between blood meals, giving 30 per cent survival from meal to meal. In East Africa Walker[60] obtained a daily survival rate of 0.93 in *C. cornutus* and 0.80 in *C. imicola* (= *C. pallidipennis* auct.), making *C. cornutus* potentially the better vector of bluetongue virus.

Seasonal Changes in Population

It has already been pointed out that, in temperate regions, many species have one generation a year with the adults usually emerging in the summer. Other species may have several generations, and *C. obsoletus* has been reported as having two generations in the north of England[24] and three generations in southern England with a generation time of seven weeks.[5] In the warm summers of north-eastern Colorado the generation time of *C. variipennis* may be as short as two weeks and seven generations are completed in the year.[2] In the tropics generations are likely to overlap and adults be present all the year round. In Kenya, Walker[61] found that the five species he was studying were present all the year round, and although the populations fluctuated, there was no clear correlation with rainfall.

It is commonplace for coastal species to show a lunar periodicity, determined by the tides. In Oceania *C. peleliouensis* has two peaks of emergence each month, corresponding to the neap tides.[12] Similar tidal dependence has been shown for *C. subimmaculatus, C. austeni, L. spinosifrons, C. furens* and *C. barbosai*. Although *L. becquaerti* is coastal in distribution, the numbers of this species biting were more dependent upon rainfall than tidal movements.

Medical and Veterinary Importance

Species of *Culicoides* are economically important as vectors of arboviruses to livestock (see Chapter 24), and of blood-dwelling Protozoa to poultry (see Chapter 27). They also transmit filarial worms of low pathogenicity to man and livestock (see Chapter 32). To most people biting midges are synonymous with acute discomfort and irritation on calm, humid summer days. In spite of their small size they often cause severe local reaction. Species of *Lasiohelea* and *Leptoconops* produce particularly persistent reactions, which may blister and weep serum from the site of the bite in sensitive people. The impact of midges is greatest on newcomers to an infested area and hence the greater sensitivity of tourists to the local pest species. Control of biting midges has been essential in many areas for the development of an expanding tourist industry. In many parts of the world the midge problem is a coastal one and hence the popular, but misleading name of 'sandflies'. 'Sandflies' infest coastal areas of the Caribbean, eastern USA and South America, coastal areas of Australia, the Pacific islands and islands of the Indian Ocean.

Populations of biting midges reach pest proportion in the northern temperate regions, extending to high latitudes. In the highlands of Scotland *C. impunctatus* can make life miserable for residents and visitors. In Siberia *Lasiohelea sibirica* hampered construction of the Krasnoyarsk Power Station.[23] Reference has already been made to biting midges at high altitudes in Tibet (p. 139), and Spencer Chapman in his book *The Jungle is Neutral* (BT Reprint Society, London 1950, p.62), describing personal experiences of guerrilla warfare in Malaya, gave pride of place to biting midges as troublesome nocturnal pests.

References

1. Atchley, W.R., Wirth, W.W., Gaskins, C.T. and Strauss, S.L. (1981). A bibliography and keyword index of the biting midges (Diptera: Ceratopogonidae). *United States Department of Agriculture, Science and Education Administration, Bibliographies and Literature of Agriculture No. 13*
2. Barnard, D.R. and Jones, R.H. (1980). *Culicoides variipennis*: seasonal abundance, overwintering, and voltinism in northeastern Colorado. *Environmental Entomology* 9: 709-12
3. Becker, P. (1961). Observations on the life cycle and immature stages of *Culicoides circumscriptus* Kieff. (Diptera, Ceratopogonidae). *Proceedings of the Royal Society of Edinburgh B 67*: 363-86
4. Bidlingmayer, W.L. (1961). Field activity studies on adult *Culicoides furens. Annals of the Entomological Society of America 54*: 149-56
5. Birley, M.H. and Boorman, J.P.T. (1982). Estimating the survival and biting rates of haematophagous insects, with particular reference to the *Culicoides obsoletus* group (Diptera, Ceratopogonidae) in southern England. *Journal of Animal Ecology 51*: 135-48
6. Buxton, P.A. (1960). British Diptera associated with fungi. III. Flies of all families reared from about 150 species of fungi. *Entomologist's Monthly Magazine 96*: 61-94
7. Campbell, M.M. and Kettle, D.S (1975). Oogenesis in *Culicoides brevitarsis* Kieffer (Diptera: Ceratopogonidae) and the development of a plastron-like layer on the egg. *Australian Journal of Zoology 23*: 203-18
8. _____ and Kettle, D.S. (1976). Numbers of adult *Culicoides brevitarsis* Kieffer (Diptera: Ceratopogonidae) emerging from bovine dung exposed under different conditions in the field. *Australian Journal of Zoology 24*: 75-85
9. Carter, H.F., Ingram, A. and Macfie, J.W.S. (1921). Observations on the ceratopogonine midges of the Gold Coast with descriptions of new species. Part I. *Annals of Tropical Medicine and Parasitology 14*: 187-210
10. Das Gupta, S.K. (1964). *Culicoides (Trithecoides) anophelis* Edwards (Insecta: Diptera:

Ceratopogonidae) as an ectoparasite of insect vectors. *Proceedings of the Zoological Society 17*: 1-20

11. Davies, J.B. (1969). Effect of felling mangroves on emergence of *Culicoides* spp. in Jamaica. *Mosquito News 29*: 566-71

12. Dorsey, C.K. (1947). Population and control studies of the Palau gnat on Peleliu, Western Caroline Islands. *Journal of Economic Entomology 40*: 805-14

13. Downes, J.A. (1955). Observations on the swarming flight and mating of *Culicoides* (Diptera: Ceratopogonidae). *Transactions of the Royal Entomological Society of London 106*: 213-36

14. _____ (1962). What is an arctic insect? *Canadian Entomologist 94*: 143-62

15. _____ (1978). Feeding and mating in the insectivorous Ceratopogoninae (Diptera). *Memoirs of the Entomological Society of Canada 104*: 1-62

16. Duval, J., Rajaonarivelo, E. and Rabenirainy, L. (1974). Écologie de *Styloconops spinosifrons* (Carter, 1921) (Diptera, Ceratopogonidae) sur les plages de la côte Est de Madagascar. *Cahiers ORSTOM Entomologie Médicale et parasitologie 12*: 245-58

17. Dyce, A.L. (1969). Biting midges (Diptera: Ceratopogonidae) reared from rotting cactus in Australia. *Mosquito News 29*: 644-9

18. _____ (1969). The recognition of nulliparous and parous *Culicoides* (Diptera: Ceratopogonidae) without dissection. *Journal of the Australian Entomological Society 8*: 11-15

19. Edwards, F.W. (1926). On the British biting midges (Diptera, Ceratopogonidae). *Transactions of the Entomological Society of London 74*: 389-426

20. Edwards, P.B. (1977). Biology and bionomics of the biting midge *Culicoides subimmaculatus* Lee and Reye (Diptera: Ceratopogonidae) and other coastal *Culicoides* in southeast Queensland. Ph.D. thesis, University of Queensland, Brisbane, Australia

21. Fox, I. and Hoffman, W.A. (1944). New neotropical biting sandflies of the genus *Culicoides* (Diptera: Ceratopogonidae). *Puerto Rico Journal of Public Health and Tropical Medicine 20*: 108-11

22. Fredeen, F.J.H. (1969). *Culicoides (Selfia) denningi*, a unique river-breeding species. *Canadian Entomologist 101*: 539-44

23. Gornostaeva, R.M. (1967). The diurnal activity of attacks of *Lasiohelea sibirica* Bujan midges in the area of Krasnoyarsk hydropower station construction. *Meditsinskaya Parazitologiya i Parazitarnye Bolezni 36*: 11-17

24. Hill, M.A (1947). The life-cycle and habits of *Culicoides impunctatus* Goetghebuer and *Culicoides obsoletus* Meigen, together with some observations on the life-cycle of *Culicoides odibilis* Austen, *Culicoides pallidicornis* Kieffer, *Culicoides cubitalis* Edwards and *Culicoides chiopterus* Meigen. *Annals of Tropical Medicine and Parasitology 41*: 55-115

25. Howard-Bury, C.K. (1922). *Mount Everest, the Reconnaissance, 1921*. Edward Arnold, London

26. Ismail, M.T. and Kremer, M. (1980). L'effet du repas sanguin sur la production de phéromone par les femelles de *C. nubeculosus* (Diptera). *Annales de Parasitologie 55*: 455-66

27. Jamnback, H. (1965). The *Culicoides* of New York State (Diptera: Ceratopogonidae). *New York State Museum and Science Service Bulletin 399*: 1-154

28. Jobling, B. (1953). On the blood-sucking midge *Culicoides vexans* Staeger, including the description of its eggs and the first-stage larva. *Parasitology 43*: 148-59

29. Jones, R.H., Potter, H.W. and Baker, S.K. (1969). An improved larval medium for colonized *Culicoides variipennis*. *Journal of Economic Entomology 62*: 1483-6

30. Kettle, D.S. (1951). The spatial distribution of *Culicoides impunctatus* Goet. under woodland and moorland conditions and its flight range through woodland. *Bulletin of Entomological Research 42*: 239-91

31. _____ (1960). The flight of *Culicoides impunctatus* Goetghebuer (Diptera, Ceratopogonidae) over moorland and its bearing on midge control. *Bulletin of Entomological Rsearch 51*: 461-89

32. _____ (1969). The biting habits of *Culicoides furens* (Poey) and *C.barbosai* Wirth and Blanton. I. The 24-h cycle, with a note on differences between collectors. *Bulletin of Entomological Research 59*: 21-31

33. _____ (1977). Biology and bionomics of bloodsucking ceratopogonids. *Annual Review of Entomology 22*: 33-51

34. _____ and Elson, M.M. (1976). The immature stages of some Australian *Culicoides* Latreille (Diptera: Ceratopogonidae). *Journal of the Australian Entomological Society 15*: 303-32

35. _____ and Lawson, J.W.H. (1952). The early stages of British biting midges *Culicoides* Latreille (Diptera: Ceratopogonidae) and allied genera. *Bulletin of Entomological Research 43*: 421-67

36. _____ and Linley, J.R. (1967). The biting habits of *Leptoconops bequaerti*. I. Methods; standardisation of technique; preference for individuals, limbs and positions. *Journal of Applied Ecology 4*: 379-95

37. _____ and Linley, J.R. (1969). The biting habits of some Jamaican *Culicoides*. I. *C.barbosai* Wirth and Blanton, *Bulletin of Entomological Research 58*: 729-53

38. _____ and Linley, J.R. (1969). The biting habits of some Jamaican *Culicoides*. II. *C.furens* (Poey). *Bulletin of Entomological Research 59*: 1-20

39. _____ Wild, C.H. and Elson, M.M. (1975). A new technique for rearing individual *Culicoides* larvae (Diptera: Ceratopogonidae). *Journal of Medical Entomology 12*: 263-4

40. Khamala, C.P.M. (1975). Investigations of seasonal and environmental influences on biting and immature populations of *Culicoides cornutus* in Kenya, East Africa. *East African Journal of Medical Research 2*: 283-92

41. Kitaoka, S. and Morii, T. (1964). Chicken-biting ceratopogonid midges in Japan with special reference to *Culicoides odibilis* Austen. *National Institute of Animal Health Quarterly 4*: 167-75

42. Kremer, M., Ismail, M.T. and Rebholtz, C. (1979). Detection of a pheromone released by females of *Culicoides nubeculosus* (Diptera, Ceratopogonidae) attracting the males and stimulating copulation. *Mosquito News 39*: 627-31

43. Laurence, B.R. and Mathias, P.L. (1972). The biology of *Leptoconops (Styloconops) spinosifrons* (Carter) (Diptera, Ceratopogonidae) in the Seychelles Islands, with descriptions of the immature stages. *Journal of Medical Entomology 9*: 51-9

44. Lawson, J.W.H. (1951). The anatomy and morphology of the early stages of *Culicoides nubeculosus* Meigen (Diptera: Ceratopogonidae=Heleidae). *Tansactions of the Royal Entomological Society of London 102*: 511-70

45. Linley, J.R. (1966). Field and laboratory observations on the behavior of the immature stages of *Culicoides furens* Poey (Diptera: Ceratopogonidae). *Journal of Medical Entomology 2*: 385-91

46. _____ (1968). Autogeny and polymorphism for wing length in *Leptoconops becquaerti* (Kieff.) (Diptera: Ceratopogonidae). *Journal of Medical Entomology 5*: 53-66

47. _____ and Adams, G.M. (1972). A study of the mating behaviour of *Culicoides melleus* (Coquillett) (Diptera: Ceratopogonidae). *Transactions of the Royal Entomological Society of London 124*: 81-121

48. _____ and Carlson, D.A. (1978). A contact mating pheromone in the biting midge, *Culicoides melleus*. *Journal of Insect Physiology 24*: 423-7

49. _____ and Davies, J.B. (1971). Sandflies and tourism in Florida and the Bahamas and Caribbean area. *Journal of Economic Entomology 64*: 264-78

50. _____ Evans, H.T. and Evans, F.D.S. (1970). A quantitative study of autogeny in a naturally occurring population of *Culicoides furens* (Poey) (Diptera: Ceratopogonidae). *Journal of Animal Ecology 39*:169-83

51. _____ and Kettle, D.S. (1964). A description of the larvae and pupae of *Culicoides furens* Poey and *Culicoides hoffmani* Fox (Diptera: Ceratopogonidae). *Annals and Magazine of Natural History Series 13,7*: 129-49

52. Marks, E.N. and Reye, E.J. (1982). *An Atlas of Common Queensland Mosquitoes with a Guide to Common Queensland Biting Midges.* Queensland Institute of Medical Research, Brisbane, Australia

53. Megahed, M.M. (1956). A culture method for *Culicoides nubeculosus* (Meigen) (Diptera: Ceratopogonidae) in the laboratory, with notes on the biology. *Bulletin of Entomological Research 47*: 107-14

54. Nathan, M.B. (1981). Transmission of the human filarial parasite *Mansonella ozzardi* by

Culicoides phlebotomus (Williston) (Diptera: Ceratopogonidae) in coastal north Trinidad. *Bulletin of Entomological Research 71*: 97-105

55. _____ (1981). A study of the diurnal biting and flight activity of *Culicoides phlebotomus* (Williston) (Diptera: Ceratopogonidae) using three trapping methods. *Bulletin of Entomological Research 71*: 121-8

56. Parker, A.H. (1950). Studies on the eggs of certain biting midges (*Culicoides* Latreille) occurring in Scotland. *Proceedings of the Royal Entomological Society of London A 25*: 43-52

57. Reuben, R. (1963). A comparison of trap catches of *Culicoides impunctatus* Goetghebuer (Diptera: Ceratopogonidae) with meteorological data. *Proceedings of the Royal Entomological Society of London A 38*: 181-93

58. Saunders, L.G. (1964). New species of *Forcipomyia* in the *Lasiohelea* complex described in all stages (Diptera, Ceratopogonidae). *Canadian Journal of Zoology 42*: 463-82

59. Smith, L.M. and Lowe, H. (1948). The black gnats of California. *Hilgardia 18*: 157-83

60. Walker, A.R. (1977). Adult lifespan and reproductive status of *Culicoides* species (Diptera: Ceratopogonidae) in Kenya, with reference to virus transmission. *Bulletin of Entomological Research 67*: 205-15

61. _____ (1977). Seasonal fluctuations of *Culicoides* species (Diptera: Ceratopogonidae) in Kenya. *Bulletin of Entomological Research 67*: 217-33

62. Williams, R.W. (1964). Observations on habitats of *Culicoides* larvae in Trinidad, W.I. (Diptera: Ceratopogonidae). *Annals of the Entomological Society of America 57*: 462-6

63. Winder, J.A. (1978). Cocoa flower Diptera: their identity, pollinating activity and breeding sites. *PANS 24*: 5-18

64. Wirth, W.W., Ratanaworabhan, N.C. and Blanton, F.S. (1974). Synopsis of the genera of Ceratopogonidae (Diptera). *Annales de Parasitologie Humaine et Comparée 49*: 595-613

9 PSYCHODIDAE — PHLEBOTOMINAE (SANDFLIES)

The phlebotomine sandflies are a well-defined group of species, which are sometimes accorded family rank as the Phlebotomidae, but more frequently are regarded as a subfamily, Phlebotominae, of the Psychodidae.[20] Psychodids are small nematoceran flies with long antennae, pendulous palps, and hairy bodies and wings (Figure 9.1). Their venation is characterised by more or less parallel, longitudinal veins, the radial sector 3- or 4-branched, and the media 4-branched (Figure 9.2).

Plebotomine sandflies are brownish, long-legged flies with narrow bodies; narrow, lanceolate wings, less than 3 mm long, which are held erect above the body; the radial sector is 4-branched; and the palps 5-segmented

Figure 9.1: Lateral View of Female *Phlebotomus*

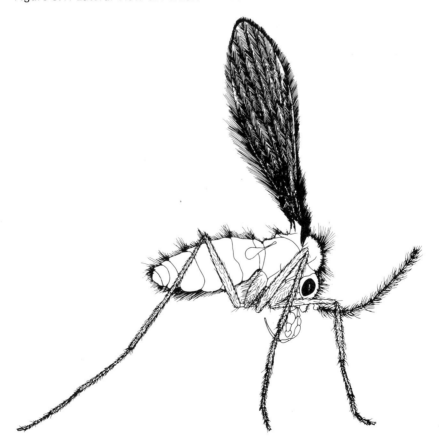

Figure 9.2: Wing Venation of a Phlebotomine Sandfly (above) and a Psychodine (below)

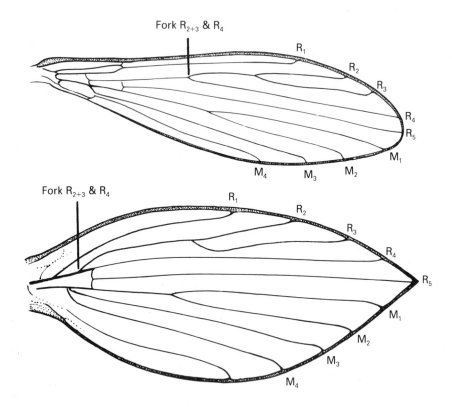

(Figure 9.1). The fork of R_{2+3} and R_4 occurs about the middle of the wing (Figure 9.2). The mouthparts are moderately long with functional mandibles in the females which are haematophagous. Mandibles are absent in the males, which are not blood-sucking. Phlebotomines are primarily inhabitants of the warmer areas of the world although they extend as far as 50°N in central Asia.

The majority of the other psychodids are in the Psychodinae, and are dark, squat flies with broad, oval wings held roof-like over the body at rest. The fork separating veins R_{2+3} and R_4 occurs towards the base of the wing (Figure 9.2). The mouthparts are not piercing and they do not feed on blood. The antennae bear cupuliform whorls of hairs. Psychodine larvae feed on organic material, and some are important in facilitating filtration in the clinker beds of sewage works by keeping them free from accumulating organic matter. The larvae have a posterior siphon, and secondary annulations on the body, which bear tergal plates.

About 600 species of phlebotomines have been described and included in five genera. About half of the species are contained in the genus *Lutzomyia*, a third in *Sergentomyia* and the majority of the remainder in the genus *Phlebotomus* with a small number of species in *Brumptomyia* and about five species in *Warileya*.[20] Phlebotomines are a geologically old group, being identified from the Lower Cretaceous, about 120 million years ago. They therefore originated before the mammals and must have fed originally on reptiles. This ancient origin has led to the evolution of different genera in the Old and New Worlds. *Phlebotomus* and *Sergentomyia* are confined to the Old World and *Lutzomyia*, *Brumptomyia* and *Warileya* to the New World, mainly the Neotropical region.[18]

Life Cycle

Egg

Phlebotomine eggs measure 300 to 400 µm long by 90 to 150 µm wide (Figure 9.3). They are white, when laid, but in a few hours darken to various shades of brown to black, according to the species.[1] In the laboratory *P. longipes* lays an average of 52 eggs in a batch with a range of 11 to 95[13] and *L. vexator occidentis* matures 70 eggs but only deposits 40, retaining the other 30.[4] Females in a laboratory colony of *L. longipalpis* behave similarly. They mature an average of 80 eggs (max. 146) but lay only 50 (max. 136), retaining the others in the abdomen.[16] Substantial egg retention is an artefact induced by laboratory conditions because females with retained eggs are rare in the field. The eggs of 13 species, examined by EM scanning, have sculptured chorions which probably act as plastrons when the eggs are covered by water.[31] Both eggs and larvae of *L. v. occidentis* need contact with water and are unable to survive even in a saturated atmosphere.[4]

Larva

The larva which emerges from the egg passes through 4 instars before pupating. The mature larva is greyish white with a dark head and no secondary annulations on the body (Figure 9.4). The antennae are small and leaf-like. The thorax is not differentiated from the abdomen although the abdominal segments bear ventral pseudopods, i.e. unjointed evaginations from the body, which are used for progression. The body segments bear characteristic pinnate hairs, the function of which is unknown. A diagnostic feature of phlebotomine larvae is the possession of two or four long caudal setae. First instar larvae have only one pair of caudal setae, but 2nd to 4th instars have two pairs.[1] The larva is amphipneustic with spiracles opening on the prothorax and the 8th abdominal segment (Figure 9.4).[1] The head bears chewing mouthparts, which the larva uses to feed on

Figure 9.3: Phlebotomine Egg Showing Ornamentation on the Chorion

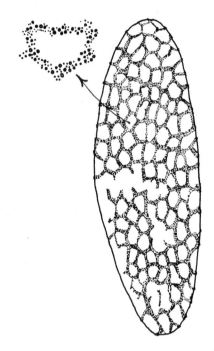

Source: From Abonnenc[1]

decaying organic matter, leaf mould, insect bodies and, when living in animal burrows, faeces of the host animal. Larvae of *P. longipes* have been reared in the laboratory on autoclaved rabbit faeces, and on a diet mainly composed of powdered liver or yeast.[13]

Pupa

The pupa stands upright being secured to the substrate by the larval exuviae, which is retained at the end of the abdomen.[17] Therefore all the larval setal characters are available for identification of the pupa. The pupa is exarate with legs and wings free from the body (Figure 9.5). It has short prothoracic respiratory horns. (The long horns of the culicid and ceratopogonid pupae are adaptations to an aquatic environment.) Although phlebotomines have terrestrial larvae and pupae they are very sensitive to desiccation. Pupae of *L. v. occidentis* are independent of free water, but require a relative humidity of 75 to 100 per cent for survival.[4]

Development is slow and in the laboratory *P. longipes* took over 3 months to produce adults from eggs at 18-20°C, and 7 to 8 weeks at 28-29°C.[11] The latter figure may be high as the same species reached the adult stage from the egg in 6 to 7 weeks at 25°C,[13] but the difference could

Figure 9.4: A, Lateral View of a Larva of a Phlebotomine; B, Dorsal View of Larval Head (numbers 1-9 refer to setae); C, Lateral View of Terminal Abdominal Segments

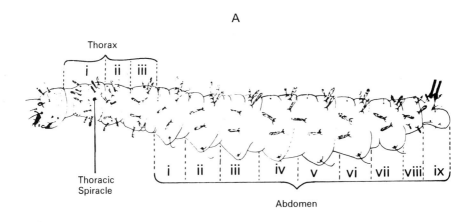

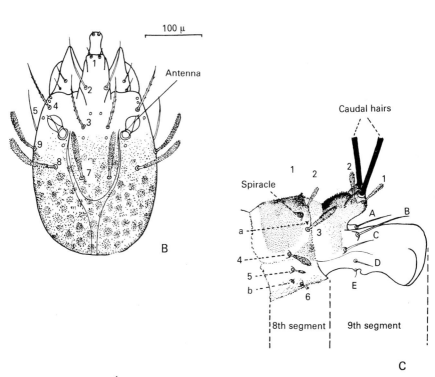

Source: From Abonnenc[1]

Figure 9.5: Pupa of a phlebotomine

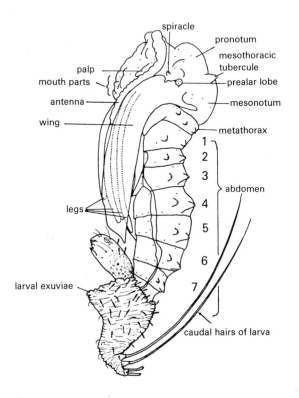

Source: From Abonnenc[1]

have been due to improved larval feeding. *P. papatasi* and *P. caucasicus* took 6 to 7 weeks to develop at 25-26°C in the absence of diapause, but 7 to 9 months when the larvae entered diapause.[7]

Adult

The 16 segmented antennae are pilose in both sexes, showing no sexual dimorphism. Males are, however, easily recognised by the possession of large terminalia of which the claspers (coxite and style) and surstyle are particularly prominent (Figure 9.6). Absence of plumosity on the male antenna suggests that phlebotomines do not swarm and that the sexes find each other by a different means. Hertig[14] has reported mating occurring in flight, but Ashford[3] has observed mating dances of *Phlebotomus orientalis* on horizontal white surfaces in the last few minutes of daylight before dark.

Figure 9.6: Lateral View of Terminal Segments of the Abdomen of a Male
Phlebotomus

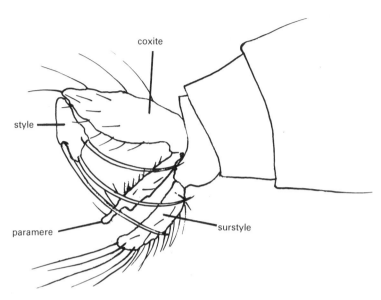

Male *P. orientalis* land and run around in all directions, stopping periodically to shake their wings before running on. Females land and behave
similarly until quickly paired with a male. Presumably sexual recognition is
achieved by pheromones emitted when the wings are shaken.

Male *L. v. occidentis* emerge, on average, earlier than the females and
rotation of the male terminalia is completed 12 hours after emergence.[4]
Mating in this species often occurs shortly after the female has fed or while
still feeding, but, when *L. v. occidentis* feeds on cold-blooded hosts,
feeding is protracted, taking an hour.[4] Spermatozoa are sometimes injected
directly into the spermathecal ducts,[14] and are stored in paired spermathecae of unusual appearance. The ducts are moderately long and
Abonnenc distinguished three main groups among Afrotropical phlebotomines: spermathecae with annulated walls; with tomentose or folded
walls; and with smooth walls.[1]

The palps are 5-segmented and, as in the Ceratopogonidae, the 3rd
segment bears sensilla. The maxillae are hooked at the tip in mammal-
feeding *Phlebotomus* and *Lutzomyia*, and ridge-tipped in reptile-feeding
Sergentomyia.[19] In the female the cibarium often bears teeth, which are
valuable in identification (Figure 9.7).

As in other blood-sucking Nematocera only the females are haematophagous, but both sexes feed on plant juices. Males of *P. orientalis* and *P.
longipes* have been observed apparently feeding on leaves and stems of
plants.[3] When *L. longipalpis* feeds on free sugar solutions the ingested fluid

Figure 9.7: Cibarium and Pharynx of — A, Female *Phlebotomus papatasi*; B, Male *P. papatasi*; and C, *Sergentomyia queenslandi*

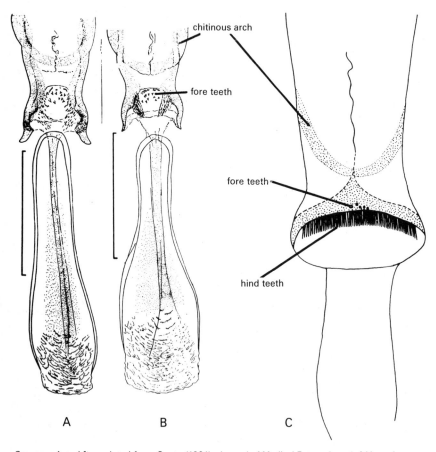

chitinous arch

fore teeth

fore teeth

hind teeth

A   B   C

Sources: A and B reprinted from Quote (1964). *Journal of Medical Entomology 1*: 241

passes to the crop, but when sugar solutions are imbibed by piercing a membrane they pass directly to the midgut.[23] Blood passes directly to the midgut, and unexpectedly engorgement is not stimulated by the presence of ATP as in other blood-feeding insects.[23] The midgut consists of a narrow, anterior cardiac portion, and a broad, sac-like posterior portion. A peritrophic membrane is secreted around the blood meal, and its structure may be important in the development of the pathogenic protozoan, *Leishmania*. In *P. longipes* the peritrophic membrane develops within 24 h of feeding, reaches a maximum at the end of 48 h, before breaking up on the third day, and finally is excreted with the residue of the blood meal after six to seven days.[12]

Genera[17]

The Old World genera *Phlebotomus* and *Sergentomyia* are separated from the New World genera by having the 5th palpal segment the longest, no post spiracular setae, and no posterior bulge to the cibarium.[17] In the New World genera palpal segment 3 is usually the longest, post spiracular setae are present, and there is a posterior bulge to the cibarium. Old World phlebotomines are savanna and desert species, associated with areas of low rainfall, whereas New World phlebotomines are inhabitants of forests and occur in areas of higher rainfall.

Phlebotomus

This mammal-biting genus reaches its maximum development in the warmer temperate and subtropical regions with hot summers and cold winters. It is characterised by the absence of cibarial teeth in the female (Figure 9.7A) and by the possession of erect hairs on the hind borders of abdominal tergites 2 to 6 (Figure 9.1).

Sergentomyia

This is the dominant genus in the Old World tropics of Africa, India and Australia, where its species feed on reptiles and amphibia. The genus is characterised by the possession of cibarial teeth in a posterior transverse row in the female (Figure 9.7C) and recumbent setae on abdominal tergites 2 to 6.

Lutzomyia

This genus is mainly Neotropical in distribution but a few species occur in the south of the Nearctic region. They feed on both mammals and reptiles. Species of *Lutzomyia* are characterised by having a transverse row of hind teeth and one or more rows of fore teeth on the cibarium of the female.

Brumptomyia

This genus is associated with armadillos, on which presumably they feed. The female cibarium bears four longitudinal rows of teeth.

Bionomics of Phlebotominae

Lewis[17] remarks that 'Adults [sandflies] are often hard to find and larvae usually impossible'. Consequently there are fewer observations on the bionomics of Phlebotominae than on the Culicidae or Ceratopogonidae. They are likely to show a comparable range of behaviour and ecology, and currently these aspects are receiving much attention. It has already been mentioned that mammal-feeding is largely confined to *Phlebotomus* and

Lutzomyia, and these genera are the vectors of disease to man and domestic animals.

In arid savanna and desert areas phlebotomines seek a favourable microclimate, and are often found in the burrows of rodents or in termitaria. Breeding often takes place in these microhabitats, and the females feed on their mammalian occupants or in the close vicinity. This habit, coupled with the short flight range, characteristic of the subfamily, leads to local concentrations of phlebotomines and the diseases they transmit, and is a good example of the concept of focality or nidality of disease, enunciated by Pavlovsky.[22]

Most species are exophilic but a few, and these are the most important, have become endophilic in human dwellings and anthropophilic, e.g. *P. papatasi* in the Mediterranean and Middle East to longitude 80 E; *P. sergenti* in Iran; *P. argentipes* in India; and *L. longipalpis* in north-east Brazil.[18] In Ethiopia *P. longipes* is exophilic and a cattle feeder, but in Addis Ababa it has become endophilic and attacks man near cattle sheds.[18] *P. pedifer,* a sibling species of *P. longipes,* is a cave dwelling species, which on Mt Elgon in Kenya fed largely (87 per cent) on cattle that entered the cave.[21] Most of the remaining feeds (9 per cent) were taken from hyraces. *P. orientalis* in Ethiopia is exophilic, but markedly anthropophilic;[3] and *L. wellcomei* in Brazil is largely anthropophilic (65 per cent), but also feeds regularly on rodents (25 per cent).[32] Another forest dwelling phlebotomine *L. flaviscutellata* is zoophilic, feeding on ground dwelling rodents of the genera *Oryzomys* and *Proechimys.*[29] *P. caucasicus* lives in the burrows of the giant gerbil *Rhombomys opimus,* on which it feeds.

On man, phlebotomines feed on exposed areas of skin, and these are the sites for the development of ulcers of cutaneous leishmaniasis. Feeding is mainly nocturnal and crepuscular. In Belize, biting of ten species of *Lutzomyia* was at its highest between 18.00-24.00 h and a few species continued biting until 06.00 h.[33] In Ethiopia the feeding of *P. orientalis* on man began after sunset, and rapidly reached a peak from which it declined and ceased when the temperature reached 16°C, which in the highlands was rarely more than 4 hours after sunset.[3] Some species, e.g. *P. papatasi,* will feed during the day under shaded conditions indoors, and others will feed if disturbed from their resting places.

Phlebotomines rest by day in dark, cool, humid niches where the microclimate is favourable for survival, e.g. *L. betrani* rests in caves.[34] *P. longipes* occurs in a variety of cavities including caves, tree holes and burrows.[3] Three closely-related species of the subgenus *Paraphlebotomus* are associated with rodent burrows in the USSR. *P. mongolensis* is found in oases where the conditions are relatively cool and humid, *P. caucasicus* in loess desert and *P. andrejevi* in very hot sandy deserts. The three species differ in their spiracular indices which is largest in *P. mongolensis* and smallest in *P. andrejevi.* Reduction in spiracular index would be an adaptation to an increasingly arid environment.[8]

Phlebotomines have a characteristic hopping flight and, if disturbed, quickly settle again a short distance away. In the open they are very sensitive to wind speed and feed only under near calm conditions. Perhaps to avoid higher wind speeds many species tend to fly close to the ground in the open. Even under forest conditions 80 per cent of the blood meals of *L. olmeca olmeca* are taken near the ground;[33] while *L. trapidoi* rests in the lower layers by day, and ascends into the canopy at night to feed on arboreal vertebrates.[6] *L. trinidadensis* takes 60 per cent of its feeds at 13 m, and less than 5 per cent of them at ground level.[33]

Most species are unable to develop eggs without a blood meal, e.g. *P. longipes*,[11] *L. californica*,[4] *L. longipalpis*,[16] and *L. trapidoi*;[5] but autogeny occurs in some other species, e.g. *P. papatasi*[10] and *L. gomezi*.[15]

Oviposition presumably occurs in soil, in burrows, in leaf litter on the forest floor, and around the bases of forest trees, particularly those with buttress roots, situations where larvae are found later. *P. papatasi* breeds in a range of sites, with greatest numbers being reared from the burrows of *Rhombomys opimus* and cattle sheds (more than 1,000 individuals per site), and less from burrows of *Meriones erythrourus* and unoccupied store rooms (100 to 250 per site).[2] Rutledge and Ellenwood[25,26,27] carried out a detailed analysis of the breeding sites of phlebotomines on the forest floor in Panama. *L. trapidoi* was the dominant species and favoured hillside and streams in the vicinity of large lianas (*Orouparia* and *Sabicea*) while *L. pessoana* was associated with hilltops and larger trees, e.g. *Anacardium.*

The slow rate of development, already referred to, will limit the number of generations which may be produced each year. Palaearctic species are often bivoltine, e.g. early summer eggs of *P. papatasi* and *P. caucasicus* develop without diapause, but late summer eggs give rise to diapausing larvae thus producing two generations per annum.[7] Ward and Killick-Kendrick[30] have reported diapausing eggs in a species of *Lutzomyia* provisionally referred to as *L.* sp. 260.44. In cooler climates species overwinter in the larval stage, which may be a true diapause or temperature induced cessation of growth.[7,15] Perhaps as an adaptation to survival in a hostile environment emergence of a generation may be extended by delaying hatching of eggs and eclosion of adults from pupae.[1,18] Abundance of *Lutzomyia* species seems to be dependent on rainfall and temperature. Numbers of *L. flaviscutellata* declined during the rains (January to May) and then increased to reach a peak in December to January.[28]

In the laboratory there is high mortality of females at and after oviposition. Few *L. longipalpis* survive oviposition,[16] and only 19 per cent of *L. lainsoni* survive to feed once more, and 2 per cent to feed twice more.[30] Survival in the field must be higher because Detinova[9] has recorded finding individual *P. papatasi*, which had completed six ovarian cycles. Dillick-Kendrick[15] notes that in nature infected *P. ariasi* can survive at least 29 days.

The flight range of phlebotomines is short, usually a matter of 100 to 200 m, but they may disperse 1 km or more. Mark-release-recapture experiments with *P. ariasi* showed that this species dispersed a maximum distance of 750 m from the point of release, and of 1 km between the extreme points of recapture.[24] When 20,000 marked *L. trapidoi* were released at ground and canopy (30 m) levels in forest, 90 per cent of those recaptured were taken within 57 m of the point of release, and only four individuals were collected at the limit of observations (200 m).[6]

Medical and Veterinary Importance

Phlebotomines are rarely present in sufficient density to reach pest proportions and their importance is as vectors of various pathogens, the most important of which are species of *Leishmania* causing cutaneous, visceral and mucocutaneous leishmaniasis of man (see Chapter 29). These diseases are widely but patchily distributed throughout the warmer areas of the world. They are mostly zoonoses in which, in the Neotropical region, man becomes involved by entering the focus of the disease and hence infections are confined to forest workers. Some species of *Leishmania* also infect dogs, and domestic foci of disease may develop in association with endophilic vectors.

Other diseases of which phlebotomines are vectors include bartonellosis, a disease of man living in certain high altitude valleys in the Andes of South America (see Chapter 25); and sandfly or papatasi fever, a virus disease spread by *P. papatasi* throughout much of its range (see Chapter 24). This virus is particularly interesting because there is evidence of transovarian transmission from one generation of *P. papatasi* to the next. Phlebotomines are also implicated in the transmission of vesicular stomatitis, a virus disease of cattle and horses (see Chapter 24).

Phlebotomines are highly susceptible to DDT, and in areas where the vector is endophilic, house spraying with DDT for malaria control dramatically reduced phlebotomine populations and the diseases they spread. Reinfestation is slow and may take up to three years after the cessation of spraying.

References

1. Abonnenc, E. (1972). Les phlébotomes de la région Éthiopienne (Diptera, Psychodidae). *Mémoires ORSTOM 55*: 1-289
2. Artem'ev, M.M., Flerova, O.A. and Belyaev, A.E. (1972. Quantitative evaluation of the productivity of breeding places of sandflies in the wild and in villages. *Meditsinskaya Parazitologiya i Parazitarnye Bolezni 41*: 31-5
3. Ashford, R.W. (1974). Sandflies (Diptera: Phlebotomidae) from Ethiopia: taxonomic

and biological notes. *Journal of Medical Entomology 11*: 605-16
4. Chaniotis, B.N. (1967). The biology of Californian *Phlebotomus* (Diptera: Psychodidae) under laboratory conditions. *Journal of Medical Entomology 4*: 221-33
5. _____ (1975). A new method for rearing *Lutzomyia trapidoi* (Diptera: Psychodidae) with observations on its development and behaviour in the laboratory. *Journal of Medical Entomology 12*: 183-8
6. _____ Correa, M.A., Tesh, R.B. and Johnson, K.M. (1974). Horizontal and vertical movements of phlebotomine sandflies in a Panamanian rain forest. *Journal of Medical Entomology 11*: 369-75
7. Dergacheva, T.I. (1972). The duration of development of the preimaginal stages of some species of sandflies (Diptera: Phlebotomidae) as observed in the laboratory. *Meditsinskaya Parazitologiya i Parazitarnye Bolezni 41*: 536-42
8. _____ (1974). The ecological relations of certain species of the subgenus *Paraphlebotomus* as observed in the Karshinskaya Steppe. *Zoologicheskii Zhurnal 53*: 1661-8
9. Detinova, T.S. (1968). Age structure of insect populations of medical importance. *Annual Review of Entomology 13*: 427-50
10. El Kammah, K.M. (1972). Frequency of autogeny in wild-caught Egyptian *Phlebotomus papatasi* (Scopoli) (Diptera: Psychodidae). *Journal of Medical Entomology 9*: 294
11. Foster, W.A., Tesfa-Yohannes, T.M. and Tecle, T. (1970). Studies on leishmaniasis in Ethiopia. II. Laboratory culture and biology of *Phlebotomus longipes* (Diptera: Psychodidae). *Annals of Tropical Medicine and Parasitology 64*: 403-9
12. Gemetchu, T. (1974). The morphology and fine structure of the midgut and peritrophic membrane of the adult female, *Phlebotomus longipes* Parrot and Martin (Diptera: Psychodidae). *Annals of Tropical Medicine and Parasitology 68*: 111-24
13. _____ (1976). The biology of a laboratory colony of *Phlebotomus longipes* Parrot and Martin (Diptera: Phlebotomidae). *Journal of Medical Entomology 12*: 661-71
14. Hertig, M. (1949). The genital filament of *Phlebotomus* during copulation. *Proceedings of the Entomological Society of Washington 51*: 286-8
15. Killick-Kendrick, R. (1978). Recent advances and outstanding problems in the biology of phlebotomine sandflies. *Acta Tropica 35*: 297-313
16. _____ Leaney, A.J. and Ready, P.D. (1977). The establishment, maintenance and productivity of a laboratory colony of *Lutzomyia longipalpis* (Diptera: Psychodidae). *Journal of Medical Entomology 13*: 429-40
17. Lewis, D.J. (1973). Phlebotomidae and Psychodidae. pp. 155-79 in *Insects and Other Arthropods of Medical Importance*, K.G.V. Smith (ed.), British Museum (Natural History), London
18. _____ (1974). The biology of the Phlebotomidae in relation to Leishmaniasis. *Annual Review of Entomology 19*: 363-84
19. _____ (1978). Phlebotomine sandfly research. pp. 94-9 in *Medical Entomology Centenary Symposium Proceedings*, S. Willmott (ed.), Royal Society of Tropical Medicine and Hygiene, London
20. _____ Young, D.G., Fairchild, G.B. and Minter, D.M. (1977). Proposals for a stable classification of the phlebotomine sandflies (Diptera: Psychodidae). *Systematic Entomology 2*: 319-32
21. Mutinga, M.J. (1975). The animal reservoir of cutaneous leishmaniasis on Mount Elgon, Kenya. *East African Medical Journal 52*: 142-51
22. Pavlovsky, E.N. (1964). *Natural Nidality of Transmissive Diseases with Special Reference to the Landscape Epidemiology of Zooanthroponoses*. Nauka, Leningrad
23. Ready, P.D. (1978). The feeding habits of laboratory-bred *Lutzomyia longipalpis* (Diptera: Psychodidae). *Journal of Medical Entomology 14*: 545-52
24. Rioux, J.A., Killick-Kendrick, R., Leaney, A.J., Turner, D.P., Bailly, M. and Young, C.J. (1979). Écologie des leishmanioses dans la sud de la France. 12. Dispersion horizontale due *Phlebotomus ariasi* Tonnoir 1921. Expériences préliminaires. *Annales de Parasitologie Humaine et Comparée 54*: 673-82
25. Rutledge, L.C. and Ellenwood, D.A. (1975). Production of phlebotomine sandflies on the open forest floor in Panama: the species complement. *Environmental Entomology 4*: 71-7

26. _____ and Ellenwood, D.A. (1975). Production of phlebotomine sandflies on the open forest floor in Panama: hydrologic and physiographic relations. *Environmental Entomology 4*: 78-82

27. _____ and Ellenwood, D.A. (1975). Production of phlebotomine sandflies on the open forest floor in Panama: phytologic and edaphic relations. *Environmental Entomology 4*: 83-9

28. Shaw, J.J. and Lainson, R. (1972). Leishmaniasis in Brazil: VI. Observations on the seasonal variations of *Lutzomyia flaviscutellata* in different types of forest and its relationship to enzootic rodent leishmaniasis (*Leishmania mexicana amazonensis*). *Transactions of the Royal Society of Tropical Medicine and Hygiene 66*: 709-17

29. _____ Lainson, R. and Ward, R.D. (1972). Leishmaniasis in Brazil: VII. Further observations on the feeding habitats of *Lutzomyia flaviscutellata* (Mangabeira) with particular reference to the biting habits at different heights. *Transactions of the Royal Society of Tropical Medicine and Hygiene 66*: 718-23

30. Ward, R.D. and Killick-Kendrick, R. (1974). Field and laboratory observations on *Psychodopygus lainsoni* Fraiha and Ward and other sandflies (Diptera, Phlebotomidae) from the Transamazônica highway, Pará State, Brazil. *Bulletin of Entomological Research 64*: 213-21

31. _____ and Ready, P.A. (1975). Chorionic sculpturing in some sandfly eggs (Diptera: Psychodidae). *Journal of Entomology A 50*: 127-34

32. _____ Shaw, J.J., Lainson, R. and Fraiha, H. (1973). Leishmaniasis in Brazil: VIII. Observations on the phlebotomine fauna of an area highly endemic for cutaneous leishmaniasis in the Serra Dos Carajas, Pará State. *Transactions of the Royal Society of Tropical Medicine and Hygiene 67*: 174-83

33. Williams, P. (1970). Phlebotomine sandlfies and leishmaniasis in British Honduras (Belize). *Transactions of the Royal Society of Tropical Medicine and Hygiene 64*: 317-64

34. _____ (1976). The phlebotomine sandflies (Diptera: Psychodidae) of caves in Belize, Central America. *Bulletin of Entomological Research 65*: 601-14

10 SIMULIIDAE (BLACKFLIES)

Simuliids are often known as blackflies. They are small, dark, stout-bodied, hump-backed Nematocera (Figure 10.1). They are larger than blood-sucking ceratopogonids and have wing lengths of 1.5 to 6.0 mm. Simuliids are largely diurnal and vision plays an important role in their behaviour. In the female the individual elements (ommatidia) of which the eyes are composed are small (10-15 μm) and the eyes are well separated above the antennae, i.e. the female is dichoptic (Figure 10.2). In the male the eyes are larger and are broadly contiguous above the antennae, i.e. the male is holoptic, and the lower ommatidia are similar to those of the female but the upper ones are greatly enlarged, measuring 25-40 μm (Figure 10.2). The antennae are the same in both sexes and consist of small, globular segments, compacted together to give a beaded appearance (Figure 10.2). The number of antennal segments ranges from 9 to 12 but the commonest number is 11; occasionally there are 10 (*Austrosimulium*) and rarely there

Figure 10.1: Lateral (left) and Dorsal (right) Views of a Female *Simulium*

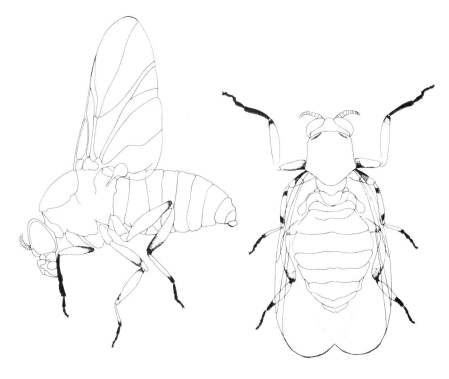

Figure 10.2: Front View of Heads of Male (left) and Female (right) *Simulium*

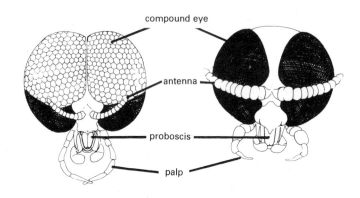

are 9 or 12.[15] The 5-segmented, pendulous palps are considerably longer than the short proboscis and carry a sense organ on the third segment. In males and in a few species in which the females do not bite, the mandibles and maxillae are not toothed.

The wings are short and broad with a large anal lobe (Figure 10.3). The venation is characteristic with well-developed radial veins along the anterior margin of the wing and weaker median and cubital veins posteriorly. In spite of its weak appearance the wing is highly efficient and in still air simuliids are capable of flying in excess of 100 km.[29] The radial sector may be unbranched or have two branches. Between the median (M_2) and the cubital (Cu_1) veins there is a forked submedian fold.[15] The male terminalia are compact and relatively inconspicuous, particularly when compared to the prominent terminalia of male phlebotomines. The female has a single subspherical spermatheca.

According to Crosskey,[16,17] 1,270 species of Simuliidae have been described, and he assigns them to 19 genera of which only four, *Simulium*, *Austrosimulium*, *Prosimulium* and *Cnephia*, are of economic importance. The largest and most important genus is *Simulium* with 1,000 species arranged in 38 subgenera. The next largest genus is *Prosimulium* with about 12 per cent of the species in the family; *Austrosimulium* with 2 per cent; and the remaining 6 per cent distributed among 16 other genera, of which the largest are *Metacnephia* and *Gigantodax*.[15] Although simuliids are distributed widely throughout the world, *Austrosimulium* is restricted to Australia and New Zealand and *Prosimulium* and *Cnephia* to the Holarctic region. Species of *Simulium* occur in all zoogeographical regions with the greatest number (366) being found in the Palaearctic, a large number (257) in the Neotropical, rather fewer (155) in the Afrotropical and Oriental (110) regions and least in the Australian (78) and Nearctic

Figure 10.3: Wing of Female *Simulium* (× 50). Rs, radial sector

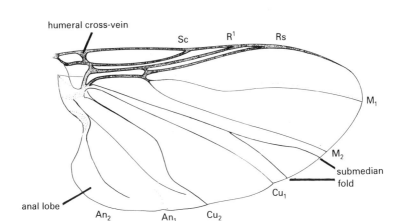

(75).[17] The Simuliidae is rich in species complexes and that of *S. damnosum* has been considered briefly in Chapter 6.

In *Simulium* the antennae have 11 segments; the radial sector is unbranched, and there are both spiniform setae and hairs on the costa. *Prosimulium* also has 11 antennal segments, but the radial sector is branched, and the costa bears only hairs and has no spiniform setae. *Austrosimulium* has 10-segmented antennae, an unbranched radial sector; and spiniform setae and hairs on the costa. Species identification is difficult and uses, among other characters, the structure of the male and female terminalia, the pupal respiratory organ, and the larval head. Peterson and Dang[44] list the morphological characters of the Simuliidae.

Life Cycle

A generalised life cycle will be given in this section and variations on the basic pattern will be considered in the bionomics section later. In their early stages simuliids are limited to fluvial ecosystems, breeding in running, often swiftly running, water. The eggs are laid in batches of 150-600 on objects in or near running water or directly into the water. It is not uncommon for communal egg masses to be formed by several females ovipositing in close proximity. Presumably this aggregation is induced by a pheromone emitted by the ovipositing female. Eggs are either dropped directly into the water and sink to the bottom or are laid on emergent objects close to the waterline, where they are either directly wetted by water or are in the splash zone. Hinton[28] states that as far as he knows egg laying does not occur below the surface.

Egg

Eggs are 100 to 400 µm long and ovoid-triangular in shape. Their surface is comparatively smooth, lacking the patterned chorion found in the eggs of *Culicoides* and culicids. Williams[57] considers that the gelatinous substance in which the eggs are embedded is formed by adherent outer membranes of the individual eggs, i.e. their exochorions. The apparent egg 'shell' is the inner egg membrane or endochorion and the chorionic plastron is poorly developed. A well-developed plastron would not be necessary in eggs laid near the surface of running water where the oxygen tension would be high. Simuliid eggs are sensitive to desiccation; even those of *A. pestilens*, which survive for many months in wet river deposits, desiccate rapidly when exposed to relative humidities of 96 per cent or less.[11] Eggs laid near the surface hatch when the embryo has completed development, a matter of days under favourable conditions. Other species produce dormant eggs in which the adverse conditions of summer and/or winter are passed.[13]

Larva

The egg hatches to produce a larva, much of whose behaviour revolves around the secretion of silk by the long salivary glands, which are longer than the larva (Figure 10.4). The larva spins a web of silk on the substrate, which is continued into a silken thread on which the larva drifts downstream with the current in search of a suitable object on which to settle. When this has been found the larva spins a patch of silk on the selected site and anchors itself to the silk by its posterior circlet of hooks (posterior sucker in Figure 10.4). Larvae remain near the surface of the water and are usually found at depths less than 300 mm. The larva can change its location by drifting downstream again on a silken thread, or by looping over the surface using the posterior circlet and the hooks on the anterior proleg to retain a hold on secreted silk. Some species disperse further from the oviposition site than others. Larvae of *S. ornatipes* are more sessile than those of *A. bancrofti*, which move from the quieter waters of the oviposition site to rapids.[12] In very large rivers, with fast-flowing water, larvae have been found at depths of several metres.[13]

The larva has a distinct, sclerotised head with paired, simple eyes, and an elongated hour-glass shaped body, in which the thorax and posterior part of the abdomen are broader than the anterior segments of the abdomen (Figure 10.4). The head bears a pair of cephalic fans, homologous structures to the mouth brushes of the Culicidae. They do not create a current but filter water passing over the larva. Larvae are anchored posteriorly and extended in the direction of the current with the head leading. The body is twisted through 90-180° so that the fans and mouthparts face towards the surface of the water (Figure 10.5). The water current is divided by the proleg and directed towards the fans. A sticky secretion produced by the cibarial glands enables the fans to capture fine particles,

Figure 10.4: Lateral View of a Mature Larva of *Simulium ornatum*

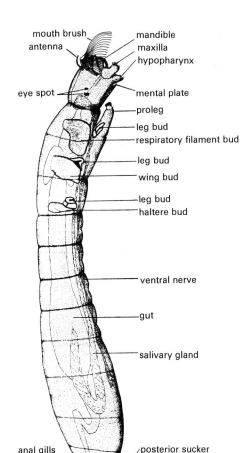

mouth brush
antenna
mandible
maxilla
hypopharynx

eye spot
mental plate
proleg
leg bud
respiratory filament bud

leg bud
wing bud

leg bud
haltere bud

ventral nerve

gut

salivary gland

anal gills
posterior sucker

Source: Reproduced with permission from Smart, J. (1944). *The British Simuliidae*, Scientific
Publication No.9. Freshwater Biological Association, Ambleside, Cumbria, U.K.

which are transferred to the cibarium by the mandibular brushes.[13]

Chance[9] has found that although simuliid larvae ingest particles up to 350 μm the most commonly ingested particles are 10-100 μm. In practice this means that simuliid larvae can be reared in the laboratory on bacteria, which, in certain streams, may form an important element in the feeding of blackfly larvae.[24] Wotton[59] has shown that simuliid larvae are capable of ingesting particles of colloidal size (0.091 μm). Algae pass apparently unchanged through the blackfly gut but diatoms may form as much as 50

Figure 10.5: A, Larva of *Simulium*; B, Larva in Feeding Posture in a Current (arrows indicate direction); C, Attitude of Larva in Response to Sudden Increase in Current Velocity or Disturbance — head close to substrate in position to attach silken thread. ba, anal gills; dp, posterior circlet; di, imaginal discs of developing adult structures; pa, proleg; pm, cephalic fans; pv, ventral papillae

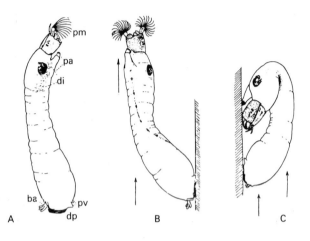

Source: From Grenier, P. (1948). *Physiologia Comparata et Oecotogia 1*: 232

per cent of the gut contents and are digested.[35] Ladle[36] found that larvae of *S. ornatum* and *S. equinum* ingested particles with a maximum diameter of 25-30 μm, with diatoms forming the main food early in the year and small particles of detritus predominating later in the year. Filter-feeding larvae may also browse and a few species, e.g. *Twinnia biclavata*, do not filter-feed but graze on the substrate.[13,15]

Simuliid larvae are often particularly abundant where the water current accelerates, as at rapids, and where presumably larvae will strain a greater volume of water in a fixed period of time. Heavy larval concentrations are to be found at the outflows of large lakes, where the water will be rich in phytoplankton for larval food. This was true of the Ripon Falls in Uganda, where the Nile flowed out from Lake Victoria. Breeding was eliminated when a dam was built and the falls were submerged.

The larva has a single anterior proleg, surmounted by a circlet of hooks and the abdomen ends in a posterior circlet (Figure 10.4). The anus opens dorsally of the posterior circlet, and from it may be extruded the rectal 'gills', which probably, by analogy with the anal papillae of culicid larvae, are concerned with chloride extraction from the water. There is often an X-shaped anal sclerite between the anus and the posterior circlet. Movement of water over the body surface provides the larva with adequate dissolved oxygen for respiration. In deoxygenated water larvae detach and drift downstream. Larvae pass through six to nine instars and the number is not constant even within a species; *P. mixtum* may have six or seven larval instars.[13] Simuliid larvae reach a length of 4-12 mm, and being reasonably large and aggregated, are easily seen on submerged objects. Phoretic larvae of the subgenera *Lewisellum* and *Phoretomyia* of the genus *Simulium*, have microsculptured cuticles, which differentiate them from all except two species of free-living larvae.[58]

The mature larva is actually a pharate pupa within the larval skin, and may move to a different site before pupating. Pupae of *A. bancrofti* occur on the downstream side of submerged substrates.[12] The pharate pupa spins a slipper-shaped cocoon with the closed end directed upstream and the open end downstream (Figure 10.6). The alignment prevents the cocoon being torn off the substrate by the current. Construction of the cocoon takes about an hour and then the larval skin is shed.

Pupa

The head and thorax of the pupa are combined into a single cephalothorax, and there is a segmented abdomen (Figure 10.6). The latter bears spines and hooks which engage with the threads of the cocoon and retain the pupa in place. The cephalothorax bears a pair of elongate, branched pupal gills, which trail downstream of the cocoon. They are homologous with the

Figure 10.6: Pupa and Cocoon of *Simulium simile*. From left to right: dorsal view of pupa in cocoon; ventral view of pupa removed from cocoon; lateral view of cocoon. Current of water flows up the page

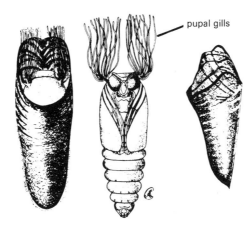

pupal gills

Source: Reproduced by permission of the Minister, Supply and Services, Canada. From Cameron, A.E. (1922). Agriculture Canada Entomological Bulletin No. 20: *The Morphology and Biology of a Canadian Cattle-infesting Blackfly, Simulium simile Mall. (Diptera: Simuliidae)*

respiratory horns of the Culicidae and Ceratopogonidae, but they do not have open spiracles. The tubular branches of the gill bear vertical struts which support a very thin, outer, minutely perforated, trilaminate epicuticle and an inner fine meshwork. The enclosed air-filled space around the struts functions as a plastron, and Hinton[27] considers that the water-air interface will be about 50 per cent of the total plastron area. The shapes of the cocoon and gills are important characters in the identification of species.

The pupa, which does not feed, becomes progressively darker as the adult develops within, but the mature pupa takes on a silvery appearance as a film of air is secreted between the pharate adult and the pupal cuticle. When the pupal exuviae splits, the adult floats up to the surface in a bubble of air and immediately takes flight. Alternatively the newly emerged adult crawls up some emergent object to reach the air.[15] The length of the life cycle varies with the species and environmental conditions. Some species in temperate regions have one generation a year, while continuous breeding occurs in tropical species, and the larval stage of *S. damnosum* can be completed in as little as eight days. For that reason the Onchocerciasis Control Programme in West Africa treats breeding sites weekly.[54] The life cycle from egg to adult can be completed in less than two weeks.

Adult

Adult emergence occurs predominantly in the daytime, depending on light and temperature. In *S. damnosum* 60-90 per cent of the day's emergence has occurred by midday and there is no emergence at night. At 24-28°C peak emergence of *S. damnosum* occurs at 06.00-09.00 h and when the water temperature is lower (20-24°C) the peak is reached later in the morning between 09.00-12.00 h.[56]

Mating. Mating occurs in close association with the breeding site, and in a few species occurs on the ground,[22] but in the large majority of species it occurs on the wing when males form small swarms in association with visual markers. In *A. pestilens* male swarms orientate to *Callistemon viminalis* along the banks of the semi-permanent stream in which it breeds.[42] Male simuliids recognise the female from distances up to 50 cm and pursue the female and attempt to couple. There appears to be no contact pheromone because males will attempt to mate with other males and with individuals of other species.[56] In some species male swarms and mating occur in close proximity to the feeding sites of the females, which, in *S. ornatum* and *S. erythrocephalum*, are respectively the navel and ears of cattle.[56] During mating a 2-chambered spermatophore is transferred to the female.

Feeding. Crosskey[15] considers that ornithophilic species probably predominate in the Simuliidae. Ornithophilic and mammalophilic species are distinguished morphologically by the shape of the claws. In mammal feeders the claws are simple but in bird feeders they are toothed. This must be an adaptation to holding and penetrating feathers. Simuliids are exophilic, exophagic and largely diurnal, although Davies and Williams[20] collected ten species in light traps in Scotland, mainly *S. ornatipes* and *S. tuberosum*. Some species will enter the natural openings of the body, nose, ear and eye; behaviour which is particularly worrying to livestock. As in other blood-sucking Nematocera both males and females feed on nectar, which is stored in the crop, and only the females are haematophagous with blood passing directly to the midgut.

Some species are autogenous for the first batch of eggs, but most species require a blood meal for maturation of the ovaries. When feeding, the female simuliid anchors its proboscis to the host by small hooks on the labrum and hypopharynx. The maxillae are protruded alternately, penetrating downwards and anchoring the proboscis more firmly. The mandibles cut into the skin with rapid scissor-like movements, penetrating to a depth of about 400 µm. Blood is ingested, using the cibarial and pharyngeal pumps. Blood feeding takes about 4-5 min.[56]

Bionomics

The bionomics of the Simuliidae have been reviewed by Crosskey,[15] Colbo and Wotton (immature stages)[13] and Wenk (adults).[56]

Oviposition

S. damnosum females oviposit communally in the short period between tropical sunset and darkness. Dense swarms of females lay their eggs on vegetation trailing in the water achieving densities of two to three thousand eggs per square centimetre.[53] *A. pestilens* also forms swarms of ovipositing females which scatter their eggs over the surface of the water, where they become incorporated in the sandy river bed and can survive two and a half years, providing they are kept permanently damp.[11,42] Dalmat[18] found that in Guatemala *S. ochraceum* dropped its eggs directly into the water; *S. callidum* laid its eggs one at a time on the inclined surfaces of rocks; and *S. metallicum*, in fast-flowing water, laid its eggs on leaves without landing, and in slower flowing water actually landed. Eggs of *S. argyreatum* can withstand dryness during autumn and winter when the temperatures are low, and they and the eggs of *S. pictipes* resist frost and ice to survive the winter and hatch in the spring.[34,50]

Breeding Sites

Simuliids breed only in running water, ranging from torrential mountain streams to slowly moving lowland rivers. In Newfoundland Lewis and Bennett[40] found that the most significant factors affecting the distribution of simuliid larvae were current velocity, substrate type and water depth. Grunewald[26] investigated the distribution of larvae of the *S. damnosum* complex and found that their breeding sites could be classified on the pH and conductivity of the water.

Some species have a phoretic association with crabs, prawns or mayflies in Africa and the Himalayan region.[13] Larvae and pupae of *S. nyasalandicum* and *S. woodi* occur on the sides, the chelipeds, and the basal segments of the walking legs of the crab *Potamon (Potamonautes) pseudoperlatum*. They also occur on other species of crab.[48,49] Eggs are not laid on the crab and the young larva must find its own phoretic partner.[21] The most important of these phoretic simuliid species is *S. neavei*, a vector of onchocerciasis (see Chapter 31). *S. woodi* occurs in small, heavily shaded, forest streams but in general such areas have a poor blackfly fauna with a marked increase in species occurring at the forest edge, and where there are breaks in the canopy.[12,13]

When eggs are deposited in dense masses it is essential that the first instar larvae disperse. Larvae drift downstream attached to a silken thread or they can break the thread and drift with the current.[13] Larvae drift throughout the 24 hours and early instars of *A. bancrofti* show a diurnal tendency with a greater proportion of older instars drifting at night.[12]

Biting Habits

The females of most simuliids require a blood meal to develop eggs but a few, including *S. argyreatum*, are autogenous.[50] *A. pestilens* feeds on man and many mammals and is probably an opportunist feeder, which may be related to the fact that it remains close to the breeding site.[31] The closely related *A. bancrofti* is more selective and Hunter and Moorhouse[31] found that it did not bite any of the four mammals, including man, and two bird species tested. In Scotland Davies *et al.*[19] found that *S. tuberosum* fed on a wide range of hosts including man, other mammals and birds; while *S. latipes* fed largely on birds; and *S. reptans* and *S. monticola* took over 90 per cent of their feeds on bovines.

The gonotrophic cycle is remarkably short, being completed in 24 h in *A. pestilens*,[31] and in two days in *S. metallicum*.[47] In *S. damnosum* the first cycle from blood meal to oviposition takes three or four days and thereafter eggs are laid at intervals of four to five days, the additional time being required for nectar feeding before the blood meal.[56]

Simuliids are essentially diurnal species and in open sunny situations *S. damnosum* tends to have a bimodal pattern of activity with peaks around 09.00 h in the morning and 17.00 h in the afternoon, but in shaded areas biting is more evenly distributed throughout the day.[33] The circadian rhythm of biting activity varies with the age of the flies, with parous females feeding earlier in the day than nullipars.[38] Although mainly diurnal, ten species of simuliids were taken in light traps in Scotland;[20] three different species were trapped in Norway;[46] and Service[52] collected large numbers (3,600 per night) of ovipositing *S. squamosum*, a member of the *S. damnosum* complex, in light traps in Ghana. Activity of simuliids is influenced by barometric pressure,[55] and in Ghana the numbers of simuliids biting increase with rising humidity and lowering barometric pressure.[14]

Host Finding

Working with seven species of simuliids, mainly *S. venustum*, in Canada Bradbury and Bennett[6] proposed a three-stage model of host finding. Long-range attraction was initiated by host odour leading to an upwind response of the fly. Nearer the host, orientation was to carbon dioxide emitted by the host, and within 1.8 m orientation was visual. The visual component is supported by the fact that *S. erythrocephalum*, which feeds on the ears of cattle, will attack protruding parts of a dummy; and *S. ornatum*, which feeds near the navel, attacks the flat underparts of a model.[56] Most (93 per cent) *S. damnosum* land on the ankles of man, but then ascend the leg and feed on the calves. After landing, other stimuli, such as odour, sweat and other chemicals, are likely to be involved in probing. The ornithophilic species, *S. euryadminiculum*, is strongly attracted to extracts of the uropygial gland of the common loon (*Gavia immer*).[4] Simuliids can discriminate between colours of the same reflectance with *S. venustum* being attracted to blue, *P. mixtum* to black and *S. vittatum* to black, red and blue but not to yellow.[5]

Dispersal

Adult females of many species of simuliids disperse far from their breeding sites. Hocking[29] has shown by laboratory experiments that *S. venustum* is capable of flying 116 km in still air, following a sugar meal. In the field, Baldwin *et al.*[1] found that this species dispersed on average 9-13 km, but a few individuals covered 35 km in two days. Females of *S. arcticum* dispersed for distances of at least 150 km from the Athabasca River in western Canada in sufficient numbers to be a pest.[10]

Wenk[56] distinguishes different categories of dispersal in *S. damnosum*. There is linear dispersal along river courses in the gallery forest of the West African savanna; radial dispersal in the savanna during the rainy season, and in the forest region throughout the year; and differential dispersal, when nullipars disperse further than parous females, which tend to remain near the breeding sites.

Only parous females can transmit *Onchocerca volvulus*, and if they stay close to the breeding site then transmission of onchocerciasis will be concentrated in the vicinity of rivers and streams.[23,37] There is also wind-borne dispersal of blackflies, and Garms *et al.*[25] found that flies which invaded the Onchocerciasis Control Programme in West Africa were parous flies, many of which were infected with *Onchocerca* larvae. This indicates that, under certain conditions, parous females can disperse as widely, if not more widely, than nullipars.

Response to Varying Conditions

Simuliids have to survive periods when the temperature is too low to sustain normal activities, and when rivers cease to flow in the dry season, which may be indeterminate in length. Larvae of *P. mixtum* and *P. fuscum* grow actively during the winter at temperatures near freezing point,[39] and larvae of *P. mysticum* are dormant below 4°C, when they reduce their respiratory rates substantially and replace trehalose in the haemolymph by high polyhydric alcohols. When the temperature rises above 4°C the reverse process is rapidly completed and growth resumes.[41]

S. latipes was taken in light traps in Scotland in every month of the year in 1957, and in other years was present from March or April to November.[20] Perhaps this species has overwintering adults, which can be active or dormant, depending upon the temperature.

Simuliids living in the severe climate of high latitudes show various adaptations to survival, involving reducing the time spent in the adult stage, which is the most vulnerable to low temperatures and high winds. Eight out of the nine species restricted to the Canadian tundra are autogenous and have reduced mouthparts, e.g. *S. baffinense*; the females do not need to seek a blood meal and indeed are unable to feed. The risk to the species' survival if the males had to swarm, is avoided by mating occurring on the ground where adults cluster near the breeding site. As an adaptation to that behaviour the eyes of the male are sometimes dichoptic as in the female, e.g. *Gymnopsis dichopticus*. As a further adaptation a species may be both autogenous and parthenogenetic with the adult female becoming gravid in the pupa, e.g. *P. ursinum*, and there is virtually no free adult life.[22]

Aridity poses other problems. *A. pestilens* survives a dry season of uncertain length as viable eggs deep in the moist, sandy beds of transient rivers.[11] Eggs of *C. pecuarum* laid in April remained dormant until November and then developed and hatched in December. This carried the species over the summer months when many breeding places ceased to flow.[8] Adult *S. damnosum* are regarded as having a maximum life span of three to four weeks[37] but this does not explain their appearance before the rivers begin to flow again after the dry season. Have these adults arrived from unidentified breeding sites which have persisted during the dry season? Or have these adults been aestivating?[14]

Many species of *Simulium* have several generations a year. Where such species overwinter as growing larvae, as in *S. monticola*, there are likely to be large size differences between adults produced in the different seasons.

Winter larvae produce larger adults than summer larvae. Changes in the total biovolume of the adult were found to be inversely related to mean water temperature.[43] In addition size was also influenced by the quantity of food available and the photoperiod.

Medical and Veterinary Importance

Simuliids are important as pests in their own right and also as vectors of pathogens. Vectors need not be present in high enough density to be regarded as pests. The most serious human disease associated with simuliids is onchocerciasis or river blindness, due to infection with the filarial worm *Onchocerca volvulus*. This disease exists in the Afrotropical and Neotropical regions and is dealt with in Chapter 31. Simuliids are also vectors of other *Onchocerca* spp to livestock, e.g. *O.gutterosa* in cattle (see Chapter 32). Simuliids also transmit blood-dwelling Protozoa of the genus *Leucocytozoon* among birds including domestic poultry (see Chapter 27). Simuliids play only a minor role in the transmission of arboviruses, but there is evidence that they are involved in the transmission of Venezuelan equine encephalitis in certain locations in Colombia, where more isolations of the virus were made from simuliids than from mosquitoes (11 cf. 8; 4 cf. 2).[51] They can also act as mechanical vectors of myxomatosis among rabbits.[32]

Simuliids have a well-deserved reputation as pests, particularly of livestock, in many areas of the world. Along the lower reaches of the Mississippi River *C. pecuarum* caused the death of large numbers of livestock prior to 1897. This loss was reduced as the flooding of the river was contained by the building of levees, but even as late as 1931 the deaths of more than a thousand mules was attributed to *C. pecuarum*.[7] Flood control has now eliminated *C. pecuarum* as a pest.

In Yugoslavia and Rumania the production of vast numbers of the Golubatz fly, *S. columbaschense* (sometimes spelt *S. columbaczense*), in the 1930s, caused thousands of deaths of livestock over a very wide area. Baranov established that this was a new species of simuliid which bred in the Danube at the Iron Gate at Golubatz, from which it dispersed 100-250 km.[2,3] Outbreaks of pest proportions required dry, warm weather and low water levels in the Danube in spring, creating extensive breeding sites. Environmental changes have eliminated *S. columbaschense* as a pest.[17]

Even when the numbers of simuliids biting do not cause deaths, livestock are less thrifty, with lower weight gains in beef cattle and decreased milk production in dairy cattle. Following the floods of 1974, *A. pestilens* reduced milk yields by up to 15 per cent in parts of Queensland.[30] More recently a haemorrhagic syndrome, associated with some deaths, has occurred among immigrants to forested areas along the Transamazon highway in Brazil, and has been attributed to intense biting of simuliids.[45]

Crosskey[17] lists 43 species of Simuliidae, which are pests and/or vectors of disease to man or domestic animals. Of these 37 are species of *Simulium,* four of *Austrosimulium* and one each of *Prosimulium* and *Cnephia.* This excludes *C. pecuarum* and *S. columbaschense.* Most of these species are pests but ten are involved in human disease, two in bovine onchocerciasis, and six as vectors of *Leucocytozoon.*

References

1. Baldwin, W., West, A.S. and Gomery, J. (1975). Dispersal patterns of blackflies (Diptera: Simuliidae) tagged with ^{32}P. *Canadian Entomologist 107*: 113-8
2. Baranov, N. (1935). New information on the Golubatz fly, *S. columbaczense. Review of Applied Entomology B 23*: 275-6
3. _____ (1937). Contribution to the knowledge of the Golubatz fly. V. (Study of the epidemiology of the fly in 1936). *Review of Applied Entomology B 25*: 249-50
4. Bennett, G.F., Fallis, A.M. and Campbell, A.G. (1972). The response of *Simulium* (*Eusimulium*) *euryadminiculum* Davies (Diptera: Simuliidae) to some olfactory and visual stimuli. *Canadian Journal of Zoology 50*: 793-800
5. Bradbury, W.C. and Bennett, G.F. (1974). Behaviour of adult Simuliidae (Diptera). I. Response to color and shape. *Canadian Journal of Zoology 52*: 251-9
6. _____ and Bennett, G.F. (1974). Behavior of adult Simuliidae (Diptera). II. Vision and olfaction in near-orientation and landing. *Canadian Journal of Zoology 52*: 1355-64
7. Bradley, G.H. (1935). Notes on the southern buffalo gnat *Eusimulium pecuarum* (Riley) (Diptera: Simuliidae). *Proceedings of the Entomological Society of Washington 37*: 60-4
8. _____ (1935). The hatching of eggs of the southern buffalo gnat. *Science 82*: 277-8
9. Chance, M.M. (1970). The functional morphology of the mouthparts of blackfly larvae (Diptera: Simuliidae). *Quaestiones Entomologicae 6*: 245-84
10. Charnetski, W.A. and Haufe, W.O. (1981). Control of *Simulium arcticum* Malloch in northern Alberta, Canada. pp. 117-32 in *Blackflies,* Marshall Laird (ed.), Academic Press, London
11. Colbo, M.H. and Moorhouse, D.E. (1974). The survival of eggs of *Austrosimulium pestilens* Mack. and Mack. (Diptera, Simuliidae). *Bulletin of Entomological Research 64*: 629-32
12. _____ and Moorhouse, D.E. (1979). The ecology of pre-imaginal Simuliidae (Diptera) in south-east Queensland, Australia. *Hydrobiologia 63*: 63-79
13. _____ and Wotton, R.S. (1981). Preimaginal blackfly bionomics. pp. 209-26 in *Blackflies,* Marshall Laird (ed.), Academic Press, London
14. Crisp, G. (1956). *Simulium and Onchocerciasis in the Northern Territories of the Gold Coast.* H.K. Lewis, London
15. Crosskey, R.W. (1973). Simuliidae. pp. 109-53 in *Insects and Other Arthropods of Medical Importance,* K.G.V. Smith (ed.), British Museum (National History), London
16. _____ (1981). Simuliid taxonomy — the contemporary scene. pp. 3-18 in *Blackflies* Marshall Laird (ed.), Academic Press, London
17. _____ (1981). Geographical distribution of Simuliidae. pp. 57-73 in *Blackflies,* Marshall Laird (ed.), Academic Press, London
18. Dalmat, H.T. (1955). The blackflies (Diptera, Simuliidae) of Guatemala and their role as vectors of onchocerciasis. *Smithsonian Miscellaneous Collections 125*: 1-425
19. Davies, L., Downe, A.E.R., Weitz, B. and Williams, C.B. (1962). studies on black flies (Diptera: Simuliidae) taken in a light trap in Scotland. II. Blood-meal identification by precipitin tests. *Transactions of the Royal Entomological Society of London 114*: 21-7
20. _____ and Williams, C.B. (1962). Studies on black flies (Diptera: Simuliidae) taken in a light trap in Scotland. I. Seasonal distribution, sex ratio and internal condition of

catches. *Transactions of the Royal Entomological Society of London 114*: 1-20
21. De Meillon, B. (1957). The bionomics of the vectors of onchocerciasis in the Ethiopian geographical region. *Bulletin of the World Health Organisation 16*: 509-22
22. Downes, J.A. (1962). What is an arctic insect? *Canadian Entomologist 94*: 143-62
23. Duke, B.O.L. (1975). The differential dispersal of nulliparous and parous *Simulium damnosum. Tropenmedizin und Parasitologie 26*: 88-97
24. Fredeen, F.J.H. (1964). Bacteria as food for blackfly larvae (Diptera: Simuliidae) in laboratory cultures and in natural streams. *Canadian Journal of Zoology 42*: 527-48
25. Garms, R., Walsh, J.F. and Davies, J.B. (1979). Studies on the reinvasion of the Onchocerciasis Control Programme in the Volta River basin by *Simulium damnosum* s.1. with emphasis on the south-western areas. *Tropenmedizin und Parasitologie 30*: 345-62
26. Grunewald, J. (1976). The hydrochemical and physical conditions of the development of the immature stages of some species of the *Simulium (Edwardsellum) damnosum* complex (Diptera). *Tropenmedizin und Parasitologie 27*: 438-54
27. Hinton, H.E. (1976). The fine structure of the pupal plastron of simuliid flies. *Journal of Insect Physiology 22*: 1061-70
28. _____ (1981). *Biology of Insect Eggs 2*: 734-5, Pergamon Press, Oxford
29. Hocking, B. (1953). The intrinsic range and speed of flight of insects. *Transactions of the Royal Entomological Society of London 104*: 223-345
30. Hunter, D.M. and Moorhouse, D.E. (1976). The effects of *Austrosimulium pestilens* on the milk production of dairy cattle. *Australian Veterinary Journal 52*: 97-9
31. _____ and Moorhouse, D.E. (1976). Comparative bionomics of adult *Austrosimulium pestilens* Mackerras and Mackerras and *A.bancrofti* (Taylor) (Diptera, Simuliidae). *Bulletin of Entomological research 66*: 453-67
32. Joubeit, L. and Monnet, P. (1975). Vérification expérimentale du rôle des simulies (*Tetisimulium bezzii* Corti, 1914 et *Odagmia* group *ornatum*) dans la transmission du virus myxomateux en Haute-Provence. *Revue de Médecine Vétérinaire 126*: 617-34
33. Kaneko, K., Saito, K. and Wonde, T. (1973). Observations on the diurnal rhythm of the biting activity of *Simulium damnosum* in Omo-Gibe and Gojjeb Rivers, south-west Ethiopia. *Japanese Journal of Sanitary Zoology 24*: 175-80
34. Kurtak, D. (1974). Overwintering of *Simulium pictipes* Hagen (Diptera: Simuliidae) as eggs. *Journal of Medical Entomology 11*: 383-4
35. Kurtak, D.C. (1979). Food of black fly larvae (Diptera: Simuliidae): seasonal changes in gut contents and suspended material at several sites in a single watershed. *Quaestiones Entomologicae 15*: 357-74
36. Ladle, M. (1972). Larval Simuliidae as detritus feeders in chalk streams. *Memorie dell'Instituto Italiano di Idrobiologia 29 (Supplement)*: 429-39
37. Le Berre, R. (1966). Contribution à l'étude biologique et écologique de *Simulium damnosum* Theobald, 1903 (Diptera, Simuliidae). *Mémoires ORSTOM 17*: 1-204
38. Lewis, D.J. (1956). Biting times of parous and nulliparous *Simulium damnosum. Naiure, London 178*: 98-9
39. Lewis, D.J. and Bennett, G.F. (1974). The blackflies (Diptera: Simuliidae) of insular Newfoundland. II. Seasonal succession and abundance in a complex of small streams on the Avalon Peninsular. *Canadian Journal of Zoology 52*: 1107-13
40. _____ and Bennett, G.F. (1975). The blackflies (Diptera: Simuliidae) of insular Newfoundland. III. Factors affecting the distribution and migration of larval simuliids in small streams on the Avalon Peninsular. *Canadian Journal of Zoology 53*: 114-23
41. Mansingh, A. and Steele, R.W. (1973). Studies on insect dormancy. I. Physiology of hibernation in the larvae of the blackfly *Prosimulium mysticum* Peterson. *Canadian Journal of Zoology 51*: 611-8
42. Moorhouse, D.E. and Colbo, M.H. (1973). On the swarming of *Austrosimulium pestilens* Mackerras and Mackerras (Diptera: Simuliidae). *Journal of the Australian Entomological Society 12*: 127-30
43. Neveu, A. (1973). Variations biométriques saisonnières chez les adultes de quelques espèces de Simuliidae (Diptera, Nematocera). *Archives de Zoologie Expérimentale et Générale 114*: 261-70
44. Peterson, B.V. and Dang, P.T. (1981). Morphological means of separating siblings of

the *Simulium damnosum* complex (Diptera: Simuliidae). pp. 45-56 in *Blackflies*, Marshall Laird (ed.), Academic Press, London

45. Pinheiro, F.P., Bensabath, G., Costa, D., Maroja, O.M., Lins, Z.C. and Andrade, A.H.P. (1974). Haemorrhagic syndrome of Altamira. *Lancet 1*: 639-42

46. Raastad, J.E. and Mehl, R. (1972). Night activity of black flies (Diptera, Simuliidae) in Norway. *Norsk Entomologisk Tidsskrift 19*: 172-3

47. Ramirez-Pérez, J., Rassi, E., Convit, J. and Ramirez, A. (1976). Importancia epedemiológica de los grupos de edad en las poblaciones de *Simulium metallicum* (Diptera: Simuliidae) en Venezuela. *Boletin de la Oficina Sanitaria Panamericana 80*: 105-22

48. Raybould, J.N. (1968). Studies on the immature stages of the *Simulium neavei* Roubaud complex and their associated crabs in the Eastern Usambara Mountains in Tanzania. I. Investigations in rivers and large streams. *Annals of Tropical Medicine and Parasitology 63*: 269-87

49. _____ and Yagunga, A.S.K. (1969). Studies on the immature stages of the *Simulium naevei* Roubaud complex and their associated crabs in the Eastern Usambara Mountains in Tanzania. II. Investigations in small heavily shaded streams. *Annals of Tropical Medicine and Parasitology 63*: 289-300

50. Rühm, W. (1975). Freilandbeobachtungen zum Funktionskreis der Eiablage verschiedener Simuliidenarten unter besonderer Berüchsichtigung von *Simulium argyreatum* Meig. (Dipt. Simuliidae). *Zeitschrift für Angewandte Entomologie 78*: 321-34

51. Sanmartin, C., Mackenzie, R.B., Trapido, H., Barreto, P., Mullenax, C.H., Gutierrez, E. and Lesmes, C. (1973). Encefalitis equina venezolana en Colombia 1967. *Boletin de la Oficina Sanitaria Panamericana 74*: 108-37

52. Service, M.W. (1979). Light trap collections of ovipositing *Simulium squamosum* in Ghana. *Annals of Tropical Medicine and Parasitology 73*: 487-90

53. Thomson, R.C.M. (1956). Communal oviposition in *Simulium damnosum* Theobald (Diptera, Simuliidae). *Nature, London 178*: 1297-9

54. Walsh, J.F., Davies, J.B. and Cliff, B. (1981). World Health Organization Onchocerciasis Control Programme in the Volta River basin. pp. 85-103 in *Blackflies*, Marshall Laird (ed.), Academic Press, London

55. Wellington, W.G. (1974). Black-fly activity during cumulus-induced pressure fluctuations. *Environmental Entomology 3*: 351-3

56. Wenk, P. (1981). Bionomics of adult blackflies. pp. 259-79 in *Blackflies*, Marshall Laird (ed.), Academic Press, London

57. Williams, T.R. (1974). Egg membranes of Simuliidae. *Transactions of the Royal Society of Tropical Medicine and Hygiene 68*: 15-16

58. _____ (1978). Cuticular microsculpture in larval blackflies (Diptera, Simuliidae). *Journal of Anatomy 127*: 214-5

59. Wotton, R.S. (1976). Evidence that blackfly larvae can feed on particles of colloidal size. *Nature, London 261*: 697

11 TABANIDAE (HORSEFLIES, DEER FLIES, CLEGS)

Tabanids are large, stout-bodied Brachycera (Figure 11.1), ranging in wing length from 5 to 25 mm. The large, bean-shaped head is much broader than long and the eyes are particularly well-developed, as befits predominantly diurnal creatures. As in the Simuliidae, the sexes can be differentiated on eye size with the males being holoptic and the females dichoptic. The frons, separating the eyes in the female, is wider in *Haematopota* (cleg) than in *Tabanus* (horsefly). The eyes are often brilliantly coloured, being spotted in *Chrysops*, with zigzag bands in *Haematopota*, and unicolorous or horizontally banded in *Tabanus*.[31] The eye colours disappear shortly after death.

The palps are 2-jointed with the second segment being particularly prominent. The antennae are porrect, i.e. stiffly projecting forwards, and consist of scape, pedicel and flagellum. The 3rd segment of the antenna, i.e. 1st of the flagellum, is greatly enlarged. The number of flagellar segments varies from four to eight. The mouthparts are adapted for both blood-sucking and lapping (see Chapter 4). Both sexes feed on nectar and in most species the female also feeds on blood but in some species the females have reduced mandibles and are solely nectar feeders. This occurs particularly in the Pangoniinae.

The wing venation is very well developed with all wing veins obvious (Figure 11.2). The venation is characteristic, but not diagnostic, similar venations occurring in related brachyceran families. Both the radius and the media are 4-branched with R_4 and R_5 straddling the apex of the wing. The discal cell is located more or less in the centre of the wing. The anal cell may be open or closed, i.e. the first anal vein may join Cu_1 before the wing margin. The squamae are large and obvious. The stout legs end in three pads because the empodium is pad-like and similar to the pulvilli (Figure 2.11).

Classification

More than 3,000 species of Tabanids have been described. The classification of Mackerras[28] is generally accepted[9,30,31] and is followed here. Four subfamilies are recognised on the basis of the male and female terminalia. One of these, the Scepsidinae, includes only four species of coastal, non-blood-sucking tabanids of which three are found in eastern Africa and one in South America. The Pangoniinae are of little economic importance but the Chrysopsinae, main genus *Chrysops*, and the Tabaninae, main genera

Figure 11.1: A, *Pangonia ruppellii* Female ×2; B, *Chrysops dispar* Female ×3.5; C, *Haematopota vittata* ×3

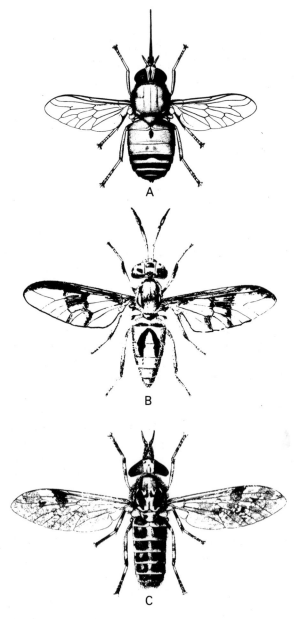

Sources: A and C from Castellani, A. and Chalmers, A.J. (1913). *A Manual of Tropical Medicine.* Baillière Tindall, London. B from Patton, W.S. and Cragg, F.W. (1913). *Textbook of Medical Entomology.* Christian Literature Society for India, London.

Figure 11.2: Wing of *Chrysops australis* ($\times$ 10)

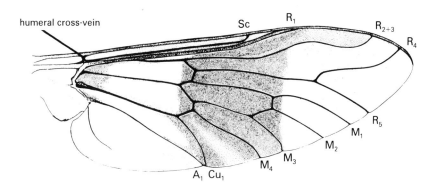

Tabanus and *Haematopota*, are of considerable economic significance. These three genera and the Pangoniinae may be distinguished by the following characters.

Pangoniinae

Head with functional ocelli; proboscis longer than head and may exceed length of insect (Figure 11.1A); antennae with seven or eight segments in the flagellum; a pair of large spurs apically on the hind tibiae (all tabanids have apical spurs on the mid tibiae) (Figure 11.3); wings clear or dusky. Largely tropical or subtropical in distribution.

Chrysops

Head with functional ocelli; proboscis not longer than head (Figure 11.1B); antennal flagellum with five segments; apical spurs on hind tibiae are small, and may be hidden in hair; wings usually with costal region dark and a single, broad, transverse, dark band (Figure 11.2). Mainly Holarctic and Oriental.

Tabanus

Head with, at most, vestigial ocelli; proboscis shorter than head; antennal flagellum with five segments; no apical spurs on hind tibiae; wings usually clear but may be dark or banded. Worldwide.

Haematopota

As for *Tabanus* but only four segments in the antennal flagellum and wings mottled (Figure 11.1C). Palaearctic, Afrotropical, Oriental. Absent from Australia and rare in the Americas.

Figure 11.3: Hind Tibia of a Pangonine

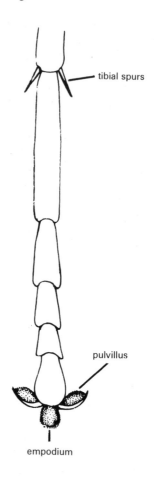

Biology and Life Cycle

Egg

Eggs are laid in masses of special design on leaves or rocks or debris over-hanging water. An egg mass may contain 200 to 1,000 eggs. Eggs of *Chrysops* are often laid in a single layer, and those of *Tabanus* and *Haematopota* stratified into three to four and two to three layers, respectively.[9] The creamy white eggs darken with age and are dark grey to black at hatching, which occurs in four or more days depending on temperature.[17]

Larva

The larva emerges from the egg using a hatching spine and moults soon after emergence. The 2nd-stage larva does not feed and is postively phototactic, moving over the surface of the substrate in close association with water.[9] After three to six days it moults into the 3rd instar which is negatively photactic and it burrows into the substrate, where it will spend many months. The number of moults is variable even in the same species and 7 to 11 instars may occur during larval development.[9]

The mature larva is a greyish white, soft bodied, cylindrical grub (Figure 11.4). In common with the larvae of other Brachycera the head is reduced and retractile into the thorax. It bears a pair of simple eyes and a pair of piercing mandibles. The larvae of *Tabanus* and *Haematopota* are carnivorous and cannibalistic whereas those of *Chrysops* feed on plant remains.[31] Consequently, *Chrysops* larvae are often found in considerable density compared to carnivorous larvae. The larval thorax and abdomen merge imperceptibly. Ventral abdominal pads and smaller, dorsal pads facilitate movement of the larva.

The larva is metapneustic with the spiracles opening at the end of a siphon, located dorsally on the 8th abdominal segment. The siphon is variable in shape, being short and conical in *H. pluvialis*,[7] and moderately long and blunt in *T. septentrionalis*.[6] Graber's organ is an internal structure, located dorsally of the gut and anterior to the siphon. The function of Graber's organ is unknown, and it appears as a longitudinal row of small, paired, dark bodies. The number of pairs is approximately related to the number of moults which the larva has undergone, but this relationship is not consistent.[7,9]

Pupa

At pupation the larva moves to the edge of aquatic habitats or to the surface of edaphic habitats. *T. biguttatus*, which breeds in temporary ponds, has an interesting pattern of behaviour at pupation, which is designed to avoid being exposed to predators and parasites when the pond dries out and the mud cracks. The larva comes near to the surface, and then descends on a spiral course to a depth of 8-10 cm, isolating a central core of mud. It then moves upwards on the outside of the core, and near the surface burrows into the core, hollowing out the interior to form a pupal cell. The entrance to the cell is blocked to deter predators. When the mud dries the soil cracks at the line of weakness made by the spiral but the mud cell remains intact. At emergence the pupa rasps its way through the cap of the cell and the adult emerges.[25,32]

The tabanid pupa is obtect (Figure 11.5) and with limited movement. There is no compound cephalothorax but head, thorax and abdomen are distinct. Respiration occurs through kidney-shaped, thoracic spiracles and seven pairs of abdominal spiracles on short, lateral projections (Figures 11.5A, B). The abdominal segments are each fringed with a row of stout bristles and the terminal segment bears a spiny aster (Figure 11.5C). The

Figure 11.4: Ninth Larval Instar of *Haematopota pluvialis*, (× 4). a.t., anal tubercle; d.p., dorsal pseudopod; h.c., head capsule; l.p. lateral pseudopod; l.v.p., lateroventral pseudopod; m.v.p., medioventral pseudopod; sph., siphon; I to XI, body segments of larva

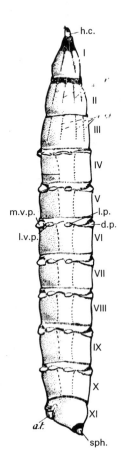

Source: From Cameron[7]

function of these spines is to give the pupa purchase, to enable it to move up and down in the substrate or pupal cell, permitting it to move away from adverse conditions at the surface, and to move up for emergence at the appropriate time. The head is often rugose and is used to effect escape from the soil. The pupal stage lasts about one to three weeks.

Adult

The newly emerged female mates before seeking a blood meal. Males form

Figure 11.5: Pupa of a Female *Haematopota pluvialis*. A, ventral view (×8); B, lateral view of head, thorax and first abdominal segment (×7); C, view of pupal aster from behind (×15). ant, antenna; a.sp.l, a.sp.VII, first and seventh abdominal spiracles; ast., aster; f.l., first femur; lb, labium; le., labrum; md., mandible; mx., maxilla; mx.p., maxillary palp; pl., pleuron; sp.f., spinous abdominal fringe; ster., sternum; ta.1, ta.2, ta.3, first, second and third tarsi; th.sp., thoracic spiracle; tb.1, tb.2, first and second tibiae; tr.2, second trochanter; w., wing

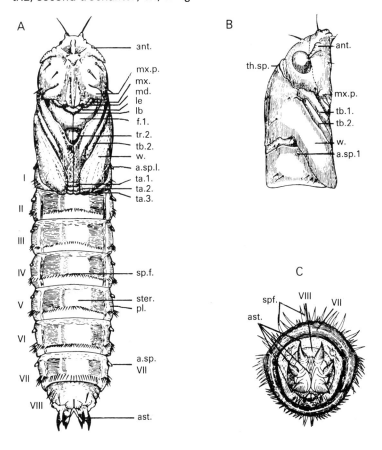

Source: From Cameron[7]

swarms, usually early in the morning, and virgin females entering the swarms are seized by the males with copulation beginning in the air and insemination being completed on the ground, taking about five minutes. In forests, male swarms occur above the canopy. Recognition of the female by the male is apparently visual, and the male has very well-developed eyes. The mated female seeks a blood meal which is required in most species for the development of the ovaries, although some species, e.g. *T. nigro-vittatus*[4] and *T. iyoensis*,[40] are autogenous in mainly haematophagous genera, and some genera, e.g. *Pangonia*[9] and *Scaptia*,[29] have many flower-feeding, non-blood-sucking species.

Most species are diurnal, but a few, e.g. *T. paradoxus*,[9] are nocturnal. Activity is higher on warm, sunny days with low wind speeds. European species have a temperature threshold of 13° to 15°C and reach maximum activity at 25°C, providing that the wind speed is less than 4 m/s.[9] Tabanids have evolved in close association with the ungulates,[31] and feed mainly on mammals and only rarely on birds. In feeding, the female will imbibe 20 to 200 mg of blood[9] but the loss of blood from the host is frequently greater, as the mouthparts of the tabanid make a relatively large puncture, which continues to ooze blood after the mouthparts have been withdrawn.

Bionomics

Oviposition

Gravid female tabanids are selective of the plants on which they oviposit. Thus *C. discalis* oviposits only on *Scirpus americanus* and not on other plants,[15] while various species of *Chrysops* selected *Pontederia cordata* and three other plants for oviposition out of 13 common plants in the site of oviposition at the lake edge.[14] In the field *T. taeniola* laid an average of 259 eggs.[16] The eggs of *C. discalis* hatched in five to six days and the young larvae dispersed widely from the site of hatching, being carried by water movement as they floated at the surface. Mature larvae of *C. discalis* have been found 10 m from the shore in shallow, alkaline lakes under 60 cm of water and at a depth of 5 to 10 cm in the underlying mud.[15]

Breeding Sites and Immature Stages

Three broad divisions of breeding sites have been recognised depending on the proportion of water which they contain. *Chrysops* larvae are generally hydrobionts, occurring in the wettest situations; *Tabanus* larvae are hemi-hydrobionts, occurring in soil near water; while *Haematopota* larvae are edaphic, being found in soil.[9,38] Lane[26] found no immature tabanids in woodland litter and soil, but this was to be expected, since he found no larvae of *Haematopota*. He found *Chrysops* larvae to be associated with large amounts of decaying organic matter, on which presumably they fed; *Hybomitra* in mosses; larvae of *Sylvius* in sand and silt above the margins of flowing water; while larvae of *Tabanus* were generally more widely distributed, with those of *T. punctifer* occurring in every semiaquatic habitat except tree holes. Within a habitat larvae may be generally distributed as are those of *C. fuliginosus* and *T. nigrovittatus* in *Spartina* salt marshes.[13]

Larvae of *T. taeniola* pass through seven instars usually but the range is six to nine instars before pupation.[16] Although the larvae of *C. fuliginosus* are widespread through the salt marsh, adult emergences occur within 9 m of the ecotone where the influence of fresh water is apparent.[19] Pupae of *T. taeniola* were able to reach the surface from a depth of 2 m in dry sand but from only 10 cm when the sand was wet, the more natural situation.[18] Speed of development is temperature-dependent. At a constant high temperature, i.e. 32° and 35°C, *T. taeniola* completes its life cycle from egg to adult in 10 to 11 weeks but at 22°C it takes 42 weeks. This 'hibernation' is a function of temperature and season. At 32° and 35°C there is no 'hibernation' while at 22°C, 'hiberation' always occurs with the prepupal stage being prolonged. At 27°C 'hibernation' occurs in larvae, which emerge from eggs laid after August, but is absent in larvae hatching from eggs laid in May to August.[16] Pavlova[33] calculated the threshold temperatures and total day-degrees required for the development of the pupal stage of ten species of tabanids. Thresholds varied from 5.7° to 10.1°C and day-degrees from 92 to 192. For *T. autumnalis*, *H. pluvialis* and *C. relictus* the respective figures were: 8.9°, 7.2°, 8.7°C and 176, 170 and 104 day-degrees.

Adult Mating and Feeding

Males of *C. fuliginosus* become active earlier in the day than the females. Mating and blood-feeding are temperature-dependent with mating occurring at 19° to 20°C, and females becoming host-seeking at 24° to 25°C.[8] The effect of this is for mating to occur early in the morning and blood-feeding later in the day. *T. nigrovittatus* and *T. iyoensis*, which are autogenous for the first batch of eggs, require a blood meal for second and subsequent batches.[4,40]

Sugars play a large part in the survival of tabanids, although they are inadequate for egg production. With constant access to water and either blood or sugar solution *C. silacea* survived considerably longer on sugar but, of course, laid no eggs.[10] *T. taeniola* fed on sugar within a few hours of emergence but did not take its first blood meal for several days.[18] Fifty-nine to 97 per cent of *T. iyoensis* coming to take a blood meal had previously fed on sugar.[41]

Host-finding by tabanids is similar to that outlined earlier for Simuliids (p. 183) involving host odour, carbon dioxide and visual stimuli. Visual cues were the most important when the host was moving, but a stationary host was located either visually or olfactorily, the two stimuli reinforcing each other; and the catch increased when both cues were presented simultaneously.[39] Carbon dioxide was a powerful attractant, and 12 species of tabanids were attracted equally by carbon dioxide at 3.5 litres per min or by a steer, while *T. sulcifrons* and *T. fuscicostatus* were actually attracted in larger numbers to carbon dioxide than to the steer.[35] Species feed preferentially on different parts of the host. *C. fuliginosus* attacks the head of man and *C. atlanticus* attacks the upper parts of a walking man, but the lower limbs of a seated man.[1] *C. silacea* feeds on the lower limbs of man and cattle.

Adult Activity and Dispersal

The activity of tabanids is greatly influenced by meteorological conditions, especially light intensity and temperature.[34] The flight activity of three species of salt marsh tabanids responded differently to light intensity. *C. fuliginosus* was most active under very bright conditions (100,000 lux); *T. nigrovittatus* under bright, warm conditions (40,000 lux; 25°C); while *C. atlanticus* was most active under hot, overcast conditions (5,000 lux; 30°C).[11]

Burnett and Hays[5] found barometric pressure to be the most important meteorological factor influencing the flight of *T. pallidescens* and *T. fulvulus*, which formed 60 per cent of their total catch of tabanids. Both species were influenced by evaporation, but the catches of *T. fulvulus* were more closely related to changes in rate of evaporation, and those of *T. pallidescens* to the actual rate of evaporation. Three species of *Tabanus* showed marked bimodal, diurnal activity in sunny weather, but activity became irregular under cloudy conditions unless the air temperature was above 25°C, when it remained bimodal.[36] Some species, e.g. *C. fuliginosus*, and *T. taeniola*, normally have only one period of activity during the day.[1,23]

In the open, tabanids, such as *T. nigrovittatus*, remain close to the ground,[37] but in the forest many species occur in the canopy, e.g. *C. langi*, while *C. silacea* feeds in the canopy and only comes to the forest floor in clearings or when attracted by wood smoke. Wood smoke increases the biting of *C. silacea* at ground level by more than ten-fold, and that of *C. dimidiata* by nearly five-fold.[12] The richness of the canopy fauna was appreciated when a nest of *Bembix bequaerti dira* was examined. This wasp builds its nest at ground level but hunts in the canopy. The nest contained 26 species of tabanids, of which four were species new to science, two had previously been rare, and there were also the unknown males of ten more species.[30] Clearly man's limited view of the tabanid fauna from the forest floor is but a pale reflection of the teeming life of the canopy.

Tabanid flies differ in the habitats they haunt. Inaoka[21] recognised three groups: (a) species that were confined to forest; (b) those that occurred on open land; and (c) those that were widespread, i.e. eurytopic. With the extension of pasture and rice production in recent years in Hokkaido, there has been a change in the tabanid fauna from one dominated by forest/eurytopic species to an openland/eurytopic fauna, with a corresponding decrease in *H. tristis*, and an increase in *T. nipponicus*.

Although tabanid flies have an intrinsic flight range of over 50 km,[20] they are not noted for their wide dispersal. The salt marsh tabanids *T. nigrovittatus, C. fuliginosus* and *C. atlanticus* dispersed less than 200 m from the marshes from which they emerged.[19,37] *T. iyoensis* and *C. silacea* dispersed 1 to 3 km,[2,22] and *C. discalis* can be numerous 7 km from its source;[15] but these flights represent only a small fraction of the potential flight range of tabanids.

Survival

In the field, adults live a maximum of three to four weeks, and produce five to six batches of eggs.[2,16] The survival rate of *T. iyoensis* has been calculated to be 0.73 per day,[22] which gives a survival of 11 per cent after one week, and 0.13 per cent after 3 weeks. Making certain reasonable assumptions, Inoue *et al.*[22] have calculated the emergence of *T. iyoensis* in a linear habitat to be 14,000 per metre of river.

With the larval stage being very long, tabanids pass adverse conditions in that stage. Little is known about the ways in which tabanids survive drought, except for the pupal mud cells constructed by *T. biguttatus* and *T. conspicuus*,[32] but presumably larvae survive deep in soil, where the atmosphere is moist. The cold season can be passed in the larval stage, but a problem arises when the soil freezes. *T. autumnalis* overwinters as a larva at a depth of 2 to 20 cm, and 50 to 100 cm above the waterline of small lakes, where it is warmed by the winter sun. Larvae of this species can survive $-4°C$ and, as the temperature 10 cm deep in the soil remains above that threshold, the larvae survive. After cold acclimatisation, 60 per cent of *T. autumnalis* larvae can survive $-6°C$. *C. caecutiens* larvae remain in the soil below water, where they are protected by a layer of ice.[3]

Medical and Veterinary Importance

The role of tabanids as vectors of disease has been reviewed by Krinsky.[24] Tabanids are biological vectors of three species of filaroid worms: *Elaeophora schneideri*, the arterial worm of sheep; *Loa loa*, the cause of Calabar or fugitive swellings in man in West Africa; and *Dirofilaria roemeri*, a parasite of macropodid marsupials (see Chapter 32). Tabanids are also biological vectors of the blood-dwelling sporozoan, *Haematoproteus metchnikovi*, of turtles, and there is evidence that tabanids may be biological vectors of *Trypanosoma theileri*, a benign parasite of cattle (see Chapters 27 and 29).

The mouthparts of tabanids are particularly well suited to the mechanical transmission of blood-dwelling pathogens from host to host (p. 53). This ability is enhanced when the species is a determined feeder, passing readily from host to host as, for example, does *T. taeniola*.[42] Leclercq[27] has summarised the extensive experiments of Nieschultz made between 1925 and 1930, on the mechanical transmission of *Trypanosoma evansi*, which causes Surra in camels and horses (see Chapter 29). Species of *Tabanus* were more efficient vectors than those of *Chrysops* and *Haematopota*, and all tabanids were better vectors than mosquitoes or biting Muscids, such as *Stomoxys*. The probability of transmission occurring declined rapidly with time between successive feeds on an infected and a susceptible host. It was as high as 0.5, when the two feeds were separated by less than 15 min, but declined to 0.04, 0.003, 0.001 and 0.0003 when the intervals were 1,3,6 and 24 hours, respectively.[27]

Tr. evansi and *Tr. vivax viennei* are only transmitted mechanically, and tabanids are the most important of the mechanical vectors; but it is more difficult to evaluate the importance of mechanical transmission where there are alternative routes of infection. Thus the role of tabanids in the transmission of pathogenic trypanosomes in the tsetse fly (*Glossina*) areas is unknown. With regard to other diseases there is evidence that tabanids are important mechanical vectors of *Anaplasma marginale* to cattle; of *Francisella tularensis*, the causative organism of tularaemia, to man and domestic stock; and of *Bacillus anthracis*, which causes anthrax in man and animals. Tabanids are also the vectors of two viral diseases, equine infectious anaemia and hog cholera, and they may play a significant role in the transmission of the rinderpest virus.

Independent of their role in spreading disease, when tabanids are abundant, they worry stock and make them less thrifty. Indeed in some areas, e.g. Fraser Island, Queensland, tabanids can be so great a nuisance as to prevent the pleasurable use of recreational areas by man.

References

1. Anderson, J.F. (1973). Biting behavior of salt marsh deerflies. *Annals of the Entomological Society of America 66*: 21-3
2. Beesley, W.N. and Crewe, W. (1963). The bionomics of *Chrysops silacea* Austen 1907. II. The biting rhythm and dispersal in rainforest. *Annals of Tropical Medicine and Parasitology 57*: 191-203
3. Boshko, G.V. and Shevtsova, N.P. (1975). Hibernation of tabanid larvae in the Ukrainian SSR. *Vestnik Zoologii 5*: 71-4
4. Bosler, E.M. and Hansens, E.J. (1974). Natural feeding behavior of adult saltmarsh greenheads, and its relation to oogensis. *Annals of the Entomological Society of America 67*: 321-4
5. Burnett, A.M. and Hays, K.L. (1974). Some influences of meteorological factors on flight activity of female horse flies (Diptera: Tabanidae). *Environmental Entomology 3*: 515-21
6. Cameron, A.E. (1926). Bionomics of the Tabanidae (Diptera) of the Canadian prairie. *Bulletin of Entomological Research 17*: 1-42
7. _____ (1934). The life history and structure of *Haematopota pluvialis* Linné (Tabanidae). *Transactions of the Royal Society of Edinburgh 58*: 211-50
8. Catts, E.P. and Olkowski, W. (1972). Biology of Tabanidae (Diptera): mating and feeding behavior of *Chrysops fuliginosus*. *Environmental Entomology 1*: 448-53

9. Chvala, M., Lyneborg, L. and Moucha, J. (1972). *The Horse Flies of Europe (Diptera, Tabanidae).* Entomological Society of Copenhagen, Copenhagen
10. Crewe, W. and Beesley, W.N. (1963). The bionomics of *Chrysops silacea* Austen 1907. I. The longevity and food requirements of the adult fly. *Annals of Tropical Medicine and Parasitology 57*: 1-6
11. Dale, W.E. and Axtell, R.C. (1975). Flight of the salt marsh Tabanidae (Diptera), *Tabanus nigrovittatus, Chrysops atlanticus* and *C. fuliginosus.* Correlation with temperature, light, moisture and wind velocity. *Journal of Medical Entomology 12*: 551-7
12. Duke, B.O.L. (1959). Studies on the biting habits of *Chrysops.* VI A comparison of the biting habits, monthly biting densities and infection rates of *C. silacea* and *C. dimidiata* (Bombe form) in the rain forest at Kumba, Southern Cameroons, U.U.K.A. *Annals of Tropical Medicine and Parasitology 53*: 203-14
13. Dukes, J.C., Edwards, T.D. and Axtell, R.C. (1974). Distribution of larval Tabanidae (Diptera) in a *Spartina alterniflora* salt marsh. *Journal of Medical Entomology 11*:79-83
14. Foster, C.H., Renaud, G.D. and Hays, K.L. (1973). Some effects of the environment on oviposition by *Chrysops* (Diptera: Tabanidae). *Environmental Entomology 2*: 1048-50
15. Gjullin, C.M. and Mote, D.C. (1945). Notes on the biology and control of *Chrysops discalis* Williston (Diptera: Tabanidae). *Proceedings of Entomological Society of Washington 47*: 236-44
16. Hafez, M., El-Ziady, S. and Hefnawy, T. (1970). Biological studies of the immature stages of *Tabanus taeniola* P. de B. (Diptera: Tabanidae) in Egypt. *Bulletin de la Société Entomologique d'Egypte 54*: 465-93
17. _____ El-Ziady, and Hefnawy, T. (1970). Studies on the feeding habits of *Tabanus taeniola* P. de B. (Diptera: Tabanidae). *Bulletin de la Société Entomologique d'Egypte 54*: 365-76
18. _____ El-Ziady, S. and Hefnawy, T. (1970). Biological studies on *Tabanus taeniola* P. de B. adults (Diptera: Tabanidae). *Bulletin de le Société Entomologique d'Egypte 54*: 327-44
19. Hansens, E.J. and Robinson, J.W. (1973). Emergence and movement of the saltmarsh deerflies *Chrysops fuliginosus* and *Chrysops atlanticaus.* *Annals of the Entomological Society of America 66*: 1215-8
20. Hocking, B. (1953). The intrinsic range and speed of flight of insects. *Transactions of the Royal Entomological Society of London 104*: 223-345
21. Inaoka, T. (1975). Habitat preference of tabanid flies in Hokkaido based upon the collection of female adults. *Journal of the Faculty of Science Hokkaido University Series VI Zoology 20*: 77-92
22. Inoue, T., Kamimura, K. and Watanabe, M. (1973). A quantitative analysis of dispersal in a horse fly *Tabanus iyoensis* Shiraki and its application to estimate the population size. *Research on Population Ecology 14*: 209-33
23. Kangwagye, T.N. (1973). Diurnal and nocturnal biting activity of flies (Diptera) in western Uganda. *Bulletin of Entomological Research 63*: 17-29
24. Krinsky, W.L. (1976). Animal disease agents transmitted by horse flies and deer flies (Diptera: Tabanidae). *Journal of Medical Entomology 13*: 225-75
25. Lamborn, W.A. (1930). The remarkable adaptation by which a dipterous pupa (Tabanidae) is preserved from the dangers of fissures in drying mud. *Proceedings of the Royal Society of London B 106*: 83-7
26. Lane, R.S. (1976). Density and diversity of immature Tabanidae (Diptera) in relation to habitat type in Mendocino County, California. *Journal of Medical Entomology 12*: 683-91
27. Leclercq, M. (1952). Introduction à l'étude des tabanides et revision des espèces de Belgique. *Mémoires de l'Institut Royale des Sciences Naturelles de Belgique 123*: 1-80
28. Mackerras, I.M. (1954). The classification and distribution of Tabanidae (Diptera). I. General Review. *Australian Journal of Zoology 2*: 431-54
29. _____ (1955). The classification and distribution of Tabanidae (Diptera). II. History; morphology; classification: subfamily Pangoniinae. *Australian Journal of Zoology 3*: 439-511
30. Oldroyd, H. (1952-7). *Horseflies of the Ethiopian Region. I. Haematopota and*

Hippocentrum. II. Tabanus and related genera. III. Chrysopinae, Scepsidinae, Pangoniinae. British Museum (Natural History), London

31. _____ (1973). Tabanidae (horseflies, clegs, deerflies etc.). pp. 195-208 in *Insects and Other Arthropods of Medical Importance*, K.G.V. Smith (ed.), British Museum (Natural History), London

32. Parsons, B.T. (1971). Construction of mud cylinders by species of the genus *Tabanus* (Dipt. Tabanidae). *Entomologist's Monthly Magazine 107*: 89-90

33. Pavlova, R.P. (1974). Influence of the temperature of the surrounding environment on the length of the pupal phase of tabanids. *Parazitologiya 8*: 243-8

34. Polyakov, V.A. and Polyakov, M.A. (1973). Statistical analysis of the influence of environmental factors on the flight of tabanids in the conditions of Chukotka. *Sel'skokhozyaistvennaya Biologiya 8*: 690-4

35. Roberts, R.H. (1972). Relative attractiveness of CO_2 and a steer to Tabanidae, Culicidae and *Stomoxys calcitrans*. *Mosquito News 32*: 208-11

36. Sasakawa, M., Yoshida, A., Yamouchi, T. and Kuriyama, M. (1969). Studies on the bionomics and control of the horseflies attacking the grazing Japanese cattle. III.Diurnal biting activity in cloudy weather and control of the flies by trapping. *Review of Applied Entomology B 61*: 2360 (1973)

37. Schultze, T.L., Hansens, E.J. and Trout, J.R. (1975). Some environmental factors affecting the daily and seasonal movements of the salt marsh greenhead *Tabanus nigrovittatus*. *Environmental Entomology 4*: 965-71

38. Soboleva, R.G. and Bodrova, Yu.D. (1973). The breeding places of gadflies (Diptera: Tabanidae) in the southern part of the Maritime Territory. *Entomological Researches in the Far East, Issue 2 Diptera of the Far East* 57-77

39. Vale. G.A. and Phelps, R.J. (1974). Notes on the host-finding behaviour of Tabanidae (Diptera). *Arnoldia, Rhodesia 6*: 1-6

40. Watanabe, M. and Kamimura, K. (1971). Observations on the autogeny of horsefly, *Tabanus iyoensis* Shiraki. *Japanese Journal of Sanitary Zoology 22*: 170-6

41. _____ and Kamimura, K. (1975). Nectar sucking behaviour of *Tabanus iyoensis* (Diptera: Tabanidae). *Japanese Journal of Sanitary Zoology 26*: 41-7

42. Wiesenhutter, E. (1975). Research into the relative importance of Tabanidae (Diptera) in mechanical disease transmission. II Investigation of the behaviour and feeding habits of Tabanidae in relation to cattle. *Journal of Natural History 9*: 385-92

12 GLOSSINIDAE (TSETSE FLIES)

The tsetse flies form a well-defined taxonomic group which has previously been included in the Muscidae as a separate subfamily, Glossinae, or with the blood-sucking muscids in the Stomoxinae, but is now regarded as a separate family, the Glossinidae. Tsetse flies are readily recognised. They are medium to large brown flies, 6 to 14 mm long, excluding the proboscis. The long, forwardly directed proboscis is sheathed by equally long palps (Figure 12.1). The antenna has the typical cyclorrhaphan structure with an elongated 3rd segment but is distinctive in that the rays of the arista are feathered and are only present on the dorsal side (Figure 12.2). When viewed laterally the 3rd segment bears a fringe of hairs, the length of which is a specific character. The eyes are dichoptic in both sexes. The wings are folded scissor-like at rest and extend a short distance beyond the end of the abdomen. The wing venation is characterised by the discal cell being

Figure 12.1: Female *Glossina fuscipes* Seen from Above, Resting on a Vertical Surface

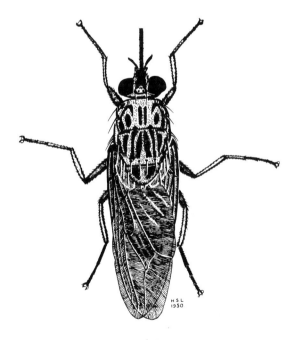

Source: From Buxton[12]

Figure 12.2: Antennae of *Glossina*. A, *G. palpalis* (× 50); B, *G. nigrofusca* (× 40); C, *G. morsitans* (× 45). *a, b, c,* first, second and third antennal segments; *d,* arista

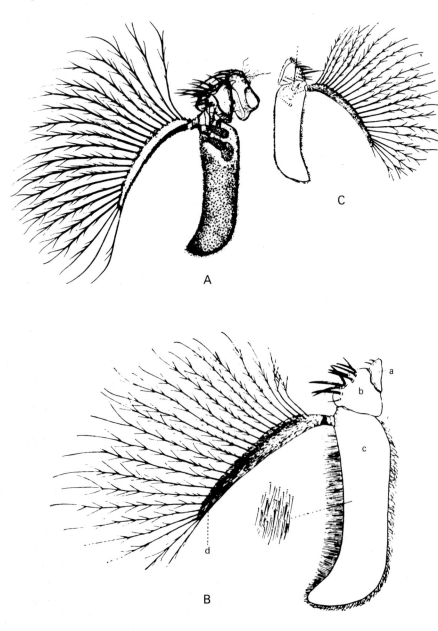

Source: From Buxton[12]

Figure 12.3: Wing of *Glossina* × 15

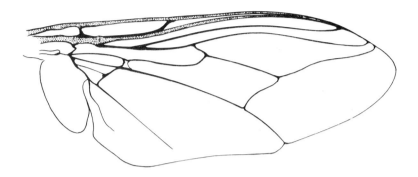

'hatchet' shaped (Figure 12.3). The abdomen of the male bears posteriorly on its ventral surface a button-like structure, the folded male terminalia. This is absent in the female. Both sexes are haematophagous and therefore both are potential vectors of trypanosomiasis to man and domestic animals.

Classification

Only one genus, *Glossina*, is included in the Glossinidae. At the present day *Glossina* is confined to the Afrotropical region but in the past it occurred in the Nearctic since four species of fossil *Glossina* have been found in beds of Miocene age in Colorado. The genus *Glossina* contains 30 living taxa, 22 species and eight subspecies.[41] The species are assigned to three subgenera (*Glossina, Nemorhina, Austenina*), which were formerly referred to respectively as *morsitans, palpalis* and *fusca* groups, named after the commonest species in each group. The status of the subspecies is unresolved but there is evidence of genetic incompatibility causing sterility when subspecies of *G. morsitans* are cross-mated.[15]

The subgenus *Glossina* contains five species of which two, *G. morsitans* and *G. pallidipes*, are of major economic importance, and *G. swynnertoni and G. austeni* are of local significance. They are small to medium sized tsetse, 6 to 11 mm long, with distinct bands on the abdomen (except in *G. austeni*); the distal segments of the hind tarsus are dark dorsally; and the male claspers are swollen distally. They are species which are commonly found in savanna woodland and evergreen thickets, except for *G. austeni*, which is restricted to coastal forest and relict forest. Although *G. morsitans* ranges widely in tropical Africa the other four species in the subgenus occur only in East Africa.

Potts[41] recognises three zoogeographical regions when discussing tsetse distribution: West Africa, which is approximately Africa north of the Bay of Biafra; Central Africa, which extends from West Africa eastwards to the Sudan and south to Namibia and includes the densely forested belt west of the western Rift Valley; and East Africa, which is Africa east of the previous region and includes the countries bordering the Indian Ocean and extends west to Angola and the lakes of the western Rift Valley.

The subgenus *Nemorhina* also contains five species of which three, *G. palpalis*, *G. fuscipes* and *G. tachinoides*, occur in riverine and lakeside habitats and are particularly important as vectors of human trypanosomiasis. They are small to medium sized tsetse, 6 to 11 mm long, with dorsum of abdomen dark brown (except in *G. tachinoides*, which has a banded abdomen of the *morsitans* type), all hind tarsi dark dorsally, and male claspers not swollen distally but joined by a membrane. The subgenus occurs mainly in West and Central Africa, extending eastwards to the shores of Lake Victoria. *G. tachinoides* is largely restricted to West Africa and *G. fuscipes* to Central Africa.

The 12 species of the subgenus *Austenina* are, except for *G. brevipalpis* and *G. longipennis*, forest dwelling species and have little contact with man or his livestock, and therefore are of little economic importance, except when man moves his cattle into forested areas, as for example in western Uganda.[1] *Austenina* are large tsetse, 9 to 11 mm in length, with strong bristles on the pteropleuron as well as on the sternopleuron, and in which male claspers are neither swollen distally nor joined by a membrane. In the other subgenera, *Glossina* and *Nemorhina*, there are no strong bristles on the pteropleuron.[41]

Life Cycle

Tsetse flies are viviparous, the female producing fully grown larvae. Each ovary is composed of two polytrophic ovarioles. Ovaries and ovarioles produce ova alternately, beginning with the right ovary. Since the relict body left in the ovariole after ovulation can be easily recognised it is possible to age (physiologically) tsetse flies accurately over the first four cycles by observing the condition of the ovaries and the contents of the uterus.[47] Using these criteria 14 different stages can be recognised, covering the equivalent of 40 days of adult life at 25°C. The technique has been elaborated to enable female flies to be classified up to 80 days.[13] The egg passes down the common oviduct to the uterus (Figure 12.4), where its micropyle comes opposite the opening of the spermathecal duct. The release of sperm is regulated by a sphincter on the spermathecal duct, which opens at ovulation but is closed during the rest of the breeding cycle.[45]

Figure 12.4: Reproductive Organs of Female *Glossina*. Dotted line in uterus indicate position of larva with its anterior end lying near the duct from the uterine or milk glands

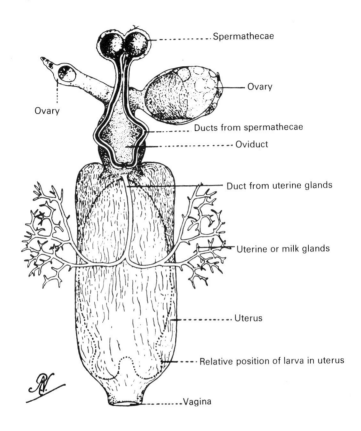

Source: From Buxton[12]

Larva

The larva emerges from the egg by means of a labral tooth, and is then nourished by secretions of the uterine gland, which are discharged on to the oviductal shelf (Figure 12.4). The larva is held in position by the choriothete, which secretes a sticky material. Although the chorion and exuviae may adhere to the sticky material the choriothete plays no role in hatching or ecdysis as originally believed.[44] As the larva grows in size the role of the choriothete declines and the 2nd instar larva is held in place by uterine ridges, and the 3rd instar by the walls of the uterus, which are stretched by the bulk of larva. A fully-grown 3rd instar larva at deposition weighs more than the containing female. At 25°C the egg stage lasts four days, and the three instars, 1, $1\frac{1}{2}$ and $2\frac{1}{2}$ days, respectively, in a nine-day developmental cycle. (All times quoted in this chapter will refer to 25°C unless stated otherwise.)

The larva grows steadily throughout its time in the uterus feeding on secreted 'milk'. To meet the growing larval needs the uterine gland goes through a cycle during which its cells increase in volume a hundredfold, i.e. $\times 4.6$ linearly. Maximum size of the cells is reached about two-thirds of the way through pregnancy, just before the larva reaches the 3rd instar.[33] The secretion is mainly composed of acidic lipids at first but changes later to protein. The fully-grown larva contains a great deal of unassimilated food material in its gut, which comprises two-thirds of the live weight of the larva. Perhaps that is why there is no open connection between the midgut and the hindgut of the larva, to avoid loss of nutrients through the anus. At deposition the larval gut contains 80 per cent of the fat, 70 per cent of the water and 50 per cent of the protein in the whole larva.[30]

Symbionts. Fimbriated, Gram-negative bacteroids occur free in the tubules of the uterine gland, but not intracellularly.[32] They could be passed to the larva with the 'milk', and be the source of the symbiotic bacteroids, which occur intracellularly in the mycetome of the anterior midgut of the adult. However, similar bacteroids have been described as being intra-cellular in the ovaries of *G. austeni.*[24] It is still an open question whether the symbionts are transferred to the ovum in the ovary, or to the larva with the 'milk', and it is possible that both routes may be effective in view of the importance of symbionts to reproduction in *Glossina.* Tsetse flies whose symbionts have been reduced by antibiotics have reduced fecundity and fertility.[23]

Respiration. The 1st and 2nd instar larvae respire through posterior spiracles, which become elaborated into polypneustic lobes in the 3rd instar (Figure 12.4 and 12.5a). In each lobe there are three airchambers which open via numerous supernumerary stigmata. The 2nd instar tracheal system is persistent and remains within the 3rd instar system, except pos-teriorly, where it opens to the exterior between the polypneustic lobes. The three outer chambers are connected individually to the inner air chambers by felt chambers. The felt chambers act as pistons, and when they are drawn forwards air enters the supernumerary stigmata, and, at the same time, air is driven forwards between the 2nd and 3rd instar tracheae, back-wards through the 2nd instar tracheae, and out through the 2nd instar spi-racles. Reversal of air flow is prevented by the stigmata being closed by valves.[6]

Pupa. The polypneustic lobes darken and harden 24 to 48 hours before the larva is deposited (Figure 12.5). The length of free larval life is influenced

Figure 12.5: Pupa and Puparium of *Glossina morsitans*. a, puparium, showing pupa by dotted lines; b, adult fly emerging from puparium, showing ptilinum; c, pupa removed from puparium

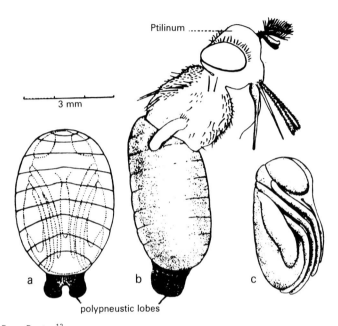

Ptilinum

3 mm

a b c

polypneustic lobes

Source: From Buxton[12]

by time of deposition, presence or absence of light, and nature of substrate. Pupariation is accelerated by darkness and mechanical stimulation of a particulate substrate. The larva is negatively phototactic, positively thigmotactic, and seeks a high humidity. It burrows rapidly into the substrate, and pupariation occurs within one to five hours of deposition.[30] During barrelleling and contraction a fluid is discharged from the anus, the function of which is uncertain, but it may include a pheromone attracting females to larviposit in the same site.[36] The puparium darkens rapidly becoming light brown in 10 min and dark brown in several hours. During this process the endocuticle of the larval cuticle is sclerotised to form the puparium. Pupal apolysis occurs two to three days later, when the pupal cuticle is formed. At first the pupa is cryptocephalic, but it becomes phanerocephalic five days later when the appendages are everted. Two days later the pupal/adult apolysis occurs, but another three weeks will elapse before adult development is complete, and the adult emerges.[30] The polypneustic lobes cease to function after pupal formation. The pupal spiracles are located in the same position as the adult prothoracic spiracles, and they continue to function until adult emergence.[7]

Adult

The adult emerges from the puparium using its ptilinum to force off the cap from the puparium (Figure 12.5b), and then to burrow upwards to the surface. The wings are expanded, but for the first ten days of its life the adult is soft to handle, and is said to be the 'teneral'. During this phase the endocuticle is secreted, the exocuticle hardened, and the proportion of myofibrils in the thoracic musculature greatly increased.[30]

Mating. Females emerge one to four days before the males, and are ready for mating when they are two to three days old, by which time they will have fed twice. Although spermatogenesis is complete well before adult emergence, males are not fully fertile until seven days old, when they will have fed several times.[30]

Males orientate to the female visually, but the initiation of a copulatory response requires the presence of a contact pheromone,[31] which appears in the cuticular waxes of the females two days before eclosion, and remains for the rest of the female's life.[26] Males responded similarly to both dead and alive conspecific females, and showed varying responses to females of other species, i.e. allospecific females, except for female *G. austeni* to which only male *G. austeni* of the seven species tested, responded.[27]

During copulation the male transfers successively a diffuse secretion, material to form the spermatophore coat, and finally the spermatozoa, some of which may be introduced directly into the spermathecal duct, but most stream into the spermathecae after cessation of copulation.[40]

Reproduction. With free access to a host for feeding a female will have a fully developed egg ready for ovulation seven to nine days after emergence, but ovulation is dependent upon copulation exceeding 60 min. Ovulation appears to be independent of any material transferred by the male but controlled by the hormones released as a result of prolonged copulation. Ovulation can be produced by several interrupted matings during which no spermatozoa are transferred. It can also be induced in a virgin female by the injection of haemolymph from a mated female.[14,48] Males may mate repeatedly, but females require only one insemination to be fully fertile. If a female is mated twice, the products of the first mating fertilise 75 per cent of the progeny.[30]

Subsequent ovulations occur within an hour of parturition, and therefore occur at nine- to ten-day intervals. Since the first ovulation occurs when the female is nine to ten days old, the first larviposition will be made at about 20 days, followed by subsequent larvipositions at ten-day intervals. Therefore a female must live for 30 days to produce two progeny as replacements for herself and her mate. Equal numbers of each sex occur at emergence. This implies that tsetse flies must be long lived if the population is not to die out, and, in fact, females survive for several months. Female *G. palpalis* have been recaptured six months after having been caught in the wild, marked and released. A reasonable average length of life is six weeks for males and 14 weeks for females.[35]

Jackson[28] calculated that the length of life of male *G. morsitans* varied from two weeks in the dry season to six weeks in the wet season. The low reproduction rate of tsetse flies implies that populations of *Glossina* will be relatively steady, changing only slowly with time. They will not be subject to rapid fluctuations common in fecund ovigerous insects such as mosquitoes and houseflies. Over a period of 16 years monthly variations in populations of *G. p. palpalis* varied by factors of 2.3 to 12.9 in any particular year, while the highest population in any one year was only 3.8 times that found in the year with the lowest population.[29]

It has already been pointed out that ovulation is hormonally controlled and there is evidence that other processes in the reproductive cycle are also under hormonal control, but the details are difficult to resolve because events overlap. Except in the first ovulation, larviposition and ovulation take place within a short time of each other. Similarly vitellogenesis of the next ovum occurs together with the secretory cycle of the uterine glands.[37]

Feeding and Digestion. When *Glossina* feeds, blood passes at first into the midgut, which has a limited capacity, and, when the midgut is distended, blood passes into the more capacious crop. Blood is transferred from the crop to the midgut, as required, by the co-ordinated action of valves, and the posterior section of the foregut, which functions as an 'oesophageal pump' (M.J. Rice, personal communication).[42] In the midgut the blood is enclosed in the peritrophic membrane, secreted at the proventriculus. In young tsetse flies the size of the meal may be limited by the development of the peritrophic membrane.

There are no air sacs to compensate for the volume of blood ingested and meal size is probably regulated by stretch receptors in the ventral wall of the abdomen, which becomes greatly distended.[30] Freshly fed *G. morsitans* and *G. pallidipes*, collected in the field, were estimated to have ingested 37 to 76 mg of blood. *G. pallidipes* ingested more than *G. morsitans* and in both species females took larger meals than males.[49] The actual size of the meal in the female will depend upon the size of the ovaries and uterus. The meal is rapidly reduced in volume by excretion of water, and within 30 min the blood in the crop will have been transferred to the midgut, and the blood meal reduced by half. This concentration of the blood meal occurs in the anterior portion of the midgut (Figure 5.4) but no digestive enzymes are secreted there. Enzymes are produced in the middle section of the midgut and include a powerful protease. Absorption of the products of digestion occurs in the posterior section of the midgut.

Digestion is 60 per cent complete in 24 hours and 90 per cent by 48 hours.[30]

Energy Production. Bursell *et al.*[10] distinguish three stages in the hunger cycle of *Glossina.* A lipogenic phase, lasting about 24 h, follows immediately after a blood meal and is accompanied by a rapid rise in oxygen consumption. The energy, which becomes available, is used for growth, for excretion of excess nitrogen, and for lipid formation, which reaches a peak 12 hours after the feed. The first lipolytic phase begins on the second day after feeding, and is marked by an increase in proline, mobilisation of the lipid reserves, and a reduced respiratory rate. The second lipolytic phase begins on the 3rd to 4th day, when digestion is complete. The rate of lipid mobilisation is reduced and the concentration of proline declines. The insect now suffers nitrogen depletion.

In flight proline can only supply the short-term energy needs of the tsetse fly. In the flight muscles proline is converted into alanine and the reverse process (alanine to proline) occurs in the abdominal fat body utilising available lipids. This process limits continuous flight to about 2 min in *Glossina.* After 2 to 3 min continuous flight the wing beat falls from 220 to 180 c/s, and is incapable of lifting a load. Teneral flies have a low wing beat because their flight muscles are underdeveloped, and consequently they cannot lift heavy loads and therefore they ingest smaller meals. The greater part of meals taken early in life is used to develop the thoracic musculature, and the build up of fat reserves is undertaken later.[10]

The times given above for the various stages in the hunger cycle are appropriate for a temperature of 25°C which may be considered optimal since, at that temperature, fat reserves are used most economically, and mortality is minimal in *G. morsitans.*[38] At 25°C the cycle of larviposition is 9 to 10 days, at 18°C it is extended to 25 days, and at 30°C it is reduced to 7 days. Similar temperature-related changes occur in the duration of the puparium before emergence of the adult tsetse fly. At 16°, 25° and 32°C the durations are 100, 30 and 20 days respectively. The relationship is linear from 18°C to 27°C, but above 27°C development is slower than expected, and thermal stress is becoming evident. One hour's exposure to 40.6°C and 6 h to 39.7°C produce death of the puparium.[30]

Bionomics of *Glossina*

The need to increase world food production and pressure for economic growth in the newly independent countries of Africa have focused attention on the tsetse fly as a constraint on agricultural development. A great deal of work has been, and is being, done on the bionomics of *Glossina,* knowledge of which is basic to the development of rational, economic control measures. Nevertheless the results of these studies are not easy to summarise. This is perhaps not surprising when it is remembered that studies are being undertaken in different ecological habitats over an area of 10,000,000 km², which is larger than the United States of America or Australia. Fortunately, a number of syntheses have been published, beginning in 1955 with Buxton's monumental *Natural History of Tsetse Flies*[12] and followed by Glover, 1961,[18] Glasgow, 1963,[17] Nash, 1969,[35] Ford, 1971,[16] and Jordan, 1974.[29]

Sampling

Tsetse flies are diurnally active blood-sucking flies which rest and feed out of doors, i.e. they are exophilic and exophagic. They are present in low density with total populations estimated to range from 4 to 18 tsetse/hectare.[35] Therefore special methods have to be used to sample such small populations and difficulties of interpretation arise because different methods selectively sample different fractions of the tsetse population. From the marked difference in lengths of life of the two sexes it is generally agreed that, although equal numbers of each sex emerge from puparia, field populations contain 70 to 80 per cent females and only 20 to 30 per cent males; yet on human or animal baits more males than females are captured, and the percentage of males may be as high as 90 per cent.[50]

The difficulty of sampling savanna-inhabiting tsetse largely arises from two features of tsetse behaviour. Firstly, man is not an attractive host, and indeed there is evidence that he is actually repellent to *G. morsitans* and *G. pallidipes*.[9,51] When an ox is used as bait not only does the catch increase many times, but a higher percentage of females are caught. The percentage of *G. longipalpis* increased from 2 per cent on a human bait to 39 per cent on an ox.[50] The second factor is that male tsetse are attracted to moving hosts, which they follow. When the host stops they settle on the ground and on the bait, but many of them make no attempt to feed. These males are said to be sexually appetitive.[16] The host is being used as a marker to bring the sexes together for mating. The most representative sample is obtained by using a stationary trap, which attracts hungry flies of both sexes, and often gives the expected high proportion (75 per cent) of females. On human bait females formed only 25 per cent of the catch of *G. pallidipes*, on cattle 38 per cent but in stationary traps 73 per cent.[50]

The relative efficiency of traps is seasonally dependent. In the cool, dry season traps are ten times as efficient as human bait for *G. tachinoides* and *G. palpalis*, but at the end of the rains human baits are four times as efficient as traps.[50] The pattern of behaviour in *G. pallidipes* changes as the female ages, and Harley[22] studied this by age grading females, caught by various methods. As few flies were caught on moving or stationary men the catches made by these two methods were pooled. Forty-eight per cent of the female flies caught on man and 39 per cent of the resting flies, i.e. flies

Table 12.1: Percentage Age Composition of Female *G. pallidipes* and
G. fuscipes Collected by Various Techniques

Collecting technique	*G. pallidipes*					*G. fuscipes*				
	A	B	C	D	E	A	B	C	D	E
Moving ox	6	11	21	37	25	33	13	16	25	13
Stationary ox	5	15	24	35	21	28	15	21	21	15
Moving vehicle	27	16	19	22	16	45	10	16	19	10
Traps	6	7	22	36	29	37	13	19	17	14
Moving man	48	6	21	12	13	33	11	14	21	21
Stationary man						22	14	22	23	19
'Resting'	39	16	20	17	8	28	14	20	23	15

Note: Column headings A, B, C, D and E indicate 0, 1, 2+3, 4+5 and 6+7 ovarian cycles
completed, respectively

Source: Data from Harley[22]

collected from vegetation where they had settled after following a party of
men, were in the first ovarian cycle (Table 12.1). This suggests that they
were attracted to the moving bait for mating. Mating occurs early in the life
of the female, and it is claimed that two-thirds of the teneral flies and all
non-teneral flies are inseminated.[17] A feeding response was shown by older
females, that had completed four or more ovarian cycles, and these formed
56 to 65 per cent of the catches on stationary or moving oxen, and in
traps.[22]

The results, obtained at the same time with *G. fuscipes*, were quite
different. The age grades of females caught by seven different techniques
(moving ox, man or vehicle; stationary ox, man or trap and resting flies)
were not markedly different. Females in the first cycle constituted 22 to 46
per cent of the catch and those in the second cycle 10 to 15 per cent, which
remained virtually unchanged thereafter. Paired data for females in cycles 3
and 4, 5 and 6, 7 and 8, i.e. females that had completed 2 or 3, 4 or 5 and 6
or 7 cycles, ranged, respectively, from 14 to 22 per cent, 17 to 25 per cent,
and 10 to 21 per cent (Table 12.1).

Activity Cycle

Tsetse flies are active by day and Brady[5] has shown that in *G. m. morsitans*
six out of seven unrelated behavioural responses were bimodal, with
morning and evening peaks separated by a decline of activity at noon. This
pattern is comparable to the activity pattern of their hosts.[16] Two of the
responses of *G. m. morsitans* are truly circadian rhythms, which persist
under constant conditions.[5] Such rhythms are modified by environmental
conditions, and the bimodal response is temperature dependent, being
bimodal at 22°C, but reduced to a single morning peak at 19°C.[3] The

feeding response is reduced by high illumination (25,000 lux), while the phototactic response to light varies with temperature. At 26°C *G. m. morsitans* is positively phototactic, but at 34 to 38°C it seeks the dark, and the threshold for this response is lowered by 2.2°C for a ten-fold increase in illumination.[25]

Field observations indicate specific differences in activity patterns, with *G. pallidipes* showing increased feeding activity throughout the day and reaching a peak in the evening. This pattern applies to catches made off man in a fly round, and off an ox, but the pattern of captures in a stationary, unbaited trap showed a maximum after midday. *G. f. fuscipes* showed a midday peak with low activity both in the morning and in the late afternoon. On the contrary, *G. brevipalpis* had peaks before dawn and after sunset.[21] Activity patterns are also modified by environmental conditions in the field. *G. longipalpis* is inactive below 22°C,[50] while *G. pallidipes* feeds at temperatures between 18 to 32°C.[16] Eclosion of *G. morsitans* occurs in the same temperature range (18°–32°C), and produces a bimodal pattern in summer, when midday temperatures exceed 32°C, and a unimodal pattern in winter, when the temperature remains below 32°C.[39] In the hot season *G. m. morsitans* is active early in the day, becoming inactive when the temperature reaches 32°C; in the cool season activity begins later in the day, and in the wet season activity is more evenly distributed throughout the day.[29]

Host Finding

Host finding by tsetse flies involves visual and chemosensory stimuli. In the laboratory *G. m. morsitans* shows a bimodal rhythm of response to a visual stimulus with peak activity in the morning and afternoon being five times that at midday.[2] The response increases steadily with time since the last feed until flies become moribund after five days' starvation. Visual responsiveness correlated most closely with the flies' total bodyweight (r = 0.89).[4] As might be expected, gravid females were only half as responsive as males to visual stimuli.

The attraction of odour from oxen, hidden out of sight in an underground pit, to *G. pallidipes* and *G. m. morsitans* increased with the number of oxen, and attracted rather more females than males of both species.[52] These species differ in their visual responsiveness. *G. pallidipes* was eight times as responsive as *G. m. morsitans* to a stationary, compared to a mobile, host. The percentage of females of both species on a stationary bait was 70 per cent but it dropped to 40 and 60 per cent for *G. m. morsitans* and *G. pallidipes*, respectively, on a moving bait. Only hungry flies were attracted to a stationary host, while 10 to 25 per cent of those attracted to a moving bait had fed recently.[51]

Host Selection

Teneral flies are low in energy reserves, particularly if their puparia have been exposed to high temperatures, and the mortality of teneral flies is high in the first week of adult life.[20] They need a blood meal in the minimum time, and young *G. morsitans* will feed on man, although usually man is repellent to this species. Hunger overcomes repellency and nonteneral flies feeding on man have less energy reserves than those feeding on cattle which, in turn, have less energy reserves than those in swarms following a host.

The length of the feeding cycle is usually two to three days but can be extended in the absence of hosts to five or possibly more days. Hungry flies readily attack man and it was the presence of such flies in open woodland, where hosts were readily visible, which gave rise to the concept of 'feeding grounds' in early tsetse ecology.[16] This concept has little validity now.

Choice of host is only partly a matter of availability. *G. swynnertoni* and *G. morsitans* were feeding on warthog, giraffe and buffalo, in an area where zebra, wildebeeste and impala formed 80 per cent of the available hosts.[29] Only one of the identified blood meals had been taken from the more abundant mammals. This may be due in part to the reaction of the mammalian host to the presence of the flies, because *G. morsitans* and *G. pallidipes* are said to avoid mammals, such as baboons, impala and man, which resist attack, and to feed on relatively quiescent animals, such as pigs and cattle.[9]

Species of *Nemorhina* are opportunist feeders and frequently feed on reptiles, including crocodiles, and *G. f. fuscipes* feeds readily on monitor lizards (*Varanus* ssp).[29] Change of habit, plus the preference of *Glossina* for warthog, operates against the success of tsetse control by game eradication. The larger game are relatively easy to exclude or shoot, but the tsetse population may not be markedly affected.[53]

Evolution of Feeding Preferences

Ford[16] has outlined a possible evolution of tsetse flies based on their feeding preferences. The genus probably arose in Mesozoic and would have fed on large reptiles. This ancestral habit is reflected in the *Nemorhina*, which inhabit riverine and lacustrine environments and feed largely on reptiles. With the decline of reptiles in the Tertiary and the emergence of mammals it is postulated that tsetse flies transferred their feeding to early mammals, which would have included the Suidae or pigs, and the ancestors of large mammals, such as hippopotami, which predominated in the Eocene and Oligocene. Pigs were, and still largely are, inhabitants of forest, to which the subgenus *Austenia* of *Glossina* is largely restricted. The ancestors of the subgenus *Glossina* moved into the savanna with the ancestors of the savanna-dwelling warthog. Ruminants, such as antelope,

giraffe and buffalo, only became dominant in the Plicocene, and the shift of
tsetse to these hosts is relatively recent. Evidence for this is to be found in
their response to infection with trypanosomes (see Chapter 29).

Data on the blood meals of *Glossina* on wild hosts, i.e. excluding man
and domestic animals, are summarised in Table 12.2. Species of *Nemorhina* feed largely on reptiles, which are common in their riverine and
lakeside habitats. Forest dwelling species can be separated into those that
feed mainly on pigs, e.g. *G. (G.) austeni, G. (A.) tabaniformis,* and those
that feed mainly on bushbuck with some feeding on bushpig, e.g. *G. (G.)
pallidipes, G. (A.) fusca.* The savanna species of subgenus *Glossina* feed
largely on warthog, buffalo and large bovids. Lastly there are the specialised feeders among the *Austenina,* which have adapted to feeding on large
mammals, which frequent thickets and secondary forest.

Habitats

The broad classification of habitats of *Glossina* has been given in the
previous section. There is a trend towards survival in habitats of increasing
aridity. *Austenina* species inhabit humid forests, and even *G. (A.) brevipalpis,* which extends into dry regions of East Africa, requires a relative
humidity in excess of 70 per cent for its puparium to survive to produce an

Table 12.2: Summary of Blood Meal Analyses, Excluding Man, Domestic
Animals and Blood Meals Not Fully Identified

Habitat	Host	%
Lacustrine and riverine feeders	Reptiles	56
subgenus *Nemorhina*	Bushbuck	22
	Remainder	22
Forest thicket or forest edge feeders		
A. *G. (G.) austeni*	Bushpig and forest hog	74
G. (A.) tabaniformis	Remainder	26
B. *G. (G.) pallidipes*	Bushbuck	61
G. (A.) fusca	Bushpig	12
	Remainder	27
Savanna feeders		
G. (G.) morsitans	Warthog	57
G. (G.) swynnertoni	Buffalo	21
	Giraffe, kudu and remainder	22
Specialised East African *Austenina*		
G. (A.) brevipalpis	Elephant, rhino, hippo, buffalo	71
G. (A.) longipennis	Bushpig	18
	Remainder	11

Source: Adapted from Ford[16]

adult, and, as a result, it is restricted to residual or secondary forest. The puparia of the savanna species, *G. swynnertoni* and *G. m. centralis*, can complete development in humidities as low as 10 per cent. Other species of the subgenus *Glossina* and those of *Nemorhina* have intermediate requirements. Rather contrary to this view is that the species best adapted to aridity, *G. longipennis*, is a member of the forest-dwelling subgenus *Austenina*, and its puparia are 'completely viable at 0% RH'.[7] Of course, this series can be reversed and be read as a movement from arid to more humid habitats. Puparia are found in holes in the ground, under logs, under fallen leaves and bark, and in tufts of grass. In the hot season the microclimate under logs becomes too hot for the survival of puparia of *G. m. centralis* and they are deposited in holes in the ground, which are more humid.[29]

Tsetse are considered to concentrate in favourable habitats in the dry season. This is marked in *G. m. submorsitans* during the hot, dry season in northern Nigeria but is less evident in the less extreme climate of the south.[29] In Zimbabwe in the hot, dry season the sexually appetitive males concentrate in riverine areas, but other adults are more evenly distributed.[8] Removal of selected vegetation, which formed the dry season resting sites for *G. palpalis* in northern Ghana, virtually eliminated this species, but success was dependent in part on the severity of the dry season.[34] At one time considerable attention was paid to the vegetation in which tsetse were found, but it is now considered that the observed tsetse-vegetation associations reflect habitat selection by the host rather than by the tsetse.[16] *G. tachinoides* has adapted to a peridomestic mode of life in southern Nigeria, where its puparia are deposited in areas of human activity and in lantana thickets. *G. f. fuscipes* has also established a population in lantana, away from its typical lacustrine habitat.[29]

Resting Places

Bursell and Taylor[11] calculate that female *G. m. morsitans* spend on average only 5 min per day in flight, and the more active males about 15 min in the hot season and more than twice as long in the cold season. Consequently most of their time is spent resting. Knowledge of resting places is essential to any estimate of absolute numbers of tsetse and for their control by the application of insecticides to their resting places. The daytime and nocturnal resting places are different. *G. m. morsitans* rests on branches, boles and rot holes of trees by day, and at night on twigs and leaves.[29] This may be an adaptation to avoid nocturnal predators. By day tsetse could see an approaching predator, and by night detect the vibration caused by a predator on an easily disturbed leaf or twig. *G. pallidipes* occupies similar resting places but nearer the ground, i.e. mostly below 3m whereas *G. morsitans* extends up to 6m and on occasions to 12m. Both species show a change in resting site during the day in the hot season, when they move from branches to rot holes and boles.[29,50]

Another response to harsh conditions is for tsetse to rest nearer the ground. In the Cameroons the behaviour of *G. tachinoides* is temperature dependent. Above 30°C it rests nearer the ground, and when the temperature exceeds 35°C it moves to a cooler site. In intense heat, it seeks the shelter of dense stands of *Mimosa nigra*.[19] This response has an effect on control measures. The severity of the hot dry season in West Africa increases with distance from the coast. In the severer climate it is sufficient to treat vegetation with insecticides to a height of 1.5 m to control *G. m. submorsitans*, whereas nearer the coast, treatment must be applied up to 3.6 m.[29]

Dispersal

The average time spent by a male *G. m. morsitans* in flight each day is very short. Bursell and Taylor[11] calculated that, flying at 11 km/h for 18 min, a male *G. m. morsitans* would fly a distance of 3.3 km. However, such a flight is not made in one direction, but is composed of a series of short, random flights, each occupying about 5 s. For male *G. m. morsitans* the average length of a step was determined to be 15.9 m and the number of steps per day as 208. The effect of such a large number of short, random movements is to disperse male *G. f. fuscipes* 338 m/d, and the average of 13 observations on four species, mostly *G. morsitans*, was 252 m/d.[46] These are average figures and Hargrove[20] considers that in the first week of life male *G. morsitans* disperse only a short distance and that this rises steadily as the flies age, to reach a peak in the fourth to sixth weeks, after which dispersion declines rapidly in older flies.

Such modest dispersal is consistent with the long-term extension of *G. morsitans* in Nigeria, where its spread along the cattle routes has been calculated at 5 km per year or about 100 m per week. This is about half the rate of dispersal (180 m per week) observed for individual flies.[43] Nevertheless, when continued over many years tsetse have considerable potential as invaders of suitable uninfested areas. In that way they maintain continual pressure to extend their limits. The detailed distribution of *Glossina* is changing continually as new areas are invaded and established areas vacated.

Medical and Veterinary Importance

Tsetse flies are probably never present in sufficient density to pose a biting fly problem. Their very great economic importance resides in their role as biological vectors of pathogenic trypanosomes, which cause severe disease in man and domestic animals. Two forms of *Trypanosoma brucei*, *T. b. gambiense* and *T. b. rhodesiense*, cause sleeping sickness in man in West and Central Africa and are transmitted, respectively, by tsetse flies of the subgenera *Nemorhina* and *Glossina.* Devastating epidemics of sleeping sickness have occurred in the past. Animal trypanosomiases, sometimes referred to as nagana, are caused by several species of *Trypanosoma* (see Chapter 29) and are associated with tsetse flies of the subgenus *Glossina.* Wherever there are tsetse flies it is impossible to keep cattle without regular chemotherapy. Trypanosomiasis has inhibited the development of a cattle-raising industry in much of tropical Africa, and even today, cattle ranching is impractical in much of Africa's savanna lands.

References

1. Bikingi-Wataaka, S.C.U. (1975). The incidence of trypanosomes in *Glossina fusca congolensis* in Bunyoro District, western Uganda. *East African Journal of Medical Research 2*: 13-16
2. Brady, J. (1972). The visual responsiveness of the tsetse fly *Glossina morsitans* Westw. (Glossinidae) to moving objects: the effect of hunger, sex, host odour and stimulus characteristics. *Bulletin of Entomological Research 62*: 257-79
3. _____ (1974). The pattern of spontaneous activity in the tsetse fly *Glossina morsitans* Westw. (Diptera, Glossinidae) at low temperatures. *Bulletin of Entomological Research 63*: 441-4
4. _____ (1975). 'Hunger' in the tsetse fly: the nutritional correlates of behaviour. *Journal of Insect Physiology 21*: 807-29
5. _____ (1975). Circadian changes in central excitability — the origin of behavioural rhythms in tsetse flies and other animals? *Journal of Entomology A 50*: 79-95
6. Bursell, E. (1955). The polypneustic lobes of the tsetse larva (*Glossina*, Diptera). *Proceedings of the Royal Society of London B 144*: 275-86
7. _____ (1958). The water balance of tsetse pupae. *Philosophical Transactions of the Royal Society of London B 241*: 179-210
8. _____ (1966). The nutritional state of tsetse flies from different vegetation types in Rhodesia. *Bulletin of Entomological Research 57*: 171-80
9. _____ (1973). Entomological aspects of the epidemiology of sleeping sickness. *Central African Journal of Medicine 19*: 201-14
10. _____ Billing, K.C., Hargrove, J.W., McCabe, C.T. and Slack, E. (1974). Metabolism of the bloodmeal in tsetse flies (a review). *Acta Tropica 31*: 297-320
11. _____ and Taylor, P. (1980). An energy budget for *Glossina* (Diptera: Glossinidae). *Bulletin of Entomological Research 70*: 187-96
12. Buxton, P.A. (1955). *The Natural History of Tsetse Flies.* H.K. Lewis, London
13. Challier, A. (1965). Amélioration de la methode de détermination de l'age physiologique des glossines. Etudes faites sur *Glossina palpalis gambiensis* Vanderplank 1949. *Bulletin de la Société de Pathologie Exotique 58*: 250-9
14. Chaudhury, M.F.B. and Dhadialla, T.S. (1976). Evidence of hormonal control of ovulation in tsetse flies. *Nature, London 260*:243-4
15. Curtis, C.F. (1972). Sterility from crosses between subspecies of the tsetse fly *Glossina morsitans. Acta Tropica 29*: 250-68
16. Ford, J. (9171). *The Role of the Trypanosomiases in African Ecology* ; *a Study of the Tsetse Fly Problem.* Clarendon Press, Oxford
17. Glasgow, J.P. (1963). *The Distribution and Abundance of Tsetse.* Pergamon Press, Oxford
18. Glover, P.E. (1961). *The Tsetse Problem in Northern Nigeria.* Patwa News Agency, Nairobi
19. Gruvel, J. (1975). Lieux de repos de *Glossina tachinoides* w. *Revue d'Elevage et de Médecine Vétérinaire des Pays Tropicaux 28*: 153-72

20. Hargrove, J.W. (1981). Tsetse dispersal reconsidered. *Journal of Animal Ecology 50*: 351-73

21. Harley, J.M.B. (1965). Activity cycles of *Glossina pallidipes* Aust. *G. palpalis fuscipes* Newst. and *G. brevipalpis* Newst. *Bulletin of Entomological Research 56*: 141-60

22. _____ (1967). The influence of sampling method on the trypanosome infection rate of catches of *G. pallidipes* and *G. fuscipes*. *Entomologia Experimentalis et Applicata 10*: 240-52

23. Hill, P., Saunders, D.S. and Campbell, J.A. (1973). The production of 'symbiont-free' *Glossina morsitans* and an associated loss of female fertility. *Transactions of the Royal Society of Tropical Medicine and Hygiene 67*:727-8

24. Huebner, E. and Davey, K.G. (1974). Bacteroids in the ovaries of a tsetsefly. *Nature, London 249*: 260-1

25. Huyton, P.M. and Brady, J. (1975). Some effects of light and heat on the feeding and resting behaviour of tsetse flies, *Glossina morsitans* Westwood. *Journal of Entomology A 50*: 23-30

26. _____ Langley, P.A., Carlson, D.A. and Coates, T.W. (1980). The role of sex pheromones in initiation of copulatory behaviour by male tsetse flies, *Glossina morsitans morsitans*. *Physiological Entomology 5*: 243-52

27. _____ Langley, P.A., Carlson, D.A. and Schwarz, M. (1980). Specificity of contact sex pheromones in tsetse flies, *Glossina* spp. *Physiological Entomology 5*: 253-64

28. Jackson, C.H.N. (1941). The analysis of a tsetse-fly population. *Annals of Eugenics 10*: 332-69

29. Jordan, A.M. (1974). Recent developments in the ecology and methods of control of tsetse flies (*Glossina* spp.) (Dipt., Glossinidae) — a review. *Bulletin of Entomological Research 63*: 361-99

30. Langley, P.A. (1977). Physiology of tsetse flies (*Glossina* spp.) (Diptera: Glossinidae): a review. *Bulletin of Entomological Research 67*: 523-74

31. _____ Pimley, R.W. and Carlson, D.A. (1975). Sex recognition pheromone in tsetse fly *Glossina morsitans*. *Nature, London 254*: 51-3

32. Ma, W.C. and Denlinger, D.L. (1974). Secretory discharge and microflora of milk gland in tsetse flies. *Nature, London 247*: 301-3

33. _____ Denlinger, D.L., Järlfors, U. and Smith D.S. (1975). Structural modifications in the tsetse fly milk gland during a pregnancy cycle. *Tissue and Cell 7*: 319-30

34. Morris, K.R.S. (1946). The control of trypanosomiasis by entomological means. *Bulletin of Entomological Research 37*: 201-50

35. Nash, T.A.M. (1969). *Africa's Bane: the Tsetse Fly*. Collins, London

36. _____ Trewern, M.A. and Moloo, S.K. (1976). Observations on the free larval stage of *Glossina morsitans morsitans* Westw. (Diptera ; Glossinidae): the possibility of a larval pheromone. *Bulletin of Entomological Research 66*: 17-24

37. Nkouka, É. (1976). Variations de la neurosécrétion cérébrale au cours du cycle génital d' un insecte vivipare, *Glossina fuscipes fuscipes* (Diptères, Muscidae). *Comptes Rendus Hebdomadaires des Séances de l'Académie des Sciences 282*: 557-60

38. Phelps, R.J. and Burrows, P.M. (1969). Puparial duration in *Glossina morsitans orientalis* under conditions of constant temperature. *Entomologia Experimentalis et Applicata 12*: 33-43

39. _____ and Jackson, P.J. (1971). Factors influencing the moment of larviposition and eclosion in *Glossina morsitans orientalis* Vanderplank (Diptera: Muscidae). *Journal of the Entomological Society of Southern Africa 34*: 145-57

40. Pollock, J.N. (1974). Anatomical relations during sperm transfer in *Glossina austeni* Newstead (Glossinidae, Diptera). *Transactions of the Royal Entomological Society of London 125*: 489-501

41. Potts, W.H. (1973). Glossinidae (Tsetse-flies). pp. 209-49 in *Insects and Other Arthropods of Medical Importance*, K.G.V. Smith (ed.), British Museum, Natural History

42. Rice, M.J. (1970). *A Study of the Innervation, Structure and Function of the Anterior Alimentary Canal of the Adult Tsetse Fly (Glossina austeni) and other Diptera*. Ph.D. thesis, University of Birmingham

43. Riordan, K. (1976). Rate of linear advance by *Glossina morsitans submorsitans* Newst.

(Diptera, Glossinidae) on a trade cattle route in south-western Nigeria. *Bulletin of Entomological Research 66*: 365-72

44. Roberts, M.J. (1973). Observations on the function of the choriothete and on egg hatching in *Glossina* spp. (Dipt., Glossinidae). *Bulletin of Entomological Research 62*: 371-4

45. _____ (1973). The control of fertilisation in tsetse flies. *Annals of Tropical Medicine and Parasitology 67*: 117-23

46. Rogers, D. (1977). Study of a natural population of *Glossina fuscipes fuscipes* Newstead and a model of fly movement. *Journal of Animal Ecology 46*: 309-30

47. Saunders, D.S. (1960). The ovulation cycle in *Glossina morsitans* Westwood (Diptera: Muscidae) and a possible method of age determination for female tsetse flies by the examination of their ovaries. *Transactions of the Royal Entomological Society of London 112*: 221-38

48. _____ and Dodd, C.W.H. (1972). Mating, insemination and ovulation in the tsetse fly *Glossina morsitans. Journal of Insect Physiology 18*: 187-98

49. Taylor, P. (1976). Blood-meal size of *Glossina morsitans* Westw. and *G. pallidipes* Austen (Diptera: Glossinidae) under field conditions. *Transactions of the Rhodesia Scientific Association 57*: 29-34

50. Thomson, R.C.M. (1968). *Ecology of Insect Vector Populations.* Academic Press, London

51. Vale, G.A. (1974). The responses of tsetse flies (Diptera: Glossinidae) to mobile and stationary baits. *Bulletin of Entomological Research 64*: 545-88

52. _____ and Hargrove, J.W. (1975). Field attraction of tsetse flies (Diptera: Glossinidae) to ox odour; the effects of dose. *Transactions of the Rhodesia Scientific Association 56*: 46-50

53. Wilson, V.J. (1975). Game and tsetse fly in eastern Zambia. *Occasional Papers of the National Museums and Monuments of Rhodesia B 5*: 339-404

13 MUSCIDAE (HOUSEFLIES, STABLEFLIES)

The Muscidae is a family of cyclorrhapous flies which includes the house-flies and the blood-sucking stableflies. The medically important members of the family are dark coloured medium-sized flies, whose immature stages occur in fermenting organic material of vegetable origin and are often associated with the dung of herbivorous mammals.

Classification

Seven subfamilies are recognised,[2] of which three are of medical import-ance. They are the Muscinae, the Stomoxinae (= Stomoxyinae) and the Fanniinae. The Stomoxinae are haematophagous and may be readily recognised by their possession of an elongate, sclerotised proboscis, which is always visible (Figure 13.1C, D). Wing vein iv is gently curved towards vein iii (Figure 13.2). This subfamily includes the stablefly. *Stomoxys calcitrans* (Figure 13.1C) and the hornfly, *Haematobia irritans irritans.* In the other two subfamilies the mouthparts are of the lapping type and can be folded into a subcranial cavity. In the Muscinae vein iv is strongly bent forwards towards vein iii (Figure 13.2), and the lower squama is broad with its posterior margin almost straight and at right angles to the long axis of the body. This subfamily includes the housefly, *Musca domestica*, and the Australian bushfly, *Musca vetustissima.* In the Fanniinae vein iv either runs straight to the wing margin, as in *Fannia* (Figure 13.4), or it is gently bent towards vein iii. The lower squama is narrow with a rounded posterior margin. This subfamily includes the lesser housefly, *Fannia canicularis.*

Flies and other animals, which live closely with man are said to be synanthropic. Greenberg[7] recognises various forms of synanthropy. Eusynanthropes are flies which can complete their entire development within the residences of man and his domestic animals. Many of these species have become cosmopolitan, spreading throughout the world with man. *M. domestica* is an endophilic eusynanthrope which is trophically and microclimatically related to man and his domestic habitats. Exophilic eusynanthropes, such as *Lucilia sericata* (Calliphoridae) and *F. canicularis*, are less closely related to man both trophically and microclimatically. Symbovines are linked with man through the excreta of domestic herbivores and fall into two groups. Symbovines, such as *S. calcitrans*, are associated with stabled domestic animals, and others, e.g. *H. irritans exigua*, associated with domestic animals in pasture. Hemisynanthropes operate

Figure 13.1: A, *Musca domestica*; B, *Musca vetustissima*; C, *Stomoxys calcitrans*; D, *Haematobia exigua*

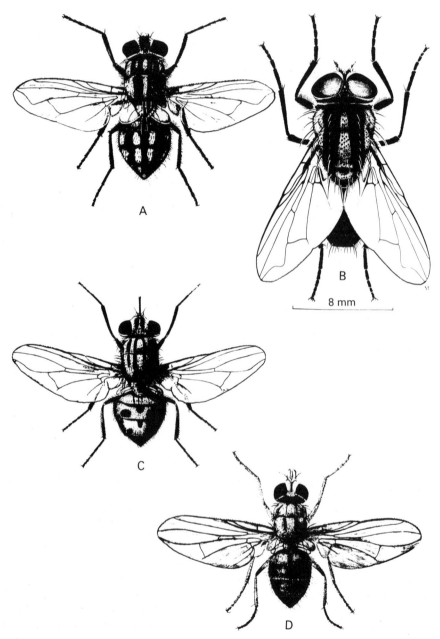

Sources: A, C and D from Patton, W.S. and Cragg, F.W. (1913). *Textbook of Medical Entomology.* Christian Literature Society for India, London. B from Colless and McAlpine[2]

Figure 13.2: Wings of *Musca domestica* (above) (× 20), and *Stomoxys calcitrans* (× 17)

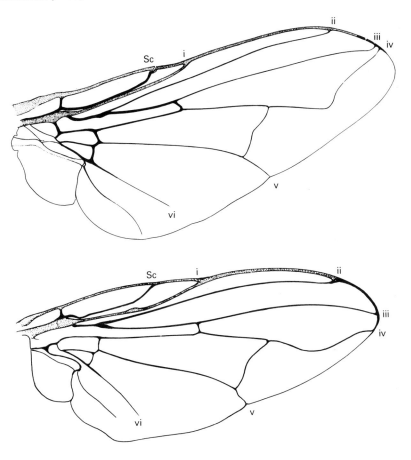

independently of man but interact with him when he enters their habitat, e.g. *Hydrotaea irritans.*

Musca domestica (Housefly)[4,20,25]

This widely distributed species is likely to prove to be a species complex. It is recognised by the presence of four dark, longitudinal stripes or vittae on the mesonotum (Figure 13.1A). The arista is plumose with branches above and below. The arrangement of bristles on the thorax includes two or three dorsocentrals on the prescutum and four on the scutum; a single acrostichal bristle on the scutum; three sternopleurals, one anterior and two posterior.

Life Cycle

The pearly-white eggs are long and narrow, measuring about 1.20 × 0.25 mm. Under optimal conditions (37°C) they hatch in about eight hours to give rise to legless, saprophagous larvae (maggots). There are three larval instars. The first two instars last about 24 h, and the third instar for three or more days.

Figure 13.3: A, Third Stage Maggot of *Musca domestica*. B, view of maggot from behind; C, anterior spiracle; D, posterior spiracles; E, puparium, showing pupal respiratory horns; F, posterior spiracles of third stage larva of *Stomoxys calcitrans*

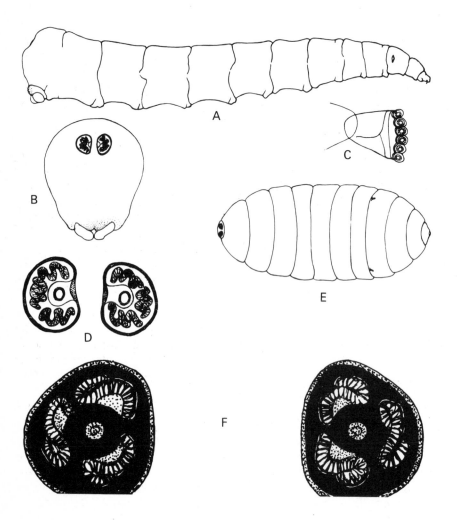

Larva. The third stage larva (Figure 13.3) measures 6-12 × 1-2 mm, and has 12 visible segments (one head segment, three thoracic and eight abdominal).[4] On the ventral side of the first segment there is a mouth surrounded by two oral lobes, transversed by parallel tubes which converge on the mouth, and function in a comparable manner to the pseudotrachae of the labellum of the adult fly. A pair of retractable mouth-hooks can be extended through the mouth and are used for progression and tearing at the substrate. In *Musca* the mouth-hooks are closely apposed, with the right one being markedly larger than the left. The head is retracted into the thorax and the dark, sclerotised cephalopharyngeal skeleton can be seen through the translucent body of the larva. The mouth-hooks are attached to this skeleton.

Respiration is amphipneustic with fan-shaped anterior spiracles on the second segment and dark, flat, plate-like spiracles on the posterior surface of the body. The anterior spiracles are undeveloped in the 1st instar larva, and have five to seven openings in the 3rd instar. In the 3rd instar larva the posterior spiracles are D-shaped with three sinuous slits and a button in the middle of the straight side of the D (Figure 13.3D). The button is the scar left at the moult from 2nd to 3rd instar. There is only one opening in the posterior spiracle in the 1st instar and two in the 2nd.

Pupa. The fully grown larva ceases to feed, and empties its gut to become a prepupa, which moves into drier conditions and buries itself into the substrate, where it pupates. The last larval skin is retained around the pupa as the puparium (Figure 13.3E). Immediately after moulting the puparium is creamy white, the colour of the larva, but it steadily darkens through shades of reddish brown until the mature puparium is almost black. The external larval structures can be recognised on the outside of the puparium, which measures 4-6 × 2-2.5 mm. The larval spiracles are non-functional and the pupa respires through pupal horns which pierce the puparium between the fifth and sixth segments.[10]

When the adult fly has completed its development within the pupa, it emerges from the puparium by using its ptilinum to force off a hemispherical cap from the anterior end of the puparium. Using its ptilinum (Figure 12.5) the fly makes its way up to the surface of the soil when the ptilinum is withdrawn into the head, and the frontal suture closed. The body of the fly is expanded by taking air into the gut, and the wings extended by pumping haemolymph through the veins. This ability of the newly emerged fly to move up to the surface of the soil can render the burying of infested material ineffective as a measure of fly control. Flies are able to emerge from material buried under 1.2 m of clay, loam or sand because most of the prepupae move to within 30 cm of the surface before pupating, and from this distance adults can easily reach the surface.[25]

Adult. Adult *M. domestica* are diurnal, and activity is favoured by high temperatures and low humidities, but, as the name housefly implies, they are more active in shade than in sunlight. Females emerge before the males, and mating takes place soon after emergence. Males will mate on the day of emergence, but the response of females is highest on the third day after emergence.[24] Maturation of the eggs depends upon the female having access to a diet of protein, and a batch of eggs may be laid as early as 54 h after emergence of the female.[19]

The ovipositing female deposits her eggs in clumps in cracks and crevices of a suitable medium, and sometimes the whole batch may be deposited in a single clump. By inserting the eggs into a moist medium the female protects them from desiccation. The original, ancestral breeding site was probably horse dung, but houseflies now breed in the dung of a wide range of herbivores, in fowl manure, in fermenting kitchen waste, and in rubbish tips.[20] Indeed separate populations of *M. domestica* may develop in association with stabled animals, and breed in urine and dung-contaminated stable refuse,[4,7] but *M. domestica* does not breed in cow dung, which is the main source of other species of *Musca*.

Temperature and Development

The duration of the larval instars is a function of the temperature and the quality of the larval medium. When dung quality is not limiting, the development time of the larval stages is 145 day-degrees above a threshold of 12°C and up to an optimum of 36°C, above which development is adversely affected. This relationship implies that at 22°C, i.e. 10°C above the threshold, the larval duration would be 14.5 days. Activity of the prepupa is optimal at 29°C. Susceptibility to high temperatures is lowest in the egg and highest in the pupa, and all stages are killed by exposure to 50°C or higher. This knowledge is used in fly control. Part of the rationale for the tight-packing of refuse dumps containing organic material is the attainment of temperatures lethal to the immature stages of the housefly through the fermentation and decay of the organic material.

Population Growth

On the average a female will mature 120 eggs in a batch (range 100-150) and deposit four to six batches of eggs during a lifetime of two to four weeks in summer.[10] Patton and Evans[19] recorded a particularly fecund female which laid 2,387 eggs in 21 batches over a period of 31 days after emergence. This is obviously exceptional. Nevertheless, the potential rate of increase of houseflies is enormous. *M. domestica* is an r-type species with power of rapid multiplication. Using conservative rates of development and fecundity Howard, cited by Hewitt,[10] calculated that, over the northern hemisphere summer, a single female ovipositing on 15 April would have produced 5.6×10^{12} progeny by 10 September, if they had all lived. Obviously they do not, but the species potential for exploiting favour-able conditions is outstanding. With a cycle from egg to egg of three weeks, ten to twelve generations can be produced a year in the warmer temperate regions of the world. In colder regions breeding will be restricted to the warmer months, and the winter passed as slowly growing larvae and pupae, some of which will survive to emerge, when warmer conditions return.[24]

Houseflies and Disease

Horseflies have adapted to living with man, feeding and breeding on his food, his organic wastes and his faeces. The movement of houseflies between faeces and food makes them ideal candidates as transmitters of human disease. A vast literature has developed on this subject and was summarised by West[25] for work published before 1950. Greenberg has given a full list of the organisms which have been recovered from house-flies,[7] and a detailed consideration of their relationship to human and animal diseases in a later publication.[8] In addition work on *M. domestica* has been consolidated in an annotated bibliography by West and Peters.[26]

Pathogens Involved

Houseflies have been found to harbour about 100 different pathogens and charged with transmitting 65 of these.[6] The pathogens recovered from flies range from viruses to helminths, and include the polio virus, the viruses of infectious hepatitis, the bacteria associated with cholera (*Vibrio*), enteric infections caused by species of *Salmonella* and *Shigella*, pathogenic *Escherichia coli*, haemolytic streptococci, *Staphylococcus aureus*, agents of trachoma, bacterial conjunctivitis, anthrax, diptheria, tuberculosis, leprosy and yaws. In addition flies can carry the cysts of Protozoa, including those of *Entamoeba histolytica* which causes amoebic dysentery, and the eggs of the threadworm *Trichuris trichiura*, and the hookworm *Ancylostoma duodenale* and of other nematodes and cestodes.

The housefly is the biological vector and intermediate host of certain cestodes of poultry, and of nematodes, which cause habronemiasis in horses (see Chapter 32). Fly larvae have only a tenuous association with myiasis, the invasion of living tissue by dipterous larvae. When they occur in an advanced stage of myiasis in sheep they do not feed on living tissue, but on the exudate and matted wool.[20] In this connection it is of interest that fly larvae were only found in carcasses when the vegetable contents of the gut were exposed.[9]

The recovery of pathogens from houseflies does not necessarily involve them in the transmission of disease. There are other routes of infection and, depending upon circumstances, houseflies may play a major, or minor or no role at all in disease transmission. A comparison between two groups of towns in Texas, one of which was sprayed with DDT for housefly control and the other left untreated, produced a reduction in acute diarrhoeal infection of children, with infections due to *Shigella* declining, but those due to *Salmonella* were much less affected.[6]

Methods of Transmission

There are three ways in which houseflies can disseminate pathogens. The surface of the body of the fly, particularly its legs and proboscis, can be contaminated; pathogens can be regurgitated on to food via the vomit drop; or pass through the gut of the fly and be deposited in the faeces. Infective material picked up on the body hairs and tarsi of houseflies may survive only a short period. They will be subject to the cleaning behaviour of the fly, in which it seeks to rid itself of foreign material, and organisms exposed on the surface will be subject to desiccation, particularly in flight, and to UV sterilisation in sunlight.[8] Greater survival would be expected for organisms trapped between the lobes of the labellum. There is a minimum number of pathogens needed to infect a human being, but a lesser number of organisms deposited into a medium, e.g. milk, in which they can multiply, can reach an infective density. The infective dose to a man is 10^5 virus particles and 10^6 for bacteria. Only the latter could multiply in human food; viruses require a host cell.[6]

When the housefly feeds the filtering function of the pseudotracheae will exclude protozoal cysts and eggs of helminths, but the fly can ingest larger particles directly through the prestomum at the distal end of the food canal. The vomit drop is formed from the contents of the crop, which represents the most recently taken in food. The vomit drop is therefore an important method of disseminating pathogens. Small pathogens pass out freely with the vomit drop, but larger cysts and eggs are laid back by the pseudo-tracheae.[8] The contents of the crop are passed to the midgut, and viable cysts and eggs appear in the fly's faeces.

Pathogens and the Fly's Gut Fauna

Pathogens that pass through the gut of the adult housefly have the opportunity to multiply before being deposited in the faeces. Their ability to develop an infection in the housefly depends upon the number ingested. When inputs were below 10^3 *Salmonella*, no organisms appeared in the fly's faeces. A higher intake is required in the presence of the fly's normal gut flora. Interspecific antagonism may lead to the rapid elimination of *Salmonella*,[8] and rapid multiplication of *Salmonella* occurs in houseflies freed from their normal gut flora. In comparison with the green blowfly *Lucilia sericata*, the housefly was a superior host for *Salmonella*.[8]

The fermenting material in which housefly larvae live is teeming with bacteria. For growth, fly larvae require micro-organisms or some product of micro-organisms. On emergence the adult fly is virtually free from micro-organisms. Several factors account for this change. Firstly, in the prepupa the fly larva ceases to feed, and reduces the microbe population to less than 1 per cent, completely eliminating a substantial population of *Salmonella*. There are two main reasons for this elimination. There is competition from the fly's normal commensal bacterium, *Proteus mirabilis*, and high mortality in the midgut. Most of the fly's intestinal tract is alkaline but the midgut is strongly acid with a pH of 3.0-3.5. Passage through the midgut reduces the microbial population to less than 2 per cent. The speed with which this reduction takes place indicates the existence of another factor other than pH in producing mortality. In the alkaline rectum the *Proteus* population may recover but *Salmonella* rarely does so. The microbial population is further reduced at pupation when the linings of the fore and hindgut and most of their contents are shed.[6]

Musca vetustissima (Australian Bushfly)

The *Musca sorbens* complex of species is widely distributed in the tropics and subtropics of the Afrotropical, Oriental and Australian regions. There are at least two different populations in tropical Africa and a third in Australia, assigned to a separate species *M. vetustissima*.[18,20] This account will be based on *M. vetustissima*, which has been studied in depth by Hughes and his colleagues.[11] The Oriental populations have not been studied in the same detail.

Flies of the *M. sorbens* complex have two broad, dark longitudinal vittae on the scutum (Figure 13.1B). The wings are clear with very white squamae, and the first abdominal segment is black. The proboscis is of the normal lapping type with small prestomal teeth. The female is dichoptic and the male nearly holoptic. The primary breeding site of members of the *M. sorbens* complex is cow dung.

Life Cycle and Bionomics

The eggs of *M. vetustissima* are larger than those of *M. domestica*, measuring 1.7×0.3 mm.[4] They have the typical muscine shape with a hatching strip on the concave surface, which functions as a plastron facilitating respiration when the eggs are in water. Eggs of *M. vetustissima* will hatch in water but not if totally immersed in faeces, when the plastron is unable to function. The eggs are very susceptible to desiccation and some die when exposed to 90 per cent RH for only one hour. Development is rapid being completed in 7 h at 32°C and 17 h at 21°C. Larval growth is even more rapid than in *M. domestica*, the three instars being completed in 8 h, 10 h and 49 h, respectively, at 32°C. For rapid development larvae need access to moist dung for feeding, and air to which they expose the posterior spiracles for respiration. The 3rd instar larva is very similar to that of *M.*

domestica, being of comparable size, with the right mouth-hook longer than the left, with about six openings in the anterior spiracle, and three sinuous slits in the posterior spiracle.

Mature larvae are sensitive to exposure to excess water, and no pupation occurs in waterlogged soil. Even temporary waterlogging reduces survival of pupae, particularly if exposed early in their lives before the respiratory horns have pierced the puparium. Prepupae leave the dung between midnight and dawn, and bury themselves into the substrate, where they pupate at depths of 20-30 mm. Moving from the dung during the hours of darkness must reduce predation. *M. vetustissima* is a pioneer species in dung, and larval survival is inversely related to population density. The duration of the pupal stage is about 80 per cent of that of the combined larval stages, taking 3 days at 39°C and 18 days at 18°C. Eclosion occurs in the few hours around dawn, which is appropriate for a diurnally active adult. The adults are active by day and roost at night.

Females develop faster than males and emerge first. Mating occurs on the third day after emergence at 27°C and it is believed that a second mating occurs after the second ovarian cycle. Copulation is a long process lasting about 80 min during which spermatozoa are transferred together with an oviposition stimulant and monocoitic substances, which temporarily restrict further mating. The female requires a protein meal to develop the ovaries. In the field females have been found which have completed four ovarian cycles. Wild flies develop 4-48 eggs in a cycle, the number of eggs maturing being reduced in each subsequent cycle. Ovarian development depends upon the nutritional state of the female, and where that is inadequate fewer eggs are matured. The female is attracted to fresh cow dung to which it flies upwind and deposits its eggs in crevices in the dung. Oviposition occurs during daylight and an ovipositing female attracts other gravid females, probably through the emission of an egg-laying pheromone.

Adult survival is inversely related to temperature, being eleven days at 29°C, during which four ovarian cycles can be completed, and seven or more weeks at 12°C, the threshold temperature for development. Survival is dependent on the adult having access to free water, and an easily metabolised energy source such as sugar. They are active in temperatures up to 35°C and windspeeds of 8 km/h. They can be displaced hundreds of kilometres in a day on hot, strong winds, and are also regularly dispersed via human transport.

They are mainly nuisance flies, feeding at the eyes, mouths and wounds of domestic animals and man, and also on dung. They settle out of the wind, and can be present on the backs of men in large numbers. Their wide dispersal from the pastures in which they originate allows them to be a pest in the suburbs of large cities.

Phenology

Several features of the bushfly biology determine its seasonal distribution. There is no diapausing stage in the life cycle, and the temperature threshold for activity, and immature and adult development is 12°C. At low temperatures all stages may survive for a long time but temperatures below freezing are lethal. The effect of this is that the bushfly dies out in the southern parts of Australia during the winter. Rapid development of the immature stages, and high fecundity in the females, is dependent on the quality of bovine dung available. In addition temporary waterlogging reduces survival of both prepupae and pupae. The net result of these different responses is that the bushfly population increases dramatically after the wet season when the cattle are feeding on rapidly growing grasses and producing rich dung.

The bushfly populations are highest in the north in the autumn following the summer rains and decline in the winter and spring as the pasture deteriorates. They move south on warm winds and are able to exploit the spring flush of vegetation following the winter rains in the south of Australia. There, bushfly populations reach a peak in late spring and early summer, and then wane as the summer dry season advances. Like many other Australian animals the bushfly is nomadic, moving around to exploit favourable conditions.

Control

In view of its wide dispersal local control measures will be ineffective against the bushfly. The ready availability of bovine dung to bushflies in Australia results partly from the absence, over the greater part of the country, of any dung beetles able to cope with bovine dung. To redress this situation a range of dung beetles has been introduced into Australia, of which one of the first was *Onthophagus gazella.* This species has proved to be highly effective over a limited area of the country, successfully competing with bushflies for bovine dung, and spreading widely from the centres of release. The effect of competition between *O. gazella* and *M. vetustissima* in the laboratory has been reported by Bornemissza.[1]

Stomoxinae[27]

Species of *Stomoxys* can be recognised by their palps being less than half the length of the proboscis (Figure 4.6), and the sternopleuron having one posterior bristle. In *Haematobia* the palps, which are grooved internally, are as long as the proboscis, and the sternopleuron has both an anterior and a posterior bristle. In both *Stomoxys* and *Haematobia*, but not in all Stomoxinae, the arista carries hairs only on the dorsal side.

Stomoxys calcitrans (Stablefly or Biting Housefly)

In *S. calcitrans* there are four dark, longitudinal vittae on the thorax, the lateral ones being interrupted at the suture (Figure 13.1C). The pattern is similar to that found in *M. domestica.* The abdomen has a grey and dark brown pollinosity, forming a pattern of light spots on a darker background. This pattern is characteristic but variable.

The life cycle of *S. calcitrans* is that of a typical muscid fly. The elongate, white egg hatches into a saprophagous maggot, which undergoes three moults before forming the pupa. In the third stage larva the right mouth-hook is larger than the left, the anterior spiracles have about six openings, and the posterior spiracles have three S-shaped slits surrounding a central button[4] (Figure 13.3F). At 26.7°C the egg stage lasts 23 h, and the three instars 23 h, 27 h and approximately 7 days respectively.[16] At 30-31°C the pupal stage lasts five days. The female is anautogenous, requiring several blood meals to complete ovarian development. Both sexes are haemato-phagous, and Parr[17] reports that in *S. calcitrans* the average blood meal (25.8 mg) is three times the average bloodweight (8.6 mg).

S. calcitrans bites by day, commonly with peak activity in the early morning and late afternoon, a bimodal pattern of activity common to many diurnal insects. Individual *S. calcitrans* may feed more than once a day, biting their host low down. They attack the ankles of man, and the belly, lower body and limbs of domestic stock, particularly cattle and horses. In summer the adults survive for three to four weeks, and considerably longer in the cooler times of the year.[23]

The number of eggs matured by an individual female *S. calcitrans* has been variously recorded as less than 200 or up to 600,[23] and even as many as 820 eggs in 20 ovipositions.[27] The eggs are not cemented together, and the female may scatter eggs throughout a suitable medium. Stableflies breed in straw contaminated with the urine and dung of cattle and horses. Their larvae are not found in pure faeces, but in animal bedding, lawn cuttings and rotting vegetables. The dung of equines is particularly attrac-tive, compared to that of ruminants,[27] but in Uganda the breeding sites of *S. calcitrans* are characterised by the presence of rotted cattle manure, rotten straw, grass or leaves, and shade.[17] In lakeside and coastal areas of the USA, *S. calcitrans* may breed in large numbers in shoreline deposits of aquatic vegetation, and constitute a major nuisance to holidaymakers.[7,8] Pupation occurs in the drier parts of stable refuse.[4]

Economic Importance. S. calcitrans is a cosmopolitan synanthrope, which worries stock particularly around stables, but less so in pastures where it is rarer. It may reduce milk yield by 25 per cent, or as much as 40-60 per cent.[8] *S. calcitrans* can affect the behaviour of wild animals. Fosbrooke[5] reports that a severe outbreak of *S. calcitrans* in the Ngorongoro Crater in

Tanzania in 1962 led to a change in behaviour of lions, which climbed trees to avoid being bitten.

Pathogens. A large number of pathogens have been recorded from *S. calcitrans* and have been listed by Greenberg.[7] Stableflies act as both biological and mechanical vectors of disease. *S. calcitrans* is the intermediate host of nematode worms, including *Setaria cervi*, a parasite of cattle, and several species of *Habronema*, parasites of horses.[8] Stableflies are persistent biters, and often engage in interrupted feeding. This, together with the fact that they feed more than once per day, fits them to be mechanical vectors of blood-dwelling pathogens. They contribute to the spread of trypanosomiasis, especially of *Trypanosoma evansi*, the causative agent of surra, which occurs in a wide range of hosts.[27] The role of *S. calcitrans* in the transmission of other infectious diseases, e.g. anthrax, is less clear. It has been accused of transmitting the virus of fowl pox but as Zumpt[27] points out *S. calcitrans* does not feed readily on poultry, and is unlikely therefore to be a vector.

Stomoxys nigra

S. nigra occurs in the Afrotropical and Oriental regions. In Mauritius it is an important pest and a mechanical vector of surra among equines and cattle.[14] It breeds in the decaying trash of canefields, which dominate the agricultural scene on the island.[22] The seasonal fluctuations in numbers of *S. nigra* are closely associated with the sugar cane harvest (late June to end of December). The population increases from July to September, with a plateau from October to December, a decline in numbers from January to April, and a crisis period between May and July.[21]

Haematobia irritans

H. irritans is a small, brownish, obligate parasite of cattle, variable in colour being darker in northern and paler in southern populations[27] (Figure 13.1D). An annotated bibliography of both subspecies of *H. irritans* and other species of *Haematobia* has been produced by Morgan and Thomas.[13] The two subspecies are *H. irritans irritans*, the horn fly, and *H. i. exigua*, the buffalo fly. The former subspecies developed in the western Palaearctic region, being introduced into the Nearctic in the late nineteenth century, from which it has spread to Central America and the Hawaiian Islands. *H. i. exigua* occurs in the Oriental and Australian regions, being introduced to Australia from Timor via Melville Island in 1838 on imported water buffalo,[23] where it has established itself in the tropical northern area and spread southwards into the subtropics.

H. irritans has a typical muscid life cycle. The eggs are bright yellowish-brown in colour. They hatch in 18-24 h, and are followed by three larval instars, and a pupa within a puparium. The larva is a small, slender maggot with the right mouth-hook larger than the left, the anterior spiracle with about five lobes and the posterior spiracle with three very sinuous slits similar to those of *M. domestica*, except that the curves are more sharply angled. The duration of the larval stages is three to five days and a similar time is spent in the pupa. Pupation occurs at the dung pat or in nearby soil.[23] In the northern temperate regions *H. irritans* overwinters as a diapausing pupa.

Both sexes are haematophagous and feed mainly on cattle and buffaloes, and occasionally on other animals, including man, when closely associated with bovines. They rest on cattle, being present in the greatest numbers on the withers, shoulders and flanks, but also on the neck, ribs and back.[23] They do not walk over the surface of the bovid but fly to change position. There is a single mating which occurs on the host. They take frequent small blood meals. The female oviposits only into fresh dung and leaves the host, when dung is dropped, to deposit small batches of eggs (12-20) on to the underside of the dung pat in a few minutes before returning to its host.

Figure 13.4: Male *Fannia canicularis*

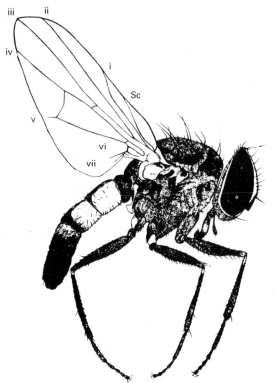

Source: Reproduced with permission from Zumpt, F. (1965). *Myiasis in Man and Animals in the Old World*. Butterworths, London

In spite of the adults apparently being sedentary on cattle, the spread of both subspecies indicates considerable powers of dispersion. Adult *H. i. irritans* disperse mainly at night, and adult *H. i. exigua* have invaded Magnetic Island, seven kilometres off the Queensland coast.[3] The distribution of *H. i. exigua* fluctuates with time. Early workers forecast that the buffalo fly would spread through the coastal areas of Queensland to northern New South Wales. Its limits are set in part by the need for an annual rainfall of 500 mm, and a temperature of 22°C for effective reproduction. In addition the immature stages require a moisture content of 68 per cent in dung.[20] In the early 1950s the buffalo fly had reached Gympie, about 200 km north of Brisbane, but by the early 1970s it had retreated northwards, and its southern limit was Gladstone, 500 km north of Brisbane. During the 1970s the buffalo fly spread southwards again and in 1981 was established in Brisbane and some distance further south. It looks as if the early forecasts will be shown to be correct.

Economic Importance. It is considered that 100-300 buffalo flies per beast can be tolerated without adverse effect but densities of 500-1,000 and up to 5,000 are found, which must affect productivity leading to lower weight gains in beef cattle, and lower milk yield in dairy herds. *H. i. irritans* is the intermediate host of *Stephanofilaria stilesi*, a parasite of cattle in North America,[27] but the sedentary nature of *H. irritans* on cattle would operate against either subspecies being important mechanical vectors of pathogens.

Other Muscids

Hydrotaea irritans

This fly is known as the headfly of sheep in Scotland and in Denmark as the plantation fly. It worries domestic stock and man by attacking the mouth, nose, ears, eyes and wounds to feed on secretions, becoming facultatively haematophagous.[7] Third instar larvae of the Hydrotaeini are predatory on other maggots in dung.[20] Greenberg[7] ascribes the same habit to *H. irritans* but Nielsen *et al.*[15] were unable to get gravid females to oviposit into dung; but large numbers of eggs were deposited in *Sphagnum*, where they hatched.

The main haunts of *H. irritans* are spruce and pine plantations and mixed forest with brushwood. The adults are active under calm, humid, sultry conditions particularly before and after rain, when their attacks can be intolerable.[15] The threshold temperature for activity is about 12°C, similar to that for *M. vetustissima*, and activity ceases at windspeeds above 3.6 km/h.[15] Activity is bimodal with peaks in the morning and evening. Adults concentrate on faeces and carrion where, presumably, they acquire the necessary protein for ovarian development. This species is important as

Figure 13.5: Third Stage Larvae of *Fannia canicularis* (right) and *F. scalaris* (left)

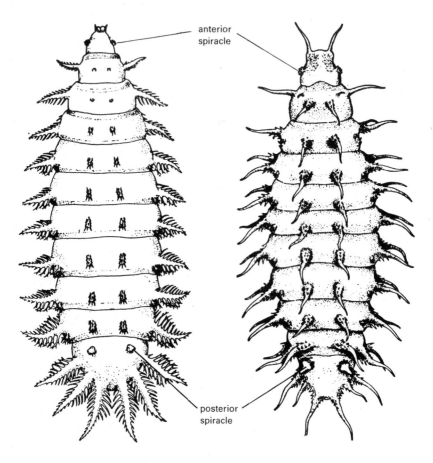

Source: From Hewitt, C.G.(1912). *Parasitology 5*: 164

a mechanical vector of bacterial pathogens, in particular *Corynebacterium pyogenes*, the cause of mastitis in cattle.[15]

Fannia

Species of *Fannia* are small to medium-sized muscid flies with bare arista, and a characteristic venation, in which vein iv is straight, vein vi is short and vein vii curved so that if extended it would intersect with an extended vein vi (Figure 13.4). The larvae are flattened, tapering anteriorly and bearing prominent lateral processes on most segments[12] (Figure 13.5). The anterior spiracles are prominent and the posterior ones elevated with three lobes in the mature larva. Two species are of minor importance:

F. canicularis (the lesser housefly) and *F. scalaris* (the latrine fly). *F. canicularis* is a worldwide, endophilic synanthrope and *F. scalaris* is an exophilic synanthrope, which has an Holarctic distribution.[7]
They breed in decaying animal and vegetable matter, especially faeces, including human faeces. *F. canicularis* breeds in chicken manure and *F. scalaris* in semi-fluid faeces of man and pigs.[7] The larvae of *F. canicularis* have long lateral and dorsal processes with short basal spines; and those of *F. scalaris* have short dorsal processes and pinnate lateral processes[12] (Figure 13.5). The adults are more abundant in the cooler months, declining in the summer, and where necessary the species overwinter as pupae buried 50-80 mm in the soil.[8] *F. canicularis*, which is attracted indoors, does not readily settle on human food, and is therefore less annoying than *M. domestica*. Both *F. canicularis* and *F. scalaris* have been recorded as causing intestinal myiasis in man, probably as the result of eating infested vegetables or fruit.[8]

References

1. Bornemissza, G.F. (1970). Insectary studies on the control of dung breeding flies by the activity of the dung beetle, *Onthophagus gazella* F. (Coleoptera: Scarabaeinae). *Journal of the Australian Entomological Society 9*: 31-41
2. Colless, D.H. and McAlpine, D.K. (1970). Diptera. pp. 656-740 in *The Insects of Australia*, sponsored by the CSIRO Division of Entomology, Melbourne University Press
3. Ferrar, P. (1969). Colonisation of an island by the buffalo fly, *Haematobia exigua*. *Australian Veterinary Journal 45*: 290-2
4. _____ (1979). The immature stages of dung-breeding muscoid flies in Australia, with notes on the species, and keys to larvae and puparia. *Australian Journal of Zoology Supplementary Series 73*: 1-106
5. Fosbrooke, H.A. (1963). The stomoxys plague in Ngorongoro, 1962. *East African Wildlife Journal 1*: 124-6
6. Greenberg, B. (1965). Flies and disease. *Scientific American 213 (1)*: 92-9
7. _____ (1971). *Flies and Disease. I. Ecology, Classification and Biotic Associations.* Princeton University Press, Princeton, New Jersey
8. _____ (1973). *Flies and Disease. II. Biology and Disease Transmission.* Princeton University Press, Princeton, New Jersey
9. Hepburn, G.A. (1943). Sheep blowfly research. V. Carcases as sources of blowflies. *Ondersterpoort Journal of Veterinary Science and Animal Industry 18*: 59-72
10. Hewitt, C.G. (1914). *The Housefly*. Cambridge University Press, Cambridge
11. Hughes, R.D., Greenham, P.M., Tyndale-Biscoe, M. and Walker, J.M. (1972). A synopsis of observations on the biology of the Australian bushfly (*Musca vetustissima* Walker). *Journal of the Australian Entomological Society 11*: 311-31
12. James, M.T. (1947). The flies that cause myiasis in man. *Miscellaneous Publications, United States Department of Agriculture 631*: 1-175
13. Morgan, C.E. and Thomas, G.D. (1974). Annotated bibliography of the horn fly, *Haematobia irritans*(L.), including references to the buffalo fly, *H.exigua* (de Meijere), and other species belonging to the genus *Haematobia*. *Miscellaneous Publications, United States Department of Agriculture 1278*: 1-134
14. Moutia, A. (1928). Surra in Mauritius and its principal vector, *Stomoxys nigra*. *Bulletin of Entomological Research 19*: 211-16
15. Nielsen, B.O., Nielsen, B.M. and Christensen, O. (1971). Bidrag til plantagefluens,

Hydrotaea irritans Fall., biologi (Diptera, Muscidae). *Entomologiske Meddelelser 39*: 30-44

16. Parr, H.C.M. (1962). Studies on *Stomoxys calcitrans* (L.) in Uganda (Diptera). II. The morphological development of the cephalopharyngeal sclerites of *S. calcitrans. Journal of the Entomological Society of Southern Africa 25*: 73-81

17. _____ (1962). Studies on *Stomoxys calcitrans* (L.) in Uganda, East Africa. II. Notes on life-history and behaviour. *Bulletin of Entomological Research 53*: 437-43

18. Paterson, H.E. and Norris, K.R. (1970). The *Musca sorbens* complex: the relative status of the Australian and two African populations. *Australian Journal of Zoology 18*: 231-45

19. Patton, W.S. and Evans, A.M. (1929). *Insects, Ticks, Mites and Venomous Animals of Medical and Veterinary Importance. I. Medical.* Grubb, Croydon

20. Pont, A.C. (1973). Studies on Australian Muscidae (Diptera). IV. A revision of the subfamilies Muscinae and Stomoxyinae. *Australian Journal of Zoology Supplementary Series 21*: 129-296

21. Ramsamy, M. (1978). *Some Aspects of Stable Fly (Stomoxys nigra Macquart) Control by the Sterile Insect Release Method.* Ph.D. thesis, University of London

22. _____ (1981). Development of a sampling plan for estimating the absolute population of *Stomoxys nigra* Macquart (Diptera, Muscidae) in Mauritius. *Insect Science and its Application 1*: 133-7

23. Roberts, F.H.S. (1952). *Insects Affecting Livestock.* Angus and Robertson, Sydney

24. Sacca, G. (1964). Comparative bionomics in the genus *Musca. Annual Review of Entomology 9*: 341-58

25. West, L.S. (1951). *The Housefly.* Comstock Publishing Company, New York

26. _____ and Peters, O.B. (1973). *An Annotated Bibliography of Musca domestica* Linnaeus. Dawsons of Pall Mall, London

27. Zumpt, F. (1973). *The Stomoxyine Biting Flies of the World (Diptera: Muscidae).* Gustav Fischer Verlag, Stuttgart

14 CALLIPHORIDAE, SARCOPHAGIDAE (BLOWFLIES) AND MYIASIS

Lucilia
Chrysomyia
Cochliomyia

Sarcoph
Wohl

The subject of myiasis will be dealt with in this and the succeeding chapter. This division is somewhat arbitrary. Myiasis is the invasion of living tissue of animals by the larvae of Diptera. The Calliphoridae and Sarcophagidae are large families in which the adults have functional mouthparts. A few species are obligatory agents of myiasis; rather more are facultative agents but the majority of the species breed in carrion. The next chapter will deal with a number of highly specialised families, each containing relatively few species. In these families the mouthparts of the adult are non-functional and the larvae are obligatory endoparasites of mammals often parasitising specific hosts.

dead decaying flesh

Classification

Adult Calliphoridae and Sarcophagidae have a row of bristles on the meropleuron and one or more bristles on the pteropleuron. The closely related Tachinidae have those same two characters but they are stout-bodied, strongly bristled flies with a prominent subscutellum, whose larvae are endoparasites of insects. The Calliphoridae are medium to large, metallic (Figure 14.1) or testaceous flies and the Sarcophagidae are grey-black, non-metallic, medium to large flies with prominent stripes on the mesonotum (Figure 14.9)

The Calliphoridae is divided into several subfamilies of which two, the Calliphorinae and Chrysomyinae, are of medical and veterinary importance. The Calliphorinae may be distinguished by well-developed bristles on the mesonotum (Figure 14.1); the radial stem vein (stem of veins i, ii and iii) is bare (Figure 14.2); and there are either two notopleural bristles and two anterior plus one posterior sternopleural bristles, or three notopleurals and one plus one sternopleurals. The external posthumeral is located lateral to the level of the presutural. In the Chrysomyinae the bristles on the mesonotum are poorly developed (Figure 14.3); there is no external posthumeral bristle, and the stem vein bears a row of hairs posteriorly. These two subfamilies contain all those involved in myiasis; the other subfamilies parasitise earthworms, snails, or live in association with ant or termite nests.[11]

The Chrysomyinae contain the important genera *Cochliomyia* and *Chrysomya*. Species of *Cochliomyia* are green to violet-green blowflies with three prominent black, longitudinal vittae on the mesonotum and

Figure 14.1: Male *Calliphora stygia*

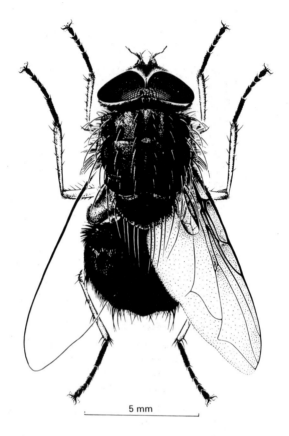

5 mm

Source: From Colless and McAlpine[11]

short palps, and those of *Chrysomya* are green to bluish-black blowflies with transverse bands or two narrow vittae or both on the mesonotum. *Cochliomyia* is restricted to the New World and *Chrysomya* to the Old World.

The Calliphorinae includes the greenbottles, *Lucilia*; the bluebottles with blue thorax and abdomen, some *Calliphora*; the brown blowflies with blue thorax and brown abdomen, other *Calliphora*; and the testaceous blowflies, *Cordylobia* and *Auchmeromyia*.[23]

The Sarcophagidae includes the subfamily Sarcophaginae, containing the genera *Sarcophaga* and *Wohlfahrtia* with usually four notopleural and three sternopleural bristles. In *Sarcophaga* the arista is plumose and the abdomen has a tesselated pattern of silver grey and black markings, which varies with the angle of the incident light (Figure 14.9A). In *Wohlfahrtia*

Figure 14.2: Wing of *Lucilia cuprina* (× 15)

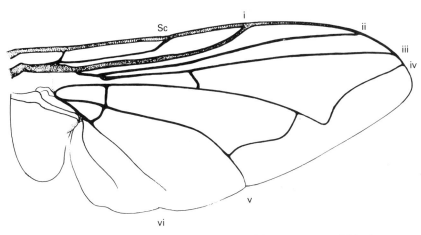

the arista is bare and the abdomen is grey with a pattern of black spots which are unaffected by the angle at which they are viewed (Figure 14.9B).

Much work has been done on the physiology of blowflies and Dethier[12] has summarised work on the adult black blowfly, *Phormia regina*, in his book *The Hungry Fly*.

Myiasis[49,50]

The various forms of myiasis may be classified from an entomological or a clinical point of view. Entomologically flies may be classified into three groups: obligatory or specific; facultative or semi-specific; and accidental. An example of an obligatory agent of myiasis is *Chrysomya bezziana*, the larvae of which are found in wounds; *Lucilia cuprina* is a facultative agent, which both causes myiasis in sheep and also breeds in carrion. Eggs or maggots of *Musca domestica* or *Sarcophaga* consumed with food and which survive in the alimentary tract, can be regarded as accidental agents of myiasis. The group of facultative myiasis agents may be further refined into primary flies which initiate myiasis, secondary flies which are unable to initiate myiasis but which readily participate once an animal has been infested, and tertiary flies which become involved in myiasis at a late stage when the host animal is almost dead. *L. cuprina* is a primary fly and *Chrysomya rufifacies* a secondary fly. Many carrion-breeding blowflies may act as tertiary flies.

The ability of calliphorid maggots to feed on decaying organic matter of animal origin was turned to good use by Baer,[2] who used maggots in the treatment of chronic osteomyelitis before the advent of antibiotics.

Figure 14.3: Female *Chrysomya bezziana*

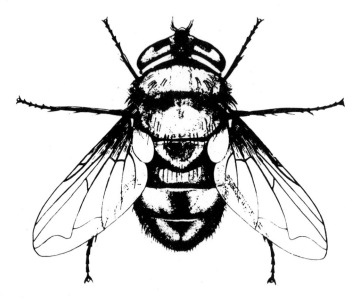

Source: From Zumpt[50]

Clinically myiasis can be classified on the tissue and part of the body affected. Dermal and subdermal myiasis includes wound or traumatic myiasis and furuncular myiasis in which a boil-like condition is produced, e.g. *Cordylobia anthropophaga*. Nasopharyngeal myiasis, including aural and ocular myiases, involves invasion of the head cavities of the outer ear, nose, mouth and accessory sinuses. Intestinal and urogenital myiases involve invasion of the alimentary tract or the urogenital system. The last category, sanguinivorous, is atypical and includes blood-sucking larvae of Diptera. West[49] gives a long table classifying the different species involved in myiasis on both clinical and entomological grounds and includes their geographical distribution.

Chrysomyinae

The Chrysomyinae includes two important species, *Chrysomya bezziana* in the Old World and *Cochliomyia hominivorax* in the New World, which are obligatory agents of myiasis. Their larvae are armed with broad, encircling bands of spines, which give them an undulating outline (Figure 14.4) and the common name of screw-worms. The posterior spiracles consist of three straight slits surrounded by an incomplete peritreme with an indistinct

Figure 14.4: Third Stage Larva of *Chrysomya bezziana*. A, lateral view of larva; B, posterior spiracles; C, view of larva from behind

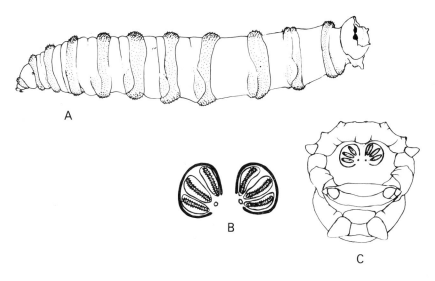

button in the unsclerotised zone. *Chrysomya rufifacies* in the Australian and Oriental regions and *Ch. albiceps* in the Palaearctic and Afrotropical regions are facultative agents of myiasis. Their larvae have a row of fleshy tubercles and are known as hairy maggots. *Cochliomyia macellaria* is a minor secondary fly in myiasis and more important as a fly of the market place where it oviposits on meat. *Ch. marginalis* and *Ch. megacephala* are common Old World bazaar flies.[17]

Chrysomya bezziana

Ch. bezziana is widely distributed in the Afrotropical and Oriental regions extending as far south as Papua New Guinea, but not to Australia. It attacks a wide range of hosts, but there are few records from wild animals. In Papua New Guinea feral pigs have a low infestation rate with *Ch. bezziana*,[34] but a more realistic picture is probably given by infestations among animals in a zoo in Malaysia, where in a period of 15 years there were 91 attacks on 21 species of mammals, resulting in 12 deaths.[44] The economic importance of *Ch. bezziana* stems from it causing myiasis in cattle. Cases of human myiasis are common in the Oriental region but rare in Africa.[50]

Females are attracted to wounds, several days old, for oviposition[32] and eggs are laid on the upper, dry side of wounds.[40] Oviposition occurs in the late afternoon, two to three hours before dusk when 100-250 eggs are deposited in a single batch, and they hatch 12-16 h later.[40,42] The importance of this timing and location of oviposition enables egg development to be completed in the hours of darkness. Eggs exposed to more than two hours' solar radiation suffer a high mortality and all are dead after six hours' exposure. There is also a low hatch when eggs are kept moist, hence the value of ovipositing on the dry upper edge of the wound.[40] Eggs are deposited in a shingle-like mass, giving the inner eggs protection from solar radiation.

Larvae feed initially on blood and serum and later lacerate tissue with their mouth-hooks. They bunch together and tunnel deeply (15 cm) into the host's tissue causing considerable destruction. Several females may oviposit at the same site, probably attracted by pheromones emitted by the first ovipositing female. As a result 3,000 larvae may occur in a wound.[42] In six to eight days the larvae are fully developed, leave the host as prepupae, and pupate in the ground, the pupal period lasting eight to ten days.[42]

The female is autogenous, developing the first batch of eggs without a protein meal, and the male is equally unattracted to protein baits.[39] Peak sexual activity occurs on the third day and the female is gravid in six to eight days.[34] The female can take in sufficient protein to mature a second batch of eggs in 13 s, and this can be done while ovipositing the first batch.[43] In the field few females lay more than two batches of eggs[41] The population of *Ch. bezziana* is very low, of the order of one to 200/25 ha.[34] They range widely and labelled females have deposited egg masses 50 km from their point of release.[25,41]

In domestic stock the areas most susceptible to attack by *Ch. bezziana* are the navels of newborn animals, surgical wounds produced during castration, docking and de-horning, and tick bites; the condition is complicated by secondary infections.[6] Preventive measures include delaying surgery to the cooler season of the year when *Ch. bezziana* is less active, dressing wounds, and twice weekly inspection of livestock.[6]

Cochliomyia hominivorax (= Callitroga americana)

An annotated bibliography of *C. hominivorax* has been produced by Snow *et al.*[37] Its distribution extended from the USA to southern Brazil, until a large-scale eradication programme reduced its distribution in the USA. The closely related *C. macellaria* has a rather wider distribution from southern Canada to Chile and Argentina.[18] Like *Ch. bezziana*, the eggs of *C. hominivorax* are laid in batches on the dry surfaces at the edge of wounds, two to ten days old. They hatch in 11-21 h and the larvae bunch together to feed with their posterior spiracles exposed. They are fully developed in four to eight days, leave the host in the morning (09.00-14.00) and pupate in the surface layers of the soil.[18] Prepupae bury themselves rather deeper in cold weather and if they are exposed to temperatures below 9.5°C for three months they die. They also require a soil moisture of less than 16 per cent.[32]

The adults emerge around dawn (04.00-07.00). Females mate only once and after a preoviposition period of five to ten days deposit batches of about 300 eggs. A particularly fecund female may produce nearly 3,000 eggs.[18] Their activity is reduced by hot, dry conditions, strong winds and by rain, but increases after rain.[32] They feed on wounds, dung and fresh meat, presumably to obtain protein for ovarian development.[18]

C. hominivorax is active all the year round in areas where the temperature is above 16°C,[21] and during the summer disperses widely from its overwintering areas moving 56 km per week[3] and a maximum of nearly 300 km.[22] Populations of *C. hominivorax* in Texas are depressed in the summer, increase in the autumn and are low in the winter. These fluctuations follow the incidence of myiasis.[32] In the USA populations of *C. hominivorax* overwinter in the south, especially in Texas. Control of *C. hominivorax* is complicated by the fact that it causes myiasis not only in cattle but in wild animals including opossums, cottontail and jack rabbits and the white tailed deer *Odocoileus virginianus texanus*.[27]

C. hominivorax has become famous among entomologists as being the first insect to be controlled and, on occasions, eradicated by the use of the sterile male release technique. This technique, which was originally proposed by Knipling,[24] requires the release of sterilised flies in numbers which will swamp the wild population. *C. hominivorax* was a good test insect to use because its populations are much lower than those of other pest insects, e.g. a few hundred per 250 ha, cf. thousands or hundreds of thousands.[28] The initial technical problem was to develop a technique for sterilising flies without markedly reducing their ability to compete with normal wild males. This was achieved by irradiating five-day-old pupae at a dosage of 5,000 r.[10]

The first trial on Sanibel Island showed that the technique had possibilities but the island was only 3 km off the Florida coast and subject to reinfestation from the mainland.[28] The main demonstration was made on Curaçao in the Netherlands Antilles and was outstandingly successful. A sterilising dose of 7,500 r was used because this prevented oviposition in sterilised females.[4] Sterilised adult flies were distributed by aircraft once a week. A release of 100 sterilised males per 250 ha per week for six weeks produced 15 per cent sterility among egg batches laid on wounded goats. From 9 August to 3 October 1954 the entire island was treated at an average rate of 435 males per 250 ha per week and in eight weeks all egg masses deposited were sterile; and from early October only two sterile egg batches were laid in the next three months. The screw-worm had been eradicated from Curaçao.[4]

This success was followed firstly by the eradication of *C. hominivorax* from Florida in 1959,[9] and secondly by the institution of a sterile male release programme along the USA-Mexico border to control the local population and prevent reintroduction from Mexico. This mammoth programme involved the production of 100,000,000 sterile male flies per week and their release along a barrier 400 km wide and more than 3,000 km in length.[1,38] It was highly successful from its initiation in 1962 through to 1971, with cases being reduced from 50,000 in 1960 to 153 in 1970.[1]

In 1972 a major outbreak occurred with nearly 100,000 cases being reported.[38] This has been attributed to the inadvertent selection of a non-competitive ecotype during mass rearing.[8] A new strain of flies has been established for mass production and the programme revised with the intention of shifting the barrier further south, which would substantially reduce its length. The success of the new programme is shown by the fact that in Texas in 1976 there were nearly 30,000 cases of myiasis but only 39 in 1977.[38] *C. hominivorax* also reappeared in Curaçao with a relatively high incidence of cases in man.[36,45] This reintroduction is not attributed to wind carriage of adult flies but to the introduction of infested cattle from South America.

Control of *C. hominivorax* has had unexpected consequences. The screw-worm attacked both deer and cattle and was an important factor in limiting the deer population. Control of the screw-worm fly has led to a substantial increase in the deer population. Deer and cattle are parasitised by the same ixodid tick, *Amblyomma maculatum*. An increase in the deer population has led to an increase in *A. maculatum* and a higher incidence of the tick on cattle. This became particularly important when control of *C. hominivorax* failed because tick bites are potential oviposition sites for the fly.

Metallic Calliphorinae

The majority of metallic Calliphorinae breed in carrion but some are facultative myiasis flies of which the most important are primary flies of the genus *Lucilia* and *Calliphora*. Calliphorine larvae are smooth-bodied maggots in which the posterior spiracles have three slits and are surrounded by a continuous peritreme ring, which includes the button (Figure 14.5). Larvae of *Calliphora* have an additional accessory sclerite between the mouth-hooks. This is lacking in *Lucilia*.

Species of *Lucilia* and *Calliphora* are the cause of cutaneous myiasis in sheep in which they may be associated with some *Chrysomya*. This condition is associated with sheep with heavily wrinkled skins, e.g. merino, and is particularly important in Australia, South Africa and Britain, being of lesser importance in New Zealand and the USA.[6] In 1969-70 sheep myiasis was estimated to have cost Australia A$28,000,000[14] and in a bad outbreak 30 per cent of a flock may die.[6]

In Australia and South Africa the main species is *L. cuprina* which is involved in 90 per cent of all strikes and was the only species present in 55-71 per cent of infestations.[20,48] *L. cuprina* is closely related to *L.*

Figure 14.5: A, Third Stage Larva of *Calliphora* (Lateral View); B, Posterior Spiracles of Larva; C, View of Larva from Behind; D, Puparium of *Calliphora*

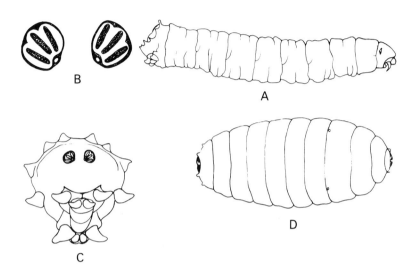

sericata, the sheep blowfly of Great Britain. In the southern hemisphere *L. sericata* plays only a minor role in sheep myiasis, being less important than species of *Calliphora* such as *C. stygia*, which is responsible for 95 per cent of strikes in New Zealand compared to 5 per cent for *L. sericata*.[31,47,50]

Lucilia cuprina

Gravid female *L. cuprina* lay their eggs in carrion or on sheep. They are attracted to sheep which have areas of soiled fleece or are suffering from bacterial decomposition of the fleece in fleece rot. The eggs are deposited in a cluster of 100-300, depending upon the size of the female. For development they require a temperature above 30°C, which will be present on the skin and in the fleece of sheep, and a humidity of more than 90 per cent.[14] Under these conditions the eggs hatch in 8-12 h. *L. cuprina* is diurnal in activity and hence eggs laid in the mid-afternoon complete their development during the night when humidities are high. Eggs placed at skin level failed to hatch unless the area was kept saturated.[14] Fertility of the eggs is of the order of 70-86 per cent.

The process by which *L. cuprina* orientates to sheep and suitable oviposition sites is complicated, involving visual, olfactory and gustatory stimuli. The visual response to living sheep was clearly demonstrated in the field when about 50 *L. cuprina* were paying attention to a blowfly-infested sheep, but when the sheep died they left within ten minutes. Later these or other *L. cuprina* returned to oviposit in the corpse.[33] In exploring a sheep for oviposition the female probes potential sites with her proboscis, feeds, and then shuffles backwards, probing with her ovipositor, thrusting it deep within the fleece. There are taste receptors on the ovipositor, and this probing process is repeated before each egg is deposited.[33]

Oviposition is referred to as 'blow' and the establishment of larvae on the host as 'strike'. The newly hatched larvae are very susceptible to desiccation and move down to the skin to feed on the protein-rich exudate produced by a skin irritated by fouling and fleece rot.[14] Second and third stage larvae attack the skin causing and extending lesions. The mature third stage larvae drop from the host at night and burrow into the soil to a depth of 1-2 cm where they pupate, providing the temperature is above 10°C and the humidity low. There is no larval diapause as occurs in *L. sericata*, which is adapted to a cooler climate. The pupal stage lasts 6 days at 30°C and 25 days at 15°C with a survival of 75-95 per cent.[14] At the height of the season (October-February) survival of 1st instar larvae to adults is 20-25 per cent and the larval and pupal stages occupy two to three weeks out of a generation time of three to four weeks. There are about eight generations a year.

The female needs to feed on protein to complete ovarian development and this can be obtained from carrion, from scalded sheep, wounds and to a lesser extent, dung. Males take in protein all their life and in view of the low density in which *L. cuprina* occurs in the field, sources of protein may serve to bring the sexes together. The female mates relatively late in the first ovarian cycle and in the field females that have completed more than three cycles are rare, although seven cycles may be completed in the laboratory. Both sexes need access to a source of carbohydrate, e.g. nectar, honeydew, during adult life.[14]

Bionomics of L. cuprina

L. cuprina is an early coloniser of fresh sheep carcasses but even so fewer adults are produced than from living sheep. Under optimal conditions the average emergence of *L. cuprina* from a sheep carcass was 304 out of a total emergence of more than 36,000 calliphorids, and in less favourable conditions only four out of 10,000.[46] This failure is attributed to competition from other blowflies, especially *C. augur* in spring and *Chrysomya rufifacies* in summer, the adverse affect of high temperature generated in carcasses, and predation. Prepupae leaving a carcass are subject to predation by beetles and within the carcass by *Ch. rufifacies*. In contrast about 90 per cent of the flies bred from struck sheep were *L. cuprina*, averaging 1,220 adults per strike.[46] In eastern coastal Australia *L. cuprina* also breeds in refuse.[14]

Population densitites of *L. cuprina* are low but comparable to that of its host. Densities of females which have completed one ovarian cycle, and could therefore have attacked sheep, range from 0.2 at the start of the season to 22/ha, which compares with a sheep density of 10/ha.[14] Dispersal of the adults is probably affected by the habitat. In favourable areas adult flies disperse only a few kilometres. This is supported by the existence of localised insecticide-resistant populations which spread slowly.[14]

In Australia the various species of blowflies attacking sheep have different seasonal and geographical distributions. Species of *Calliphora* are commoner south of 25°S and *L cuprina* north of 30°S. Although *L. cuprina* is the main sheep blowfly, *C. stygia* is important in the southern half of Australia and Tasmania, *C. augur* in the south-east and *C. nociva* in the south-west.[31] Adult *C. stygia* may be present in warm periods in winter when the bulk of its population is present as prepupae and pupae. It has been calculated that 10 per cent of strikes are initiated by *C. stygia* but it also occurs in strikes commenced by other species.

C. augur is ovoviviparous depositing 50 eggs which hatch immediately. This species has more varied breeding sites, causing myiasis in birds and other mammals. *C. augur* and *C. nociva* are associated with wound myiases.[31] *Ch. rufifacies* has a higher temperature threshold than *L. cuprina* and is most abundant in the hottest months of the year. As an adaptation to its larvae being predacious *Ch. rufifacies* oviposits in carcasses a few days old when other blowflies have established themselves. It does not leave the carcass as a prepupa but pupates in or on it.[31]

The Effect on Sheep

The common site of blowfly attack on sheep is the breech, tail and crutch area, where the wool has been fouled and remains moist from faeces and urine. Less common sites are the prepuce of rams and wethers, i.e. pizzle strike; poll strike on the dorsum of the head where there is excessive skin folding; body strike in wet seasons particularly in poor, dense pasture; and wound strike. Young sheep are more susceptible because of their tender skin.[6]

The predisposition to strike can be offset by keeping the fleece short in susceptible areas. Removal of the fleece around the breech is only effective for about six weeks. More permanent protection is given by Mules' operation in which woolled skin is removed in a strip from both sides of the breech with the intention of increasing the width of the woolless area. This procedure reduces breech strike by 80-90 per cent.[6]

In untreated infestations the maggots do not burrow deeply but spread out causing increasing damage to the skin, and death eventuates from toxaemia, loss of skin, and secondary bacterial infection.[6] Suppression of helminth infections can reduce breech strike from 50 per cent to 5 per cent by reducing fouling of the breech.[30]

Mules' operation was developed in 1931 but was replaced by insecticidal protection using at first arsenicals, and then the chlorinated hydrocarbon insecticides, DDT, BHC and dieldrin. So successful was the last named that an article was published in *Rural Research* in December 1957 with the title 'Defeat of the Sheep Blowfly'. This was premature and followed, 13 years later, with another article in June 1970 'Blowfly — A Warning'. Resistance to the chlorinated hydrocarbons was followed by the use of organo-phosphorus compounds, and when these failed, carbamates. *L. cuprina* has become resistant to these compounds and in the period 1966-73 the period of protection provided by organophosphorus compounds was reduced from 16 to 9 weeks, and for carbamates from 14 to 4 weeks.[35] Conse-quently Mules' operation has been reintroduced and attention given to other means of combating *L. cuprina*, especially genetic techniques.[14]

Testaceous Calliphorinae

Two species of testaceous calliphorines, which are endemic to the Afro-tropical region, cause myiasis in man. They are *Auchmeromyia luteola*, the Congo floor maggot, and *Cordylobia anthropophaga*, the Tumbu or mango fly. The adults may occur in huts or houses and be distinguished by the second visible abdominal segment being obviously longer than the third segment in *A. luteola*, and the two segments being of similar length in *C. anthropophaga*. The eyes of male *A. luteola* are widely separated and those of *C. anthropophaga* almost contiguous.[23]

Auchmeromyia luteola (see Figure 14.6)

Adult *A. luteola* have lapping mouthparts and feed on faeces, particularly human faeces, and fermenting fruit while the larvae are haematophagous.[50] A female lays batches of about 50 eggs, and in her lifetime may lay a total of 300 eggs in six batches. They are laid in dry, dusty soil or sand in the earth floor of huts and hatch in 36-60 h at 26-28°C and 50-60 per cent RH.[50] There are three larval stages (Figure 14.7) which feed at night on the inhabitants of the hut, sleeping on the ground. the larvae are unable to climb vertical surfaces and protection against being bitten is provided by a bed raising the occupant 10 cm above ground level. There are at least two feeds in each larval instar and 6-20 feeds in the development of an indi-vidual larva. The pupal stage lasts 11 days at 28.5°C, and in the laboratory the generation time is ten weeks giving five generations per annum.[15]

Each blood meal takes about 20 min. When feeding the larva attaches itself almost at right angles to the skin and makes an incision with the mouth-hooks and the toothed maxillary plates in front of them.[50] Blood is said to be taken in by contractions of the crop in which the blood is stored before being passed to the foregut and on to the convoluted midgut lined with a peritrophic membrane, digestion being completed in the rectum.[7] There are two unusual features in this description made nearly 80 years

Figure 14.6: *Cordylobia anthropophaga* Female (above) × 4; *Auchmeromyia luteola* Female (below) × 3

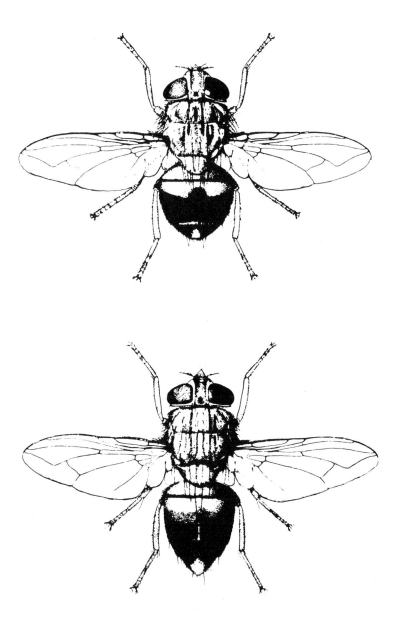

Source: From Castellani, A. and Chalmers, A.J. (1913). *A Manual of Tropical Medicine*. Baillière Tindall, London

Figure 14.7: Third Stage Larva of *Auchmeromyia luteola*. A, dorsal view; B, ventral view; C, posterior view

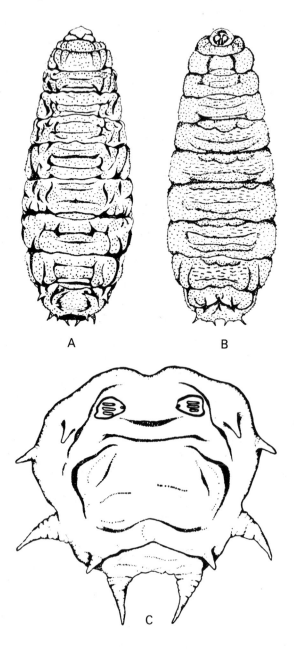

A

B

C

Source: From Zumpt[50]

ago. Firstly, the crop is usually a storage organ and not a sucking apparatus and the rectum is usually lined with cuticle and the site of the absorption of water and salts but not of digestion. Garrett-Jones[15] considers that larvae will feed daily, but in the field digestion is slow and at least five days would elapse between blood meals.

Larvae of *A. luteola* are associated with man and also with warthogs, *Phacochoerus aethiopicus*, and aardvarks, *Orycteropus afer*.[50] In the Serengeti National Park larvae and adults of *A. luteola* were common in culverts in the complete absence of man; 98 per cent of the feeds were on suids, and those meals which could be identified to species were from warthogs.[7] A small number of larvae had also fed on hyenas, probably the spotted hyena, *Crocuta crocuta*, and are the first records of *A. luteola* feeding on a hairy mammal.[7]

A high incidence of *Trypanosoma brucei* is found in the spotted hyena and the potential of *A. luteola* larvae to act as vectors was investigated.[7,16] There was no evidence of cyclical development of the trypanosome which remained viable for only 21 h in larvae but there was some evidence that *Auchmeromyia* larvae might act as mechanical vectors.[16] There are four other species of *Auchmeromyia* of which *A. bequaerti* also occurred in the Serengeti culverts. Larval populations die out if the ground is damp or wet but areas are rapidly repopulated when they dry out.

Cordylobia anthropophaga (see Figure 14.6)

The account given here is based on that of Blacklock and Thompson.[5] Adult *C. anthropophaga* are diurnal with peaks of activity in the early morning (07.00-09.00) and late afternoon (16.00-18.00). They seek shade, being more able to resist cold and damp than exposure to sunlight. They feed on fermenting fruit and, given the opportunity, liver. Females mate soon after emergence and may mate several times on the first day. Two batches of eggs are laid. The first contains about 300 eggs and the second 100-200. Oviposition takes about 30 min and the female seeks out dry sand soiled by urine and excreta for oviposition and avoids too moist sand. The female lives about two weeks.

The egg is rather smaller than those of other muscoid flies, measuring 0.8 mm. The eggs hatch in 24-48 h and the larva remains buried in the sand until responding to vibrations, heat and carbon dioxide, which could signify the arrival of a host. The larva then raises its front end in the air and searches around for a host. On a suitable host the larva will penetrate the unbroken skin and bury itself in less than a minute. It will penetrate the skin of many different mammals and also fowl but it does not develop in the last-named. The larva develops in a boil-like swelling in the skin. The swelling has an opening through which the larva breathes using the posterior spiracles in which there are three slightly sinuous slits in a weakly sclerotised peritreme (Figure 14.8). The three larval stages are completed in eight days, and then the prepupa (Figure 14.8) leaves the host and pupates in the ground. The puparium is tolerant of dry conditions but killed by continuous exposure to 37°C.

The main hosts of *C. anthropophaga* are black and brown rats and among domestic animals, dogs, particularly puppies. Larvae penetrate the feet, genitals, tail and axillary regions of their host. On man lesions are found mainly on areas of the body covered by clothing and are commoner in children. Breeding of *C. anthropophaga* continues throughout the year and the seasonal nature of human infections, which are more numerous in the wet season, is attributed to rat burrows being flooded and rats being more closely associated with human habitations. Females will oviposit on soiled or inefficiently washed clothing or bedding and hence larvae are distributed over the areas of the body covered by clothing. The boil-like swelling causes considerable discomfort as the larva increases in size and there is a copious exudate of serum, blood and larval faeces. The danger of infestation from clothing can be avoided by drying clothes in full sunlight out of contact with the ground, and then ironing the clothing to kill any eggs or larvae before storing in covered receptacles.

As a result of air transport persons infected with *C. anthropophaga* are arriving in many parts of the world, including Australia;[29] and a case has been reported of an infection in a woman who has never been to Africa and who had appeared to have acquired the infection in Spain.[26] It is possible that a focus of *C. anthropophaga* could be established outside tropical Africa.

Sarcophagidae[23,50]

The Sarcophagidae are viviparous or ovoviviparous producing either 1st instar larvae or eggs which hatch immediately on deposition. This gives members of this family considerable advantage in competing for carrion with calliphorids which are oviparous. The mature sarcophagid larva has its posterior spiracles recessed in a posterior depression and hidden from view (Figure 14.10). The spiracles have three slits which are orientated more or less dorsoventrally and surrounded by an incomplete peritreme. Two species, *Wohlfahrtia magnifica* and *Wohlfahrtia vigil*, are obligatory agents of myiasis.

Wohlfahrtia magnifica

W. magnifica is adapted to the desert areas of North Africa, Asiatic Russia and Asia Minor where it causes wound myiasis in man and domestic stock including horses, donkeys, cattle, buffalo, sheep, goats, pigs and even geese. According to Zumpt[50] there are no records of this species from wild animals. Adults occur in fields and orchards where they feed on flowers.

Figure 14.8: Third Stage Larva of *Cordylobia anthropophaga,* Ventral View (above); Posterior Spiracles of Larva (below)

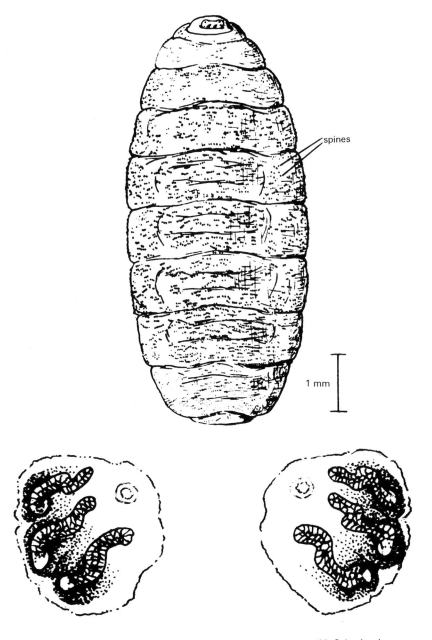

spines

1 mm

Source: Larva from Bertram, D.S.(1938). *Annals of Tropical Medicine 32*: 433. Spiracles drawn from various sources

Figure 14.9: A, *Sarcophaga haemorrhoidalis*, Adult Male; B, *Wohlfahrtia magnifica*, Adult Female

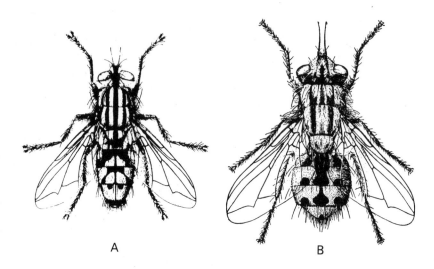

A   B

Source: From James[23]

They are active during the bright, hot period of the day from 10.00 to 16.00 h. Females larviposit in wounds and body openings, ear, nose and eyes. A female may contain 120-170 larvae. Once deposited the larvae grow rapidly, burrow into the tissues and cause extensive damage which may prove fatal.

Infection of the ears can lead to deafness, loss of an eye and cause severe damage to the tissue of the nasal region. The larvae are full grown in six to seven days when they leave the host and pupate in the ground, over-wintering as pupae in regions with a cold winter. The larvae are extremely hardy pupating and producing normal adults after one hour's exposure to 95 per cent alcohol. They survive for considerable time in concentrated hydrochloric acid and corrosive sublimate.

Wohlfahrtia vigil

This species is an obligatory myiasis fly, occurring in North America where it is a parasite of mink. Larvae are deposited in groups and can only penetrate thin skin, and for that reason human cases are restricted to young babies in whom they cause a furuncular myiasis. Prevention is easy by fly-screening prams containing sleeping infants when left out of doors.

Wohlfahrtia opaca

W. opaca, which may be a subspecies of *W. vigil*,[13] also causes human furuncular myiasis in North America.[19] In both species the larvae penetrate the unbroken skin causing boil-like swellings on exposed parts of the body. There are usually 12-14 lesions and rarely as many as 40.

Other Sarcophagids

The genus *Sarcophaga* is widely distributed throughout the world and contains hundreds of species which are very difficult to identify. They develop in carrion, excrement and any kind of decomposing organic matter. A number of species has been associated with myiasis, usually as tertiary flies or as accidental agents, but some species of *Sarcophaga* are facultative agents of myiasis as is *W. nuba*.

Figure 14.10: Third Stage Larva of *Sarcophaga*. A, lateral view; B, posterior spiracles; C, hind view

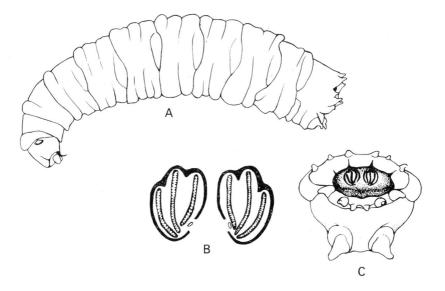

References

1. Anon. (1973). The screw worm strikes back. *Nature, London 242*: 493-4
2. Baer, W.S. (1931). The treatment of chronic osteomyelitis with the maggot (larva of the blowfly). *Journal of Bone and Joint Surgery 13*: 438-75
3. Barrett, W.L. (1937). Natural dispersion of *Cochliomyia americana. Journal of Economic Entomology 30*: 873-6
4. Baumhover, A.H., Graham, A.J., Bitter, B.A., Hopkins, D.E., New, W.D., Dudley, F.H. and Bushland, R.C. (1955). Screw-worm control through the release of sterilised flies. *Journal of Economic Entomology 48*: 462-6
5. Blacklock, B. and Thompson, M.G. (1923). A study of the tumbu-fly, *Cordylobia anthropophaga* Grünberg in Sierra Leone. *Annals of Tropical Medicine and Parasitology 17*: 443-502

6. Blood, D.C., Henderson, J.A. and Radostits, O.M. (1979). *Veterinary Medicine — A Textbook of the Diseases of Cattle, Sheep, Pigs and Horses*. Baillière Tindall, London
7. Boreham, P.F.L. and Geigy, R. (1976). Studies on the genus *Auchmeromyia* Brauer and Bergenstamm (Diptera: Calliphoridae). *Acta Tropica 33*: 74-87
8. Bush, G.L., Neck, R.W. and Kitto, G.B. (1976). Screw-worm eradication: inadvertent selection for noncompetitive ecotypes during mass rearing. *Science 193*: 491-3
9. Bushland, R.C. (1975). Screwworm research and eradication. *Bulletin of the Entomological Society of America 21*: 23-6
10. _____ and Hopkins, D.E. (1953). Sterilisation of screw-worm flies with X-rays and gamma-rays. *Journal of Economic Entomology 46*: 648-56
11. Colless, D.H. and McAlpine, D.K. (1970). Diptera. p. 656-740 in *The Insects of Australia*, sponsored by the CSIRO Division of Entomology, Melbourne University Press
12. Dethier, V.G. (1976). *The Hungry Fly*. Harvard University Press, Cambridge, Massachusetts
13. Eads, R.B. (1979). Notes on muscoid Diptera of public health interest. *Mosquito News 39*: 674-5
14. Foster, G.G., Kitching, R.L. Vogt, W.G. and Whitten, M.J. (1975). Sheep blowfly and its control in the pastoral ecosystem of Australia. *Proceedings of the Ecological Society of Australia 9*: 213-29
15. Garrett-Jones, C. (1951). The Congo floor maggot, *Auchmeromyia luteola* (F.), in a laboratory culture. *Bulletin of Entomological Research 41*: 679-708
16. Geigy, R. and Kauffmann, M. (1977). Experimental mechanical transmission of *Trypanosoma brucei* by *Auchmeromyia* larvae. *Protozoology 3*: 103-7
17. Greenberg, B. (1971). *Flies and Disease. I. Ecology, Classification and Biotic Associations*. Princeton University Press, Princeton, New Jersey
18. Hall, D.G. (1948). *The Blowflies of North America*. The Thomas Say Foundation, USA
19. Haufe, W.O. and Nelson, W.A. (1957). Human furuncular myiasis caused by the flesh fly *Wohlfahrtia opaca* (Coq.)(Sarcophagidae: Diptera). *Canadian Entomologist 89*: 325-7
20. Hepburn, G.A. (1943). Sheep blowfly research I. A survey of maggot collections from live sheep and a note on the trapping of blowflies. *Onderstepoort Journal of Veterinary Science and Animal Industry 18*: 13-17
21. Hightower, R.G. and Adams, A.L. (1969). Dispersal and local distribution of laboratory-reared sterile screw-worm flies released in winter. *Journal of Economic Entomology 62*: 259-61
22. _____ Adams, A.L. and Alley, D.A. (1965). Dispersal of released irradiated laboratory-reared screw-worm flies. *Journal of Economic Entomology 58*: 373-4
23. James, M.T. (1947). The flies that cause myiasis in man. *United States Department of Agriculture Miscellaneous Publication 631*: 1-175
24. Knipling, E.F. (1955). Possibilities of insect control or eradication through the use of sexually sterile males. *Journal of Economic Entomology 48*: 459-62
25. Lamb, K.P., Sands, D.P.A. and Spradbery, J.P. (1978). Assay of Old-World screw-worm fly, *Chrysomya bezziana*, labelled with ^{32}P. *Entomologia Experimentalis et Applicata 23*: 55-65
26. Laurence, B.R. and Herman, F.G. (1973). Tumbu fly (*Cordylobia*) infection outside Africa. *Transactions of the Royal Society of Tropical Medicine and Hygiene 67*: 888
27. Lindquist, A.W. (1937). Myiasis in wild animals in southwestern Texas. *Journal of Economic Entomology 30*: 735-40
28. _____ (1955). The use of gamma radiation for control or eradication of the screw-worm. *Journal of Economic Entomology 48*: 467-9
29. Moorhouse, D.E. (1982). Personal communication
30. Morley, F.H.W., Donald, A.D., Donnelly, J.R., Axelsen, A. and Waller, P.J. (1976). Blowfly strike in the breech region of sheep in relation to helminth infection. *Australian Veterinary Journal 52*: 325-9
31. Norris, K.R. (1959). The ecology of sheep blowflies in Australia. pp. 514-44 in *Biogeography and Ecology in Australia*, A. Keast, R.L. Crocker and C.S. Christian (eds.), Junk, Den Haag

32. _____ (1965). The bionomics of blow flies. *Annual Review of Entomology 10*: 47-68
33. Rice, M.J. (1982). Personal communication
34. Sands, D.P.A. (1979). Personal communication in an address to the Entomological Society of Queensland, 10 September 1979
35. Shanahan, G.J. and Roxburgh, N.A. (1974). Reduction in period of protection from artificial flystrike by organophosphorus and organophosphorus-carbamate resistant larvae of *Lucilia cuprina. Australian Veterinary Journal 50*: 177-8
36. Snow, J.W., Coppedge, J.R. Baumhover, A.H. and Gorsira, R. (1978). The screwworm *Cochliomyia hominivorax* (Diptera: Calliphoridae) reinfests the island of Curaçao, Netherlands Antilles. *Journal of Medical Entomology 14*: 592-3
37. _____ Sienbenaler, A.J. and Newell, F.G. (1981). *Annotated Bibliography of the Screw-worm Cochliomyia hominivorax* (Coquerel). United States Department of Agriculture, Science and Education Administration, Agricultural Reviews and Manuals ARM-S-14
38. _____ and Whitten, C.J. (1979). Status of the screwworm (Diptera: Calliphoridae) control program in the southwestern United States during 1977. *Journal of Medical Entomology 15*: 518-20
39. Spradbery, J.P. (1979). The reproductive status of *Chrysomya* spp. (Diptera: Calliphoridae) attracted to liver-baited blowfly traps in Papua New Guinea. *Journal of the Australian Entomological Society 18*: 57-61
40. _____ (1979). Daily oviposition activity and its adaptive significance in the screw-worm fly, *Chrysomya bezziana* (Diptera: Calliphoridae). *Journal of the Australian Entomological Society 18*: 63-6
41. _____ (in press). The Old World screw-worm fly, *Chrysomya bezziana*. In *Cattle Diseases, a Course for Field Veterinarians*, Universiti Portanian, Malaysia
42. _____ Sands, D.P.A. and Bakker, P. (1976). Evaluation of insecticide smears for the control of screw-worm fly, *Chrysomya bezziana*, in Papua New Guinea. *Australian Veterinary Journal 52*: 280-4
43. _____ and Schweizer, G. (1979). Ingestion of food by the adult screw-worm fly, *Chrysomya bezziana* (Diptera, Calliphoridae). *Entomologia Experimentalis et Applicata 25*: 75-85
44. _____ and Vanniasingham, J.A. (1980). Incidence of the screw-worm fly, *Chrysomya bezziana*, at the Zoo Negara, Malaysia. *Malaysian Medical Journal 7*: 28-32
45. Tannahill, F.H., Coppedge, J.R. and Snow, J.W. (1980). Screwworm (Diptera: Calliphoridae) myiasis on Curaçao: reinvasion after 20 years. *Journal of Medical Entomology 17*: 265-7
46. Waterhouse, D.F. (1947). The relative importance of live sheep and of carrion as breeding grounds for the Australian sheep blowfly *Lucilia cuprina. Council for Scientific and Industrial Research (Australia) Bulletin 217*: 1-31
47. _____ and Paramonov, S.J. (1950). The status of two species of *Lucilia* (Diptera, Calliphoridae) attacking sheep in Australia. *Australian Journal of Scientific Research B 3*: 310-36
48. Watts, J.E., Muller, M.J., Dyce, A.L. and Norris, K.R. (1976). The species of flies reared from struck sheep in south-eastern Australia. *Australian Veterinary Journal 52*: 488-9
49. West, L.S. (1951). *The Housefly.* Comstock Publishing Company, New York
50. Zumpt, F. (1965). *Myiasis in Man and Animals in the Old World.* Butterworths, London

15 OESTRIDAE, HYPODERMATIDAE, GASTEROPHILIDAE AND CUTEREBRIDAE

The members of the four families to be dealt with in this chapter are moderately large, bee-like flies with vestigial mouthparts and small eyes, giving a large interocular space. Their stout, thick larvae are obligatory endoparasites of mammals, and are referred to as grubs.

The Oestridae develop in the nasopharyngeal cavities of Perissodactyla and Artiodactyla, although one species (*Tracheomyia macropi*) parasitises the red kangaroo, and another (*Pharyngobolus africanus*) the African elephant.[45] Two species are of importance: *Oestrus ovis*, which parasitises sheep and goats, and *Rhinoestrus purpureus*, a parasite of equines. Adult oestrids have a distinct postscutellum, large squamae and the apical cell is closed by vein iv joining vein iii before the wing margin (Figure 15.2). The larvae have well-developed mouth-hooks and the posterior spiracles are large plates with numerous small openings (Figure 5.3).

The Hypodermatidae are dermal parasites of Artiodactyla, Lagomorpha and Rodentia. Two species of *Hypoderma* are important parasites of cattle. This family is sometimes treated as a subfamily of the Oestridae with which

Figure 15.1: Female *Oestrus ovis*(× 5)

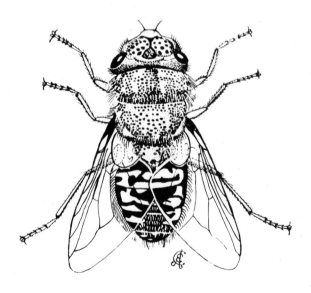

Source: From Cameron, A.E. (1942). *Transactions of the Highland and Agricultural Society*

they share the following characters: distinct postscutellum, large squamae and the posterior spiracles of the larvae with numerous small openings (Figure 15.6). They differ in having the apical cell of the wing open, i.e. vein iv meets the wing margin independently of vein iii (Figure 15.5), and by the larva having only rudimentary mouth-hooks (Figure 15.6).

The Gasterophilidae are mainly parasites of the alimentary tract of Equidae, but three species have been described from Asiatic and African rhinoceroses, and two species from the African elephant and one from the Indian elephant. Species of *Gasterophilus* (sometimes misspelt without the 'e' as *Gastrophilus*) are important parasites of horses and donkeys. In the adult gasterophilid the postscutellum is undeveloped, the squamae small and the apical cell wide open because vein iv does not bend towards vein iii (Figure 15.9). The larva has well-developed mouth-hooks and the posterior spiracles open by three bent slits in a shallow concavity.

The Cuterebridae are dermal parasites of rodents and rabbits with one species, *Dermatobia hominis*, parasitising wild and domestic animals including cattle and man. In Cuterebrids the postscutellum is undeveloped, the squamae large and the apical cell narrowed by vein iv turning towards vein iii (Figure 15.12), but not joining it. In the larva the mouth-hooks are well developed (Figure 15.14) and the posterior spiracles, which are deeply sunk, have three straight slits.

For further information, particularly on entomological aspects of these families, the reader is referred to James[24] and Zumpt;[45] and for information on their veterinary importance to Blood *et al.*[7] and Seddon and Albiston.[38] The account which follows has drawn extensively on these four works.

Oestrus ovis (Sheep Nostril Fly)

Five species are included in the genus *Oestrus* of which four are parasites of antelopes and only one, *Oestrus ovis*, parasitises sheep and goats. It does not occur in antelopes.[22] A comprehensive list of the literature on *O. ovis* is given by Papavero[30] in which he lists references from 1686 to 1973. *O. ovis* is considered to be a Palaearctic species which now has a worldwide distribution having been taken throughout the world by man with his livestock.

Adult *O. ovis* have black pits dorsally between the eyes on the frons and black tubercles on the mesonotum and scutellum (Figure 15.1). The mesonotum is yellow-brown with yellow hairs. The abdomen is black with an irregular pattern of lighter marking which varies with the angle of illumination.

Life Cycle

The female is ovoviviparous and matures about 500 eggs, which are

Figure 15.2: Wing of *Oestrus ovis* ($\times$ 10)

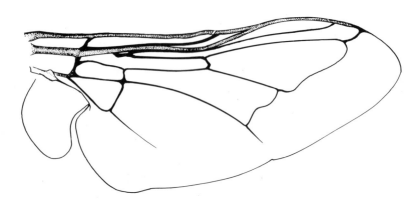

deposited in small batches of less than 50 at a time. Sheep react to the presence of female *O. ovis* by pushing their noses into the soil or into the fleece of others in the flock. They may run about erratically. When an opportunity presents itself *O. ovis* deposits larvae into the nasal cavity. They may develop there for a month before moving into the frontal, and sometimes the maxillary sinuses, where the larvae complete their development. The mature larva moves forward, is sneezed out by the host, burrows into the soil and pupates.

The 1st instar larva has gently curved mouth-hooks and 22-25 terminal spines arranged in two groups. These characters enable this larva to be separated from that of the 1st instar of *Rhinoestrus purpureus* which also causes temporary myiasis, especially ocular myiasis, in man. The mature 3rd instar larva is about 25 mm long, white or yellowish in colour with darker transverse dorsal bands and transverse rows of spines on the ventral surface of each segment (Figure 15.3). The posterior spiracles are exposed, flat, D-shaped plates with the button enclosed by the numerous small openings.

Bionomics

Development of the 1st instar larva may be delayed, and individuals from the same larviposition may spend from one to nine months in the 1st instar. This plays a role in the overwintering cycle. The pupal stage lasts 1-2 months depending upon temperature. Bukshtynov[9] found a steady increase in development from 12.5-35°C with adult emergence occurring after 14 days at the highest temperature. Rogers and Knapp[34] found that temperatures above 32°C were fatal. Breev *et al.*[8] found that there was increased pupal mortality at a constant temperature of 34°C, but that a fluctuating daily temperature of 21-38°C did not affect mortality. The same authors

Figure 15.3: Third Instar Larva of *Oestrus ovis*. A, dorsal view; B, ventral view; C, posterior view

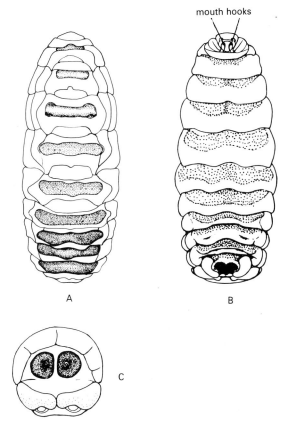

calculated a threshold of 12°C for pupal development, and its duration to be 243 day-degrees for males and 279 for females.

In areas with warm winters year-round breeding of *O. ovis* would be possible, but in many sheep areas there is a definite cool season and two generations per annum are considered to occur. In Pretoria there is no larviposition by *O. ovis* in the three winter months July-September.[20] The common pattern in the northern hemisphere is that adults emerge in late spring in June, mate and larviposit, with the larvae developing rapidly and mature 3rd instars leaving the host in July and August. These pupate to produce an autumn generation larvipositing in September and October. These larvae may remain in the 1st instar for a long period before developing to become mature larvae in March, when they leave the host, pupate and remain dormant until emergence in June.[34] Mortality among the immature stages has been calculated at 90-94 per cent in the first generation and 99 per cent in the second generation.[34]

Veterinary Importance

High infestations of *O. ovis* in sheep are commonly recorded, e.g. 73 per cent in Pretoria,[20] more than 90 per cent in Kentucky,[34] with an average infestation, respectively, of 15 and 22 larvae per sheep. Infestation with *O. ovis* is regarded as relatively benign.[38] Annoyance by adult *O. ovis* causes sheep to lose valuable grazing time, and the presence of larvae irritates the mucosa, resulting in a mucopurulent discharge and difficult snoring respiration.[7] Merino rams treated against infestation showed reduced nasal discharge and increased weight gain.[21]

Although the main host of *O. ovis* is sheep and goats, infestation occasionally occurs in dogs.[38] In man *O. ovis* is associated with myiasis of the eye region and 80 such cases were treated in two years at a clinic in Benghazi.[13] Larvae do not complete their development in either man or dog.

Rhinoestrus

Eleven species of *Rhinoestrus* have been described of which four are restricted to equines and seven are host specific for a wide range of wild animals including giraffe, warthog, bushpig and antelope. Of the four species in equines, one is restricted to zebras. One, *R. usbekistanicus*, parasitises horses and donkeys in the Palaearctic region, and occurs in zebras in Africa. *R. latifrons* parasitises domestic horses in Central Asia and adjoining regions. The most important species is *R. purpureus* which parasitises horses, donkeys and their cross-breeds.

Rhinoestrus purpureus (see Figure 15.4)

The Palaearctic species has been introduced into the Afrotropical and Oriental regions where it occurs sporadically. Rastagaev[32] found that in Mongolia and Buryat ASSR, virtually all (98-99 per cent) horses were infested with *R. purpureus* with infestations ranging from 34-731 larvae in a single host. There is one generation per year. The female matures 700-800 eggs which are deposited as larvae in batches of 8-40 at a time into the nostrils or eyes of a horse. This species causes ocular myiasis in man; and the 1st instar can be separated from that of *O. ovis*, which also causes this condition, by the possession of more strongly curved mouth-hooks and only 8-12 terminal hooklets in a single row. In the third-stage larva the spiracles are crescent-shaped and do not completely surround the button. As with *O. ovis* 1st instar larvae may remain in the nasal cavity for periods of several months before moving to the sinuses to complete their development.

Figure 15.4: Female *Rhinoestrus purpureus*

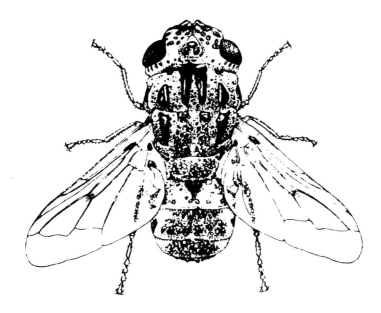

Source: From Zumpt[45]

Hypoderma (Warble Flies)

Six species are included in the genus *Hypoderma* by Zumpt.[45] Two species, *H. bovis* and *H. lineatum*, are parasites of cattle, and the other four, including *H. diana*, are parasites of deer. The cattle species are bumble bee-like flies (Figure 15.5) with reddish-yellow pile at the end of the abdomen. In *H. bovis* the hairs on the prescutum are variously described as whitish-yellow or reddish-yellow contrasting with those on the scutum which are black. In *H. lineatum* the hairs on the scutum and prescutum are white and yellow with a predominance of white on the prescutum and yellow on the scutum. *H. bovis* and *H. lineatum* are widespread in the northern hemisphere between the latitudes of 25° to 60°N. They have not established themselves in the southern hemisphere, although frequently introduced in infested cattle, but there has been a recent record of genuine endemic cases in Chile.[5] The following account will deal jointly with *H. bovis* and *H. lineatum*.

Biology and Life Cycle of H. bovis and H. lineatum

A female will lay several hundred eggs, which are firmly attached to the host's hair. The base of the egg is connected to an attachment organ by a

Figure 15.5: Female *Hypoderma lineatum* (× 4)

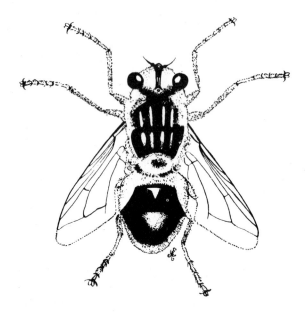

Source: From Cameron, A.E. (1942). *Transactions of the Highland and Agricultural Society*

flexible petiole. The attachment organ has a central groove filled with adhesive and a pair of adhesive-coated lateral flanges, which nearly meet around the hair. The adhesive solidifies and firmly attaches the egg to the hair, and the flexible petiole enables the egg to adjust its alignment and reduce stress.[12]

H. bovis causes cattle to gad and lays its eggs while in flight or when walking over the host. It attaches its eggs singly on the rump and upper parts of the hind leg. Ovipositing *H. lineatum* do not disturb the host, and several eggs are deposited in line along the shaft of a single hair. It oviposits on the legs and lower parts of the body on resting and standing cattle. The eggs of both species hatch in about four days, and the larvae crawl down the hair and penetrate the skin. The exact route taken by migrating larvae in the host is not known with certainty. Several months elapse before the larva reaches its final site on the back of the host.

Migrating larvae of *H. lineatum* are found in the wall of the oesophagus, and those of *H. bovis* in the epidural fat of the spinal canal, with most larvae being found in the region of the lumbar and posterior thoracic vertebrae. It has been suggested that larvae reach the spinal canal by migrating along nerve trunks or through muscles. Although it is considered that most larvae of *H. bovis* migrate via the spinal canal, that may not be the only route as the larval densities there are lower than on the back.[2]

Early in the year the larvae move to their final site on the back in an area 25 cm either side of the mid-line from shoulder to tail where the cysts or warbles, from which the flies get their popular name, are formed.[44] The larva is now more than 10 mm long but still in the 1st instar, and moults into the 2nd soon after reaching the back. The larva cuts a hole in the skin through which it respires and develops through the 3rd instar to the prepupa.

The mature larva is about 30 mm long, with a convex ventral surface and a flat dorsal surface (Figure 15.6). Most of the body segments carry on their ventral surfaces an anterior row of larger, backwardly-directed spines and a posterior band of smaller, forwardly-directed spines.[45] The spines are less well developed on the dorsal surface. In *H. lineatum* the spiracles are flat, crescent-shaped and with a considerable gap between the arms of the crescent surrounding the button\ (Figure 15.6D). In *H. bovis* the posterior spiracles are funnel-shaped with a much smaller gap between the arms (Figure 15.6C). In addition the openings on the posterior spiracles of *H. bovis* are more numerous and more densely packed than in *H. lineatum.* After several weeks, varying from four to eleven,[5,17,45] the yellowish-brown prepupa forces its way through the breathing hole in the skin and drops to the ground, where it moves around actively seeking cover; but Gregson[17] observed only prepupae of *H. bovis* burrowing beneath loose soil.

Dropping of prepupa from cattle occurred early in the morning in southern England[5] but nearer noon under colder Canadian conditions.[17] In Canada prepupae may be covered by snow and exposed to subzero temperatures. Early in life, puparia can survive cooling to $-15°C$, and following loss of water late puparia can survive $-28°C$.[17] At 20°C pupal development of *H. lineatum* is independent of humidity over the range 0 to 98 per cent and that of *H. bovis* optimal at 76 per cent RH.[17] The duration of the pupal stage varies from three to ten weeks depending upon external conditions. Adult *H. lineatum* appear about four weeks earlier than *H. bovis.*[5]

There is one generation a year, and Beesley[3] has summarised the life cycles of both species for southern England (Figure 15.7). With some minor adjustment on timing the main features will apply to other locations. Adult *H. lineatum* are on the wing from late March to the end of May. First-stage larvae are migrating from April until September, and can be found in the oesophagus from September to March with the peak from November to January. Warbles appear in the back from January to April, with a maximum in February and March, and prepupae leave the host and pupate from March to early May.

The timing of *H. bovis* is slightly later with adults being present from June to mid-September; migrating larvae from June to November, arriving in the spinal canal from November to May (main period December to March); warbles from March to July and pupae from May to August.

Figure 15.6: Third Instar Larva of *Hypoderma lineatum*. A, ventral view; B, dorsal view; enlarged posterior spiracles of *Hypoderma bovis* (C) and *H. lineatum* (D)

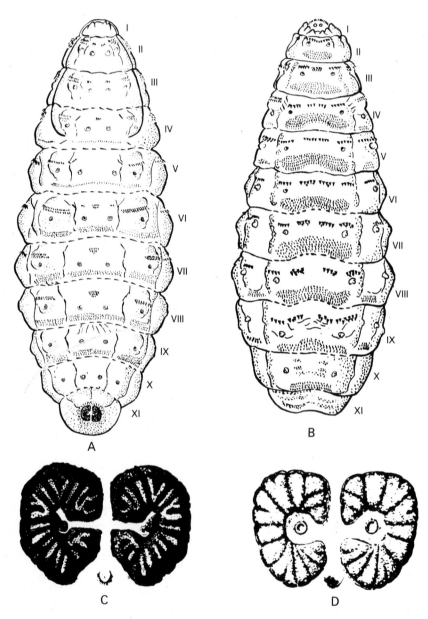

Source: A and B from Cameron, A.E.(1937) *Transactions of the Highland and Agricultural Society.* C and D from James[24]

Knowledge of this cycle is important in the timing of control measures. Systemic insecticides should be used in the early autumn, when adult activity has ceased and larvae are subcutaneous.[7]

Adults are active on sunny days when the temperature is about 18°C.[45] Being unable to feed they are short-lived, living only three to five days. In the presence of suitable hosts they probably do not fly very far, but marked flies have been recovered 300 m from the point of release after 95 min; and flight mill studies in the laboratory indicate that *H. lineatum* is capable of flying up to 16 km.[17] Adults emerge early in the day (07.30-08.30) and mate within one hour of emergence.[17]

Veterinary Importance

Some idea of the intensity of infestation is given by the data of Rich,[33] who

Figure 15.7: Annual Life Cycles of *Hypoderma lineatum* and *H. bovis* in Southern England

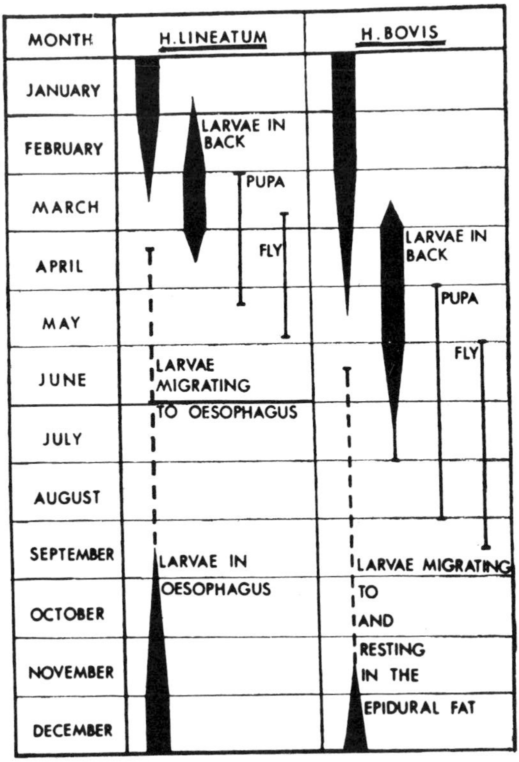

Source: From Beesley[3]

examined over 6,000 beasts in a nine-year period (1956-64) in Canada, of which 67 per cent were infested, with the number of warbles ranging from 0-229 per individual beast. The overall average number of warbles was 14.3 per beast examined and 20.8 per infected beast. The larvae were not identified to species but, on other evidence, the ratio of *H. lineatum* to *H. bovis* was estimated as 3:1. The mortality of larvae in warbles was estimated by Gregson[17] as 51 and 59 per cent in two consecutive years, and the emergence of adult *H. lineatum* from dropped larvae varied from 8-80 per cent depending upon location.

Infestations with immature stages have been determined by Beesley[1,2,3] by examining bovine gullets and spines. In the three seasons (1957-60) nearly 7,000 gullets were examined of which 7 per cent were infested with 6.6 larvae per infested gullet (September-February); and in the next four seasons (1960-64) during the main period (November-January) the infestation rate was lower, 3.8 per cent in more than 5,000 beasts, but the number of larvae (7.0) per infested gullet remained virtually unchanged. In the same area, living *H. bovis* larvae were found in 23.5 per cent of bovine spines during November 1960-April 1961 with 2.3 larvae per infested spine.[2] In 1963 and 1964 the number of larvae per infested spine remained of the same order, 2.2 and 3.1, respectively, but for comparable months the percentage of cattle infested was similar in 1963 and lower in 1964.[3]

Losses due to *Hypoderma* arise from a number of causes. There is the disturbance called 'gadding', caused by actively ovipositing flies, especially *H. bovis*. It reduces weight gain and produces losses of 10 to 15 per cent in milk production.[6] The passage of larvae results in the formation of jelly-like tracks in muscle which have to be removed at the abattoir.[44] In addition the breathing holes made by larvae weaken the hide for use as leather. The cost has been estimated at £1,000,000 per annum on 1976 prices in England.[44]

Destruction of larvae can result in the collapse of an infested beast from anaphylactic shock. It has been shown that anaphylactic shock can be produced by two successive injections of haemolymph of third stage larvae, but midgut fluid of 1st instar larvae is toxic and a single injection can be fatal.[4] To avoid these reactions systemic insecticides should not be used between mid-November and mid-March when larvae are in the spinal canal or oesophagus.[44] The advent of systemic insecticides has not affected the incidence of warble infestation in England and Wales which was 36 per cent in 1941 and 42 per cent in 1974. During that period both Northern Ireland and Eire mounted warble fly eradication programmes and reduced their infestations to 0.05 per cent in 1974 in Eire and 0.11 per cent in 1973 in Northern Ireland.[5,6] It is important that a programme should be continued to the stage of eradication because populations are able to recover. An isolated herd, in which the number of grubs per head had been reduced from 30 to 0.2 by the application of control measures, rose to 10.2 in two generations when treatment was relaxed.[5]

On rare occasions humans who are closely associated with cattle become infested with *Hypoderma* and suffer from a creeping myiasis due to wandering 1st instar larvae, abscesses, and on occasions the eye may be invaded and destroyed.[45] *Hypoderma* larvae do not complete their development in humans. Sometimes the infestation of abnormal hosts by *Hypoderma* larvae can be fatal. Invasion of the brain of a horse by *H. bovis* in the USA led to its death.[18]

An attempt was made to introduce reindeer into Scotland. The introduced animals were quarantined to prevent the introduction of the reindeer warble fly, *Oedemagena tarandi*, but when a small number of reindeer was released into a 100 ha paddock six became infested with the deer warble fly, *Hypoderma diana*, and two died.[25] Infestation of unusual hosts, if successful, can be more dangerous than in the normal host.

Gasterophilus (Stomach Bots of Equines)

Nine species of *Gasterophilus* have been described from equines of which six parasitise domestic horses and donkeys, two are restricted to zebras and the host of one species is unknown.[45] Of the six horse parasites *G. nigricornis* has the most limited distribution, occurring in the southern Asiatic part of the Palaearctic region, and *G. intestinalis* is the most important and most widely distributed horse bot. The other four species, *G. nasalis, G. haemorrhoidalis, G. pecorum* and *G. inermis*, also parasitise zebras.[45]

G. intestinalis (Figure 15.8) was originally a Palaearctic species which has been introduced to many parts of the world by man with his horses. It is now the most important horse bot in the USA[14] and in Australia.[38] The next commonest is *G. nasalis*, followed by *G. haemorrhoidalis*, and both are widely distributed. In Mongolia and Buryat ASSR, east of Lake Baikal, all six species are present and virtually all horses are parasitised. The relative proportions of the species, based on larval numbers, was *G. intestinalis* (40 per cent), *G. haemorrhoidalis* (20 per cent), *G. nasalis* and *G. pecorum* (10-15 per cent) and *G. inermis* and *G. nigricornis* (5-8 per cent).[32]

Biology and Life Cycle

In the northern temperate regions there is one generation per annum, but in areas of the world with continuous warm temperatures there may be continuous breeding. In a typical life cycle the eggs are laid on the host; the 1st instar larvae are found in the tissues of the oral cavity; the 2nd and 3rd instars are attached to the intestinal tract for many months, before the prepupae are voided in the faeces and pupate inside puparia. Some of the specific variations on this pattern will be considered.

Figure 15.8: Male *Gasterophilus intestinalis* (left), and Lateral View of Female *G. intestinalis* (right)

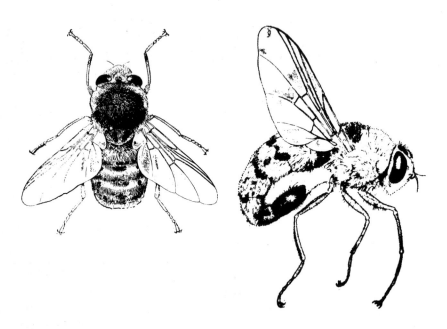

Source: From Zumpt, after Grunin[45]

Egg. Fecundity is roughly correlated with the size of the adult. *G. haemorrhoidalis* matures about 160 eggs, *G. nasalis* and *G. inermis* 300 to 500 eggs, *G. intestinalis* 400 to 700, and the largest species, *G. pecorum,* 1,300 to 2,400 eggs.[45] The eggs are laid in specific locations. *G. pecorum* lays its glossy black eggs in batches of 10 to 15 on vegetation, mainly grasses; the dark eggs of *G. haemorrhoidalis* are laid on the hairs around the lips; and the yellowish eggs of *G. nasalis, G. inermis, G. intestinalis* laid, respectively, on the intermandibular space below the jaws, on the cheeks and on the front legs.[7,45] The eggs of *G. haemorrhoidalis* have a long corrugated stalk-like pedicel, and the flanges which attach the eggs of *G. intestinalis* and *G. nasalis* to the hairs extend for half the length of the egg or the full length, respectively (Figure 15.10). It is possible, therefore, to identify gasterophilid eggs to species.

The method of attachment of the egg of *G. intestinalis* is similar to that described for *Hypoderma* above.[12] There is an attachment groove filled with an adhesive material produced by or from the follicle cells, and lateral extensions which completely surround the hair. The egg is waterproofed by layers of wax on the outer surface of the vitelline membrane surrounding the ovum and on the inner membrane of the endochorion of the eggshell.

Figure 15.9: Wing of *Gasterophilus intestinalis* (× 15)

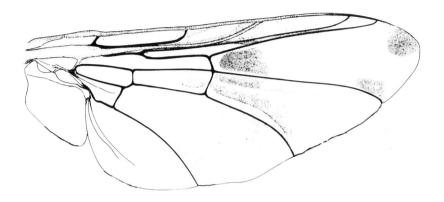

The egg respires through a free air space between the inner membrane and an outer tanned protein layer of the endochorion.[40]

Eggs of *G. pecorum* and *G. intestinalis* do not hatch until ingested by a horse or stimulated by warmth, moisture and friction. At 25-30°C embryonic development of *G. intestinalis* is completed in two to four days, but no hatching occurs for another three to six days, giving a minimum period for larval emergence of five to ten days.[39] The viability of embryonated eggs was inversely related to humidity and temperature from 10-30°C. At 10°C eggs are viable for eight weeks at 100 per cent RH and for 12 weeks at 25 per cent RH.[39] Eggs laid late in the autumn will retain the ability to hatch for several months until the advent of subzero temperatures. Viability of field-collected eggs remained virtually unchanged until the end of December after which it rapidly diminished at a time when minimum daily temperatures were below − 10°C.[39]

Larva. Eggs of *G. inermis* hatch spontaneously and the larvae burrow into the cheek of the horse causing a condition known as 'summer dermatitis'.[45] Eggs of *G. nasalis* also hatch spontaneously and the larvae migrate towards the mouth and enter the oral cavity between the lips.[43] Eggs of *G. intestinalis* hatch under the stimulus of the horse's tongue and burrow into the mucous membrane of the tongue,[45] but they, and larvae of *G. nasalis*, have been found in the alveolar space between the teeth and below the gum line, where they cause necrosis and pus formation.[37,41] In this location the larvae spend up to a month and develop to the 2nd instar. Eggs of *G. haemorrhoidalis* hatch under the stimulus of moisture and burrow into the epidermis of the lip, migrating into the mouth through the subepithelial layer.[45]

The 2nd and 3rd instars are free in the intestinal tract attached to the

Figure 15.10: Eggs of *Gasterophilus* Species. A, *G. intestinalis*; B, *G. nasalis*; C, *G. haemorrhoidalis*

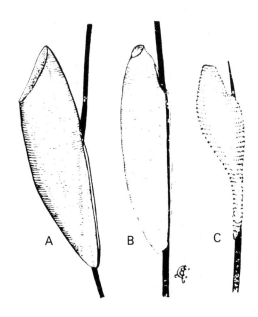

Source: From Cameron, A.E. (1942). *Transactions of the Highland and Agricultural Society*

wall of the gut by well-developed mouth-hooks. Species have different distributions. The larvae of *G. pecorum* occur on the soft palate and at the root of the tongue, but older 3rd instars pass to the stomach; those of *G. intestinalis* are in the cardiac region of the stomach; and *G. nasalis* in the pyloric region of the stomach.[7,45] Larvae of *G. haemorrhoidalis* occur in the fundus of the stomach, the duodenum and 3rd instars re-attach in the rectum where they may occur with *G. inermis*.[45]

In an area where all six horse-infesting species were present, Rastagaev[32] found 7 per cent of larvae in the oral cavity, 56 per cent in the stomach, 25 per cent in the intestine and 12 per cent in the rectum. The distribution within the stomach was 83-92 per cent in the cardiac region, 7-15 per cent in the fundus and 1 to 2 per cent in the pylorus. Most larvae have two rows of stout spines anteriorly on most segments but in *G. nasalis* there is only one row (Figure 15.11). In the other common horse bots, the spines are sharply pointed in *G. haemorrhoidalis*, and blunt in *G. intestinalis*.[45] In all species the two posterior spiracles are united along their inner margins.

Larvae feed on tissue exudates and do not draw blood. Larvae of *G. haemorrhoidalis* contain haemoglobin but it is produced by the larva itself. Larvae pupate in the soil and the duration of the pupal stage varies with temperature. For *G. intestinalis* it is eight weeks at 21°C and 18-20 days at 27-32°C and the most favourable conditions tested were 29°C and 80-92 per cent RH with no pupation occurring at 5°C, and pupation but no eclosion at 38°C.[26] There was 77 per cent survival from prepupa to adult among 269 prepupae of several species.[32]

Adult. Adult gasterophilids are bee-like flies with hairy head and thorax but few bristles (Figure 15.8). In the female more abdominal segments are exposed than is usual in the Cyclorrhapha and the abdomen is characteristically recurved ventrally. The wing of *G. pecorum* is very dark, that of *G. intestinalis* has a broad transverse median band and dark areas at the end of vein iv and the wing apex (Figure 15.9). The wings of *G. nasalis* and *G. haemorrhoidalis* are hyaline with the two cross-veins near the middle of the wing, almost meeting on vein iv in *G. nasalis* but widely separated in *G. haemorrhoidalis.*

The adults are diurnal with peak activity occurring in the early afternoon in warm, sunny weather; and with no activity on cloudy days, in strong winds or in heavy rain.[32] Adults are short-lived and, given favourable conditions, may live only one day.[10] They do not feed and the mouthparts are greatly reduced. The maxillary palps are less reduced and carry sensilla which Faucheux[16] has not found in other Cyclorrhapha, and he considers

Figure 15.11: Larvae of *Gasterophilus*. A, *G. nasalis* (× 3); B, *G. intestinalis* (× 4); C, *G. haemorrhoidalis* (× 3)

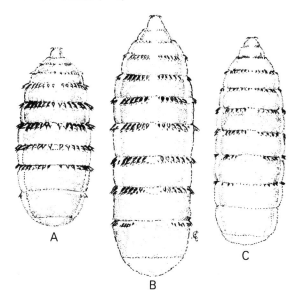

Source: From Cameron, A.E. (1942). *Transactions of the Highlands and Agricultural Society*

them to function as olfactory receptors, being used to seek out the gasterophilids' equine hosts.

Adult gasterophilids buzz, a habit shared by other 'oestrids'. This is
associated with endothermic heat production which may raise the temperature of the thorax 12°C above ambient, and is the prelude to flight.[23] Heat
loss is controlled by insulation provided by the thoracic hair, and by
restricting haemolymph circulation to the abdomen.[23] The preferred
ambient temperature for flight is 20-24°C when the thoracic temperature is
31-32°C. The energy required to produce this heat would exhaust the fly's
energy reserves in a few hours, supporting a very short adult life.

Mating occurs in the vicinity of horses when solitary hovering males will
establish and defend a territory, of either a single horse or a small group of
horses. Mating also occurs on hilltops where the males hover and aggres-
sively pursue passing objects, presumably in search of females. Males can
hover in winds of 15-20 km/h and are active at temperatures of 19-34°C.
Individuals can hover for half an hour without landing; males make contact
with a female on the wing, couple, and sink to the ground where copulation
is completed in three to four minutes.[10]

Veterinary Importance

Horses are infested with gasterophilid larvae all the year round and a
typical pattern has been described by Drudge *et al.*[14] for Kentucky in the
USA. Virtually all horses are infested with *G. intestinalis* and 81 per cent
with *G. nasalis*. The average number of *G. intestinalis* varies from a low of
50 in September to a high of 229 in March, and the corresponding figures
for *G. nasalis* are 14 in September and 82 in February. Second instar *G.
intestinalis* from the previous season continue to reach the stomach until
April, and are not voided in large numbers as prepupae until August, when
3rd instars of the present season will begin to arrive having reached the
stomach as 2nd instars in July.

A similar overlap in generations occurs with *G. nasalis* when prepupae
of the previous year's egg laying are voided from March to August, and
2nd instars of the new generation reach the stomach in July and become
3rd instars in five to seven weeks, before the previous generation's infestation has been exhausted. Hatching of the eggs of *G. nasalis* is not delayed
and consequently horses become infected only between May and November. Eggs of *G. intestinalis* can remain viable for long periods and although
oviposition only extends from early May till late October the acquisition of
infection is almost a year-long process with the exception of April.[14] This is
somewhat at variance with other work in Kentucky in which no viable eggs
of *G. intestinalis* were recovered in the field after the end of January.[39]

In the presence of ovipositing gasterophilids, horses become more difficult to control and may injure themselves. Infestations with second- and
third-stage larvae are usually in the hundreds with maximal infestations

reaching nearly 1,500.[14,32] In Kentucky only one horse out of 476 was infested with more than 500 *G. nasalis* while 13 had more than 500 *G. intestinalis.*[14] In Ireland lower maximal infestations were found in examinations of 2,500 horses. The maximum recorded for *G. nasalis* larvae was 120 and for *G. intestinalis* was 513.[19]

Considerable swelling occurs around the point of attachment of the *Gasterophilus* larva, leaving a ring-like swelling when the larva is removed. Heavy infestations result in chronic gastritis, loss of condition and in rare cases, perforation and death.[7] In a survey in eastern Australia Waddell[42] found 64 per cent of horses infested with *G. intestinalis*; 19 per cent had ulcers in the oesophageal region of the stomach, and 92 per cent of the ulcerated stomachs were associated with infestations of *G. intestinalis.* Ulcers are most common in early summer when the deeply-imbedded third-stage larvae are almost fully grown. It is postulated that infestation with *G. intestinalis* may lead to subserosal abscess formation and death by peritonitis.

Very occasionally larvae of *Gasterophilus* penetrate the human skin and cause a creeping myiasis in which the larva tunnels in the epidermis causing considerable irritation as the larva advances up to 20 mm a day. The infestation may end spontaneously or the larva may be excised.[24] Experimentally it has been shown that the 1st instar larva of *G. nasalis* cannot penetrate the intact skin; that *G. intestinalis* can penetrate damaged human skin; and that 1st instar larvae of the other four species of horse bots, including *G. haemorrhoidalis* and *G. pecorum,* can penetrate intact human skin.[31]

Dermatobia hominis [11]

Dermatobia hominis is the only species in the genus. It is a bluebottle-like fly with yellow to orange head and legs, and a feathered arista (Figure 5.12). It is endemic to the Neotropical region where it occurs from 18°S to 25°N, being associated with moist, cool tropical highlands between 160-2,000 masl, especially the coffee growing areas between 600-1,000 masl.[11,28] It causes cutaneous myiasis in a wide range of mammalian hosts, and is particularly important as a parasite of cattle. It has also been reported from chickens,[28] turkeys and toucans.[11]

D. hominis has a unique method of ensuring that its progeny reach a range of hosts. The female uses other insects as carriers of its eggs. These are carefully glued on to the carrier in such a way as not to affect its flight efficiency adversely (Figure 15.13). Nearly 50 species of carriers have been reported of which about half are mosquitoes, and a third are muscoids (Anthomyiidae).[11] In Costa Rica five carrier species were involved of which the most important was *Sarcopromusca arcuata,* which carried an

Figure 15.12: Female *Dermatobia hominis*

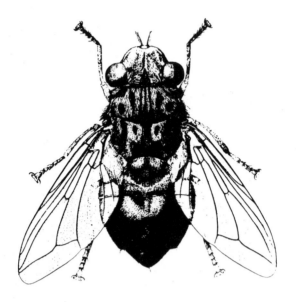

Source: From James[24]

average load of 28 eggs.[11] Fewer eggs (6-10) were laid on mosquitoes, and Mateus[28] state that there is no evidence that eggs are laid on plants or directly on hosts in the field.

A female *D. hominis* will produce 800 to 1,000 eggs.[11]. Development of the egg requires four to nine days at a temperature of 20°-30°C, but hatching is delayed until the stimulus of a sudden increase in temperature, which would occur when a carrier insect visits a warm-blooded host.[11] The larva transfers to the host, and either enters through the feeding puncture made by the carrier, or penetrates the unbroken skin, which it can do in 5-10 min.[11] Each larva penetrates individually and a boil-like swelling develops around it. The larva feeds on tissue exudate and grows slowly, requiring four to 18 weeks to complete development.[11]

The swelling has an opening through which the larva respires and secondary infections occur. Often the discharge from the opening has a foetid odour, which may attract other myiasis-causing flies.[24]

The first-stage larva is subcylindrical with small spines on segments three and four, and stouter spines on segments five to seven, arranged in two dorsal rows and one ventral row. The second-stage larva is pyriform with stout spines on the globular anterior portion and no spines on the narrower posterior part (Figure 15.14A). The third-stage larva is elongate ovate, with prominent flower-like anterior spiracles, reduced spines, and prominent

Figure 15.13: *Sarcopromusca arcuata* With the Eggs of *Dermatobia hominis* Glued to Its Abdomen (length of egg 1 mm)

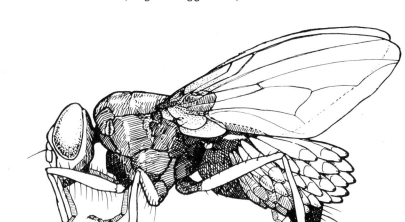

Source: From Catts[10]. Reproduced by permission of Annual Reviews Inc.

mouth-hooks (Figure 15.14B, C).[24] The posterior spiracles have three slits, no button and are sunk in a pit.[27]

The prepupae emerge from the host in the early morning, before 08.00 h, and burrow into the soil where they pupate. The pupal stage is long, taking four to eleven weeks.[111] Females mate 24 h after emergence.[28] The adults do not feed, and are comparatively inactive, living one to nine days.[28] They frequent the forest edge but will pursue large hosts 1.5 km into open cleared land.[11]

Veterinary and Medical Importance

D. hominis causes myiasis in a wide range of wild and domestic hosts, of which the most important economically is cattle.[28] The loss caused by *D. hominis* was estimated at US$260 m in the early 1970s as a result of reduced calf growth and weight gains, lowered milk yields, and hide damage.[28] Infestations in susceptible animals can exceed 1,000 warbles per beast and result in death of the host.[15] Zebu cattle are very resistant, but Holstein and Brown Swiss breeds are highly susceptible.[28] Infestation with *D. hominis* was so great in Panama at one time that the practice of purchasing cattle for fattening on readily available lush pasture, had to be abandoned in favour of purchasing fat cattle for immediate slaughter.[15]

Figure 15.14: Larvae of *Dermatobia hominis.* A, second instar larva; B, ventral view of mature third instar larva; C, dorsal view of mature third instar larva

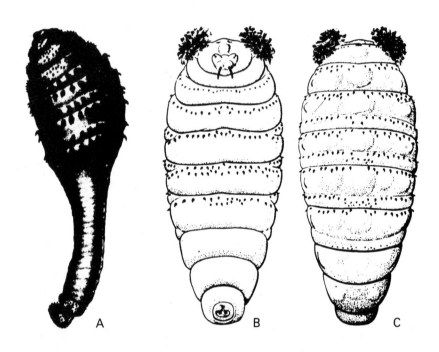

Source: From James[24]

Sheep may become heavily infested and develop severe abscesses;[15] dogs are frequently attacked; cats and rabbits less frequently attacked; and Equidae are troubled little.[24]

Man can also be a host to *D. hominis* and suffer from painful, discharging, cutaneous swellings on the body. Larvae are able to penetrate clothing and boils may be found on all parts of the body.[15] When the larva is removed, in the absence of secondary infection, the condition clears spontaneously in about a week.[35] Rarely, in very young children a larva, infesting the scalp, may penetrate the skull into the brain with fatal results. This rare condition has been reported in a five-month-old baby[36] and an 18-month-old child.[15] This is facilitated by the ossification of the skull being incomplete at that age. The long period of development of larvae in the host favours the introduction of *D. hominis* into other parts of the world. Travellers to South America have introduced *D. hominis* into Canada[35] and Australia.[29] If suitable conditions exist it is conceivable that *D. hominis* could establish itself in other parts of the tropics.

References

1. Beesley, W.N. (1961). Observations on the development of *Hypoderma lineatum* De Villiers (Diptera, Oestridae) in the bovine host. *Annals of Tropical Medicine and Parasitology 55*: 18-24
2. _____ (1962). Observations on the development of *Hypoderma bovis* de Geer (Diptera, Oestridae) in the bovine host. *Research in Veterinary Science 3*: 203-8
3. _____ (1966). Further observations on the development of *Hypoderma lineatum* De Villiers and *Hypoderma bovis* Degeer (Diptera, Oestridae) in the bovine host. *British Veterinary Journal 122*: 91-8
4. _____ (1971). Observations on the biology of the ox warble fly (*Hypoderma*: Diptera, Oestridae). V. Anaphylactoid shock in laboratory animals and calves following exposure to extracts of larvae of *Hypoderma*. *Annals of Tropical Medicine and Parasitology 65*: 567-72
5. _____ (1974). Economics and progress of warble fly eradication in Britain. *Veterinary Medical Review 4*: 334-47
6. _____ (1977). Practical relationships between the biology and control of cattle grubs. *Veterinary Parasitology 3*: 251-7
7. Blood, D.C., Henderson, J.A. and Radostits, O.M. (1979). *Veterinary Medicine — A Textbook of the Diseases of Cattle, Sheep, Pigs and Horses*. Baillière Tindall, London
8. Breev, K.A., Zagretdinov, R.G. and Minar, J. (1980). Influence of constant and variable temperatures on pupal development of the sheep bot fly (*Oestrus ovis* L.). *Folia Parazitologica 27*: 359-65
9. Bukshtynov, V.I. (1978). Determining the time of development of *Oestrus ovis*. *Veterinariya Moscow 9*: 60-2
10. Catts, E.P. (1979). Hilltop aggregation and mating behaviour by *Gasterophilus intestinalis* (Diptera: Gasterophilidae). *Journal of Medical Entomology 16*: 461-4
11. _____ (1982). Biology of New World bot flies: Cuterebridae. *Annual Review of Entomology 27*: 313-38
12. Cogley, T.P., Anderson, J.R. and Weintraub, J. (1981). Ultrastructure and function of the attachment organ of warble fly eggs (Diptera: Oestridae: Hypodermatinae). *International Journal of Insect Morphology and Embryology 10*: 7-18
13. Dar, M.S., Amer, M.B., Dar, F.K. and Papazotos, V. (1980). Ophthalmomyiasis caused by the sheep nasal bot, *Oestrus ovis* (Oestridae) larvae, in the Benghazi area of eastern Libya. *Transactions of the Royal Society of Tropical Medicine and Hygiene 74*: 303-6
14. Drudge, J.H., Lyons, E.T., Wyant, Z.N. and Tolliver, S.C. (1975). Occurrence of second and third instars of *Gasterophilus intestinalis* and *Gasterophilus nasalis* in stomachs of horses in Kentucky. *American Journal of Veterinary Research 36*: 1,585-8
15. Dunn, L.H. (1934). Prevalence and importance of the tropical warble fly, *Dermatobia hominis* Linn., in Panama. *Journal of Parasitology 20*: 219-26
16. Faucheux, M.J. (1977). Les pièces buccales vestigiales de l'imago femelle de gastrophile (*Gastrophilus intestinalis* De Geer). *Bulletin de la Société des Sciences Naturelles de l'Ouest de la France 75*: 7-10
17. Gregson, J.D. (1958). Recent cattle grub life-history studies at Kamloops, British Columbia, and Lethbridge, Alberta. *Proceedings of the 10th International Congress of Entomology 3*: 725-34
18. Hadlow, W.J., Ward, J.K. and Krinsky, W.L. (1977). Intracranial myiasis by *Hypoderma bovis* (Linnaeus) in a horse, *Cornell Veterinarian 67*: 272-81
19. Hatch, C., McCaughey, W.J. and O'Brien, J.J. (1976). The prevalence of *Gasterophilus intestinalis* and *G. nasalis* in horses in Ireland. *Veterinary Record 98*: 274-6
20. Horak, I.G. (1977). Parasites of domestic and wild animals in South Africa. I. *Oestrus ovis* in sheep. *Onderstepoort Journal of Veterinary Research 44*: 55-63
21. _____ and Snijders, A.J. (1974). The effect of *Oestrus ovis* infestation on merino lambs. *Veterinary Record 94*: 12-16
22. Howard, G.W. (1980). Second stage larvae of nasal botflies (Oestridae) from African antelopes. *Systematic Entomology 5*: 167-77
23. Humphreys, W.F. and Reynolds, S.E. (1980). Sound production and endothermy in the horse botfly, *Gasterophilus intestinalis*. *Physiological Entomology 5*: 235-42

24. James, M.T. (1947). The flies that cause myiasis in man. *United States Department of Agriculture Miscellaneous Publication 631*: 1-175
25. Kettle, D.S. and Utsi, M.N.P. (1955). *Hypoderma diana* (Diptera, Oestridae) *Lipoptena cervi* (Diptera, Hippoboscidae) as parasites of reindeer (*Rangifer tarandus*) in Scotland with notes on the second stage larva of *Hypoderma diana. Parasitology 45*: 116-20
26. Knapp, F.W., Sukhapesna, V., Lyons, E.T. and Drudge, J.H. (1979). Development of third-instar *Gasterophilus intestinalis* artificially removed from the stomachs of horses. *Annals of the Entomological Society of America 72*: 331-3
27. Kremer, M., Rebholtz, C. and Rieb, J.P. (1978). Iconagraphie des plaques stigmatiques de *Dermatobia hominis* Linné Jr (= *D.cyaniventris* Macquart 1843). *Annales de Parasitologie Humaine et Comparée 53*: 439-40
28. Mateus, G. (1975). Ecology and control of *Dermatobia hominis* in Colombia. pp. 117-23 in *Workshop on the Ecology and Control of External Parasites of Economic Importance of Bovines in Latin America*, K.G. Thompson (ed.), Centro Internacional de Agricultura Tropical, Cali, Colombia
29. Moorhouse, D.E. (1982). Private communication
30. Papavero, N. P1977). *The World Oestridae (Diptera), Mammals and Continental Drift.* W. Junk, The Hague
31. Rastagaev, Yu.M. (1978) Subcutaneous myiasis in man caused by larvae of the horse bot-fly. *Meditsinskaya Parazitologiya i Parazitarnye Bolezni 47 (6)*: 72-3
32. _____ (1979). The distribution and species composition of botflies of horses in the Buryat ASSR and the Mongolian People's Republic (Oestridae, Gasterophilidae). *Parazitologiya 13*: 547-8
33. Rich, G.B. (1965). Post-treatment reactions in cattle during extensive field tests of systemic organophosphate insecticides. *Canadian Journal of Comparative Medicine and Veterinary Science 29*: 30-7
34. Rogers, C.E. and Knapp, F.W. (1973). Bionomics of the sheep bot fly *Oestris ovis. Environmental Entomology 2*: 11-23
35. Rosen, I.J. and Neuberger, D. (1977). Myiasis *dermatobia hominis*, Linn. Report of a case and review of the literature. *Cutis 19*: 63-6
36. Rossi, M.A. and Zucoloto, S. (1973) Fatal cerebral myiasis by the tropical warble fly, *Dermatobia hominis. American Journal of Tropical Medicine and Hygiene 22*: 267-9
37. Schroeder, H.O. (1940). Habits of the larvae of *Gasterophilus nasalis* (L.) in the mouth of the horse. *Journal of Economic Entomology 33*: 382-4
38. Seddon, H.R. and Albiston, H.E. (1976). *Diseases of Domestic Animals in Australis. Part 2. Arthropod Infestations (Flies, Lice and Fleas).* Department of Health, Commonwealth of Australia
39. Sukhapesna, V., Knapp, F.W., Lyons, E.T. and Drudge, J.H. (1975). Effect of temperature on embryonic development and egg hatchability of the horse bot, *Gasterophilus intestinalis* (Diptera: Gasterophilidae). *Journal of Medical Entomology 12*: 391-2
40. Tatchell, R.J. (1961). Studies on the egg of the horse bot-fly. *Gasterophilus intestinalis* (De Geer). *Parasitology 51*: 385-94
41. Tolliver, S.C., Lyons, E.T. and Drudge, J.H. (1974). Observations on the specific location of *Gasterophilus* spp. larvae in the mouth of the horse. *Journal of Parasitology 60*: 891-2
42. Waddell, A.H. (1972). The pathogenicity of *Gasterophilus intestinalis* larvae in the stomach of the horse. *Australian Veterinary Journal 48*: 332-5
43. Wells, R.W. (1931). The method of ingress of newly hatched larvae of the throat bot of horses, *Gastrophilus nasalis* L. *Journal of Economic Entomology 24*: 1,311
44. Wright, A.I. (1979). Warble fly eradication. *Veterinary Annual 19*: 54-60
45. Zumpt, F. (1965). *Myiasis in Man and Animals in the Old World.* Butterworths, London

16 HIPPOBOSCIDAE (KEDS, LOUSE FLIES)

The Hippoboscidae are blood-sucking ectoparasites of birds and mammals, probably related to the blood-sucking muscids. They are leathery, dorsoventrally flattened flies with porrect mouthparts and robust legs ending in large recurved claws (Figure 16.1). Wings, when present, have the anterior veins strongly developed. The antennae are apparently immovable and placed far forwards in a deep antennal pit. The second antennal segment forms the greater part of the antenna and houses the greatly reduced third antennal segment in a ventral recess from which the arista protrudes.[1] The mouthparts are similar to those *Glossina* (see Chapter 4) but with the bulb of the haustellum withdrawn into the head and the narrow terminal portion concealed in grooves on the inner side of the palps. The method of reproduction is also similar to that of *Glossina* with the female being viviparous and retaining the larva within a modified common oviduct until fully grown. The female deposits an immobile prepupa which pupates where it has been deposited. The structure, physiology and natural history of this family has been reviewed by Bequaert[1] and the systematics by Maa.[8,9,10]

Classification

About 200 species are now recognised in this family and arranged in three subfamilies — Ornithomyinae, Lipopteninae and Hippoboscinae. The Ornithomyinae is the largest with over 150 species, mostly parasites of birds, but it also includes five species parasitic on wallabies and one species on lemurs in Madagascar. The Lipopteninae contains about 30 species parasitic on bovids and cervids including the economically important sheep ked, *Melophagus ovinus.* The Hippoboscinae contains eight species of which six parasitise equines and ruminants, mainly bovids; one species, *Hippobosca longipennis*, parasitises carnivores and another species is found only on ostriches.

In view of the fact that about 8 per cent of hippoboscid species occur on birds it is a pleasant surprise to find that domesticated birds, with the exception of the pigeon, are free from these blood-sucking parasites. There are no records of a hippoboscid breeding on poultry, turkeys, ducks, geese, guinea fowl or canaries. Domestic pigeons are regularly infested with *Pseudolynchia canariensis.*[1] *P. canariensis* is widely distributed geographically in the tropics and subtropics of the Old World where it is recorded from 33 genera of birds, breeding mainly on pigeons and raptors,

Figure 16.1: A, *Melophagus ovinus*, the Sheep Ked (× 11); B, *Hippobosca rufipes (× 4)*

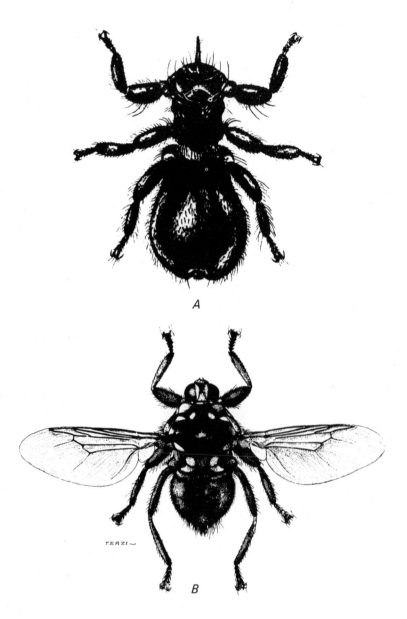

A

B

Sources: A from Patton, W.S. and Cragg, F. W. (1913). *Textbook of Medical Entomology*. Christian Literature Society for India, London. B from Castellani, A. and Chalmers, A.J. (1913). *A Manual of Tropical Medicine*. Baillière Tindall, London

but perhaps also on cuckoos.[9,10] *P. canariensis* has been introduced into the New World where it is confined to domestic pigeons.[9]

The three main genera which occur on mammals are readily distinguished. Adult *Melophagus* are wingless (Figure 16.1A), the wings being reduced to tiny, veinless, opaque knobs and there are no halteres. In *Lipoptena* the newly emerged fly has fully developed and functional wings, which break off close to the base after the final host is reached. They are said to be caducous. Adult *Hippobosca* are permanently winged (Figure 16.1B). They are distinguished from other winged genera by the pronotum being large and clearly visible, forming an easily observable neck-like segment between the mesonotum and the head. In all mammal-infesting hippoboscids the paired claws are simple while in the majority of bird-infesting species the claws have two separate teeth. Maa[8] points out that the observer must take care not to confuse the basal lobe, which is present on the claws of all hippoboscids, with a tooth. The basal lobe is distinguished by being unevenly pigmented and sclerotised, and not pointed.

Melophagus ovinus (the Sheep Ked)

Melophagus ovinus is a Palaearctic species, which has spread with sheep widely throughout the world and established itself in temperate countries, but not in the hot, humid tropics, where it is restricted to the cooler highlands. *M. ovinus* is a permanent ectoparasite on sheep with stray records on other domestic animals.[8]

Life Cycle

The life cycle of the ked has been studied in several parts of the world with substantially the same conclusions. The account which follows is based very largely on Evans.[3] The newly emerged female *M. ovinus* mates within 24 hours of emergence, but the ovaries have to be matured before an egg is available for fertilisation. This process takes six to seven days and further development within the female takes an additional seven days so that the first fully developed larva is deposited when the female is 13-14 days old. Thereafter additional larvae are deposited every seven to eight days so that in a lifetime of four to five months a female will produce about 15 larvae, a comparatively slow rate of increase for an insect. The deposited larva pupates within six hours and the duration of the pupal stage is 20-26 days. The cycle from newly emerged adult female to the emergence of an adult of the next generation is five weeks. *M. ovinus* is a permanent ectoparasite on a homoiothermic host and therefore living under very constant conditions, which accounts for the narrow range in the durations of the different stages.

Pupae develop a relatively narrow range of temperature (25°-34°C) with optimal development at 30°C. The puparia are glued to the fleece and carried away from the skin as the fleece grows. The temperature at the skin surface will be 37°C and near the surface of the fleece it will be nearer to air temperature, say 15°C. It is advantageous to the species to deposit puparia in areas of the fleece where a suitable range of temperature (25°-34°C) will be found during the three week development period of the pupa. This is found most easily in the neck region where the wool staple lies parallel to the skin, and temperature varies slowly with increasing wool length (= time). In hoggs (yearling sheep) over 50 per cent of puparia were found in the neck region while nearly 60 per cent of the adults were found on the region of the forelegs and flanks. On lambs, puparia were concentrated on the hindlegs, neck and belly although substantial numbers of adults were found on the flanks and forelegs.

Bionomics

Populations of *M. ovinus* show seasonal changes and, at the same time of the year, different levels of infestation on sheep of different ages. Populations of *M. ovinus* are at their highest in the winter and lowest in summer. At the start of the year in the northern hemisphere there is an increase in keds on both hoggs and two- and three-year-old ewes but with substantially higher infestation (x 5-6) on the hoggs.[3] Later when the sheep are penned for lambing there is a rapid rise in infestation on ewes due to

Figure 16.2: Fluctuations in Numbers of *Melophagus ovinus* on Sheep in Wales Between January and September 1946

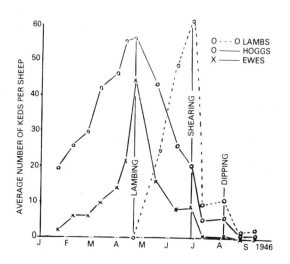

Source: From Evans[3]

transfer from hoggs as a result of their close association. After lambing (late April) the ked population on hoggs and ewes decreases sharply coincidental with a rapid rise in infestation on lambs (Figure 16.2).

This continues until shearing in late June, when 80-90 per cent of the puparia and keds may be removed with the fleece. Similar reductions (77 per cent;[17] 71-98 per cent[16]) have been reported as a result of the shearing in Wyoming, USA. In summer the ked population on lambs in Wyoming decreased by 35-69 per cent, but even so the densities of keds ranged from 36 to 66 adults per lamb.[16]

Transfer of keds from one sheep to another occurs when they move to the surface of the fleece in response to temperature. When the air temperature was 15°C only a small number of keds, average four, were on the surface of the fleece, but when the air temperature increased to 23°C the number of keds on the surface had soared to an average of 98 keds.[3] Keds are vulnerable when they are on the surface of the fleece. They may be dislodged and fall to the ground where they will survive only two to five days, and are unlikely to find another host unless sheep are densely crowded. Keds on the surface of the fleece are subject to predation by birds such as magpies and starlings.[3] They are also ingested by sheep biting their fleece, and this is probably the route by which sheep become infected with the benign trypanosome, *Trypanosoma melophagium*.

Several factors contribute to the fluctuations in natural populations of *M. ovinus*. Nelson[12,15] states that only newly emerged keds go on lambs, and that the older keds stay on the ewes and suffer considerable mortality from infection with *T. melophagium*[11] but the latter conclusion is disputed by Hoare.[7] Undoubtedly older animals have fewer keds, and in the Wyoming study[16] ked numbers increased on lambs from March to May, and then a natural decrease occurred in unshorn lambs until September, after which numbers increased to reach a maximum in February, before declining until May.

Yearlings which have lambs in March along with older sheep have similar densities of keds in the following summer and autumn as older ewes.[16] Two factors contribute to this: temperature and the development of resistance in individual sheep. Nelson and Bainborough[13] and Nelson and Hironaka[14] have shown that there are at least two factors in the development of resistance. There is a long-lasting cutaneous arteriolar vasoconstriction which reduces the ability of keds to obtain blood, and they die from starvation. The development of resistance requires adequate amounts of vitamin A in the diet. The fact that *M. ovinus* is more abundant in winter than summer and has not established itself in tropical areas, suggests that temperature may play an important part in the decline of ked populations in the summer, but no experimental work has yet been done on the effect of temperature upon population dynamics of *M. ovinus* and it must remain an open question.

Economic Importance

Infestation with *M. ovinus* does not produce any very marked change in the sheep. Presence of keds leads to wool biting and staining of the wool by the faeces of the ked. Both responses lead to down-grading of the fleece.[2] Very heavy infestations may cause severe anaemia.[2] Experiments with ked-free and ked-infested lambs showed that on a diet of alfalfa ked-free lambs gained 3.6 kg more in four months and produced 13 per cent more wool.[15] The latter was attributed to a reduction in cutaneous blood flow in lambs developing resistance. When the two groups of lambs were fed a high energy concentrate, differences in weight gain were highly significant after one month, but by four months, although the ked-free lambs had gained more than the ked-infested group, the difference was not statistically significant.[15]

Other Hippoboscids of Veterinary Importance

Geographical Distribution

Hippobosca longipennis occurs in the Afrotropical region excluding West Africa, the western Oriental and the southern Palaearctic, where it parasitises carnivores, including domestic dogs. *H. equina* is primarily an ectoparasite of horses and cattle in the Palaearctic and western Oriental regions, but has been introduced and established more widely in south-east Asia, and in some island groups in the Pacific. *H. variegata* parasitises equines and cattle in the Afrotropical and Oriental regions. No wild hosts of this species are known. *H. rufipes* occurs in the Afrotropical region, where it parasitises wild bovids and domestic cattle, and less frequently domestic and wild equines. *H. camelina* occurs where camels are present in the northern part of eastern Africa, the Mediterranean region and the southern part of the eastern Palaearctic. *Lipoptena capreoli* parasitises domestic goats in the eastern Mediterranean region and eastwards through the desert countries to north-west India.[8,10]

Studies have been made on the biology of *H. longipennis*, and the biology and ecology of *H. equina* by Hafez and his colleagues in Egypt.[4,5,6] There are many similarities between the two species of *Hippobosca* and they make an interesting comparison with studies on *M. ovinus*. Both species of *Hippobosca* are more abundant in summer and are at low numbers during the winter. Larvae are deposited off the host, in the case of *H. equina*, in crevices in mud walls of stables; and in keeping with this, *H. equina* is more abundant on stabled animals than free ranging animals in the field. The newly deposited larva is creamy in colour with the posterior end flattened and bearing dark spiracular plates. The larva pupates in four to six hours. The puparium rapidly darkens to a dark red-black colour. It is broadly oval with posterolateral spiracular lobes.

The adults are winged and fly directly to a host. The newly emerged adult does not feed in the first 24 h but thereafter feeds frequently, several times a day in the case of *H. longipennis*. Adult *H. equina* aggregate on the host in areas where the skin is thinner and comparatively hairless. On horses two thirds of the louse flies were under the tail and around the genitalia, and on cows under the tail and on the udder. On buffalo 84 per cent of *H. equina* were on the genitalia and inner thighs. The average density of *H. equina* on horses was six to ten times that on cows and buffaloes. Significantly more females than males were bred from puparia of both species of *Hippobosca*. Newly emerged adults take several days (4-11) to become sexually mature, and in *H. equina* males mature more quickly than females, but the reverse is true for *H. longipennis*.

Bionomics

The longevity of both species was about six weeks in summer (August) and eight to nine weeks in winter, with females living slightly longer than males. The interval between successive larvipositions was shorter in summer than in winter, and combined with the shorter longevity in *H. longipennis* the average number of larvae produced per female was the same all the year round; but in *H. equina* females were more fecund in winter. Both species showed a marked seasonal change in the duration of the pupa, which increased rapidly during October and November from about three weeks to more than four months. Thereafter there was a steady decline in the duration of the pupal stage from December to June. This change was not closely correlated with temperature.

From the end of November until mid-April the weekly mean temperature ranged from 13-18°C without any particular pattern, while the duration of the pupa declined more or less steadily from 130 to 33 days in *H. longipennis*, and a similar change occured in *H. equina*. The response of pupae of both species to constant temperature was similar. No adults emerged from pupae kept at temperatures above 32°C. The response over the range of 20-32°C was markedly different between 20-27°C and between 25-32°C. A change of five degrees C from 30-32°C to 25-27°C increased the duration of the pupa by 36 per cent in *H. longipennis* and 45 per cent in *H. equina*. A similar change from 25-27°C to 20-22°C increased the pupal duration by a factor of three in *H. equina* and by four in *H. longipennis*.

The number of *H. equina* on horses increased rapidly from February to reach a peak in July. This coincided with the highest percentage (57 per cent) of females with third-stage larvae in the uterus. One would have expected the population to go even higher but it did not. The population declined steadily from July to December. In spite of the high percentage of females maturing larvae and the short duration of the pupa at this time of the year, recruitment to the population of *H. equina* on domestic animals was insufficient to maintain the population, which steadily declined. The mean monthly temperature was 29.6°C, the highest of the year, in July and it is possible that there were prolonged periods with temperatures above 32°C which led to a low emergence of adults from puparia.

References

1. Bequaert, J.C. (1953). The Hippoboscidae or louse flies (Diptera) of mammals and birds. *Entomologica Americana 32, 33*: 1-442
2. Blood, D.C., Henderson, J.A. and Radostits, O.M. (1979). *Veterinary Medicine — A Textbook of the Diseases of Cattle, Sheep, Pigs and Horses.* Baillière Tindall, London
3. Evans, G.O. (1950). Studies on the bionomics of sheep ked, *Melophagus ovinus* L., in west Wales. *Bulletin of Entomological Research 40*: 459-78
4. Hafez, M. and Hilali, M. (1978). Biology of *Hippobosca longipennis* (Fabricius, 1805) in Egypt (Diptera: Hippoboscidae). *Veterinary Parasitology 4*: 275-88
5. _____ Hilali, M. and Fouda, M. (1977). Biological studies on *Hippobosca equina* (L.) (Diptera: Hippoboscidae) infesting domestic animals in Egypt. *Zeitschrift für Angewandte Entomologie 83*: 426-41
6. _____ Hilali, M. and Fouda, M. (1979). Ecological studies on *Hippobosca equina* (Linnaeus, 1758) (Diptera; Hippoboscidae) infesting domestic animals in Egypt. *Zeitschrift für Angewandte Entomologie 87*: 327-35
7. Hoare, C.A. (1972). *The Trypanosomes of Mammals.* Blackwell, Oxford
8. Maa, T.C. (1963). Genera and species of Hippoboscidae (Diptera): types, synonymy, habitats and natural groupings. *Pacific Insects Monograph 6*: 1-186
9. _____ (1966). Studies in Hippoboscidae (Diptera). *Pacific Insects Monograph 10*: 1-148
10. _____ (1969). Studies in Hippoboscidae (Diptera). Part 2. *Pacific Insects Monograph 20*: 1-312
11. Nelson, W.A. (1956). Mortality in the sheep ked, *Melophagus ovinus* (L.) caused by *Trypanosoma melophagium* Flu. *Nature, London 178*: 750
12. _____ (1958). Transfer of sheep keds, *Melophagus ovinus* (L.), from ewes to their lambs. *Nature, London 181*: 56
13. _____ and Bainborough, A.R. (1963). Development in sheep of resistance to the ked *Melophagus ovinus* (L.) III. Histopathology of sheep skin as a clue to the nature of resistance. *Experimental Parasitology 13*: 118-27
14. _____ and Hironaka, R. (1966). Effect of protein and vitamin A intake of sheep on numbers of the sheep ked, *Melophagus ovinus* (L.). *Experimental Parasitology 18*: 274-80
15. _____ and Sten, S.B. (1968). Weight gains and wool growth in sheep infested with the sheep ked *Melophagus ovinus. Experimental Parasitology 22*: 223-6
16. Pfadt, R.E. (1976). Sheep ked populations on a small farm. *Journal of Economic Entomology 69*: 313-6
17. _____ Lloyd, J.E. and Spackman, E.W. (1975). Power dusting with organophosphorus insecticides to control the sheep ked. *Journal of Economic Entomology 68*: 468-70

17 SIPHONAPTERA (FLEAS)

The Siphonaptera or fleas are wingless, ectoparasites of mammals and birds. In common with other ectoparasites, fleas are flattened to minimise damage from the host's reaction to their presence. Fleas are unique in being laterally flattened compared with lice which are dorsoventrally flattened. While lice are host specific, fleas generally parasitise a range of hosts and it is this ability to transfer from one host species to another that makes them of medical importance by transmitting disease from animals, mostly rats, to man (see Chapter 26). The adult flea is 1-6 mm long (Figure 17.1), females being larger than males of the same species, and readily recognised by their mahogany brown colour, and the habit of jumping when disturbed.

All fleas have basically the same structure and their identification is a matter for the specialist. Holland[13] states that 1,800 species and subspecies of fleas have been described and that the probable total number of species is approximately 3,000. Some idea as to the complexity of the taxonomy of the Siphonaptera is given by the history of the catalogue of the Rothschild collection of fleas in the British Museum. This collection is considered to include 85 per cent of the known species.[13] When G.H.E. Hopkins and M.

Figure 17.1: Lateral View of Female *Pulex irritans*

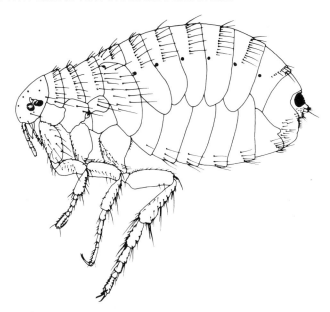

Rothschild began to catalogue the collection they estimated that it would require five volumes and take eight years.[14] Eighteen years later, when five volumes with a total of nearly 2,500 pages had been produced, they considered that another three volumes would be required to complete the catalogue but that they could do no more.[15]

Three superfamilies (Pulicoidea, Ceratophylloidea, Malacopysylloidea) are recognised within the Siphonaptera. The main fleas of medical and veterinary importance are included in the Pulicoidea with about 25 genera. The Ceratophylloidea is the largest of the superfamilies with about 150 genera, and the Malacopsylloidea is the smallest with 13 genera, and is largely Neotropical in distribution.[13] Fleas originated as parasites of mammals of which a small number of species, about 100, have become secondarily adapted to birds, mainly Passeriformes and sea birds. The main genus of fleas on birds is *Ceratophyllus*, of which about 60 species and subspecies occur in the Holarctic region parasiting many families of birds but especially the Hirundinidae, swallows and martins.[13]

Fleas occur on a wide range of terrestrial mammals, and the flea life cycle is such that they are particularly associated with mammals that spend part of their life in nests, dens, holes or caves. Fleas are therefore common on rodents, carnivores, bats and rabbits and virtually absent from free-ranging ungulates and primates. The so-called human flea, *Pulex irritans*, is a normal parasite of pigs.[13] It is considered that fleas evolved from a mecopteran-like ancestor in the late Mesozoic and have evolved with the mammals. A joint study of the zoogeographical distribution of fleas and their mammalian hosts throws light on the evolution of both groups and has been the subject of a long paper by Traub.[43]

The genus *Pulex* originated in the New World, to which most species in the genus are restricted, with the exception of *P. simulans*, which occurs in Hawaii, and *P. irritans* which is cosmopolitan. The range of hosts and variation in biology of different populations of *P. irritans* in various parts of the world, raises the question as to whether *P. irritans* is a single species or a species complex.[16]

The main fleas of medical importance are the tropical rat flea, *Xeno-psylla cheopis*, the main vector of plague and murine typhus to man; the sand-flea *Tunga penetrans*, the female of which develops as an endo-parasite under the skin of man, particularly on the feet and ankles; and *Pulex irritans* which breeds in human habitations. Fleas of veterinary importance include the sticktight flea of poultry, *Echidnophaga gallinacea*; *Ceratophyllus gallinae*, a pest of poultry and many other species of birds; and the dog and cat fleas, *Ctenocephalides canis* and *Ct. felis*.

Figure 17.2: A, Head and Thorax of *Nospsyllus fasciatus* Female; B, Antenna of Male *N. fasciatus*; C, Head and Pronotum of *Ctenocephalides felis. an.*, antenna; *anI, anII, anIII*, segments I, II and III of antenna; *al.*, clypeus; *cx.I, cx.II, cx.III,* coxae of legs; *f.*, frons; *g.c.*, genal comb; *msn.*, mesonotum; *mtepm.*, metepimeron; *mtn.*, metanotum; *mx¹ maxilla (stipes) mx.¹p.*, maxillary palp; *o.*, ocellus; *ph.*, pharynx; *pr.c.*, pronotal comb; *prn.*, pronotum; *spr.I, spr.II, spr.III,* thoracic and first abdominal spiracles; *v.*, vertex

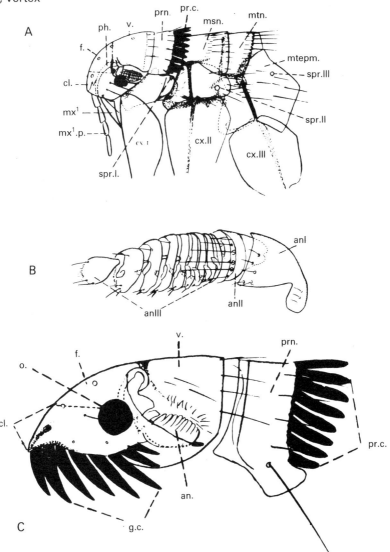

Source: From Patton, W.S. and Evans, A.M. (1929). *Insects, Ticks, Mites and Venomous Animals, Part 1: Medical.* H.R. Grubb, Croydon

Structure of Adult Flea

Fleas show many adaptations to an ectoparasitic mode of life. The antennae are recessed in a deep antennal fossa (Figure 17.2); the neck is foreshortened so that the head is sessile on the prothorax; and the body is covered with backwardly-directed setae (Figure 17.1) and, in many cases, combs. These features, together with the lateral flattening, enable fleas to move forwards easily through the pelage or feathers of their hosts. The setae and combs would impede the flea being dragged backwards by activities of the host.

Head

The antennae are 3-segmented with the third segment being elaborately developed (Figure 17.2). In many species the antennae of the males have adhesive disks on the inner surface which are used to hold the female during mating. The maxillary palps are well developed with four obvious segments. There are no compound eyes but lateral ocelli are present on either side of the head. Their development is variable, being particularly large in species of *Xenopsylla*, and reduced in many species or absent, as in the house-mouse flea *Leptopsylla segnis*.

Figure 17.3: Lateral View of Mesothorax, Metathorax and Tergum 1 of *Xenopsylla cheopis*

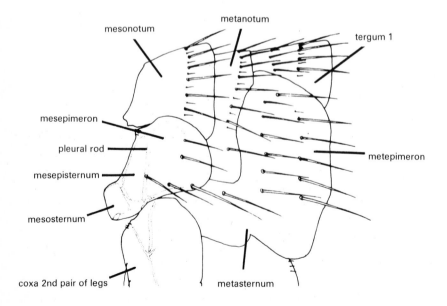

Figure 17.4: Terminal Segments of the Abdomen of the Male *Xenopsylla cheopis*

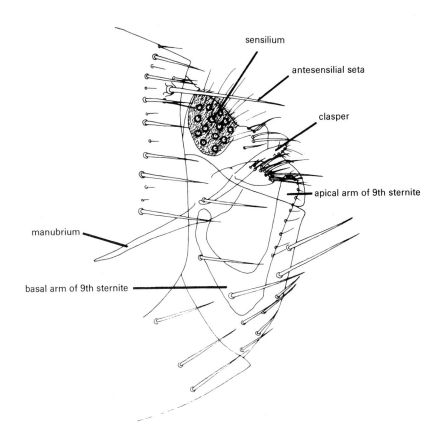

Thorax

The thorax bears three pairs of legs, of which the third pair is particularly well developed for jumping and consequently the metathorax supporting these legs is well developed. In *Xenopsylla* and some other genera the mesopleuron above the coxa of the second pair of legs is divided by the pleural rod into an anterior mesepisternum and a posterior mesepimeron (Figure 17.3). The pleural rod is absent in *Pulex* and this character enables the two genera to be distinguished.

Abdomen

The shape of the abdomen may be used to distinguish between the sexes. In female fleas both the ventral and dorsal surfaces are convex and in the male the dorsal surface is more or less flat and the ventral surface greatly curved.

Figure 17.5: Terminal Abdominal Segments of a Female *Xenopsylla cheopis*

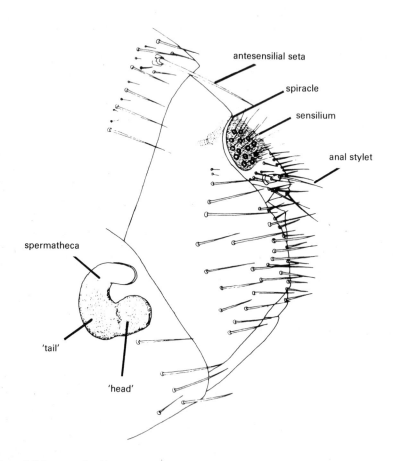

In addition male fleas may be distinguished by possession of complex copulatory apparatus posteroventrally in the abdomen. In both sexes there is a sensilium (= pygidium) posteriorly on the dorsal surface (Figure 17.4, 17.5). The antesensilial seta is immediately anterior to the sensilium.

The abdomen has ten segments of which eight are easily recognisable externally and each of these bears a pair of spiracles (Figure 17.1). In addition there are two pairs of spiracles on the thorax. The ninth abdominal segment is much modified in the male with tergum IX forming paired manubria and articulating claspers, and sternum IX forming an L-shaped clasping organ (Figure 17.4), the apical arm of which is a useful character in the separation of species of *Xenopsylla*.

There is a single spermatheca in the female (Figure 17.5). The spermathecal duct opens into the head of the spermatheca which is separated by a small constriction from the tail of the spermatheca. The relative sizes of the head and tail are useful characters in separating species of *Xenopsylla.* They are of similar size in *X. cheopis*; the head is considerably larger than the tail in *X. brasiliensis*; and the reverse is true in *X. astia.*

Combs or Ctenidia

Many fleas possess combs. The Pulicoidea are relatively combless and there are no combs in *Xenopsylla, Pulex, Echidnophaga* or *Tunga* (Figure 17.1,17.7) but there are both general and pronotal combs in *Ctenocephalides* (Figure 17.2). The pronotal comb is vertically placed with its teeth directed backwards, and although the genal comb is more or less horizontal, its teeth are directed backwards. Combs are better developed among the Ceratophylloidea where there may be metathoracic and abdominal combs present. Combs are particularly well developed in fleas that parasitise bats.[13] In *Ceratophyllus* and *Nosopsyllus*, genera in the Ceratophylloidea, only the pronotal comb is developed (Figure 17.2). The number of spines in the pronotal comb varies with the type of host. In bird fleas, e.g. *Ceratophyllus* spp, the spines are narrower and more numerous, exceeding 24, while in parasites of mammals, e.g. *Nosopsyllus* spp, the spines are broader and less numerous, less than 24.[13]

Life Cycle (see Figure 17.6)

Egg

The female flea produces two to six relatively large (0.3-0.5 mm) whitish, oval eggs per day. A female *P. irritans* may produce 400 eggs in her lifetime.[4] The eggs of *X. cheopis* are sticky, and those of *T. penetrans* and *E. gallinacea* are quite dry.[40] Eggs are deposited in the nest, or on the host from where they fall to the ground. Development is not delayed, and the eggs hatch in a few days providing the humidity is above 70 per cent. Eggs of *X. brasiliensis* at 80 per cent RH hatch in six days at 24°C and four days at 35°C,[9] and those of *E. gallinacea* somewhat more quickly, hatching in three to four days at 26°C, 85 per cent RH.[40] Eggs that lose water when exposed to low humidities (less than 70 per cent RH) are unable to recover when placed in a higher humidity.[40] The threshold temperature for egg development varies with species. For the tropical rat flea, *X. cheopis*, it is 12°C and for the temperate region European rat flea, *Nosopsyllus fasciatus*, it is 5°C.[4]

Larva (see Figure 17.6B)

The larva which hatches from the egg is nematoceran-like in appearance. It has a distinct head and 13 body segments with no distinction between thoracic and abdominal segments, and no appendages. Although the larva

Figure 17.6: Life Cycle of *Ctenocephalides felis*. A, egg; B, larva with caudal and head ends enlarged; C, pupa; D, sand-encrusted cocoon

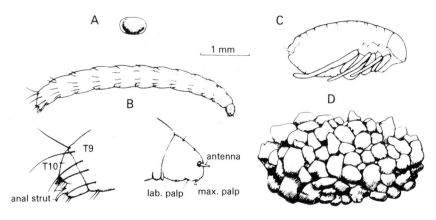

Source: From Dunnet[8]

has no eyes it is negatively phototactic burrowing into the material of the nest or substrate. The whitish, vermiform larva measures 4-10 mm when fully grown and the body segments bear a circlet of backwardly-directed bristles which, together with the anal struts on the last segment (Figure 17.6B), enable the larva to be vigorously active. There are three larval instars in most species but only two in *T. penetrans*.[40]

Larvae feed on organic debris in their environment and this is supplemented in many species by adults passing undigested blood through the anus when feeding. In *N. fasciatus* the interaction of larva and adult flea has become much closer. Larvae actively pursue and seize adult fleas with their mandibles in the region of the sensilium. The adult responds by defaecating after which the larva releases its hold on the adult and sucks the excreted faecal blood.[31] The pharynx of the larva is muscular and larvae of *N. fasciatus* imbibe blood, water and rat urine. These larvae are semi-predatory and will attack damaged adults and kill them.[31]

There are specific differences in the nutritional requirements of flea larvae of the same genus. Larvae of *X. astia* require a more nutritive diet than those of *X. cheopis* and *X. brasiliensis*.[38] Larvae of *X. cheopis* cannot develop solely on a diet of blood, and need to supplement it with food containing vitamins of the B group.[38]

Adult *Spilopsyllus cuniculi* normally defecate every 20 min, but the frequency is greatly increased shortly before egg laying, presumably to provide a more favourable environment for larval development in the rabbit burrow.[33]

Larvae of *X. cheopis* lack a closing mechanism on their spiracles,[30] and consequently they require high humidities for development. Exposure to zero per cent RH and 22°C for 24 h is lethal to larvae of *X. cheopis* but at 90 per cent RH the lethal temperature is 36°C.[28] Larvae are hygropositive and move to zones of high humidity.[44]

The length of the larval stage is dependent on temperature and humidity, and at 24°C its duration in *X. brasiliensis* increases from 12 to 25 days as the relative humidity decreases from 93 to 70 per cent.[9] At 25°C and 85 per cent RH Suter[40] found similar rates of development in four species of Pulicoidea with the larval stages being completed in one to two weeks. Bacot[4] found considerable variation in the speed of development of four species of fleas even when larvae from the same batch of eggs were reared under identical conditions. Larvae of *X. cheopis* and *P. irritans* died at 24° and 29°C when the humidity was 60 per cent.[4]

Pupa

The mature third stage larva empties its gut, enters the prepupal phase, and constructs a thin, loosely woven cocoon, which is typically ovoid, measuring about 3 mm long by 1 mm in width and height. Humphries[20] followed the development of three species of *Ceratophyllus* and *Ct. felis* within the cocoon. He found that for several days the larva remained motionless in a doubled up position. It then pupated and remained quiescent until it emerged as an adult. The main threat to adult emergence was desiccation, reducing the body volume and preventing the shedding of the pupal exuviae. If these shrunken pharate adults were liberated from the pupal exuviae they were capable of normal locomotion surviving for several days and one even took a blood meal.

Maintenance of a high water content is a key factor in the successful emergence of the adult flea. Although flea larvae readily lose water in a dry atmosphere, prepupae of *X. brasiliensis* actually gain water when maintained in an atmosphere of 50-90 per cent RH but desiccate and die at all temperatures when the humidity falls below 45 per cent. The average gain in weight before pupation is 14 per cent. The cocoon itself offers no protection against desiccation. Pupae of *X. brasiliensis* lose water but at a very slow rate.[10] If the same is true for pupae of *X. cheopis* then the rate of loss must be exceptionally low because adults emerge from pupae kept at 0 per cent RH and 30°C.[29]

Temperature is the other factor affecting development. Successful pupation and emergence of *X. cheopis* occurred at 18°-35°C and 60 per cent or higher RH, with the prepupa lasting four days at 35°C and eight days at 18°C.[29] At lower temperatures pupation was variable with none occurring at 10° and 14°C, and reduced pupation at 15°C and 80 per cent RH with many prepupal deaths.[26] As with the threshold temperature for egg development, the optimum temperature for pupal development is about 10°C higher for *X. cheopis* than *N. fasciatus*.[4]

Adult

Adults of *C. gallinae* emerge from the cocoon by using the frontal tubercle on the head to weaken the fibres of the cocoon.[20] The tubercle may be lost later in adult life. Females of *X. cheopis, X. brasiliensis, E. gallinacea* emerge three to four days before the males.[9,40] In view of the importance of water conservation to survival of the adult flea, it is of interest to learn that *C. gallinae* is able to take up water from air with a humidity in excess of 82 per cent RH but this ability is only present during the first day of adult life.[22] Edney[9,10] has shown that unfed, newly emerged adult *X. brasiliensis* are shorter lived if they have been reared at high temperatures or low humidities. The duration of the period spent in the cocoon between prepupa and the emergence of the adult varies from a week to six to twelve months. This is a major factor in the survival of flea populations during the absence of a host or adverse climatic conditions.[4]

Adult fleas are long lived. When fed regularly in captivity they survive for many months and in some cases for more than a year.[4] Unfed *S. cuniculi* can survive for nine months at $-1°C$.[33]

Unusual Life Cycle of Uropsylla tasmanica

The life cycle of the flea *Uropsylla tasmanica*, a parasite of dasyurids (marsupials), is most unusual. The eggs are cemented on to the hairs of the host and the newly emerged larvae penetrate the host's skin with their large mandibles and are endoparasitic on their host, living in burrows extending into the dermis. When mature they drop to the ground, and spin a cocoon in the normal way.[8]

Adult Behaviour and Bionomics

Host Finding

Adult fleas feed only on blood, and the newly emerged flea must find a host. This may be achieved by dispersing actively, e.g. *C. gallinae* and *C. styx*, in search of a host, or by waiting in the nest or burrow for the return of the host, e.g. *N. fasciatus* and the rabbit flea *Spilopsyllus cuniculi*. Both groups of fleas need to be able to detect a host when it is near, to orientate to it and achieve contact. Various attributes of the hosts provide stimuli to which the flea may respond. These include vibration, warmth, exhalation of carbon dioxide, characteristic odour and, in lighted situations, casting a shadow. According to Askew[2] fleas are able to detect air currents by receptors on the sensilium. Suter[40] found that three species of fleas, including *X. cheopis*, were positively phototactic when unfed but became negatively phototactic when fed. This does not occur in the female sticktight flea, *E. gallinacea*, which may remain attached to heads of poultry for several weeks.

In an olfactometer adult *X. cheopis* responded positively to the odour from a white rat at a distance of 30 cm, and distinguished between its odour and that of three other murids to which *X. cheopis* do not respond.[39] Some indication of the ability of fleas to find their hosts is given by an experiment with *S. cuniculi* in which 270 marked adults were released in an enclosed area of 1,800 m². Three rabbits released into the area had picked up 45 per cent of the marked fleas within a few days.[33] The same species was released on wild rabbits in various locations in New South Wales, Australia, for the spread of myxomatosis virus among rabbit populations. The flea has spread slowly, the fastest rate observed being 8-10 km a year.[34]

The host-finding behaviour of *C. gallinae* and *C. styx* have been studied in detail. *C. gallinae* parasitises more than 75 species of birds, while *C. styx* is restricted to the sand martin. *C. gallinae* overwinters as an adult in the cocoon and emerges in the spring in response to a sharp rise in temperature and/or tactile stimuli. The flea emerges in an old nest which will not be reoccupied. At first the newly emerged adult is negatively phototactic but after three or four days becomes positively phototactic, which, associated with negative geotaxis, ensures that the adults crawl up trees and bushes. In search of a host the flea stops periodically and faces towards the brightest source of light, and jumps when the light is suddenly obscured. Readiness to jump rises to a peak four days after emergence, coinciding with the positive response to light, but falls off later due in part to water loss.[23] In new housing estates in the west of Scotland, where trees and shrubs were scarce and small, dispersing *C. gallinae* attacked people out of doors.[17]

Adult *C. styx* emerging from old sand martin burrows, congregate in the entrance to the burrows in the spring at the time of arrival of the migrant host. Sometimes sand martins hover in front of old burrows, and *C. styx* responds to the vibration and jumps on to the hovering bird. Burrows are not reoccupied and the fleas disperse both laterally and vertically up to 34 m from the old burrow. They appear to respond to the horizontal floor of the burrow, but as they do not collect on the cliff top they must distinguish between the two horizontal surfaces, but the way in which that is done is not known.[5]

Feeding

Adult fleas are capillary feeders. Lavoipierre and Hamachi[25] studied the feeding of three species of fleas including *X. cheopis* and *P. irritans*. They found that the maxillae are used to penetrate the host's skin, and the tip of the labrum epipharynx enters a capillary from which the flea imbibes blood. Saliva is passed into the host by the salivary pump and appears as clear drops of fluid outside the capillary.[25] The saliva of *X. cheopis* contains an anticoagulant, and a material of low molecular weight which provokes allergenic activity in the host.[34]

In *Ct. canis* there are three pumps, cibarial, precerebral and post-cerebral, to convey blood to the midgut.[32] *S. cuniculi* is probably a pool feeder and at times *X. cheopis* may feed in the same manner.[34] A flea will take a blood meal in two to ten minutes, with females imbibing almost twice as much blood as males,[34] and this may explain why males feed more frequently than females.[2] Feeding is more frequent at higher temperatures as a result of accelerated physiological activity and increased rate of water loss. The latter can be replaced by drinking water and Humphries[18] has observed seven species of fleas, belonging to five genera, drinking water and increasing their weight by 13 per cent. The volume of liquid imbibed varies with its composition. When *X. cheopis* is offered distilled water, plasma or blood, it takes up liquid equal to 8, 19 and 35 per cent, respectively, of its bodyweight. The increased uptake on whole blood is attributed to the presence of ATP on the red cells.[11]

Role of Proventriculus in Feeding and Digestion

Blood passes directly to the midgut, which has the dual functions of initial storage and digestion. The proventriculus is particularly well developed, and is easily recognised in whole mounts of fleas as a mass of needle-like spines at the junction of the thorax and abdomen. Morphologically these are not true spines but modified setae.[34] Munshi[32] has studied the proventriculus of *X. cheopis* in detail. Three regions are readily discernible: a ridged, spineless anterior zone; a middle spined region; and a posterior spineless region which protrudes into the midgut. The spines are arranged in a regular series. In females there are 15 rows of 30 spines each, and in males 12 rows of 22 spines each. The most anterior spines are short being only 10 μm long. The spines steadily increase to a maximum of 70 μm in the central and posterior regions with the last two rows being somewhat shorter.

The function of the spines appears to be to keep an open passage from foregut to midgut facilitating rapid feeding. In addition the spines play a role in the fragmentation of red blood cells. Three to five peristaltic waves are followed by one antiperistaltic wave which thrusts the blood forwards against the spines. The spines do not penetrate into the midgut but only into the posterior spineless zone of the proventriculus. Other actions which contribute to breaking up the erythrocytes are the to and fro shifting movements of the proventriculus itself, and the contractile action of the posterior region of the proventriculus. The anterior half of the spined region of the proventriculus serves as an effective barrier to regurgitation.

Mating

Some fleas, especially bird fleas, mate on emergence before taking a blood meal, but most fleas, especially females, require a considerable period of feeding before mating.[34,40] The sequence of events in mating has been described by Humphries[19,21] for *C. gallinae*. The initial contact is fortuitous, and when individuals touch, recognition is achieved by a contact pheromone detected by receptors on the male palps. The pheromone is species specific and is present in both sexes.

The male erects his antennae and moves under the female grasping her with the adhesive organs on their inner surfaces. Correct alignment of the pair, and successful coupling, is probably assisted by receptors on the sensilium and the antesensilial seta. Movement of the female is inhibited by pressure of the ninth sternum of the male on hairs of the female's sensilium. The aedeagus or intromitent organ of the male is used to dilate the female's genital chamber, and one penis rod is inserted into the spermathecal duct and may reach the spermatheca. Penetration of the rod is slow, and copulation may last for up to nine hours with the average time in this species being three hours. In *S. cuniculi* the two penis rods operate together with the thicker rod, which penetrates to the female genital chamber, acting as a guide to the thinner rod which enters the spermathecal duct with sperm wound around its terminal portion.[33]

In species where the female is sessile or semi-sessile, e.g. *E. gallinacea* and *S. cuniculi*, the antennae of the male lack adhesive disks; and copulation occurs while the female is feeding.[12,35] In *E. gallinacea*, after the male is coupled with the female, it may lose all contact with the host's skin and its legs be free in the air. When, after mating, the male is returned to the host's skin it may take a blood meal. In *T. penetrans* mating occurs when the female is endoparasitic within the skin of its host. The male genitalia are modified to achieve mating with the almost inaccessible female. During copulation the male takes a blood meal from the host.[12] Geigy and Suter[12] give times of mating for *X. cheopis* (10 min), *E. gallinacea* (15 min) and *T. penetrans* (20 min).

Control of mating in *S. cuniculi* is a complex process dependent on the physiological state of the host. Maturation of the female, and maximum maturation of the male only occurs when the fleas feed on a pregnant doe rabbit or its new born young, one to ten days old.[34] The reproductive cycles of both flea and host are therefore closely co-ordinated and may be unique to *S. cuniculi*.

Reproduction

In Portugal the numbers of *S. cuniculi* on wild-caught rabbits reach a peak in February, coinciding with the hormonal cycle of the rabbits which peaks between January and March.[1] These rabbits are also parasitised by *X. cunicularis* which attains its maximum numbers in September and October. This indicates either that *X. cunicularis* reproduces independently of the hormonal cycle of its host, or that its dependency on the host cycle is completely different. The first explanation is the more likely which would bring *X. cunicularis* in line with *X. cheopis* and *X. astia*.[1]

In the tropics and subtropics it is likely that fleas breed continuously throughout the year, although it may be moderated by very hot or very dry conditions. In more temperate regions *L. segnis*, a semi-sessile parasite of the house mouse, breeds continuously throughout the year, but *X. conformis* which lives in burrows stops breeding during the winter period when only old adult fleas are present. New adults emerge from pupae in the spring.[7]

Bacot[4] pointed out that females must mate more than once if all their eggs are to be fertilised. In *E. gallinacea* egg production rose for eight days after mating to a peak of more than 20 eggs per day. Egg production then declined steadily for the next three weeks to less than five eggs per day. After a second mating egg production rose for nearly two weeks when the experiment was terminated.[40] Oviposition actually ceased when all the sperm had been used.

Fleas are anautogenous and only produce eggs when the female has access to an acceptable host. *C. gallinae* produced eggs when given the opportunity to feed on man for only 15 min per day, but *Ct. canis* required five to twelve hours per day before producing eggs.[4] Virgin female *P. irritans* developed and laid eggs when fed on blood, but the eggs were infertile.[4]

Relationship with Hosts

Some fleas are host specific; some, e.g. *C. gallinae*, infest a wide range of hosts; other have a range of hosts, which may be taxonomically related or share a common habitat.[13] Fleas that infest diurnal hosts have well developed eyes, and those that remain in the host's nest have reduced eyes, thorax and legs in keeping with their more sedentary life style.[13] The geographical distribution of a flea species is limited by the distribution of its potential hosts and also by the need for suitable larval habitats.[13]

In sticktight fleas the mouthparts are relatively much longer than they are in more mobile fleas. In *E. gallinacea* (Figure 17.7) the mouthparts are one third the length of the body, whereas in *P. irritans* and *X. cheopis* their length is only 10-20 per cent of the body length.[40] In addition the maxillae in *Echidnophaga* are strongly toothed and serve to anchor the flea in place (Figure 17.7). These adaptations are highly successful and when a chicken was artificially infested with *E. gallinacea*, 50 per cent of the females were still attached at the end of two weeks, and some remained attached for periods up to six weeks.[40]

The relationship between a flea, its host and environmental conditions is complex. Under three different sets of conditions — 16°C (60 per cent RH), 24°C (50 per cent RH) and 28°C (70 per cent RH) — populations of *L.segnis* varied according to the rodent host. On the house mouse (*Mus musculus*) and *Apodemus sylvaticus* the populations were markedly higher

Figure 17.7: Female *Echidnophaga gallinacea*

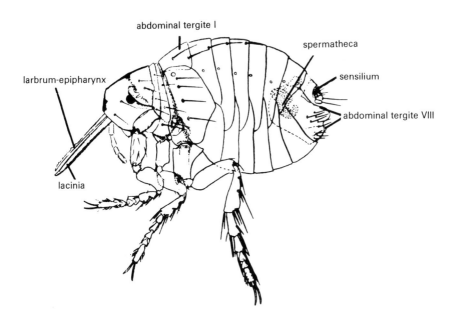

Source: From Patton, W.S. and Evans, A.M. (1929). *Insects, Ticks, Mites and Venomous Animals, Part 1: Medical.* H.R. Grubb, Croydon

at 16°C and 24°C than at 28°C; on *Apodemus agrarius* they declined at 16°C but thrived at 24°C and 28°C; while on *Mastomys natalensis* the population declined at 16° and 24°, and at 28°C produced the highest growth rate recorded for any of the nine hosts used in these experiments.[24]

Fleas have evolved together with their hosts and show certain adaptations, but there is no unanimity on their interpretation. Marshall,[27] who has examined fleas and other ectoparasites from bats in Malaysia, considers that the main structures for attachment are the claws and mouthparts, the function of the combs being not to prevent dislodgement but to protect highly mobile joints and their associated membranes. Traub [41,42] considers that the combs and bristles on fleas not only protect and aid progress through the host's pelage but maintain hold on the host. Fleas with well developed genal combs have flying or gliding hosts, or hosts that are both nocturnal and climbing, or have vast home ranges. Hosts such as hedgehogs and porcupines have fleas with bristles which are widely spaced and/or exceptionally thickened and may also have highly modified combs.

Jumping

One of the most distinctive features in the behaviour of fleas is their ability to jump. The rat flea (? *X. cheopis*) averages 18 cm, presumably horizont-ally, and a maximum of 31 cm in a single jump.[33] The hen flea, *C. gallinae*, jumps up to 24 cm horizontally and 11 cm vertically.[23] There is consider-able variation in the ability of different flea species to jump. The nest-dwelling, semi-sessile rabbit flea, *S. cuniculi*, jumps a mere 3.5 cm vertically while the human flea, *P. irritans*, was observed to jump a vertical height of 13 cm, and considered to be able to reach 20 cm.[6]

The method of jumping has been investigated by Bennet-Clark and Lucey[6] and Rothschild *et al.*[36] A flea cannot jump 'to order' when prodded, because direct muscular action is not able to deliver the required energy in the time, and over the distance involved. The flea has to be pre-set before being able to jump. Jumping is carried out by the third pair of legs with the other two pairs of legs acting chiefly as supports, at least in *X. cheopis*. The femur of the third pair of legs is rotated to a vertical position and connected to the substrate by the trochanter and tibia. On jumping the femur rotates downwards transmitting its thrust via the tibia to the sub-strate, and the flea jumps. The tarsi and claws play no part in jumping. Energy for jumping is stored in the pleural arches which are laterally placed pads of resilin. In *S. cuniculi* 2.1 ergs can be stored in each pad giving a total of 4.2 ergs, compared with 2.25 ergs required for the flea to jump 3.5 cm vertically.

The flea is pre-set by muscular contractions which engage certain cuticular catches, and compress the pleural arch. When the catches are engaged the muscle which compressed the resilin can be relaxed. The jump is initiated by the relaxation of certain muscles which enable the femur to descend, and simultaneously the muscles holding the catches in place relax, releasing the energy stored in the resilin, and arched pleural and coxal walls.[36] During jumping the flea may turn over and the legs be held out. In *N. fasciatus* the second pair of legs may extend above the dorsal surface of the body.[33] This will increase the probability of the flea holding on to a host should it encounter one during its jump.

Medical and Veterinary Importance

The most important human diseases associated with fleas are plague and murine typhus, which are dealt with in Chapters 25 and 26. A number of fleas, e.g. *P. irritans*, can achieve pest status through the irritation caused by their bites. When domestic cats and dogs are present in a house *Ct. canis* and *Ct. felis* can reach pest proportions. These fleas can also act as intermediate hosts of certain cestodes, including the dog and cat tapeworm *Dipylidium caninum*

C. gallinae and *E. gallinacea* can be important pests of poultry. Both species have a wide range of natural hosts. *C. gallinae* evolved in the

Figure 17.8: Female *Tunga penetrans*. Above, recently fertilised female with the intersegmental membrane between segments II and III beginning to be stretched. Below, gravid female, fully expanded

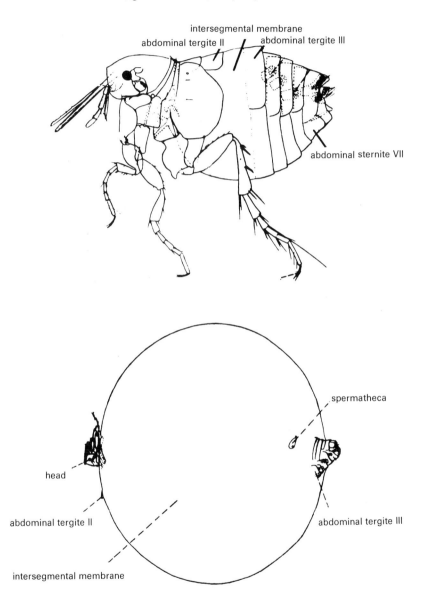

Source: From Patton, W.S. and Evans, A.M. (1929). *Insects, Ticks, Mites and Venomous Animals Part 1: Medical*. H.R. Grubb, Croydon

northern hemisphere, but has been taken round the world by man with his poultry. *E. gallinacea* is widely distributed in the warmer countries of the world, including Australia. These fleas attach themselves to the heads of poultry and may occur in clusters of 100 or more on the comb, wattles, back of the head and round the eyes and beak. This sticktight flea is a serious pest as large numbers cause a progressive anaemia and emaciation leading to lowered egg production in laying hens, and death in young birds.[37]

Tunga penetrans (Figure 17.8), the sand flea, jigger or chigoe, is an important parasite of man in the Neotropical and Afrotropical regions where people often walk about barefooted. *T. penetrans* was originally a parasite of pigs in South America and was introduced into West Africa in the middle of the nineteenth century, probably with the slave trade. It is now widespread in tropical Africa and has reached Madagascar.

The male *T. penetrans* is very small and free living. The female burrows into the skin of the feet and ankles of human beings. It begins as one of the smallest of the fleas, but then undergoes considerable hypertrophy of the abdomen, particularly the second and third abdominal segments, becoming the shape and size of a pea (17.8). Such a radical change during a stage in the life cycle has been given the name neosomy.[3] The female feeds head down and consequently the spiracles on abdominal segments 5-8 are very large, while the other abdominal spiracles are not developed. The female matures about 200 eggs which are passed out to the exterior. They hatch to produce a larva which follows the normal cycle of development for a flea. The presence of a number of adult *T. penetrans* in the foot can be crippling, and the damage to the skin can facilitate the entry of other pathogens leading to secondary infection and ulceration.

References

1. Abreu, M.H. (1980). Quelques aspects particuliers du cycle annuel d'infestation du lapin de garenne par deux especes de puces. pp. 391-6 in *Fleas*, R.Traub and H. Starcke (eds.), A.A. Balkema, Rotterdam
2. Askew, R.R. (1971). *Parasitic Insects*. Heinemann, London
3. Audy, J.R., Radovsky, F.J. and Vercammen-Grandjean, P.H. (1972). Neosomy: radical intrastadial metamorphosis associated with arthropod symbioses. *Journal of Medical Entomology 9*: 487-94
4. Bacot, A. (1914). A study of the bionomics of the common rat fleas and other species associated with human habitations, with special reference to the influence of temperature and humidity at various periods of the life history of the insect. *Journal of Hygiene 13, Plague Supplement III* 447-652
5. Bates, J.K. (1962). Field studies on the behaviour of bird fleas. I. Behaviour of the adults of three species of bird fleas in the field. *Parasitology 52*: 113-32
6. Bennet-Clark, H.C. and Lucey, E.C.A. (1967). The jump of the flea: a study of the energetics and a model of the mechanism. *Journal of Experimental Biology 47*: 59-76
7. Detinova, T.S. (1968). Age structure of insect populations of medical importance. *Annual Review of Entomology 13*: 427-50

8. Dunnet, G.M. (1970). Siphonaptera. pp. 647-655 in *The Insects of Australia*, sponsored by CSIRO Division of Entomology, Melbourne University Press, Melbourne
9. Edney, E.B. (1945). Laboratory studies on the bionomics of the rat fleas, *Xenopsylla brasiliensis*, Baker and *X. cheopis*, Roths I. Certain effects of light, temperature and humidity on the rate of development and on adult longevity. *Bulletin of Entomological Research 35*: 399-416
10. _____ (1947). Laboratory studies on the bionomics of the rat fleas, *Xenopsylla brasiliensis*, Baker and *X. cheopis*, Roths. II. Water relations during the cocoon period. *Bulletin of Entomological Research 38*: 263-80
11. Galun, R. (1966). Feeding stimulants of the rat flea *Xenopsylla cheopis* Roth. *Life Sciences 5*: 1335-42
12. Geigy, R. and Suter, P. (1960). Zur Copulation de Flöhe. *Revue Suisse de Zoologie 67*: 206-10
13. Holland, G.P. (1964). Evolution, classification, and host relationships of Siphonaptera. *Annual Review of Entomology 9*: 123-46
14. Hopkins, G.H.E. and Rothschild, M. (1953). *An Illustrated Catalogue of the Rothschild Collection of Fleas (Siphonaptera) in the British Museum (Natural History). I. Tungidae and Pulicidae*. British Museum, Natural History, London
15. _____ and Rothschild, M. (1971). *An Illustrated Catalogue of the Rothschild Collection of Fleas (Siphonaptera) in the British Museum (Natural History). V. Leptopsyllidae and Ancistropsyllidae*. British Museum, Natural History, London
16. Hopla, C.E. (1980). A study of the host associations and zoogeography of *Pulex*. pp. 185-207 in *Fleas*, R. Traub and H. Starcke (eds.), A.A. Balkema, Rotterdam
17. Hosie, G. (1980). Observations on the occurrence of *Ceratophyllus gallinae* around new housing estates in the west of Scotland. pp. 415-20 in *Fleas*, R. Traub and H. Starcke (eds.), A.A. Balkema, Rotterdam
18. Humphries, D.A. (1966). Drinking of water by fleas. *Entomologist's Monthly Magazine 102*: 200-1
19. _____ (1967). The mating behaviour of the hen flea *Ceratophyllus gallinae* (Schrank) (Siphonaptera: Insecta). *Animal Behaviour 15*: 82-90
20. _____ (1967). The behaviour of fleas (Siphonaptera) within the cocoon. *Proceedings of the Royal Entomological Society of London A 42*: 62-70
21. _____ (1967). The action of the male genitalia during the copulation of the hen flea, *Ceratophyllus gallinae* (Schrank). *Proceedings of the Royal Entomological Society of London A 42*: 101-6
22. _____ (1967). Uptake of atmospheric water by the hen flea *Ceratophyllus gallinae* (Schrank). *Nature, London 214*: 426
23. _____ (1968). The host-finding behaviour of the hen flea *Ceratophyllus gallinae* (Schrank)(Siphonaptera). *Parasitology 58*: 403-14
24. Krampitz, H.E. (1980). Host preference, sessility and mating behaviour of *Leptopsylla segnis* reared in captivity. pp. 371-8 in *Fleas*, R. Traub and H. Starcke (eds.), A.A. Balkema, Rotterdam
25. Lavoipierre, M.M.J. and Hamachi, M. (1961). An apparatus for observations on the feeding mechanism of the flea. *Nature, London 192*: 998-9
26. Margalit, J. and Shulov, A.S. (1972). Effect of temperature on the development of prepupa and pupa of the rat flea, *Xenopsylla cheopis* Rothschild. *Journal of Medical Entomology 9*: 117-25
27. Marshall, A.G. (1980). The function of combs in ectoparasitic insects. pp. 79-87 in *Fleas*, R. Traub and H. Starcke (eds.), A.A. Balkema, Rotterdam
28. Mellanby, K. (1932). The influence of atmospheric humidity on the thermal death point of a number of insects. *Journal of Experimental Biology 9*: 222-31
29. _____ (1933). The influence of temperature and humidity on the pupation of *Xenopsylla cheopis*. *Bulletin of Entomological Research 24*: 197-202
30. _____ (1934). The site of loss of water from insects. *Proceedings of the Royal Society of London B 116*: 139-49
31. Molyneux, D.H. (1967). Feeding behaviour of the larval rat flea *Nosopsyllus fasciatus* Bosc. *Nature, London 215*: 779
32. Munshi, D.M. (1960). Micro-anatomy of the proventriculus of the common rat flea

Xenopsylla cheopis (Rothschild). *Journal of Parasitology 46*: 362-72
33. Rothschild, M. (1965). Fleas. *Scientific American 213 (6)*: 44-53
34. _____ (1975). Recent advances in our knowledge of the order Siphonaptera. *Annual Review of Entomology 20*: 241-59
35. _____ and Hinton, H.E. (1968). Holding organs on the antennae of male fleas. *Proceedings of the Royal Entomological Society of London A 43*: 105-7
36. _____ Schlein, Y., Parker K. and Sternberg, S. (1972). Jump of the oriental rat flea *Xenopsylla cheopis* (Roths.). *Nature, London 239*: 45-8
37. Seddon, H.R. and Albiston, H.E. (1967). *Disease of Domestic Animals in Australia. Part 2. Arthropod Infestations (Flies, Lice and Fleas).* Department of Health, Commonwealth of Australia
38. Sharif, M. (1948). Nutritional requirements of flea larvae, and their bearing on the specific distribution and host preferences of the three Indian species of *Xenopsylla* (Siphonaptera). *Parasitology 38*: 253-63
39. Shulov, A. and Naor, D. (1964). Experiments on the olfactory responses and host-specificity of the oriental rat flea (*Xenopsylla cheopis*), (Siphonaptera: Pulicidae). *Parasitology 54*: 225-31
40. Suter, P.R. (1964). Biologie von *Echidnophaga gallinacea* (Westw.) und Vergleich mit andern Verhaltenstypen bei Flöhen. *Acta Tropica 21*: 193-238
41. Traub, R. (1972). The relationship between the spines, combs and other skeletal features of fleas (Siphonaptera) and the vestiture, affinities and habits of their hosts. *Journal of Medical Entomology 9*: 601
42. _____ (1980). Some adaptive modifications in fleas. pp. 33-67 in *Fleas*, R. Traub and H. Starcke (eds.), A.A. Balkema, Rotterdam
43. _____ (1980). The zoogeography and evolution of some fleas, lice and mammals. pp. 93-172 in *Fleas*, R. Traub and H. Starcke (eds.), A.A. Balkema, Rotterdam.
44. Yinon, U., Shulov, A. and Margalit, J. (1967). The hygroreaction of the larvae of the oriental rat flea *Xenopsylla cheopis* Rothsch. (Siphonaptera: Pulicidae). *Parasitology 57*: 315-9

18 BLOOD-SUCKING HEMIPTERA (BUGS)

Two families of Hemiptera, the Cimicidae and Reduviidae, include species which are blood-sucking. All the Cimicidae are blood-sucking, temporary ectoparasites of birds and mammals. They have oval, flattened bodies, and at first sight appear to be wingless, but they are micropterous with the forewings reduced to hemelytral pads and the hind wings absent. The Reduviidae includes many subfamilies of predacious bugs and the Triatominae which are blood-sucking on mammals and birds. The Triatominae are fully winged in the adult stage, as are other reduviids.

Cimicidae[25]

The Cimicidae is particularly well represented in the northern hemisphere. There are no native cimicids in Australia and no bird-feeding cimicids in tropical Africa or Central America. Usinger[25] recognises 74 species within the Cimicidae, arranged in 22 genera of which 12 genera are parasites of bats, nine of birds, and the genus *Cimex* which parasitises both mammals and birds. Twelve of the genera are found only in the New World, eight only in the Old World and two including *Cimex* in both.

The 16 species of *Cimex* include 13 species parasitic on bats: the *C. pipistrelli* group (7 spp) in the Palaearctic region and the *C. pilosellus* group (6 spp) in the Nearctic region; one species on birds; and *C. lectularius* and *C. hemiptera*, the bedbugs on man. *C. lectularius* is now virtually worldwide in its distribution. It is a parasite not only of man but of bats, chickens and other domestic animals. *C. hemipterus* is tropico-politan occurring in the warmer areas of the world. It is a parasite of man and chickens, but only rarely of bats. There is a third species of bedbug, *Leptocimex boueti*, which has a limited distribution in West Africa and parasitises man and bats.

Cimex lectularius and *Cimex hemipterus* [25]

External Structure (see Figure 18.1)

The two major bedbug species will be considered together and specific differences indicated. The adult bedbug measures 5-7 mm with females being slightly longer than males, and *C. hemipterus* being about 25 per cent longer than *C. lectularius*. They are red-brown in colour.

Head. The head bears long 4-segmented antennae, of which the last three

313

Figure 18.1: Female *Cimex lectularius*. Dorsal view on left and ventral view on the right

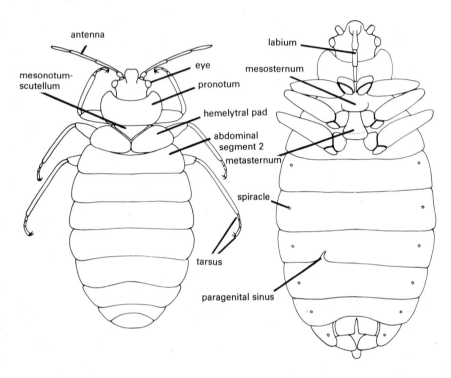

segments are long and slender, and a pair of widely separated compound eyes, laterally placed at the sides of the head. There are no ocelli; the labium has three obvious segments and is reflected backwards under the head reaching as far as the coxae of the first pair of legs.

Thorax. The prothorax is recessed anteriorly and its sides surround the posterior part of the head. In *C. lectularius* the breadth of the pronotum is more than two-and-a-half times the length of the prothorax in the midline. The mesonotum-scutellum is triangular in shape with the base adjoining the pronotum and the apex backwardly directed. Laterally there are the hemelytral pads. The tarsus has three segments, the last segment bearing a pair of simple claws. The metasternum is a more or less square, flat plate between the coxae, with rounded posterior corners. The mesosternum is rectangular being wider than it is long.

Abdomen. The abdomen is 11-segmented with segments 2 to 9 being easily recognisable dorsally. When the bedbug engorges, the abdomen greatly increases in volume by exposing the intersegmental membranes and expanding the so-called 'hunger folds', membranous areas in the mid-ventral line of the second to fifth abdominal segments. There are seven pairs of spiracles located ventrally on abdominal segments 2 to 8. Ventrally on the right side of the female there is a notch or paragenital sinus on the posterior margin of the fifth segment. It opens into the ectospermalege. There is no corresponding structure on the left side of the female. The male is similarly asymmetrical, and only the left paramere is developed at the posterior end of the abdomen (Figure 18.2). It is directed towards the left side. There is no right paramere.

Internal Structure

Certain features of the internal organs should be mentioned briefly. The midgut is divided into three ventriculi. The first is a large and bulbous zone in which the blood is stored and concentrated. This section is separated by a sphincter from the second and third ventriculi which are concerned with digestion and absorption which is so complete that only a little haematin enters the hindgut. The ganglia of the thorax and abdomen are concentrated in a single ganglionic mass in the metathorax.

Mycetome. Laterally in the abdomen between the fourth and the fifth segments there are the mycetomes, which contain symbiotic micro-organisms. Two different organisms occur in *C. lectularius,* one rod-shaped and the other 'pleomorphic'.[4] These organisms are transmitted trans-ovarially from generation to generation. Mycetomes and symbiotic micro-organisms are common in insects which only ever feed on blood. The

Figure 18.2: Ventral View of Terminalia of Male *Cimex lectularius*

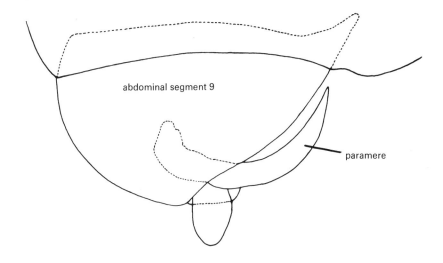

micro-organisms provide certain essential compounds effecting fertility. When *C. lectularius* is rendered nearly symbiote-free by heat treatment (37°C) only a few eggs are produced and they are infertile.[4]

Life Cycle

Egg. The female oviposits on rough rather than smooth surfaces inserting eggs into cracks and crevices. They are laid individually and held in place by a transparent cement. The eggs are white in colour, little more than 1 mm in length and less than 0.5 mm in breadth. The eggs are fertilised while still in the ovary, and the embryo has already undergone some development when the eggs are laid. The minimum time for development is four to five days at 30-35°C. No eggs hatch at 37°C or at temperatures below 13°C. Below 13°C eggs remain viable for shorter periods as the temperature approaches 0°C, and none survives for three months. Therefore in temperate climates eggs laid in the autumn are likely to have died before the temperature rises above the threshold in the spring, and consequently the species will not survive in the egg stage over the winter.[9]

Nymph. The egg has a distinct cap at one end and this is forced off when the nymph emerges. In appearance the nymph is very similar to the adult and feeds on blood in the same way. Nymphs will feed within 24 hours of emergence or of moulting to the next instar. There are five nymphal instars in the life cycle with the bodyweight increasing by 30-40 per cent at each instar. When feeding, the bug grasps the skin with its forelegs as a prelude to piercing the skin. Saliva injected during the feeding contains an anti-coagulant and the blood does not clot until it reaches the second ventriculus. Feeding takes five to ten minutes, during which time nymphs will take in two to five times their own body weight of blood. The duration of the instars is very similar for the first four instars, but the fifth is somewhat longer. At 30°C development from egg to adult takes three weeks.[25]

Mating

The method of insemination in *Cimex* is highly unusual. Males recognise another member of the same species at distances less than 15 mm, but do not distinguish between the sexes. The male climbs on to the back of the female with his head on the left side of the pronotum and the abdomen tucked under the right side of the female. There are three stages in insemination of *C. lectularius*. In the spermalege stage the male penetrates the ectospermalege and injects a mass of sperm into the adjacent meso-spermalege. The sperm becomes mobile in about 30 min and after three to four hours move into the haemocoele to being the second phase.[25]

The spermatozoa concentrate at the base of the genital apparatus near the junction of the paired and median oviducts. They penetrate into the seminal receptacle which has no direct communication with the lumen of the oviduct. The spermatozoa move up in the wall of the oviduct to the pedicel of the ovariole, and concentrate in the syncitial tissue at the distal end of the ovariole. The egg is fertilised in the ovariole before the chorion is formed. This is the intragenital phase.[25] This traumatic method of insemination may be a method of transferring nutrient materials from the male to the female which could be of value in survival of the species under adverse conditions.

Behaviour

Bedbugs are nocturnal creatures which reach peak activity before dawn. They are negatively phototactic, which combined with positive thigmotaxis ensures that they hide away in cracks and crevices during the day. In their search for hosts bedbugs respond to warmth and carbon dioxide, but not to odours. A bedbug will respond to a body which is two or more degrees above ambient temperature, but there is disagreement as to the distance from which a bug can respond with values of 3-4 cm and 150 cm being claimed.[25] Temperature receptors are probably located on the basal segments of the antennae.[15]

Adult bedbugs have a scent gland which opens ventrally on the meta-thorax on to an evaporative area. The main components of the secretion are two aldehydes which are present in the ratio of 7:3.[14] They function as alarm pheromones and cause dispersal of aggregated bugs. The receptors for this pheromone are found on the terminal segment of the antenna.[15] When alarmed bedbugs can move at a rate of 2 cm/s.[25]

Bedbugs also produce an aggregation pheromone which brings them together, when thigmotaxis will ensure that they stay grouped. The origin of this pheromone is unknown but the receptors are on the antennae. This is not a sex pheromone because the scent of males or females attracts both sexes equally. It is a pheromone to which adults are particularly sensitive, and to which 5th instars respond only slightly although they are present in the aggregations.[14] Nymphs have scent glands which open in the middorsal line on segments 3,4 and 5 of the abdomen but their function is not known.

Fecundity, Rate of Development and Survival

Fecundity. The frequency of oviposition and the number of eggs laid are dependent on the frequency with which blood meals are available. At 23°C and 75 per cent RH, newly moulted female *C. lectularius* took an average one-and-a-half times their own bodyweight of blood in their first meal and then laid nine eggs six to twelve days later. When they are fed twice a week egg laying was continuous.[9]

At 23°C and 90 per cent RH females kept with males and fed once a week, produced on the average nearly three eggs in the first week, between seven and eight eggs in the second and third weeks, and more than eight eggs in the fourth week. Thereafter egg production continued to average six to seven eggs per week for the next 13 weeks, after which it declined rapidly. Rather surprisingly, *C. lectularius* kept under the same conditions, but at 10 per cent RH, were more fecund; and averaged more than ten eggs in the fourth week, and for the next 13 weeks the average egg production was 8.6 eggs per female, cf 6.5 for females kept at 90 per cent RH.[9]

Rate of Development. Omori (cited from Usinger[25]) gives comparative data for the development of *C. lectularius* and *C. hemipterus* at various temperatures, and the survival of once-fed bedbugs of all stages at different temperatures. In all cases the performance of *C. lectularius* was superior to that of *C. hemipterus*. *C. lectularius* developed twice as fast as *C. hemipterus* at 18°C and at 33°C. This is strange when it is realised that *C. hemipterus* has a tropical and subtropical distribution. At 27°C and 30°C the two species developed at their fastest, and there was no difference between the species.

Survival. In the longevity experiments the 1st instar of both species survived for the shortest time. At all temperatures (10°, 18°, 27° and 37°) adult *C. lectularius* survived much longer than adult *C. hemipterus*. At 37°C *C. lectularius* survived considerably longer than *C. hemipterus* in all stages, and at the lowest temperature *C. lectularius* survived for almost twice as long as *C. hemipterus* in all stages.[25]

Medical Importance

The nocturnal biting of bedbugs can be debilitating to humans whose sleep is disturbed every night. The presence of bedbugs in a dwelling can be recognised from specks of faeces left by the bugs and by their smell. Although their own powers of dispersal are very limited they have been carried throughout the world by man with his possessions. The status of bedbugs as vectors of disease was summarised in 1966 by Usinger[25] when he wrote 'In summary, Cimicidae have been suspected in the transmission of many diseases or disease organisms of man and bats, but in most cases conclusive evidence is lacking.'

The position has changed more recently with the recovery of the Hepatitis B Virus from bedbugs in Africa where Hepatitis B surface antigen has been recovered from unengorged *C. hemipterus*[29] and *C. lectularius*.[10] The antigen has been shown to persist in both species for up to six weeks after a blood meal, and to be excreted in the faeces of *C. hemipterus*.[20] Virus in faeces 'could infect a susceptible person by contamination of skin lesions or mucosal surfaces, or by inhalation of dust'.[20] Earlier Newkirk *et al.*[19] had failed to detect antigen in bedbug faeces, but they found that the antigen remained in bedbugs throughout a five-week period with a suggestion of possible replication of the antigen. Replication has not been confirmed by other workers.[20]

Reduviidae — Triatominae

The Triatominae are one of about 30 subfamilies recognised within the Reduviidae.[18] Adult triatomines are large insects, commonly measuring 20-28 mm in length, and the broad abdomen 8-10 mm wide.[13] They have long, thin, 4-segmented antennae (Figure 18.4). The compound eyes are placed laterally, and there are ocelli located dorsally behind the eyes (Figure 18.4). In front of the eyes the head is narrowed and forwardly produced (Figure 18.3). The rostrum (labium) is 3-segmented and straight, not arched (Figure 18.4), and extends back to the prosternal stidulatory groove. The tarsi are 3-segmented. The forewings are hemelytra with a sclerotised basal area (corium and clavus) and a distal membranous portion (Figure 18.5). The hind wings are entirely membranous, and in repose, are folded beneath the hemelytra.

Figure 18.3: Female *Panstrongylus megistus*

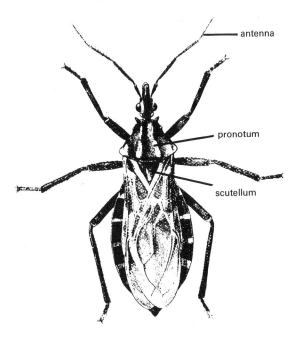

Source: From Castellani, A. and Chambers, A.J. (1913). *A Manual of Tropical Medicine*. Baillière Tindall, London

Figure 18.4: Lateral View of Head of a Reduviid

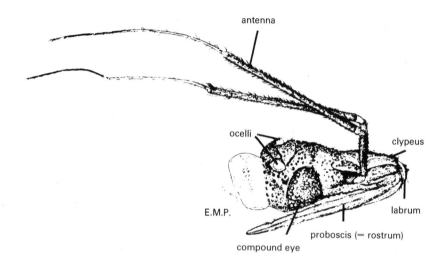

Source: From Patton, W.S. and Evans, A.M. (1929), *Insects, Ticks, Mites and Venomous Animals, Part I: Medical.* H.R. Grubb, Croydon

In the unfed state the abdomen is almost flat and the hinged dorsal and ventral connexival plates are close together and almost parallel. On feeding, the abdomen becomes greatly distended and the connexival plates rotate on the hinge and become widely separated. In some triatomines, e.g. *Rhodnius*, abdominal expansion is further increased by the unfolding of an additional longitudinally pleated membrane.[13]

The Triatominae are largely confined to the western hemisphere with one tropicopolitan species, a single species in India, and a group of seven species of *Triatoma* in south-east Asia. The subfamily has its greatest diversity in South America, extending into Central America, and to only a limited extent into the Nearctic region. Lent and Wygodzinsky,[13] who have recently revised the Triatominae, recognise 111 species classified into five tribes and 14 genera.

Biology

Life Cycle of Rhodnius prolixus

Egg. The eggs of *R. prolixus* are 2.5 mm in length with an obvious operculum at one end and within a few hours of being deposited are a bright lobster red.[24] They are laid in cracks and crevices in houses, and in wild populations they may be glued on to palm fronds.[33] A female will

Figure 18.5: Wings of a Triatomine Bug. Hemelytron (above) and hind wing (below)

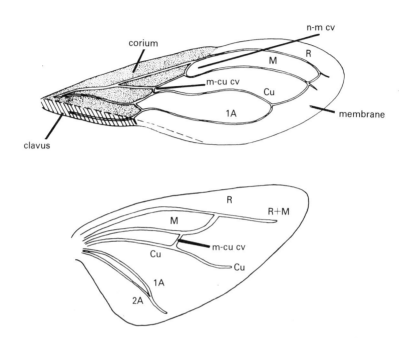

produce 200-300 eggs in her lifetime, laid in a number of batches. Uribe[24] recorded the size of egg batches as varying from one to 14 eggs with a female laying 30 to 50 batches in her lifetime; while Buxton[2] recorded up to nine egg batches per female, averaging 31 eggs per batch, and with the majority of the eggs being laid in the first four batches.

Eggs hatch over the range 16-34°C with the highest fertility occurring at 21-32°C. Fertility is also related to humidity. At 25-27°C all eggs hatched at humidities of 50 per cent RH or higher, but at 32°C a humidity of 80 per cent was required. Eggs are resistant to desiccation and 50 per cent hatch was obtained at a humidity of 20 per cent and 25°C.[5] The egg stage is relatively long, requiring 12 days at 32°C and nearly a month at 22°C.[6]

Nymph. The nymph emerges by pushing off the operculum from the egg. It is a miniature version of the adult except for the absence of wings (Figure 18.6). There are five nymphal stages all of which feed on blood. If a nymph engorges fully only one blood meal is required before moulting to the next stage. The first-stage nymph takes 12 times its own bodyweight of blood, and the other four nymphal stages six times their bodyweight, while adults take in only one-and-a-half times.[2] During development the nymph increases by 1.6 times at each moult, growing from 2.7 mm in the 1st instar

Figure 18.6: Early Stages of *Triatoma rubrofasciata*. A, egg (× 8); B, first stage nymph (× 10); C and D, second and third stage nymphs respectively (× 3)

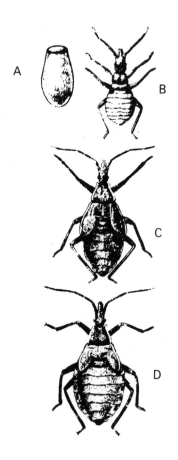

Source: From Patton, W.S. and Cragg, F.W. (1913). *Textbook of Medical Entomology*. Christian Literature Society for India, London

to 17 mm in the 5th instar.[24] In mass rearing of *R. prolixus* at 28°C and 60-70 per cent RH and fed every two weeks on hens, the life cycle from egg to adult took 80 days with 42 per cent survival.[6] The 'mortality' included deaths and individuals that did not feed which was about 18 per cent of each instar.[6] Adults live for nearly six months.[2,6]

Life Cycle of Triatoma infestans

The life cycle of *T. infestans* is very similar to that of *R. prolixus*. The eggs are white when laid and become red after about ten days.[11] At 26-27°C and

60 per cent RH the egg stage lasts about three weeks and the nymphal stages 20 weeks, with the 5th instar being the longest (seven weeks) and the 4th instar the shortest (11 days). Mortality is high in the 1st (19 per cent) and 5th (16 per cent) instars and lowest in the 3rd instar (1.6 per cent).[21]

Significantly, more females reach the adult stage than males (1.27:1.00), but the males are longer lived averaging 26 weeks compared with 16 weeks for females.[21] Egg fertility has been calculated to be 84 per cent[3] and 86 per cent,[21] which is comparable to rates of 82 per cent[2] for *R. prolixus*. On average a female lays about 150 eggs[21] to 240 eggs[3] with peak fecundity being reached eleven weeks after the first oviposition.[21]

Population Growth

Assuming a 1:1 ratio of males to females at the egg stage then about half the female eggs give rise to adults. *R. prolixus* and *T. infestans* had the shortest life cycles among nine species of Triatominae, and *T. dimidiata* and *P. megistus* took about twice as long to complete development under the same conditions.[33] Rabinovich[21] has analysed his data on *T. infestans* very fully and shown that the generation time was 31 weeks with a net reproductive rate (R_o) of 25 and an intrinsic rate of increase (r) of 0.101. That is, the population increased 25 times from one generation to the next or, put another way, a stable-aged population would increase by 10 per cent per week.

Bionomics

Feeding

Some sylvatic triatomines are aggressive in bright daylight,[33] but most triatomines are nocturnal, and in houses feed on sleeping inhabitants. For that reason they are most abundant in bedrooms, which may contain 50 per cent of the total population of *R. prolixus* in a house.[22] The stimuli that attract triatomines to a host are warmth, carbon dioxide and odour.[26,28] Sensory receptors on the antennae of *T. infestans* respond to carbon dioxide and warmth,[26] and to another component of human breath, which was probably an odour.[16] Orientation on the host and probing involves receptors on the tarsi and labium, in addition to heat receptors on the antennae.[26]

In feeding the mandibles pierce the skin and then cease to move. They are barbed and hold the insect in position. The flexible maxillae penetrate deeply and move about freely until they contact a capillary. The right maxilla is longer than the left and penetrates into the capillary, the left maxilla may enter the capillary or remain closely attached on the outside because the junction between the two maxillae is the effective functional mouth.[12]

During feeding saliva is injected containing an anticoagulant and blood is pumped into the midgut, the first section of which acts as a storage organ. Two anticoagulants have been recovered from *R. prolixus*, one from the salivary glands, the other from the gut.[8] Although the precise location of the gut anticoagulant was not stated it is probably the storage section where blood remains unclotted. This section of the midgut contains in its lumen symbionts which are important in the successful development of a triatomine.[27] In their absence development stops in the 4th or 5th instar.[1] A coagulant in this section would prevent the ingested blood clotting and trapping symbionts in the clot. It would also ensure that the blood remained fluid for easier passage into the digestive section of the midgut. In development the nymph acquires its symbionts by probing the contaminated surface of the egg from which it has emerged or from excreta of other members of the species.[1]

Most accounts of being bitten by triatomine bugs comment on the lack of pain,[12,30] although on repeated exposure some individuals had a delayed reaction 24-48 h after being bitten, and in one case a more severe response. It is possible that longer periods of exposure would produce an immediate response.[12]

Triatomines feed on a wide range of hosts, and domestic species feed on man and his domestic animals, dogs, cats and chickens, and rodents infesting the house. They will feed on more than one host, particularly if their feeding has been interrupted, and will often feed again before the previous meal has been completely digested. More than one third of *T. dimidiata* had fed on more than one host and the gut contents of one adult reacted positively to antisera of six hosts — man, dog, cat, mouse, cow and opossum.[34]

The time to take a full blood meal varies with the instar and size of the insect.[33] Wood[30] found times to engorgement among five species varying from 3-30 min with *T. protracta* being the slowest feeder. *R. prolixus* and *T. infestans* feed faster and with fewer interruptions than does *T. dimidiata*.[31] Interruptions involve the bug withdrawing its mouthparts in the course of a single meal. First instar *T. dimidiata* imbibe five times their own weight which decreases to twice the insect's weight in the 5th instar. Male and female *T. dimidiata* ingest over 40 per cent and 50 per cent, respectively, of their bodyweight at each feed and in the course of adult life a female may consume 4-10 g of blood and males about half that.[32] Fifth instar nymphs of *P. megistus* take twice as much blood as the same stage of *R. prolixus* (300 cf. 600 mg).[17] Nymphs of *T. infestans* consume about 1,000 mg of blood in developing to an adult.[33]

When a heavily infested rural house in Venezuela was demolished nearly 8,000 *R. prolixus* of all stages were recovered.[22] The information was analysed in great detail and it was calculated that in that house the feeding rate was 58 *R. prolixus* per person per day, and in 13 other houses it was nine, ranging from 0.2-33; and the loss of blood per person per month in the 13 houses ranged from 0.7-40 ml; and in the heavily infested house exceeded 100 ml.[22]

Defaecation

Infection with *T. cruzi* depends upon infective forms present in the faeces of the bug being deposited on the host and gaining access via a wound or moist mucosa. Therefore the earlier a bug defaecates during or after feeding the more likely the species is to be an efficient vector. *R. prolixus* and *T. infestans* defaecate within ten minutes of finishing a meal when the insect is still likely to be on the host and 8 per cent or *R. prolixus* defaecate during the meal. Only two-thirds of *T. dimidiata* defaecate within ten minutes of finishing a meal but, possibly because of the longer feeding time, 13 per cent defaecate during the meal.[31]

Zeledon *et al.*[31] proposed a defaecation index which, averaged for all instars and sexes, rates *R. prolixus* at 2.3, *T. infestans* at 1.1 and *T. dimidiata* 0.6. The index of *T. protracta*, which often delays defaecation, was 0.2 and for *T.rubida uhleri*, which defaecates frequently and early, 9.0 (based on data from Wood[30]). *T. rubida* frequents the nests of woodrats (*Neotoma* spp) which are sylvatic reservoirs of *T. cruzi* in the USA.[13]

Resting Places

The relationship between triatomines and man ranges from those that are totally sylvatic to those that are truly domestic. In South America many species occur in the crowns of palms but the populations are low (5-70/tree) because blood meals depend on visiting birds and mammals, and natural enemies are present. Other biotopes occupied by triatomines include bromeliads, under bark of trees, in hollow trees and fence posts and in ground burrows.[33]

R. prolixus occurs in both palms and houses, and in the latter occurs equally in the walls and roof, particularly in palm thatch roofs.[22] *T. infestans* and *P. megistus* infest cracks in unplastered mud and cane walls,[26] and are less common in mud-brick.[33] *T. dimidiata* occurs lower down than the other two species rarely being more than a metre above the floor; and in houses raised on supports it occurs on the ground or on the foundations that support the floor. Here they feed on animals that shelter under the house, and are able to enter the house at night through cracks in the floor and feed on its sleeping occupants.[34] The bugs congregate near a food source, hence the greater concentration in the walls of bedrooms. This concentration is assisted in *T. infestans* and *R. prolixus* by a pheromone in the faeces which attracts the unfed nymphs of both species. Fed nymphs are not attracted by the faecal material but their locomotory activity is arrested in its presence which leads to them congregating in the same area.[23]

Dispersal

Wild *R. prolixus* disperse mainly as ectoparasites of birds. Houses are invaded by bugs being introduced in palm fronds, in firewood and in household articles. Nearly a third of *R. prolixus* released into a house found shelter in household articles.[7] In 40 days labelled *R. prolixus* dispersed less than 4 m in houses and less than 15 m outside. Adult *R. prolixus* appear to fly very little and there was movement between palm trees and houses only when the two habitats were close together. Other workers have found some nymphs and adults of *R. prolixus* dispersing 100-500 m[33] and *P. megistus* moved 400 m from a natural to an artificial biotope.[33]

Triatomines are attracted to light which would favour their establishment in houses. There can be two-way movement between natural and artificial biotopes. The range of blood meals identified in *T. dimidiata* in natural and artificial biotopes indicated free movement between the two, with 22 per cent of the bugs in natural biotopes and some of the bugs found in houses containing opossum blood.[34]

Survival and Longevity

In the laboratory triatomines are long-lived and able to withstand long periods of starvation. The greatest resistance to starvation is shown by 4th and 5th instar nymphs which in *T. dimidiata* surived six months unfed, whereas adults survived only 4-5 months.[32] Similar powers of survival were shown by nymphs of *T. infestans* and *R. prolixus*,[33] but in the field survival of *R. prolixus* was considerably lower being measured in weeks rather than months.[7] Predation by domestic fowls, rodents and other predators was the main cause of early mortality, and Gómez-Núñez[7] calculated that *R. prolixus* had a one in four chance of successfully moving from a palm tree to an adjoining house. Perhaps as a defence against predation nymphs of *T. dimidiata* camouflage themselves by covering their bodies with debris.[34]

Medical Importance

Triatomines are of considerable medical importance as vectors of Chagas' disease caused by *Trypanosoma cruzi* on which further information is given in Chapter 29. About 66 species have been found naturally infected with *T. cruzi*,[33] belonging to eight genera and including 41 out of 63 species of *Triatoma*, nine out of 12 species of *Rhodnius* and nine out of 13 of *Panstrongylus*. The most important vectors are *T. infestans, T. dimidiata, R. prolixus* and *P. megistus*.

References

1. Brecher, G. and Wigglesworth, V.B. (1944). The transmission of *Actinomyces rhodnii* Erikson in *Rhodnius prolixus* Stål (Hemiptera) and its influence on the growth of the host. *Parasitology 35*: 220-4
2. Buxton, P.A. (1930). The biology of a blood-sucking bug, *Rhodnius prolixus*. *Transactions of the Entomological Society of London 78*: 227-36
3. Carcavallo, R.U. and Martinez, A. (1972). Life cycles of some species of *Triatoma* (Hemiptera: Reduviidae). *Canadian Entomologist 104*: 699-704
4. Chang, K.P. (1974). Effects of elevated temperature on the mycetome and symbiotes of the bed bug *Cimex lectularius* (Heteroptera). *Journal of Invertebrate Pathology 23*: 333-40
5. Clark, N. (1935). The effect of temperature and humidity upon the eggs of the bug, *Rhodnius prolixus* (Heteroptera, Reduviidae). *Journal of Animal Ecology 4*: 82-7
6. Gómez-Núñez, J.C. (1964). Mass rearing of *Rhodnius prolixus*. *Bulletin of the World Health Organization 31*: 565-7
7. _____ (1969). Resting places, dispersal and survival of Co_{60}-tagged adult *Rhodnius prolixus*. *Journal of Medical Entomology 6*: 83-6
8. Hellmann, K. and Hawkins, R.I. (1965). Prolixin-S and prolixin-G: two anticoagulants from *Rhodnius prolixus* Stål. *Nature, London 207*: 265-7
9. Johnson, C.G. (1941). The ecology of the bed-bug, *Cimex lectularius* L., in Britain. *Journal of Hygiene 41*: 345-461
10. Jupp, P.G., Prozesky, O.W., McElligott, S.E. and van Wyk, L.A.S. (1978). Infection of the common bedbug (*Cimex lectularius* L.) with hepatitis B virus in South Africa. *South African Medical Journal 53*: 598-600
11. Larrousse, F. (1927). Etude biologique et systématique du genre *Rhodnius* Stål (Hémiptères, Reduvidae). *Annales de Parasitologie Humaine et Comparée 5*: 63-88
12. Lavoipierre, M.M.J., Dickerson, G. and Gordon, R.M. (1959). Studies on the methods of feeding of blood-sucking arthropods. I. The manner in which triatomine bugs obtain their blood-meal, as observed in the tissues of the living rodent, with some remarks on the effects of the bite on human volunteers. *Annals of Tropical Medicine and Parasitology 53*: 235-50
13. Lent, H. and Wygodzinsky, P. (1979). Revision of the Triatominae (Hemiptera, Reduviidae), and their significance as vectors of Chagas' disease. *Bulletin of the American Museum of Natural History 163*: 125-520
14. Levinson, H.Z. and Bar Ilan, A.R. (1971). Assembling and alerting scents produced by the bedbug *Cimex lectularius* L. *Experientia 27*: 102-3
15. _____ Levinson, A.R., Müller, B. and Steinbrecht, R.A. (1974). Structure of sensilla, olfactory perception, and behaviour of the bedbug, *Cimex lectularius*, in response to its alarm pheromone. *Journal of Insect Physiology 20*: 1231-48
16. Mayer, M.S. (1968). Response of single olfactory cell of *Triatoma infestans* to human breath. *Nature, London 220*: 924-5
17. Miles, M.A., Patterson, J.W., Marsden, P.D. and Minter, D.M. (1975). A comparison of *Rhodnius prolixus, Triatoma infestans* and *Panstrongylus megistus* in the xenodiagnosis of a chronic *Trypanosoma (Schizotrypanum) cruzi* infection in a rhesus monkey (*Macaca mullatta*). *Transactions of the Society of Tropical Medicine and Hygiene 69*: 377-82
18. Miller, N.C.E. (1956). *The Biology of the Heteroptera*. Leonard Hill, London
19. Newkirk, M.M., Downe, A.E.R. and Simon, J.B. (1975). Fate of ingested hepatitis B antigen in blood-sucking insects. *Gastroenterology 69*: 982-7
20. Ogston, C.W. and London, W.T. (1980). Excretion of hepatitis B surface antigen by the bedbug *Cimex hemipterus* Fabr. *Transactions of the Royal Society of Tropical Medicine and Hygiene 74*: 823-5
21. Rabinovich, J.E. (1972). Vital statistics of Triatominae (Hemiptera: Reduviidae) under laboratory conditions. *Journal of Medical Entomology 9*: 351-70
22. _____ Leal, J.A. and Feliciangeli de Piñero, D. (1979). Domiciliary biting frequency and blood ingestion of the Chagas's disease vector *Rhodnius prolixus* Ståhl (Hemiptera:

Reduviidae), in Venezuela. *Transactions of the Royal Society of Tropical Medicine and Hygiene 73*: 272-83

23. Schofield, C.J. and Patterson, J.W. (1977). Assembly pheromone of *Triatoma infestans* and *Rhodnius prolixus* nymphs (Hemiptera: Reduviidae). *Journal of Medical Entomology 13*: 727:34

24. Uribe, C. (1926). On the biology and life history of *Rhodnius prolixus* Stahl. *Journal of Parasitology 13*: 129-36

25. Usinger, R.L. (1966). *Monograph of Cimicidae (Hemiptera-Heteroptera)*. The Thomas Say Foundation 7: 1-585

26. Wiesinger, D. (1956). Die Bedeutung der Umweltfaktoren für den Saugakt von *Triatoma infestans. Acta Tropica 13*: 98-141

27. Wigglesworth, V.B. (1936). Symbiotic bacteria in a blood-sucking insect, *Rhodnius prolixus* Stål. (Hemiptera, Triatomidae). *Parasitology 28*: 284-9

28. _____ (1972). *The Principles of Insect Physiology*. Chapman and Hall, London

29. Wills, W., London, W.T., Werner, B.G., Pourtaghva, M., Larouzé, B., Millman, I., Ogston, W., Diallo, S. and Blumberg, B.S. (1977). Hepatitis-B virus in bedbugs (*Cimex hemipterus*) from Senegal. *Lancet 2*: 217-9

30. Wood, S.F. (1951). Importance of feeding and defecation times of insect vectors in transmission of Chagas' disease. *Journal of Economic Entomology 44*: 52-4

31. Zeledón, R., Alvarado, R. and Jirón, L.F. (1977). Observations on the feeding and defecation patterns of three triatomine species (Hemiptera: Reduviidae). *Acta Tropica 34*: 65-77

32. _____ Guardia, V.M., Zúñiga, A. and Swartzwelder, J.C. (1970). Biology and ethology of *Triatoma dimidiata* (Latreille, 1811). I. Life cycle, amount of blood ingested, resistance to starvation and size of adults. *Journal of Medical Entomology 7*: 313-9

33. _____ and Rabinovich, J.E. (1981). Chagas' disease: an ecological appraisal with special emphasis on its insect vectors. *Annual Review of Entomology 26*: 101-33

34. _____ Solano, G., Zúñiga, A and Swartzwelder, J.C. (1973). Biology and ethology of *Triatoma dimidiata* (Latreille, 1811). III. Habitat and blood sources. *Journal of Medical Entomology 10*: 363-70

19 PHTHIRAPTERA (LICE)

The Phthiraptera or lice are wingless, dorsoventrally flattened, permanent ectoparasites of birds and mammals. They are host specific (but see p. 348) and spend their entire lives on the host. Three suborders are recognised: the Anoplura, which are blood-sucking ectoparasites of mammals; the Mallophaga, which have chewing mouthparts and feed on skin debris of birds and mammals; and the Rhynchophthirina, which includes just one species, *Haematomyzus elephantis*, which is somewhat intermediate between the other two suborders, but sometimes included in the Mallophaga. *H. elephantis* has a long, forwardly directed proboscis, which bears small cutting mandibles at its tip.[15]

Over 3,000 species of lice have been described of which the greater number are in the Mallophaga. Being host specific lice will have evolved more closely with their hosts than fleas which have a range of hosts. The subject of the evolution of lice, fleas and their hosts has been dealt with by Traub[36] and the geographical distribution of avian lice and their hosts by Clay.[9]

The species of lice parasitising domestic mammals are listed in Table 19.1. The characters distinguishing between the Anoplura and Mallophaga have been given in Chapter 2. The two suborders will be considered separately.

Table 19.1: Lice Found on Domestic Animals

Host	Anoplura	Mallophaga
Cattle	*Haematopinus eurysternus* *Haematopinus quadripertusus* *Haematopinus tuberculatus* *Linognathus vituli* *Solenopotes capillatus*	*Damalinia bovis*
Horse	*Haematopinus asini*	*Damalinia equi*
Pig	*Haematopinus suis*	None
Sheep	*Linognathus ovillus* *Linognathus pedalis*	*Damalinia ovis*
Goat	*Linognathus africanus* *Linognathus stenopsis*	*Damalinia caprae* *Damalinia crassipes* *Damalinia limbata*
Dog	*Linognathus setosus*	*Heterodoxus spiniger* *Trichodectes canis*
Cat	None	*Felicola subrostrata*

Anoplura

When Ferris[16] published his account of the Anoplura in 1951 he recognised about 250 species which he arranged in six families. When Kim and Ludwig[19] repeated the exercise in 1978 the number of species in the suborder had almost doubled and they recognised 15 families. Their Figure 1 (p. 250[19]) shows a steady increase in the number of species being described over the last 40 years with no sign of diminishing. It recalls the similar expansion in number of species of fleas described by Smit.[35] It has been postulated that there are more than 1,000 species of Anoplura of which about half have been described.[19]

The six families recognised by Ferris[16] included the Pediculidae with its medically important genera *Pediculus* and *Pthirus*; the veterinarily important Haematopinidae (*Haematopinus*) and Linognathidae (*Linognathus* and *Solenopotes*); the Hoplopleuridae, mostly parasites of rodents, but including *Pedicinus* on primates; the Echinophthiridae, parasites of marine mammals; and the Neolinognathidae, which contains one genus and two species parasitic on elephant shrews. Ten of the 15 families proposed by Kim and Ludwig[19] are based on a single genus, three have only a single species, and four families contain only two species. To the non-specialist this would seem to be excessive.

External Morphology

Anoplura are small insects, ranging from less than 0.5 mm to 8 mm in the adult and 2 mm would be an average length. The antennae are usually 5-segmented; the eyes are reduced and usually absent; and there are no ocelli (Figure 19.1). The head is prognathous with the mouth opening terminal. The highly specialised mouthparts are not visible externally and have been described in Chapter 4. There are no palps.

The three thoracic segments are fused. There is only a single tarsal segment and a single claw. When the claw is retracted it makes contact with a thumb-like process on the tibia, the enclosed space having the diameter of the hairs of the host, and enables the louse to maintain itself on an active host (Figure 19.4C). There is one pair of spiracles, the mesothoracic, on the thorax, and six pairs on segments 3-8 of the abdomen. The abdomen has nine visible segments.

The sexes can be easily distinguished. The sclerotised genitalia of the male are prominent posteriorly in the midline, and the female has two pairs of lateral gonopods and the sternal plate of the eighth segment sclerotised to varying degrees (Figure 19.2).

Internal Structure

The following account is largely based on *Pediculus* on which most work has been done. The thoracic and abdominal ganglia are fused

Figure 19.1: Two Common Human Lice — *Pediculus capitis* (left) and *Pthirus pubis* (right) from Dorsal View. Setae omitted in *P. capitis* and only selected setae shown in *P. pubis*

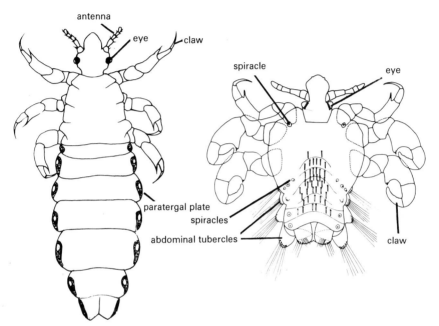

into a single ganglionic mass in the thorax. The oesophagus opens into a huge midgut dominated by a capacious ventriculus. A short narrow posterior section of the midgut connects the ventriculus to the hindgut. With the posterior section being so short the ventriculus functions as both a storage and a digestive organ. Buxton[6] comments that 'with regard to digestion nothing is known', and that still appears to be true.

Mycetome. On the ventral surface of the ventriculus there lies the mycetome, containing symbionts. In development the mycetome arises as a pouch off the midgut and symbionts, which are in the gut of the embryo, enter the mycetome. In nymphs and males they remain there throughout the life of the individual, but in females they migrate to the ovary and there is transovarian transmission of symbionts from one generation to another. In the absence of symbionts nymphs live for only a few days and females are sterile.[6] The loss of symbionts can be counteracted by a single dose of the vitamin B complex.[32]

Biology and Behaviour
Anoplura firmly attach their eggs individually to the hairs of their host, or

Figure 19.2: Ventral View of Female Terminalia (above), and Male Genitalia (below) of *Pediculus humanus*

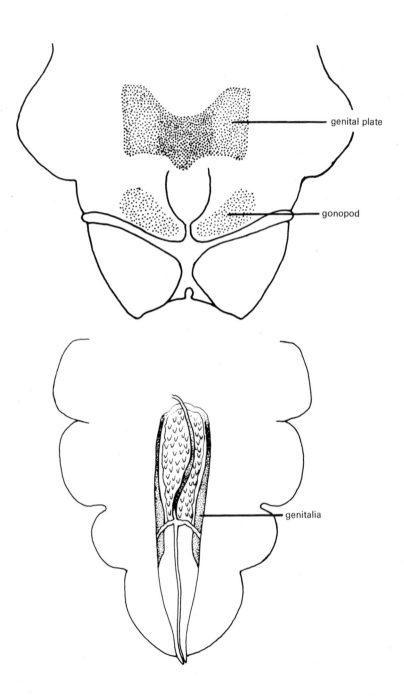

in the case of *Pediculus humanus* (Figure 19.3A), the body louse, to the clothing of its host. The eggs hatch to produce a nymph which is clearly recognisable as a small edition of the adult, living and feeding in the same way. There are three nymphal stages before the adult. All stages feed on blood and maintain contact with their host by a number of relatively simple responses.

Both *Pediculus* and *Haematopinus* respond to warmth and smell, and *Haematopinus* will distinguish between a finger and a glass rod at the same temperature.[39] Many receptors are located on the antennae, but heat receptors are more generally distributed over the body.[38] Humidity receptors are present on the antennae, and the louse avoids high humidities, but once adapted to a given humidity it turns away from higher or lower humidities. The responses of lice to stimuli are kineses and not taxes,

Figure 19.3: A, Egg of *Pediculus humanus* With Operculum Viewed From Above; B, Egg of *Pthirus pubis*

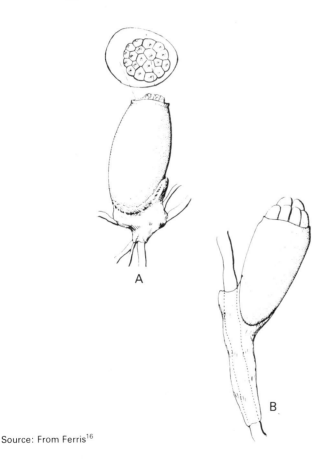

A

B

Source: From Ferris[16]

that is lice are not attracted directly to the source of the stimulus but show increased turning when they move away from the source.[38]

In addition lice are positively thigmotactic, moving less on rough surfaces, and both negatively phototactic and positively skototactic, moving towards dark objects. The preferred temperature is 29-30°C and movement into areas of higher or lower temperature results in more frequent turning of the louse to bring it back to the preferred temperature.[38] Being ecto-parasitic on warm-blooded animals lice live at a relatively high ambient temperature, and *Pediculus* does not oviposit at temperatures below 25°C.[39]

Pediculus humanus, Pediculus capitis (see Figure 19.1)

Adult *Pediculus* measure 2-3 mm in the male and 2.4-3.6 mm in the female. The simple, lateral eyes are well developed, for a louse. The legs are essentially the same size and shape; the margins of the abdomen are more or less strongly lobed, the lobes on segments 3-8 being covered by sclerotised paratergal plates; and there is a sclerotised sternal plate on the thorax.

Pediculus humanus is the human louse, and two subspecies have usually been recognised: *P. h. corporis*, the body louse, and *P. h. capitis*, the head louse. Busvine[4] has pointed out that the two forms remain distinct when both forms occur on the same individual, and although intermediate forms can be produced in the laboratory, in the field the two forms remain distinct. They should be regarded as separate species, *P. humanus* the body louse, and *P. capitis* the head louse.

Egg. The egg measures 0.8 × 0.3 mm and is glued to the hair in the case of *P. capitis* and to the inner clothing by *P. humanus*[6] (Figure 19.3A). Eggs will hatch over the temperature range 24-37°C with the highest hatching rate of 70-90 per cent occurring at 29-32°C. Outside that range the hatching rate declines reaching 10 per cent at 24° and 37°C. The percentage of eggs hatching, but not the duration of the egg stage, is affected by humidity with the highest rate occurring at 75 per cent RH. The egg stage lasts seven to ten days at 29-32°C, and the maximum time that eggs can survive unhatched is three to four weeks, which may be important when considering the survival of lice in infested clothing.

Nymph. At hatching the nymph swallows the amniotic fluid and air, forces the operculum (Figure 19.3A) off the egg and tears the vitelline membrane, using what Buxton[6] describes as 'elaborate hatching devices on a ridged area of embryonic cuticle on the front of the head'. When kept on the skin all day the three nymphal stages are passed in eight to nine days but when removed at night the duration of the nymphal stages extends to 16-19 days. Adults mate frequently throughout life, beginning soon after the final moult. Human lice survive off the host for only a few days, the duration varying inversely with the temperature, but at low temperatures lice are inactive which reduces their chance of finding another host.

Longevity and Fecundity. Three sets of data on the longevity and fecundity of *P. humanus* will be considered. When maintained as monogamous pairs on the skin permanently, the longevity of females was 34 ± 13 days and for males 31 ± 12 days. Under these conditions the preoviposition period was 24-36 h, and on average a female laid 270 to 300 eggs at a rate of nine to ten eggs per day.[6] When lice were removed from the body at night and subjected to fluctuating ambient temperatures, the longevity was very similar with that of the females being 29 ± 13 days, and of the males 31 ± 12 days.[5] The preoviposition period was two days and fecundity was greatly reduced, ranging from 80 to 212 eggs per female at a rate of three to five eggs per female per day.[5]

Evans and Smith[13] reared *P. humanus* in groups of 100 at 30°C and 30-55 per cent RH. The lice were fed twice a day on volunteers. The mean length of life was 17.6 days for both sexes with standard deviations of 8.0 (males) and 9.2 (females). The coefficients of variation (standard deviation as a percentage of the mean) are similar to those obtained by Buxton.[5,6] The average fecundity was 82 eggs per female laid at a rate of 5 eggs per female per day, and was comparable to the findings of Buxton[5] for lice removed from the body at night.

Population Dynamics. Evans and Smith[13] found that the individual instars lasted three to five days, and the total nymphal life averaged 12.8 days with a coefficient of variation of only 5 per cent. Using their observed hatching rate (87.7 per cent) and survival of nymphs to adults (86 per cent) they calculated the net reproductive rate (Ro) as 31, and the intrinsic rate of natural increase (r) at 0.111 per day. In the absence of other limiting factors the population would increase 31 times in one generation, and would double itself in six days. It might be noticed that the value for r for *P. humanus* (0.111) is similar to that obtained by Rabinovich (reference 21, p. 327) for *Triatoma infestans* for which he obtained a value of 0.101, a major difference being that the r value for *P. humanus* was per day, and for *T. infestans* per week. This is comparable to the longevity of the two forms, being weeks for lice and months for triatomines. Both Buxton[6] and Evans and Smith[13] agree that in a stable-aged population over two-thirds of the lice will be present as eggs, about a quarter as nymphs and only 6-7 per cent as adults.

Medical Importance. Infestations of *Pediculus* on man cause considerable irritation and scratching; the irritation disturbs the infested persons' rest, and the scratching leads to skin lesions and secondary infections. The medical importance of *Pediculus* does not reside in its direct effects on the human host, but in its role as the vector of epidemic typhus (*Rickettsia prowazeki*) and relapsing fever (*Borrelia recurrentis*). The transmission of these pathogens is dealt with in Chapters 25 and 26.

Pthirus pubis (see Figure 19.1)

P. pubis, the crab louse, has simple eyes and is shorter (1.5-2 mm) and broader than the more slender *Pediculus*. Its body is less than twice as long as wide. The thorax is very wide and passes imperceptibly into the short abdomen. Compared to the first pair of legs the second and third pairs are strongly developed; there is no thoracic sternal plate; the abdomen bears four pairs of lateral sclerotised tubercles; and, as a result of compression, the first three pairs of abdominal spiracles are in an almost straight, transverse row.

P. pubis occurs on the hair in the pubic and perianal regions of the body, and occasionally in the axillae, eyebrows and beard.[6] The incidence of *P. pubis* has been increasing among the human population in recent years, and pediculosis pubis, as the condition is known, is the most contagious sexually transmitted disease according to Felman and Nikitas.[14] Transmission can also occur between individuals sleeping in the same bed, one of whom is infested. A common feature of infestation with *P. pubis* is the presence of blue or slate-grey macules on the skin which are considered to be either altered patient blood pigments or substances excreted from the louse's salivary glands.[14] Fortunately *P. pubis* is not involved in the transmission of any pathogenic organisms. It has a similar life cycle to that of *P. humanus* and attaches its eggs (Figure 19.3B) to hairs in the area of infestation. *P. pubis* is considered to be less mobile than *P. humanus*, moving only 100 mm per day compared with 175 mm per hour for the latter.[14] It survives for even shorter periods off the host, dying in less than 48 hours at 15°C.[14]

Haematopinus (see Figure 19.4)

Species of *Haematopinus* are large lice measuring about 4 mm with prominent ocular points but without eyes. The thoracic sternal plate is well developed; the legs are all of similar size; the paratergal plates are strongly sclerotised on abdominal segments 2 or 3 to 8; and there is a sclerotised plate at the base of the tarsal segment, which is referred to as the pretarsal sclerite or discotibial process (Figure 19.4C).

Twenty-two species of *Haematopinus* have been described and they are all parasites of ungulates. Those occurring on domestic animals include *H. suis* on pigs; *H. asini* on equines; and three species on cattle: *H. eurysternus*, the short-nosed sucking louse; *H. quadripertusus*, the tail louse; and *H. tuberculatus*, the buffalo louse.[20]

On Cattle. Louse populations build up during the winter when the animal's

Figure 19.4: Male *Haematopinus asini*. A, in dorsal view; B, sternal plate; C, terminal segments of leg

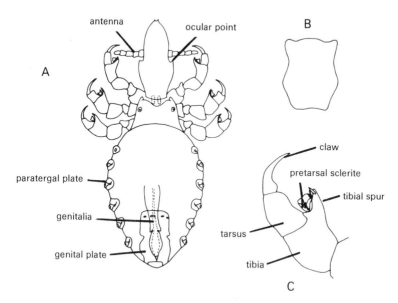

coat is longer and thicker. In Arizona cattle not given supplementary feeding lose weight during winter, and this was shown to be significantly increased when cattle had heavy infestations of *H. eurysternus*. Heavy infestations were also associated with marked anaemia. The effect was more pronounced on heifers than bulls, with heifers losing significantly more weight when moderately infested.[10]

H. eurysternus occurs on cattle worldwide. The female measures about 3.5 mm in length. The main areas of infestation are the head and neck, spreading in heavy infestations to many other parts of the body. The life cycle from egg to egg averages four weeks with females living up to 16 days and laying 35-50 eggs. *H. quadripertusus* occurs on cattle in tropical areas. It is a rather larger louse measuring 4.5 mm and occurring mainly in the tall-switch where the eggs are laid almost exclusively. The nymphs migrate to the soft skin around the anus, vulva and eyes. *H. tuberculatus* is the largest of the three measuring 5.5 mm and was originally described from the Indian buffalo. In Australia it has been found infesting camels and cattle but is not considered of any great importance.[33]

On Pigs and Horses. *H. suis* is the largest anopluran found on domestic animals and occurs in folds of the neck and jowl, and around the ears of pigs. It causes severe irritation resulting in a depressed growth rate.[34] *H. asini* is about 3.5 mm in length and favours the roots of the mane, the

Figure 19.5: A, Female *Linognathus ovillus* — dorsal view is presented in the left half and the ventral view in the right half of the illustration; B, Dorsal View of Female *Solenopotes capillatus*

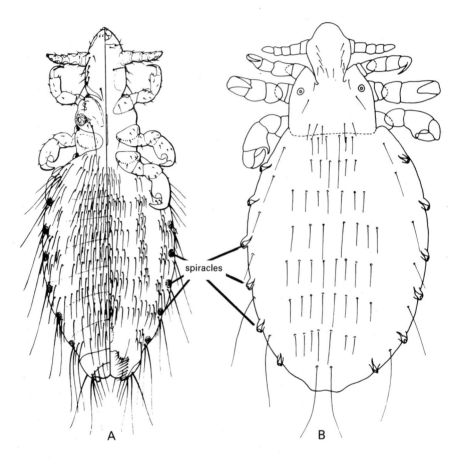

spiracles

A   B

Source: A from Ferris[16]

forelock, round the butt of the tail and above the hooves.[33] Louse populations in domestic animals are reduced at the beginning of summer by the shedding of the coat. This has least effect on populations of *H. asini* because the coarse hairs of the mane and tail to which they attach their eggs are not shed.[24]

Linognathidae (see Figures 2.14 and 19.5)

Members of this family are distinguished by the absence of eyes and ocular points; by the second and third pairs of legs, which end in large stout claws, being considerably larger than the first pair; by the thoracic sternal plate being absent or weakly developed in *Linognathus*, but distinct in *Solenopotes*; and with no paratergal plates on the abdomen. Two genera have species, which are parasitic on domestic animals, and another parasitises hyraxes.[16]

Most species of *Linognathus* are found on Artiodactyla, and a few on carnivores. More than 50 species of *Linognathus* have been described, and six occur on domestic animals. *L. setosus* parasitises dogs, particularly long-haired breeds on which it infests the neck and shoulders.[12]

On Sheep. Two species — *L. pedalis*, the foot louse, and *L. ovillus* (Figure 19.5A), the face louse — are most commonly found on sheep. Both frequent the hairy parts of the body, *L. ovillus* occurring on the face and lower jaw from which it spreads to the body,[21] and *L. pedalis* occurring on the lower hairy parts of the body, namely shanks, belly and scrotum.[33] *L. pedalis* is able to survive for several days off the host, 50 per cent being alive after seven days at 12°C and 75 per cent RH. In comparison all *L. ovillus* were dead in four days under the same conditions.[27]

The eggs of both species hatch over a relatively narrow range of temperature around 35°C, and few hatch at 38°C or higher temperatures.[25,28] During the summer months in Australia the temperature near the skin of the sheep may rise to over 45°C, and within the fleece the temperature may exceed 50°C.[30] Such conditions would have an adverse effect on louse populations.

The fact that *L. pedalis* can survive for several days off the host raises the possibility of infection being acquired from contaminated pasture.[34] On sheep *L. pedalis* is more sedentary and congregates in clusters, behaviour which does not occur in *L. ovillus*.[27] *L. stenopsis*, the goat louse, also occurs on sheep. It is larger than the other lice on sheep and can cause scabby, bleeding areas on the host.[33] *L. africanus* also parasitises domestic sheep and goats.[16]

On Cattle (Figure 2.14). *Linognathus vituli* is the long-nosed sucking louse of cattle. In a trial in New Zealand cattle with moderate infestations of *L. vituli* gained slightly more weight than the control group but the trial was conducted in winter on good pasture,[18] which means that the results are not directly comparable with those obtained with *H. eurysternus* in Arizona.[10] *L. vituli* is more common on calves and young stock, and more important among dairy cattle.[34]

Species of *Solenopotes* parasitise cervids and bovids with one species, *S. capillatus*, occurring on cattle. In *Solenopotes* the abdominal spiracles are borne on lightly sclerotised tubercles which project slightly from the body (Figure 19.5B).[16] *S. capillatus* is the smallest of the sucking lice on cattle and occurs in conspicuous clusters on the neck, head, shoulders, dewlap, back, anus and tail.[33]

Mallophaga

The Mallophaga, of which over 2,500 species have been described, are ectoparasites of birds and mammals, but mainly of birds. They are often referred to as 'biting lice', but a better term is 'chewing lice', because in popular parlance blood-sucking insects are said to bite, and the Mallophaga do not feed on blood. They feed on fragments of feathers, hair and other epidermal products.

In the Mallophaga the eyes are reduced or absent; there are no ocelli; the antennae are 3-5-segmented; the prothorax is free; and the mesothorax and metathorax may be fused. The mouthparts have been described in Chapter 4. Two divisions, the Amblycera and the Ischnocera, are recognised within the Mallophaga.

In the Amblycera the antennae are recessed in antennal grooves from which the last segment may protrude (Figure 19.6). The mandibles lie parallel to the ventral surface of the head and cut in a horizontal plane. The mesothorax and metathorax are usually separate; the antennae are 4-segmented; and the maxillary palps 2-4-segmented.

In the Ischnocera the antennae are 3- or 5-segmented, and are quite obvious because there is no antennal groove (Figures 19.8, 19.9). The mandibles are inserted more or less at right angles to the head and operate in a vertical plane. There are no maxillary palps, and the mesothorax and metathorax are fused to form the pterothorax.

Emmerson[11] lists 11 species of Mallophaga from the domestic chicken (7 Philopteridae and 4 Menoponidae), of which 7 (5 Philopteridae and 2 Menoponidae) will be briefly considered here.

Amblycera

Clay[8] considers that the Amblycera are sufficiently different from the Ischnocera to justify their elevation to a suborder comparable to the Anoplura.

There are six families in the Amblycera of which three occur on birds, and three on marsupials and New World mammals. The Boopidae are parasites of marsupials, and are distinguished from other domestic mammal-infesting lice by possessing two claws compared with one in the Anoplura and Trichodectidae (Figures 2.15 and 19.9). One species of Boopidae, *Heterodoxus spiniger*, 'occurs on domestic dogs in many parts of Australia, Africa, Asia and the Americas'.[7] Guinea pigs are frequently infested with two species of Gyropidae, *Gyropus ovalis* with an oval abdomen, broad in the middle, and *Gliricola porcelli*, a slender louse with the sides of the abdomen somewhat parallel.[12]

Several species of Menoponidae occur on domestic birds of which the most important are *Menopon gallinae*, the shaft louse (Figure 19.6), and *Menacanthus stramineus*, the chicken body louse. *M. gallinae* is about

2 mm long and lays its eggs singly at the base of a feather. It occurs on the thigh and breast feathers, and is claimed to be harmful to young fowls.[12,33] *M. stramineus* (Figure 19.7) is the commonest and most destructive louse found on chickens and has a worldwide distribution. It is up to 3.5 mm long and deposits its eggs in masses at the base of feathers especially around the vent. It occurs on the breast, thighs and around the vent, causing a marked reddening of the skin, and 'sometimes gnaws through the skin or punctures the soft quills near the base and consumes the blood that oozes out'.[12] Other species of Menoponidae occur on ducks, geese and pigeons but heavy infestations are rarely seen on these birds and little harm results.

Figure 19.6: Female *Menopon gallinae.* Dorsal view on left, and ventral view on right

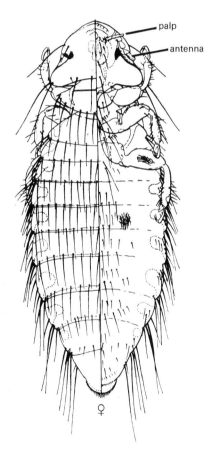

Source: From Ferris, G.F. (1924). *Parasitology 16*: 58

Figure 19.7: Female *Menacanthus stramineus*

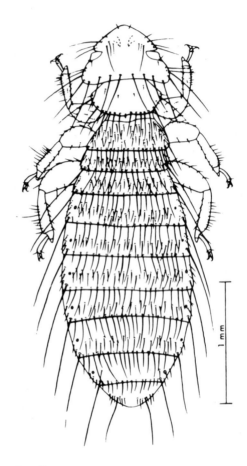

Source: From Price, in Flynn[12]

Ischnocera

Three families of Ischnocera are recognised of which two are of veterinary importance, the Philopteridae on domestic birds and the Trichodectidae on mammals. The Philopteridae have 5-segmented antennae and paired claws on the tarsi, and the Trichodectidae have 3-segmented antennae and single claws on the tarsi.

On Poultry. Five species of Philopteridae occur on poultry and have virtually a worldwide distribution. The chicken head louse, *Cuclotogaster heterographus* (Figure 19.8A), occurs on the skin and feathers of the head and neck, where the lice feed on tissue debris and occasionally ingest

Figure 19.8: Philopteridae Which Occur on Poultry. A, female *Cuclotogaster heterographus*; B, *Goniocotes gallinae* female; C, *Goniodes dissimilis;* D, *Lipeurus caponis*

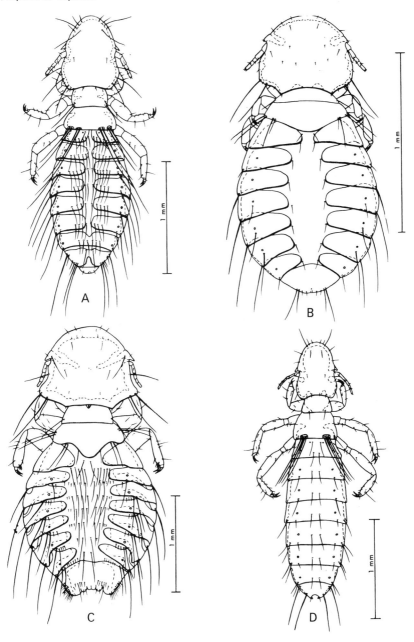

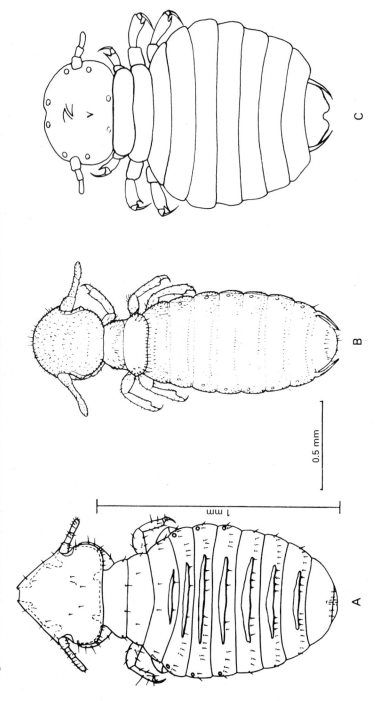

Figure 19.9: A, Female *Felicola subrostrata*; B, *Damalinia ovis*; C, *Trichodectes canis*

0.5 mm

1 mm

A

B

C

Source: A and C from Price, in Flynn.[12] B from Calaby[7]

blood. Severe infestations in young chickens are sometimes fatal.[12] The fluff louse, *Goniocotes gallinae* (Figure 19.8B), is a small louse which occurs on the down feathers anywhere on the body and generally causes little irritation. *Goniodes dissimilis* (Figure 19.8C) and *G. gigas* and about 3 mm long and brown in colour. They are among the largest lice that are found on chickens, and occur anywhere on the body. In small numbers, they have little effect on their host. *G. gigas* is more prevalent in the tropics, and *G. dissimilis* in temperate regions.[12] The fifth species, the wing louse, *Lipeurus caponis* (Figure 19.8D), is not a very active species, and occurs on the underside of the wing and tail feathers.[12,33] Other philopterids occur on turkeys, ducks, pigeons and appear to do little harm.

On Dogs and Cats. Three genera of Trichodectidae parasitise domestic animals. *Felicola subrostrata* (Figure 19.9A) is the only louse that occurs on cats. The head is triangular with the point directed forwards and notched at the apex. Ventrally there is a median longitudinal groove on the head which fits around the hair of the host. *F. subrostrata* is of minor importance, being found in large numbers only on elderly or sick cats especially if they are long-haired.[33]

Trichodectes canis (Figure 19.9C) is found on the dog and wild canids throughout the world. The head is broader than long being rectangular with rounded corners. It is found on the head, neck and tail attached to the base of hairs. Infestations are commoner on very young, very old or sick dogs. This louse can act as an intermediate host of the tapeworm *Dipylidium caninum* of which further details are given in Chapter 32.

On Sheep. Several species of *Damalinia* (Trichodectidae) occur on domestic animals. *D. ovis* (Figure 19.9B) is a small, pale species which occurs on sheep worldwide. For oviposition it requires both a suitable temperature, and fibres of an appropriate diameter to which eggs can be attached.[22] The temperature at the skin surface of sheep is 37.5°C, and this is the temperature at which maximum oviposition of *D. ovis* occurs.[22] The distribution of the eggs of *D. ovis* on sheep is governed by skin temperature. Low temperatures in certain areas of the body, e.g. legs and tail, inhibit egg laying.[23] When the thickness of the fleece was 30-100 mm most eggs (75 per cent) were laid within 6 mm of the skin surface, and even when it was 100 mm deep few eggs (5 per cent) were laid more than 12 mm from the skin surface.[23]

Eggs develop and hatch over the range 33-39°C, and are virtually independent of humidity over the range seven to 75 per cent RH.[26] Very few eggs hatch at 92 per cent RH, and this was attributed to humidity inhibiting hatching, because fully developed embryos were present in eggs which aborted.[26] In fleeces where the temperature ranged from 38°C at the skin surface to 15°C near the tip of the fleece, 69 per cent of the mobile population (nymphs and adults) were within 6 mm of the skin surface and only 15 per cent were more than 12 mm from the skin. The fleece depth varied from 25-75 mm.[31] When the tip of the fleece was shaded and warmed, adults and third-stage nymphs came to the surface. It is under these conditions that *D. ovis* spreads among a closely herded flock.[30]

Populations of *D. ovis* are limited by a number of factors including shearing, when 30-50 per cent of the population may be lost.[30] Heavy rain can cause high mortality due to soaking the fleece, immersing all stages of the louse and maintaining a high humidity during the drying out period.[29] In Australia in the summer, temperatures in a fleece exposed to the sun can reach 45°C at the skin surface in five to ten minutes with temperatures near the fleece tip being 65-70°C.[30] Such temperatures would quickly be lethal to all stages of the louse, and help to explain why louse populations are low in summer.

On Cattle. Damalinia bovis is a small, reddish-brown louse on cattle, particularly dairy cattle. This louse is commonest at the front end and on the back of cattle, spreading more widely in heavy infestations. Its effect on the host is minimal. In one experiment in New Zealand cattle developed far larger numbers of *D. bovis* than usual, and although their weight gain was less than in louse-free cattle, the difference was not significant.[18]

When two groups of Hereford cattle were fed on low and high planes of nutrition as part of an experiment with ticks it was observed that heavy infestations of *D. bovis* occurred on the low nutrition group. This was attributed to reduced self-grooming and delayed shedding of the winter coat.[37] The difference between the levels of nutrition of the two groups is shown by the fact that over a period of ten months the low nutrition group actually lost weight while the high nutrition group almost doubled in weight.

On Horses and Goats. The oviposition behaviour of *D. equi,* which occurs on horses, has been studied by Murray.[24] *D. equi* cannot attach its eggs to the coarse hairs of the face, mane and tail, and consequently it suffers a loss of population when the coat is shed. *D. caprae* parasitises the common goat and several other species occur on the Angora goat.

Effect of Lice on Domestic Animals

The effect of lice on their host is a function of their density. A small number of lice on an individual presents no particular problem other than the prospect of a future population explosion. The life cycles of all lice are very similar with the duration of the egg stage being one to two weeks, the nymphal stages occupying one to three weeks, and the total time from egg

Table 19.2: Duration (in days) of Various Stages in the Life Cycle of Various Phthiraptera

Species	Egg	Nymph	Preoviposition	Egg-Egg	Adult		Reference No.
					M	F	
Pediculus humanus	7-9	8-9	1-2	20	29	31	6
" "	5-12	13	—	22-23	18	18	13
Haematopinus asini	12-14	11-12	—	—	—	—	33
" *eurysternus*	9-19	9-16	2-7	20-41	10	16	33
" *quadripertusus*	11	—	—	—	—	—	33
" *suis*	12-14	10	—	28-33	—	—	33
" *tuberculatus*	9-13	9-11	3	—	—	—	33
Linognathus pedalis	17	21	5	43	—	—	33
" *setosus*	5-12	—	—	—	—	—	12
" *vituli*	8-13	—	—	21-30	—	—	33
Menacanthus stramineus	7	17-30	—	—	—	—	33
" "	4.5	9	—	14	—	12	12
Cuclotogaster heterographus	—	—	—	14-21	months	months	12
Goniodes gigas	7	—	—	28	19	24	12
Lipeurus caponis	—	—	—	21-35	—	—	12
Damalinia bovis	8	18	3	29	—	—	33
" *equi*	8-10	—	—	—	—	—	33
" *ovis*	9-10	21	3	34	—	—	33
" "	10	21	3-4	34	—	—	31
Felicola subrostrata	10-20	14-21	—	21-42	14-21	14-21	12
Trichodectes canis	7-14	14	—	21-28	—	30	12

Source: Mostly extracted from Emmerson *et al.*[12] and Roberts.[33]

to egg being three to five weeks (Table 19.2). Adults probably live for up to a month, although Benbrook[2] considers that the normal life-span of lice on poultry is several months.

The intrinisic rate of natural increase of *P. humanus* has been calculated at 0.111[13] and for *D. ovis* 0.065.[31] Both rates are per day and indicate a maximum rate of increase of 11.7 per cent and 6.7 per cent per day, respectively. Murray[31] states that during 'winter' when lice populations thrive, the numbers of *D. ovis* on a sheep are likely to increase from 4,000 to more than 400,000 by the spring. On sheep the main effect of lice is to lower the value of the wool crop, and this is sufficiently important for the Department of Agriculture in Western Australia to mount an intensive campaign against sheep lice.[40]

Heavy infestations of lice are associated with young animals or old animals in poor health and/or animals maintained in unhygenic conditions. Nevertheless, the irritation caused by modest populations of lice leads to animals scratching and rubbing, causing damage to fleece and hides, and heavily infested calves develop hairballs as a result of licking areas of irritation.[3] In sheep *L. pedalis* can cause lameness, and *H. suis* spreads swine-pox among pigs.[3] There is conflicting evidence on the effect of lice on production, i.e. milk, eggs, beef, and is likely to be dependent upon other factors affecting the health of the host. The host is likely to be under greater stress in winter and this may contribute to the speed with which louse populations increase.

Host Specificity of Lice

Lice are said to be host specific but the reader must have become aware in reading this chapter that some species of lice occur on more than one host species. Being permanent ectoparasites they are only accidentally divorced from their host, and then their low powers of survival and high temperature threshold for activity severely limit the probability of their finding another host. Transference from one individual host to another occurs when animals are closely herded or penned, and in the close contact of mother and young with lice transferring from mother to young within a few hours of birth, e.g. lambs can become infested with *L. pedalis* within 48 h of birth[33] and piglets have become infested with *H. suis* within 10 h of birth.[17]

Where lice occur on more than one host species the hosts are usually closely related. *L. stenopsis* and *L. africanus* occur on both sheep and goats; *T. canis* occurs on dogs and wild canids; and *H. tuberculatus* has been found not only on the Indian buffalo and cattle, but also on the more distantly related camel in Australia.[33]

Where chickens and ducks are in close contact there may be transference of chicken lice to ducks, e.g. *M. gallinae*, *M. stramineus* and *C.*

heterographus.[33] One unusual way in which lice may be spread from host to host is by carriage on another insect. Three *D. bovis* were found in a phoretic association with the hornfly, *Haematobia irritans,*[1] but the number involved was very small, and this would appear to be a very minor route for dispersing *D. bovis.*

References

1. Bay, D.E. (1977). Cattle biting louse, *Bovicola bovis* (Mallophaga: Trichodectidae), phoretic on the horn fly, *Haematobia irritans* (Diptera: Muscidae). *Journal of Medical Entomology 13*: 628
2. Benbrook, E.A. (1965). External parasites of poultry. pp. 925-64 in *Diseases of Poultry,* H.E. Biester and L.H. Schwarte (eds.) Iowa State University Press, Ames
3. Blood, D.C., Henderson, J.A. and Radostits, O.M. (1979). *Veterinary Medicine — A Textbook of the Diseases of Cattle, Sheep, Pigs and Horses.* Baillière Tindall, London
4. Busvine, J.R. (1978). Evidence from double infestations for the specific status of human head lice and body lice (Anoplura). *Systematic Entomology 3*: 1-8
5. Buxton, P.A. (1940). The biology of the body louse (*Pediculus humanus corporis*: Anoplura) under experimental conditions. *Parasitology 32*: 303-12
6. _____ (1950). *The Louse.* Edward Arnold, London
7. Calaby, J.H. (1970). Phthiraptera. pp. 376-86 in *The Insects of Australia,* sponsored by CSIRO Division of Entomology, Melbourne University Press, Melbourne
8. Clay, T. (1970). The Amblycera (Phthiraptera: Insecta). *Bulletin of the British Museum (Natural History) Entomology 25*: 75-98
9. _____ (1974). Geographical distribution of the avian lice (Phthiraptera): a review. *Journal of the Bombay Natural History Society 71*: 536-47
10. Collins, R.C. and Dewhirst, L.W. (1965). Some effects of the sucking louse, *Haematopinus eurysternus,* on cattle on unsupplemented range. *Journal of the American Veterinary Medical Association 146*: 129-32
11. Emmerson, K.C. (1956). Mallophaga (chewing lice) occurring on the domestic chicken. *Journal of the Kansas Entomological Society 29*: 63-79
12. _____ Kim, K.C. and Price, R.D. (1973). Lice. pp. 376-97 in R.J. Flynn (ed.), *Parasites of Laboratory Animals,* Iowa State University Press, Ames
13. Evans, F.C. and Smith, F.E. (1952). The intrinsic rate of natural increase for the human louse. *Pediculus humanus* L. *American Naturalist 86*: 299-310
14. Felman, Y.M. and Nikitas, J.A. (1980). Pediculosis pubis. *Cutis 25*: 482,487-9, 559
15. Ferris, G.F. (1931). The louse of elephants. *Haematomyzus elephantis* Piaget (Mallophaga: Haematomyzidae). *Parasitology 23*: 112-27
16. _____ (1951). *The Sucking Lice.* Memoirs of the Pacific Coast Entomological Society, San Francisco
17. Hiepe, T. von and Ribbeck, R. (1975). Die Schweinelaus (*Haematopinus suis*). *Angewandte Parasitologie 16: Merkblatt No. 21,* 1-13
18. Kettle, P.R. (1974). The influence of cattle lice (*Damalinia bovis* and *Linognathus vituli*) on weight gain in beef animals. *New Zealand Veterinary Journal 22*: 10-11
19. Kim, K.C. and Ludwig, H.W. (1978). The family classification of the Anoplura. *Systematic Entomology 3*: 249-84
20. Meleney, W.P. and Kim, K.C. (1974). A comparative study of cattle-infesting *Haematopinus,* with redescription of *H. quadripertusus* Fahrenholz, 1916 (Anoplura: Haematopinidae). *Journal of Parasitology 60*: 507-22
21. Murray, M.D. (1955). Infestation of sheep with the face louse (*Linognathus ovillus*). *Australian Veterinary Journal 31*: 22-6
22. _____ (1957). The distribution of the eggs of mammalian lice on their hosts. II. Analysis of the oviposition behaviour of *Damalinia ovis* L. *Australian Journal of Zoology 5*: 19-29

23. _____ (1957). The distribution of the eggs of mammalian lice on their hosts. III. The distribution of the eggs of *Damalinia ovis* (L.) on the sheep. *Australian Journal of Zoology 5*: 173-82

24. _____ (1957). The distribution of the eggs of mammalian lice on their hosts. IV. The distribution of the eggs of *Damalinia equi* (Denny) and *Haematopinus asini* (L.) on the horse. *Australian Journal of Zoology 5*: 183-7

25. _____ (1960). The ecology of lice on sheep. I. The influence of skin temperature on populations of *Linognathus pedalis* (Osborne). *Australian Journal of Zoology 8*: 349-56

26. _____ (1960). The ecology of lice on sheep. II. The influence of temperature and humidity on the development and hatching of the eggs of *Damalinia ovis* (L.). *Australian Journal of Zoology 8*: 357-62

27. _____ (1963). The ecology of lice on sheep. III. Differences between the biology of *Linognathus pedalis* (Osborne) and *L. ovillus* (Neumann). *Australian Journal of Zoology 11*: 153-6

28. _____ (1963). The ecology of lice on sheep. IV. The establishment and maintenance of populations of *Linognathus ovillus* (Neumann). *Australian Journal of Zoology 11*: 157-72

29. _____ (1963). The ecology of lice on sheep. V. Influence of heavy rain on populations of *Damalinia ovis* (L.). *Australian Journal of Zoology 11*: 173-82

30. _____ (1968). Ecology of lice on sheep. VI. The influence of shearing and solar radiation on populations and transmission of *Damalinia ovis*. *Australian Journal of Zoology 16*: 725-38

31. _____ and Gordon, G. (1969). Ecology of lice on sheep. VII. Population dynamics of *Damalinia ovis* (Schrank). *Australian Journal of Zoology 17*: 179-86

32. Puchta, O. (1955). Experimentelle Untersuchungen über die Bedeutung der Symbiose der Kleiderlais *Pediculus vestimenti* Burm. *Zeitschrift für Parasitenkunde 17*: 1-40

33. Roberts, F.H.S. (1952). *Insects Affecting Livestock*. Angus and Robertson, Sydney

34. Seddon, H.R. and Albiston, H.E. (1967). *Diseases of Domestic Animals in Australia. Part 2. Arthropod Infestations (Flies, Lice and Fleas)*. Department of Health, Commonwealth of Australia

35. Smit, F.G.A.M. (1955). Siphonaptera from Bariloche, Argentina, collected by Dr. J.M. de la Barrera in 1952-1954. *Transactions of the Royal Entomological Society of London 107*: 319-39

36. Traub, R. (1980). The zoogeography and evolution of some fleas, lice and mammals. pp. 93-172 in *Fleas*, R. Traub and H. Starcke (eds.), A.A. Balkema, Rotterdam

37. Utech, K.B.W., Wharton, R.H. and Wooderson, L.A. (1969). Biting cattle-louse infestations related to cattle nutrition. *Australian Veterinary Journal 45*: 414-6

38. Wigglesworth, V.B. (1941). The sensory physiology of the human louse *Pediculus humanus corporis* De Geer (Anoplura). *Parasitology 33*: 67-109

39. _____ (1972). *The Principles of Insect Physiology*. Chapman and Hall, London

40. Wilkinson, F.C. (1978). New policy hits hard at sheep lice. *Journal of Agriculture, Western Australia 19*: 90

20 ACARI — ASTIGMATA AND ORIBATIDA (MANGE MITES, BEETLE MITES)

The Acari (= Acarina) or mites and ticks are a group of arthropods which, apart from the parasitic species, has been largely neglected. They are widely distributed throughout the world, being mainly terrestrial; but with the Hydrachnidia (Prostigmata), a group of aquatic families, mostly in fresh water; and one marine family, the Halacaridae (Prostigmata). About 30,000 species of Acari, belonging to more than 2,000 genera, have been described; however, this is a small proportion of the half a million species which, it is believed, exist today.[22]

Classification

In recent years increasing interest has been shown in the Acari and their classification is being continually revised. The groups of Acari of medical and veterinary importance are reasonably well defined, but at the lower level of classification there is uncertainty as to whether the categories should be subfamilies and families, or families and superfamilies. The present tendency is towards using the higher categories. In a full classification of the Acari the medically and veterinarily important groups have to be integrated with the greater number of other forms.

In the latest classification Krantz[22] treats the Acari as a subclass of the Arachnida, in which he recognises two orders: the Acariformes and the Parasitiformes. He points out that his scheme is only one of a number of possible treatments and for that reason Krantz's names for the higher categories will not be adopted *in toto* but only where they are terms which have had wide usage. On the other hand these new terms may become widely adopted and they will be given in italics in parentheses after the older terms, which will be used in this text. It must also be appreciated that the same term may be used in a modified sense by different authors. Therefore when a comparable term is given in parentheses it must not be assumed that the two terms are identical, but rather that they both refer broadly to the same assemblage of organisms.

Krantz[22] characterises the Acariformes as being without visible stigmata posterior to the coxae of the second pair of legs, and with the coxae (epimeres) often fused to the ventral body wall (Figure 20.3). The Parasitiformes are defined as possessing one to four pairs of lateral stigmata posterior to the coxae of the second pair of legs, and with free coxae (Figure 23.1). The tactile and chemosensory hairs of the Acariformes contain a layer of optically active material, actinochitin, which exhibits birefringence in polarised light. Actinochitin is lacking in the Parasitiformes.[32] The Acariformes contain three suborders, the Astigmata (*Acaridida*), the Prostigmata (*Actinedida*, Trombidiformes) and the Oribatida (Cryptostigmata); the Parasitiformes have four, of which two, the Gamasida (Mesostigmata) and Ixodida (Metastigmata or Ixodides), are of medical and veterinary importance.

The Astigmata are a fairly homogeneous assemblage of slow-moving, weakly sclerotised mites. This suborder includes the economically important superfamilies Sarcoptoidea and Psoroptoidea, which cause mange and scab in domestic animals, and a number of other superfamilies containing parasites and commensals of mammals and birds. Other members of the suborder, e.g. *Acarus siro*, are pests of stored foods.

The Prostigmata are a composite of several entities. Three of the 28 superfamilies recognised by Krantz[22] are of medical or veterinary importance. The Trombidioidea include the Trombiculidae, members of which are parasitic in the larval stage on vertebrates; some are vectors of scrub typhus to man. The Cheyletoidea are a heterogeneous assemblage of nine families which are, with few exceptions, parasites of arthropods and vertebrates including man. The Pyemotoidea include a few species of Pyemotidae which cause dermatitis in man and domestic animals.

The Oribatida are soil- or humus-dwelling mites which are of minor importance as intermediate hosts of certain tapeworms of domestic animals.

The Gamasida are a large and successful group, most of which are predatory, but some are external or internal parasites of mammals, birds, reptiles and invertebrates. They range in size from 0.2 to more than 2.0 mm. Most of the gamasid mites of medical and veterinary importance are in the Dermanyssoidea.

The Ixodida or tricks are dealt with in Chapters 22 and 23.

The Astigmata and Oribatida will be dealt with in this chapter, and the Prostigmata and Gamasida in the next.

General Structure

Acarines are arachnids with a body typically composed of an anterior gnathosoma or capitulum and a posterior idiosoma (Figure 20.1), which are separated by a circumcapitular suture. The gnathosoma resembles the head of a generalised arthropod only in that the mouthparts are appended to it. The brain lies in the idiosoma. The idiosoma can be subdivided into the area of the legs, the podosoma and the area behind the fourth pair of legs, the opisthosoma. In the Acariformes the four pairs of legs are usually arranged in anterior and posterior pairs, and the areas associated with them

Figure 20.1: Divisions of the Body of a Mite

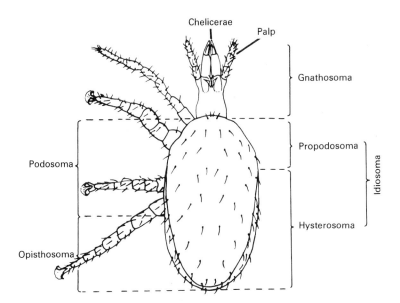

Source: From Savory T.H. (1977) *Arachnida.* Academic Press, London

referred to respectively as the propodosoma and metapodosoma. Another term in use is prosoma which includes the gnathosoma and podosoma, but excludes the opisthosoma. The gnathosoma and propodosoma are known collectively as the proterosoma while the metapodosoma and opisthosoma are referred to as the hysterosoma.

The gnathosoma bears laterally the palps and more medially the chelicerae (Figure 20.1). Typically, the palps are simple sensory appendages, which aid the acarine in locating its food. However, in some predatory Gamasida the palps are used to manipulate the prey. The palps are 1- or 2-segmented in most Astigmata and 5-segmented in the Gamasida. The chelicerae are 3-segmented in the mites and 2-segmented in the Ixodida. The chelicerae are normally chelate with the third segment being movable (Figure 20.3), but they are modified according to the feeding habits of the mite.

The legs of a typical mite are 6-segmented, seven if the pretarsus is included as a segment (Figure 20.10). The other segments are the coxa, trochanter, femur, genu, tibia and tarsus. The pretarsus bears distally the ambulacrum which may consist of paired claws, a median empodium and a median pulvillus. The empodium is variable and can be hair-like, pad-like, sucker-like or claw-like. The first pair of legs often differ from the other three pairs by being modified for special usage. Frequently they are longer and more slender, being used as sensory structures. They may also be modified in predatory species for capturing prey, and in some Rhinonyssidae (Gamasida) they function as surrogate chelicerae.

In small mites respiration may be entirely cutaneous but in larger ones gaseous exchange is facilitated by a complex tracheal system which opens to the exterior at the stigmata. In the Gamasida there is one pair of stigmata laterally located; in the Trombiculidae there are no stigmata in the larvae but one pair in the nymphs and adults, located between the bases of the chelicerae. Stigmata are absent in the Astigmata.

Transference of spermatozoa from the male to the female may be direct, as in the Astigmata; or by a complicated process known as podospermy in the Gamasida; while in the Trombiculidae the male deposits a spermatophore, which is subsequently picked up by the female.

Life Cycle

Female mites produce relatively large eggs and only a few, sometimes one or two, are laid at each oviposition. The size of the egg is conditioned by the fact that it must contain enough material to give rise to a larva which is capable of being self-sustaining. There is a minimum size for such an independent organism and it is this requirement which determines the minimum size of a mite egg.

When the egg hatches a hexapod larva emerges. Later it moults to become an octopod nymph. There may be one to three nymphal stages, usually two, before the production of the adult mite. The three nymphal stages are refered to as protonymph, deutonymph and tritonymph. One or more of these developmental stages may be inactive and non-feeding. In the Astigmata the deutonymph may be completely unlike the preceding and succeeding stages both in morphology and behaviour. Such a heteromorphic nymph is known as a hypopus. Hypopodes (plural of hypopus) are highly resistant to environmental stresses and some are adapted for dispersal by phoresy, i.e. attaching to passing animals. A true tritonymph occurs in the Oribatida and certain Prostigmata and Astigmata. Some authors, e.g. Fain,[11,13,14,15] restrict the term deutonymph in the astigmata to the hypopus and refer to the two nymphal stages in the Sarcoptoidea and Psoroptoidea as protonymph and tritonymph.

Figure 20.2: Dorsal View of Female *Sarcoptes scabiei*

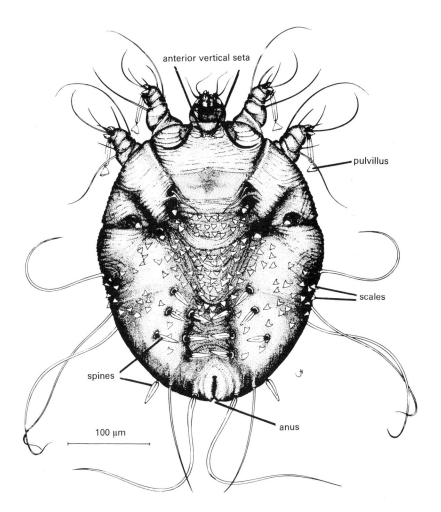

Reference to Mites and the Diseases they Cause

A major taxonomic work on mites is Krantz's *Manual of Acarology*.[22] Additional information on some families may be found in Baker and Wharton's *An Introduction to Acarology*.[3] A very old work is Hirst's *Mites Injurious to Domestic Animals*,[19] which has excellent drawings, many of which have been reproduced in later works. A wide selection of parasitic mites and the diseases they cause is given in Baker *et al.*,[2] but more detailed accounts of the diseases are given in specialist veterinary textbooks. The

Figure 20.3: Ventral View of Male *Sarcoptes scabiei*

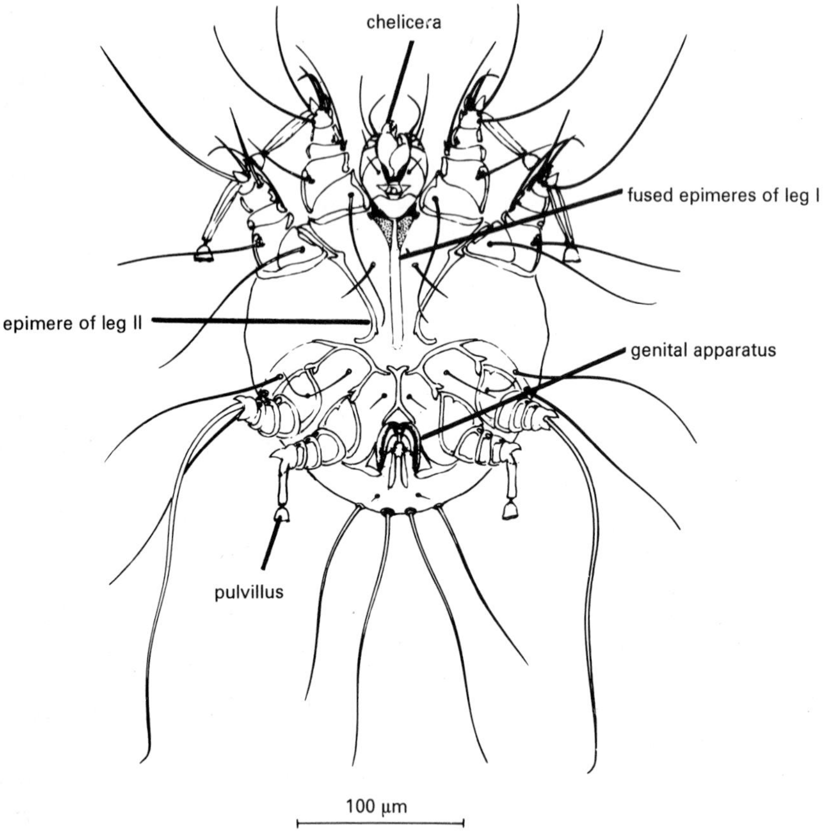

diseases of large farm animals are dealt with in Blood *et al.*,[5] and those of small domestic animals in Muller and Kirk.[25] The coverage of Yunker's chapter on 'Mites' in Flynn's *Parasites of Laboratory Animals*[40] is wider than might be expected from the title of the book.

Astigmata

The Astigmata are small, thin-skinned mites lacking obvious shields. The coxae are sunk into the body and referred to as epimeres. The empodium is claw-like, and the membranous pulvillus is stalked (Figure 20.2) or sessile. True paired claws are absent. Fertilised eggs are extruded through an anteroventral slit, the oviporus or genital opening. In both sexes the genital opening may be reinforced anteriorly by a pregenital plate or epigynium (Figure 20.3).

Sarcoptoid mites are parasitic throughout their life burrowing into the skin of mammals or birds. They are globose mites with the ventral surface somewhat flattened, the cuticle finely striated (Figure 20.2) and the chelicerae adapted for cutting and paring. Included in the Sarcoptoides are: the Sarcoptidae, which live on or in the skin of many mammals, including man; the Knemidokoptidae, skin parasites of birds; and the Teinocoptidae, parasites of bats.

The Sarcoptidae includes *Sarcoptes scabiei* and *Notoedres cati*, of which *S. scabiei* is economically the more important.

Sarcoptes scabiei (see Figures 20.2 and 20.3)

S. scabiei, the itch mite, causes scabies in man and mange in a wide range of domestic and wild mammals throughout the world. Hosts include chimpanzees and gibbons in the Primates; horses and tapirs in the Perissodactyla; domestic and wild bovids — cattle, sheep, goats, kudu and hartebeest — Old World Camels, South American llamas, pigs in the Artiodactyla; lions, foxes, wolves, dogs and ferrets among the Carnivora; rabbits and guinea pigs among the Rodentia; and koalas and wombats among the Marsupialia.

In literature from eastern Europe *S. scabiei* is sometimes referred to as *Acarus siro*. In the West *Acarus siro* is the name given to a free-living mite associated with grain and grain products. The reason for the confusion is that Linnaeus throught that the itch mite and the grain mite were identical, and in 1758 he described them as subspecies *scabiei* and *farinae* of *A. siro*. Western workers retain *A. siro* for the free-living mite and transfer *scabiei* to *Sarcoptes*, while some eastern European workers, e.g. Petrov *et al.*,[28] retain *A. siro* for the mange mite.

Fain[15] made a detailed study of *Sarcoptes* mites taken from a wide range of hosts with the intention of defining species or subspecies on the various hosts. He found that some morphological characters were stable and others were unstable. Variation in the unstable characters occurred: (a) within the same population; (b) between populations on different hosts; (c) between populations on the same host but in geographically different localities. He recognised nine different forms but concluded that these were of little taxonomic value although they might be helpful in identifying the origin, i.e. host or locality, or the degree of adaptation of a population to a host. The conclusion is that there is one species *Sarcoptes scabiei* which infests a very wide range of mammalian hosts.

The populations of *S. scabiei* infesting different mammalian species may differ more physiologically than morphologically. Populations from one host species do not readily establish themselves on another host species. Human infections with *S. scabiei* acquired from infected horses or dogs are considered to produce mild infestations which cure spontaneously.[24,25,40]

Spontaneous recovery never happens with infestations of *S. scabiei* of human origin.

Life Cycle

The following account is based on the work of Mellanby[24] on scabies in man. Females are to be found at the end of burrows in the horny layer of the skin. The burrows contain faeces and relatively large eggs, which are laid singly.

The egg hatches in three to four days giving rise to a hexapod larva, which can move on the surface of the skin practically as rapidly as the adults. Larvae find shelter, and presumably also food, by entering hair follicles. In two to three days the larva moults into an octopod protonymph, which is also to be found in hair follicles. This is followed by the deutonymph which gives rise to an adult male or immature female. At this stage both adults are about 250 μm long.

Both sexes make short burrows ($<$ 1 mm) in the skin. Pairing probably occurs on the surface of the skin, and then the female makes a permanent burrow. As the ovaries develop the female increases in size so that the mature female is about 400 μm long. The female never voluntarily leaves the burrow but, if removed undamaged from a burrow, she will construct another. The female takes about an hour to bury herself in the horny layer of the skin using her chelicerae and the 'elbows' of the first two pairs of legs. The rate of extension of the burrow varies from 0.5 to 5 mm per day.

The female takes three to four days to become mature and then lays one to three eggs a day during a reproductive period lasting about two months. The total length of the life cycle from egg to egg is of the order of 10 to 14 days during which there is a mortality of about 90 per cent, i.e. 10 per cent survival. Making certain assumptions these data can be used to calculate the growth of a population of *S. scabiei*. Assuming that a female lays two eggs a day during a reproductive life of 60 days, and that the development cycle from egg to ovigerous female is 12 days with a survival of 10 per cent and a 1:1 sex ratio, there is a 17-fold increase in the ovigerous female population in two months.

Diagnosis of Scabies or Mange

A firm diagnosis of scabies or mange must be based on recovery of mites from the affected host. In man this requires the recognition of the burrows of the female mite in the skin, removal of the mite, and its examination under suitable magnification. With animals a skin scraping is made of the infected area. The material removed may be examined directly, or preferably after disrupting the keratin by boiling for a few minutes in 10 per cent caustic soda or potash. The fluid is then centrifuged and the sediment examined. In skin scrapings males are rarer than females, and this probably reflects their being shorter-lived.

In the diagnosis of scabies it is important to appreciate the fact that the distribution of the rash on the body bears no relation to the distribution of the mites. Nearly two-thirds of the mites are to be found on the hands and wrists with the remainder being more or less equally distributed between the elbows, feet and genital area. The rash develops bilaterally being concentrated on the axillae, waist, and inner and posterior parts of the upper thighs and buttocks.

Recognition of S. scabiei (see Figures 20.2 and 20.3)

Sarcoptes scabiei may be readily identified by its size, shape and morphology. The skin is striated but dorsally bears a central patch of raised scales which extend in lesser density posterolaterally. Also on the dorsal surface there are three pairs of lateral spines about midway along the body and six or seven pairs of spines posteromedially. Dorsally on the propodosoma, behind the gnathosoma, there is a pair of anterior vertical setae, which are of taxonomic significance.

In both sexes the pretarsi of legs I and II bear empodial claws and stalked pulvilli (Figures 20.2 and 20.3); the latter are sometimes referred to as suckers. In life they function as adhesive flaps which grip the substrate and give the mite purchase for movement. The epimeres of the first pair of legs are fused in the midventral line (Figure 20.3). Legs III and IV in the female end in long setae and lack stalked pulvilli. They are located on the ventral surface and are not visible in dorsal view. In the female the oviporus is a transverse slit in the middle of the ventral surface of the body. The anus is terminal and slightly dorsal (Figure 20.2)

The male is similar to, but smaller than, the female and is distinguished by the presence of stalked pulvilli on the fourth pair of legs between which is the obvious, sclerotised genital apparatus (Figure 20.3). The nymphs are similar to the female but smaller and lack an oviporus, while the larva resembles a nymph but has only one pair of legs posteriorly.

Scabies in Man

Transmission of *S. scabiei* among a population is dependent upon prolonged and close personal contact. Under normal working conditions transmission of mites from one human being to another is highly unlikely. Slightly less unlikely is transmission by fomites, but the greatest risk is in close bodily contact under warm conditions, such as in bed, when the mite will have optimal mobility. Like other ectoparasites *S. scabiei* is virtually immobile at temperatures below 20°C. The most likely stage in the life cycle of the mite to establish a new infestation is a newly inseminated female mite whose next activity is establishing a permanent burrow.

In man there is a period of one or more months before symptoms of scabies become manifest. This appears to be a period of sensitisation during which the host does not react. Following sensitisation the host reacts strongly by scratching and thus induces secondary infections, complicating the direct effect of the mite. Scratching appears to exert a certain degree of control because, in Mellanby's work,[24] the average number of ovigerous female *S. scabiei* on an infected person was only eleven with most patients having one to five adult female mites, and only 3 per cent had more than 50 ovigerous female mites on them. The highest number found on one individual was 511. People that have been cured of scabies by treatment with an acaricide such as benzyl benzoate retain their sensitivity and, when re-infected, react immediately without a further period of sensitisation. In theory there should ultimately be a stage of tolerance reached, and this may be the case in Norwegian or crusted scabies in which there are huge numbers of mites in a host who does not itch or scratch.[24]

Mange in Animals

On animals *S. scabiei* is found more frequently on the sparsely-haired parts of the body such as the face and ears of goats, sheep and rabbits; the hock, muzzle and root of the tail in dogs and foxes; the sacral and neck regions of cattle; the head and neck of equines; and the backs of pigs. The burrowing and feeding of the mites in the skin cause irritation and consequential scratching which leads to inflammation and exudations which form crusts on the skin. If left untreated the skin wrinkles and thickens with proliferation of the connective tissue. This is followed by depilation, i.e. loss of hair. Small foci of infection do not appear to affect the health of an animal adversely but under certain conditions infestation may spread all over the body and, if untreated, cause death of domestic animals. Mange is a disease associated with animals in poor condition and therefore is commoner at the end of the winter or in the early spring.[5]

The spread of *S. scabiei* among animals is by close contact and this is facilitated by close herding of domestic animals, and in wild animals by living in family or social groups. When a case of mange is diagnosed it is necessary to treat all animals that have been in contact with the infected animal because the early stages of infection may be clinically inapparent. The length of time that *S. scabiei* can survive off its host will depend upon environmental conditions. It has been found that kraals previously occupied by infected goats were free from infestation when left unoccupied for 17 days.[8] Blood *et al.*,[5] recommend that quarters previously occupied by infected animals should either be left unoccupied for three weeks or treated with an acaricide.

Notoedres

More than 20 species of *Notoedres* have been described, most of them being parasites of tropical bats.[11] Three species are of interest to the vet-

Figure 20.4: Dorsal View of *Notoedres muris* Female

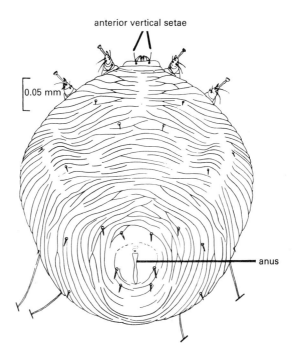

anterior vertical setae

0.05 mm

anus

Source: From Lavoipierre, M.M.J. (1964). *Journal of Medical Entomology 1*: 11. Reproduced by permission of the Editor

erinary entomologist, and one, *N. cati*, is important. *N. muris* occurs on rats throughout the world, including laboratory colonies;[40] and *N. musculi* on the house mouse in Europe.[11]

Notoedres cati[19,25,40]

N. cati is a mange mite of cats which on occasions may also infest dogs and cause a transient dermatitis in man. A morphologically identical form occurs on rabbits, but since it is difficult to transmit the cat parasite to the rabbit, two sibling species may be involved. Cats and rabbits share a predator-prey relationship in which it would be easier for the parasite to move from the prey to the predator rather than the reverse. In both hosts *N. cati* attacks the head and ears and, more rarely, in advanced cases, the legs, genitalia and perineum. In cats the infestation begins at the nape and spreads to the ears, to the head, and to the anterior region of the neck. The original lesion is the size of a pinhead but as it spreads a crust develops and hair falls out. Notoedric mange is highly contagious among cats and can prove fatal in four to six months.

Figure 20.5: Dorsal View of Anterior Half of Female *Knemidokoptes pilae*

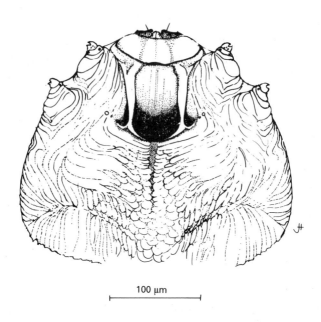

100 μm

Diagnosis is by recovery of mites from skin scrapings. *N. cati* is similar to *S. scabiei* having stalked pulvilli on legs I and II in all stages, and on leg IV in the male. It is considerably smaller, the female being 225 μm and the male 150 μm. In *N. cati* the anus is located on the dorsal surface, as in *N. muris* (Figure 20.4); there are no projecting scales, but middorsally the striae are broken into a scale-like pattern; and stout setae replace the lanceolate spines of *S. scabiei*.[2]

The life cycle of an unnamed species of *Notoedres*, probably *muris*, has been studied by Gordon *et al.*[18] In outline the life cycle is similar to that of *S. scabiei* but differs in that transmission from host to host is by larvae or nymphs. The female makes a burrow in the stratum corneum in which eggs are deposited. Larvae and nymphs may stay in the females' burrow or move on to the surface of the skin where they make small pits in which they moult. All moults may occur in the pit made by the larva, or each stage may make a separate pit. The immature female remains in the moulting pit until she has been inseminated when she forms a permanent burrow.

The cycle from egg to adult takes 17 days, and maturation and deposition of the first egg four to five days so that the generation time is three weeks. The ovigerous female lays about 60 eggs in a lifetime of two to three weeks at a rate of three to four eggs per day.

Knemidokoptidae

Twelve species of Knemidokoptidae have been described,[17] of which three are of veterinary importance. *Knemidokoptes mutans* and *Mesoknemidokoptes laevis gallinae* infest poultry, and *K. pilae* is common in caged parakeets. Female knemidokoptid mites are about 400 μm long and similar in general appearance to *S. scabiei*, but have no spines or sharp pointed scales, and no anterior vertical setae. Anteriorly on the middorsal surface there are two sclerotised, more or less parallel, longitudinal bands, which are connected posteriorly by a less well-developed transverse band (Figure 20.5). In the female the epimeres of the first pair of legs are concave laterally and do not meet in the midline (Figure 20.6). In the male the epimeres of the first pair of legs fuse in the midline and have a postero-median extension as in *S. scabiei* (Figure 20.7). Stalked pulvilli are present

Figure 20.6: Ventral View of Female *Knemidokoptes pilae*

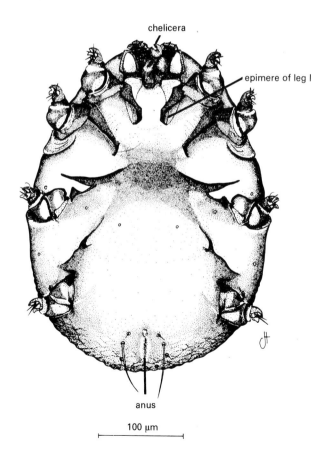

chelicera

epimere of leg I

anus

100 μm

Figure 20.7: Ventral View of Male *Knemidokoptes mutans* (× 250)

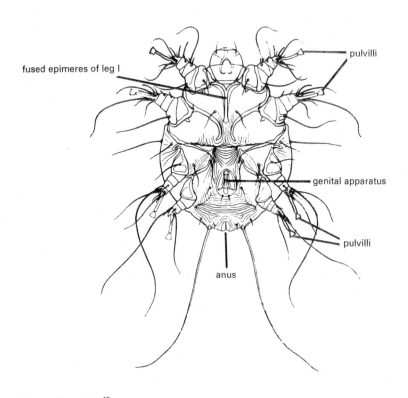

Source: From Hirst[19]

on all legs of the male and larva, but are absent in the nymphal stages and female. The female is viviparous, and there are one larval and two nymphal stages before the adult.

Knemidokoptes mutans[2,40]

K. mutans causes scaly leg in domestic poultry. At first the infestation is localised on the legs to the lower ends of the tarsus and digits, where the epidermal scales swell up and exude a whitish floury powder. This may develop into a thick, nodular, spongey crust, and in advanced cases the comb and neck may also be affected. The disease develops slowly over many months while the bird loses its appetite and wastes away. Diagnosis requires finding the adult mites on the underside of the crust where ovigerous females will be found surrounded by a proliferation of epidermal cells.

Female *K. mutans* and *K. pilae* can be distinguished from *M. laevis* by the presence middorsally of rounded or oval plaques resembling smooth scales (Figure 20.5). In *M. laevis* the dorsal surface has only regular striations, some of which may be very finely toothed (Figure 20.8). Male *M. laevis* have a pair of copulatory suckers posteroventrally, but these are absent in male *K. mutans.*

Knemidokoptes pilae

K. pilae was first recorded as the cause of scaly leg in budgerigars in Great Britain.[23] Soon afterwards it was recorded as infesting the face and base of the beak of budgerigars and a parakeet.[27] It is now known that this species occurs widely throughout the world on parakeets.[40] Separation of *K. pilae* from *K. mutans* is a matter for the specialist.

Mesoknemidokoptes laevis gallinae[2,6,40]

M. laevis causes depluming itch, characterised by the loss of feathers over extended areas of the body. *M. laevis gallinae* infests poultry, pheasants and geese while *M. laevis laevis* has only been recorded from pigeons. The mite attacks the base of the feathers on the back, head, neck, around the vent and on the breast and thighs. The condition can be diagnosed by plucking a few feathers from these areas when the mites will be found

Figure 20.8: Dorsal View of Female *Mesoknemidokoptes laevis gallinae* (× 180)

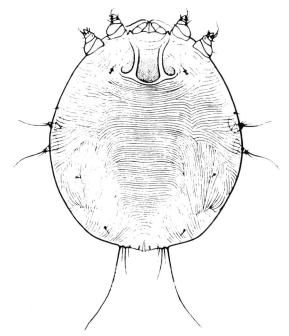

Source: From Hirst[19]

Figure 20.9: Ventral View of Female *Psoroptes ovis*

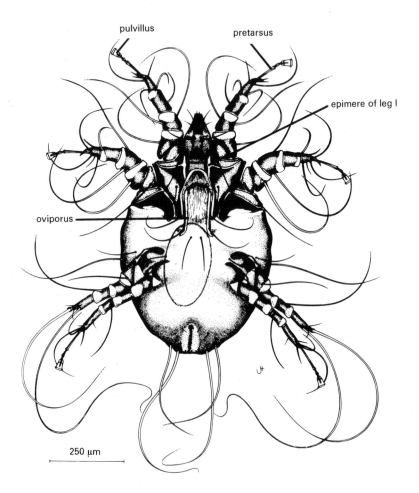

embedded in the tissue or scales at the base of the quill. This disease is more noticeable in the spring and summer.

Psoroptoidea — Psoroptidae

Krantz places seven families in the Psoroptoidea, of which five are parasites of mammals and two are free-living. The only parasitic family of veterinary importance is the Psoroptidae. Some members of the free-living family Pyroglyphidae are of medical importance because they produce powerful antigens which produce an allergic reaction among susceptible people (see p. 374).

Members of the Psoroptidae are oval, non-burrowing mites, which are parasites on the skin of mammals. They differ from most sarcoptid mites in shape, by the third and fourth pairs of legs usually being visible from above, by the epimeres of the first pair of legs not being fused (Figure 20.9), and by the absence of vertical setae on the propodosoma. There are two nymphal stages in the life cycle.

The male has prominent adanal copulatory suckers (Figure 20.10, 20.12, 20.13) which engage with copulatory tubercles on the female deutonymph (= pubescent female) (Figure 20.11). On the ventral surface of the ovigerous female, just posterior to the second pair of legs, there is an obvious inverted U-shaped oviporus through which the eggs are passed (Figure 20.9). Three genera, *Psoroptes*, *Chorioptes* and *Otodectes*, are of economic importance as parasites of domestic animals. The status of species attributed to these genera have been subjected to critical study by Sweatman.[33,34,35,36]

The most important disease caused by *Psoroptes* is scab in sheep (*P. ovis*). Three other species cause body mange in cattle and other closely related bovids, and in horses; *P. bovis* is cosmopolitan, *P. equi* occurs in England and *P. natalensis* occurs mainly in the southern hemisphere (South Africa, South America and New Zealand). Ear mange is caused by *P. cervinus* in the American bighorn sheep, and by *P. cuniculi* in equines,

Figure 20.10: Ventral View of Hysterosoma of Male *Psoroptes ovis*

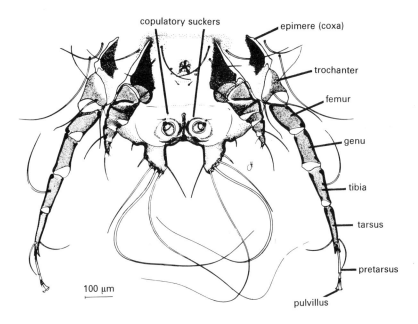

Figure 20.11: Ventral View of Hysterosoma of Female Deutonymph
(Pubescent Female) of *Psoroptes ovis*

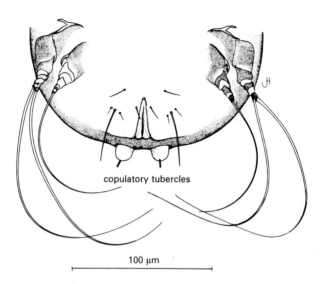

copulatory tubercles

100 µm

ovines and rabbits. *P. cuniculi* is cosmopolitan in distribution. All stages of *Psoroptes* are distinguished by sucker-like pulvilli borne at the end of long, jointed pretarsi (peduncles) (Figures 20.9 and 20.10)

Psoroptes ovis

The ovigerous *P. ovis*, 750 µm long, lays oval, glistening white eggs, about 250 µm long. The larva which emerges has pulvilli on legs I and II, and leg III terminates in two exceptionally long setae. The larva is about 330 µm long. It moults to a protonymph with pulvilli on legs I, II and IV and long setae on leg III. Legs III and IV are shorter and less stout than legs I and II. The female protonymph and deutonymph are similar but bear copulatory tubercles posterodorsally (Figure 20.11).

The adult male is readily recognisable by possession of paired adanal copulatory suckers and paired posterior lobes which carry two long and three shorter setae (Figure 20.10). Leg III is the longest, leg IV the shortest, and legs I and II markedly stouter than legs III and IV. Pulvilli are borne on legs I, II and III.

Female deutonymphs attach to males and remain so until they moult to ovigerous females, when, it is believed, insemination occurs. The legs of the ovigerous females are more or less equal with pulvilli on all except leg III which bears two long setae. A female will lay between 30 and 40 eggs at a rate of one to five eggs per day, the rate being inversely related to air temperature. She will live 11 to 42 days.[2]

In the developmental stages of the life cycle of *P. ovis* there is a period of active feeding, followed by a quiescent immobile phase prior to moulting. Under optimal conditions the quiescent phase lasts about a day and the active feeding phase about two days. The minimum duration of the life cycle from egg to egg is 11 days for *P. ovis*[7] while *P. cuniculi* and *P. equi* require about three weeks for the complete cycle..[36]

Sheep Scab. P. ovis causes a highly contagious disease of sheep and cattle. In cattle lesions appear on the withers, neck and around the root of the tail from which, in severe cases, the condition may spread to the rest of the body. In sheep lesions may occur on any part of the body but in badly affected animals they are most obvious on the sides.[5] The mites pierce the skin, leading to the exuding of serum. As the lesion increases a dry scab forms in the centre and is surrounded successively by zones of moist crust and moist reddened skin. The mites are most active in the moist areas feeding at the periphery of the scab which extends rapidly. In sheep this leads to loss of fleece, markedly reducing wool production. The disease spreads rapidly and in six to eight weeks three quarters of the body of the sheep may be covered with crusts or be denuded of wool.[2]

Active sheep scab is commoner in autumn and winter. In the summer the disease may enter a latent phase during which the skin recovers and the animals appear normal, only to relapse in the following winter. Diagnosis of sheep scab and other diseases caused by *Psoroptes* is made by finding the mites. These may be demonstrated in skin scrapings made from the moist areas at the periphery of the scabs. Identification of *Psoroptes* to species is a matter for the specialist.[36]

It is necessary to correlate the biology of *P. ovis* with the pattern of the disease. The higher oviposition rate of *P. ovis* at low air temperatures explains why scab is a cold season disease. Populations of *P. ovis* on sheep are lowest in the summer but since there is no diapausing stage, the proportions of the different stages remain more or less constant all the year round.[4] There is no particular stage which predominates during summer. it has been suggested that in summer the mites hide away in sheltered recesses on the sheep. However, Roberts *et al.*[30] found that in summer, *P. ovis* could be anywhere on the body surface, including skin invaginations.

P. ovis spreads rapidly through herds and flocks by direct contact between infested and clean animals. It is useful to know how long mites can survive off the host. The length of this period is dependent upon environmental conditions and difficult to summarise. Nevertheless no natural transmission of *P. ovis* has been reported where a minimum of ten days has elapsed between the removal of contaminated sheep and the introduction of clean ones.[39] In many countries sheep scab has been markedly reduced by the use of modern acaricides and it has been eradicated from Australia;[5] but difficulties are being experienced in the USA due in part to the existence of more viorous acaricide-resistant strains of mites;[31] and it has recently reappeared in the UK.[21]

Chorioptes

Chorioptic mange is the commonest form of mange in horses and cattle. In horses the mites occur on the lower parts of the legs and are rarely found on other parts of the body. They are a source of irritation and reduce the performance of infected horses. In cattle *Chorioptes* mites most commonly cause lesions at the base of the tail, on the perineum, and the back of the udder. Chorioptic mange is largely a winter disease and in the summer the mites are to be found on the area above the hooves on the hind legs. In cattle the damage caused by chorioptic mange is mainly aesthetic.[5] In sheep the mites affect the wool-less areas particularly the lower parts of the hind legs and scrotum, and cause a decrease in fertility.[29]

It has been customary to regard *Chorioptes* mites found on different hosts as different species or different races. Sweatman[33,34] has made a detailed biological and morphological study of *Chorioptes* and concluded that only two species are involved: *C. bovis* on horses, cattle, sheep, goats and llamas, and *C. texanus,* described originally from goats, has been found on cattle in Brazil.[9] Separation of species is a matter for the specialist. *C. bovis* and *C. texanus* are identical in all stages except for the adult male, in

Figure 20.12: Ventral View of Hysterosoma of Male *Chorioptes bovis*

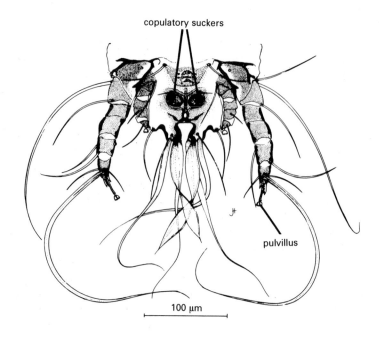

which there are differences in the lengths of setae on the paired posterior processes.[34]

Unlike *Psoroptes*, *Chorioptes* mites do not pierce the skin but feed on skin debris and it has been possible, therefore, to rear them in the laboratory on epidermal material from a range of herbivores including deer, antelopes, water buffalo, zebu, zebra and donkey, from which Sweatman[33] concluded that chorioptic mites were potentially ubiquitous. He commented that survival was less related to host species than to differences between individual hosts of the same species.

The life cycle of *C. bovis* is similar to that of *P. ovis* but at each stage *C. bovis* is considerably smaller than the corresponding stage of *P. ovis*. The ovigerous female *C. bovis* is little more than 300 µm in length, i.e. about half the size of *P. ovis* at the same stage. *Chorioptes* differs from *Psoroptes* in that the pretarsi are not jointed (Figure 20.12). Male *C. bovis* have pulvilli on all four pairs of legs, and two long broad flat setae, together with three normal setae of varying lengths, on well-developed paired posterior lobes (Figure 20.12). In the nymphal stages leg IV ends in moderately long setae.

As *C. bovis* can be reared *in vitro* more definite data can be provided on longevity and fecundity. The complete life cycle takes about three weeks, and an egg-laying ovigerous female may live for three weeks, while non-laying females and adult males may live for up to seven or eight weeks. Ovigerous females lay a total of three to 17 eggs with an average of 9.5 eggs per female (n = 56).[33]

Otodectes cynotis

Otodectes mites generally live deep in the ear canal, near the eardrum of dogs, foxes, cats and ferrets but lesions have also been seen on the body. These mites are mainly parasites of carnivores, although they have also been collected from the body of a captive white tailed deer.[35] In heavily infested cats and dogs convulsions may occur.[40]

Otodectes mites resemble *Chorioptes* in being of a similar size and having unjointed pretarsi. They can be reared *in vitro* on epidermal debris and hair from the inside of the ears of carnivores. As a result it has been shown that mites from the ears of dogs, red fox, cat and ferret are biologically and morphologically identical, and should be referred to the same species, *Otodectes cynotis*. In addition to the hosts already listed, the life cycle has been completed *in vitro* on ear debris from other carnivores including coyote, timber wolf and black bear.

The life cycle of *O. cynotis* is similar to that of other psoroptids. In the protonymph leg IV is greatly reduced and has no pulvillus. In the deutonymph leg IV is lacking, and copulatory tubercles occur in both sexes. The male has pulvilli on all four pairs of legs, and copulatory suckers, but the posterior processes are only weakly developed and the hind margin of the

Figure 20.13: Ventral View of Hysterosoma of Male *Otodectes cynotis*

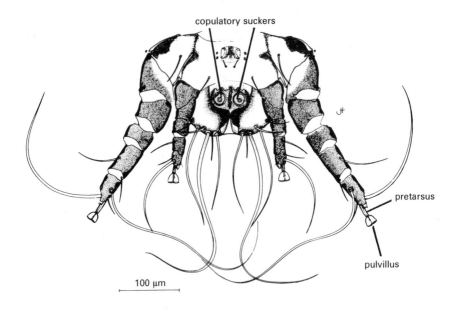

body is only slightly emarginate (Figure 20.13). In the ovigerous female leg IV is reduced and lacks a pulvillus.

Other Astigmatic Mites — Cytoditoidea

The cytoditoid mites are subdermal, respiratory or visceral parasites of birds, bats and rodents. There are four families in the Cytoditoidea of which two species, each in separate families, are of minor veterinary importance. Both occur in poultry, and are said to be in farm flocks in the USA.[40] Neither species is restricted to poultry, occurring also in wild birds.[10,16] They are the air sac mite (*Cytodites nudus*) and the fowl cyst mite (*Laminosioptes cysticola*).

Cytodites nudus

This oval mite is usually more than 500 μm long. It occurs in the linings of the air sacs and air passages of some wild birds. Small numbers of mites have no noticeable effect on the host, but in vast numbers they may cause death. They have sometimes been found within the peritoneal and thoracic cavities. Diagnosis is only possible on clinical symptoms, or by finding the mites on post mortem examination. The mites have a smooth cuticle, largely devoid of striations (Figure 20.14). They have a few short setae but no anterior vertical setae. The chelicerae are absent and the pedipalps are fused to form a soft sucking organ through which fluids exuded by the host are imbibed. The epimeres of the first pair of legs are fused into Y-shaped structures. In the female all the legs have long pretarsi bearing subglobose pulvilli, while in the male there are no pulvilli and the pretarsi are short.

Figure 20.14: Ventral View of Female *Cytodites nudus* (left) and of Male (right)

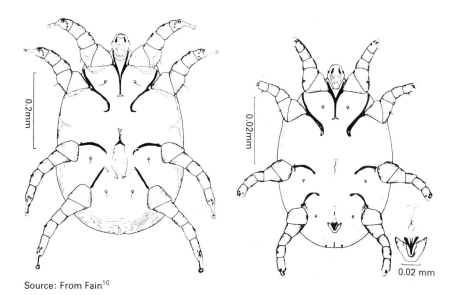

Source: From Fain[10]

Laminosioptes cysticola

L. cysticola is present in many parts of the world including North and South America, Europe and Australia. The mites may occur in millions in the cellular tissue of turkeys and chickens where they destroy the fibres. The mites bring about the formation of nodules which become calcified on the death of the mite, and reduce the market value of the carcass. *L. cysticola* is a small elongate mite about 250 μm long with smooth cuticle and few long setae (Figure 20.15). The gnathosoma is recessed on the ventral surface and not visible from above. The epimeres of the first pair of legs are fused into the usual Y-shaped structure and those of the second pair of legs meet in the midventral line and then diverge posteriorly. Legs I and II bear claw-like tarsi and legs III and IV end in long spatulate pretarsi according to Baker *et al.*[2] and Hirst,[19] but Fain[16] states that all legs end in a 'pedunculate sucker'.

Figure 20.15: Ventral View of Female *Laminosioptes cysticola*

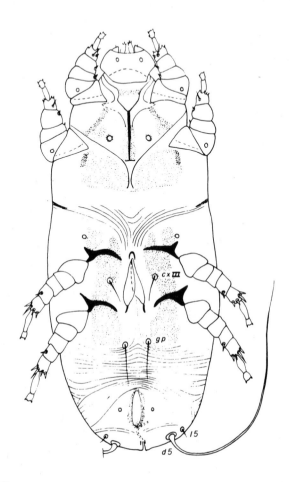

Source: From Fain[16]

Astigmatic Mites and Human Allergies

Astigmatic mites are very widely distributed being found in habitats ranging from arctic tundra to tropical rain forest, and wherever man has taken them in his food and produce.[3] They live on all kinds of organic substances and are commonly found infesting stored foods of plant or animal origin.[3] Sensitive individuals handling heavily infested produce may develop dermatitis. *Tyrophagus putrescentiae* has been associated with copra itch, *Glycyphagus domesticus* with grocer's itch, and *G. destructor* with hay itch. As a result of their adaptibility astigmatic mites are commonly found in houses, often in very large numbers. In recent years considerable interest has been taken in house mites with the discovery that the allergic material associated with house dust, and which can cause allergic rhinitis and asthma, is due to the house dust mite *Dermatophagoides pteronyssinus*[32] (Figure 20.16).

The allergen produced by *D. pteronyssinus* is not exclusive to that species being also produced by *D. farinae* and *Euroglyphus maynei.*[38] These three species are all members of the same family, the Pyroglyphidae. Different allergens are produced by the stored food mites *Acarus siro, T. putrescentiae* and *G. destructor*. In a study in which 87 allergic patients were tested for antibodies against the house dust allergen, 66 (75 per cent)

Figure 20.16: Ventral View of Female *Dermatophagoides pteronyssinus*

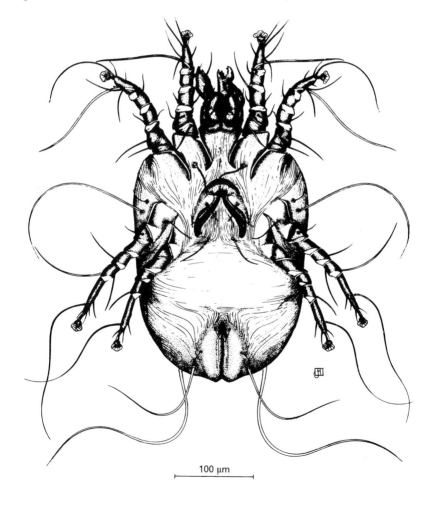

100 μm

reacted positively and all but one of these was positive for *D. pteronyssinus*. About two-thirds (42/66) also reacted to *T. putrescentiae* and 11 to *G. destructor*.[1] The allergen associated with *D. pteronyssinus* is present not only in the mite itself, but also in its secretions and excreta.[12,38] There is no doubt that *D. pteronyssinus* possesses a powerful antigen, and there is some evidence that hypersensitivity to this mite may be a factor in the aetiology of sudden infant death or cot death syndrome.[37]

D. pteronyssinus is widespread throughout the world and has been recorded from all inhabited continents.[13,32] It was present in every one of 150 houses sampled in Holland and accounted for 61 per cent of all the mites recovered from house dust.[32] Densities as high as 3,500 per gram of house dust were recorded in one house in Leiden but the average for 150 houses was 11 while in Hobart, Tasmania, the average was 27 mites per gram of house dust.[26] In Holland there was a positive correlation between increasing dampness of house and the population of mites, but this correlation was more marked for other species than for *D. pteronyssinus* (see Figure 3 in Spieksma and Spieksma-Boezeman[32]). In Europe mite populations in houses increase to a maximum in August and September.

In nature the main food of *D. pteronyssinus* is considered to be human skin scales,[38] and in the laboratory it has been reared on electric razor cuttings of human beard growth.[26] Under optimum conditions the life cycle of *D. pteronyssinus* from egg to adult is completed in about 21 days. A female will produce 25-50 eggs in a first oviposition period lasting about 20 days, and it may be followed by a less fecund second oviposition period.[38] Laboratory populations of *D. pteronyssinus* increase most rapidly at 25°C and 75 per cent RH[26] or 80 per cent RH.[38]

Fur and Feather Mites

Listrophoroid mites are found in the fur of small to medium sized mammals. Two species occur on laboratory animals: *Myocoptes musculinus* on mice and *Chirodiscoides caviae* on guinea pigs. In both species certain legs are adapted for clasping the hairs of the host. These adaptations are found on the third and fourth pairs of legs of female *M. musculinus* and on the third pair of legs of the male. The fourth pair of legs in the male is greatly enlarged but is not adapted for clasping hair. In *C. caviae* the first and second pairs of legs are modified for clinging to hair. These mites also feed at the base of the hairs and *M. musculinus* appears to feed on epidermal tissue and not on tissue fluids.[40]

The feather mites belong to three superfamilies of the Astigmata, and include a large number of species which inhabit feathers, skin or, exceptionally, the respiratory system of birds throughout the world. The majority lives on the feather surface or in the feather calamus.[22] Members of the Epidermoptidae are normally encountered on the skin of birds and one species, *Epidermoptes bilobatus*, is a common skin parasite of galliform birds and can cause a scaly skin disease in chickens.[2] Members of the Epidermoptidae have also been found to be phoretic on hippoboscid or mallophagan ectoparasites of their host.[22]

Until a few years ago it was considered that a feather mite found on pigeons, *Falculifer rostratus* (Falculiferidae), had an hypopus stage between two nymphal stages. The hypopus was thought to migrate internally through the feather follicles and come to lie in the subcutaneous or tracheal tissue where it lived and grew, until external conditions were suitable for it to return to the outside and resume its original form.[2] It is now known that the hypopus is in fact a stage in the development of a wholly different free-living nest-inhabiting mite, *Hypodectes propus* (Hypoderidae). This species produces eggs which develop directly into hypopodes which invade the tissue of the host and grow markedly in size. By the time the hypopodes leave the host they have increased tenfold in length. After leaving the host, the hypopodes moult directly into the adult stage, a most unusual life cycle, even for an acarine.[22]

Oribatida

Oribatid mites are free-living, dark coloured mites with a rigid exoskeleton from which the popular name of 'beetle' mite is derived. Apart from some rare exceptions they possess prominent club-like sensilla (pseudostigmatic or bothridial organs), which arise from large pits on the posterolateral margins of the propodosoma. In heavily sclerotised species respiration is conducted through tracheal tubes with stigmata opening at the bases of the legs. The alternative name Cryptostigmata refers to the fact that the stigmata are poorly defined and difficult to observe. Oribatid mites are primarily fungivorous or saprophagous inhabitants of the upper layers and surface litter of soil. Their economic importance lies in their being intermediate hosts of various cestodes, especially *Moniezia expansa*, the broad tapeworm of cattle.[20]

References

1. Araujo-Fontaine, A., Miltgen, F., Rombourg, H., Molet, B., Pauli, G. and Basset, A. (1974). Contribution à l'étude du rôle allergisant des acariens de la poussière. Étude immunologique des sérums des malades et des sérums des lapins hyperimmunisés. *Revue Française d'Allergologie et d'Immunologie Clinique 14*: 91-6
2. Baker, E.W., Evans, T.M., Gould, D.J., Hull, W.B. and Keegan, H.L. (1956). *A Manual of Parasitic Mites of Medical and Economic Importance.* National Pest Control Association, New York

378   *Acari — Astigmata and Oribatida*

3. Baker, E.W. and Wharton, G.W. (1959). *An Introduction to Acarology.* Macmillan, New York
4. Blachut, K., Roberts, I.H. and Meleney, W.P. (1973). Seasonal independence and relative frequency of motile stages of scab mites, *Psoroptes ovis,* on sheep. *Annals of the Entomological Society of America 66:* 285-7
5. Blood, D.C., Henderson, J.A. and Radostits, O.M. (1979). *Veterinary Medicine — A Textbook of the Diseases of Cattle, Sheep, Pigs and Horses.* Baillière Tindall, London
6. Dodd, K. (1972). The identity of *Knemidokoptes laevis* (Railliet, 1885) (Acari: Knemidokoptidae). *Acarologia 14:* 675-80
7. Downing, W. (1936). The life history of *Psoroptes communis* var. *ovis* with particular reference to latent or suppressed scab. *Journal of Comparative Pathology and Therapeutics 49:* 63-206
8. Du Toit, P.J. and Bedford, G.A.H. (1932). Goat mange — the infectivity of kraals. *18th Report of the Director of Veterinary Services and Animal Industry, Union of South Africa:* 145-52
9. Faccini, J.L.H. and Massard, C.L. (1976). O gênero *Chorioptes* Gervais, 1895, parasita de ruminantes no Brasil (Psoroptidae, Acarina). *Revista Brasileira de Biologia 36:* 871-2
10. Fain, A. (1960). Révision du genre *Cytodites* (Megnin) et description de deux espèces et un genre nouveaux dans la famille Cytoditidae Oudemans (Acarina: Sarcoptiformes). *Acarologia 2:* 238-49
11. _____ (1965). Notes sur le genre *Notoedres,* Railliet 1893 (Sarcoptidae: Sarcoptiformes). *Acarologia 7:* 321-42
12. _____ (1966). Nouvelle description de *Dermatophagoides pteronyssinus* (Trouessart, 1897) importance de cet acarien en pathologie humaine (Psoroptidae: Sarcoptiformes). *Acarologia 8:* 302-27
13. _____ (1967). Le genre *Dermatophagoides* Bogdanov 1864 son importance dans les allergies respiratoires et cutanées chez l'homme (Psoroptidae: Sarcoptiformes). *Acarologia 9:* 179-225
14. _____ (1967). Deux nouvelles espèces de Dermatophagoidinae rattachement de cette sous-famille aux Pyroglyphidae (Sarcoptiformes). *Acarologia 9:* 870-81
15. _____ (1968). Étude de la variabilité de *Sarcoptes scabiei* avec une revision des Sarcoptidae. *Acta Zoologica et Pathologica Antverpiensia 47:* 1-196
16. _____ (1981). Notes on the genus *Laminosoptes* Megnin, 1880 (Acari, Astigmata) with description of three new species. *Systematic Parasitology 2:* 123-32
17. _____ and Elsen, P. (1967). Les acariens de la famille Knemidokoptidae producterus de gale chez les oiseaux (Sarcoptiformes). *Acta Zoologica Pathologica Antverpiensia 45:* 3-145
18. Gordon, R.M., Unsworth, K. and Seaton, D.R. (1943). The development and transmission of scabies as studied in rodent infestations. *Annals of Tropical Medicine and Parasitology 37:* 174-94
19. Hirst, S. (1922). *Mites Injurious to Domestic Animals.* British Museum, Natural History, London, Economic Series No. 13
20. Kates, K.C. and Runkel, C. E. (1948). Observations on oribatid mite vectors of *Moniezia expansa* on pastures, with a report of several new vectors from the United States. *Proceedings of the Helminthological Society of Washington 15:* 10-33
21. Kirkwood, A.C. and Quick, M.P.(1981). Diazinon for the control of sheep scab. *Veterinary Record 108:* 279-80
22. Krantz, G.W. (1978). *A Manual of Acarology.* Oregon State University Book Stores, Corvallis, Oregon
23. Lavoipierre, M.M.J. and Griffiths, R.B. (1951). A preliminary note on a new species of *Cnemidocoptes* (Acarina) causing scaly leg in a budgerigar (*Melopsittacus undulatus*) in Great Britain. *Annals of Tropical Medicine and Parasitology 45:* 253-4
24. Mellanby, K. (1943). *Scabies.* Oxford University Press, London
25. Muller, G.H. and Kirk, R.W. (1976). *Small Animal Dermatology.* W.B. Saunders, Philadelphia
26. Murton, J.J. and Madden, J.L. (1977). Observations on the biology, behaviour and ecology of the house-dust mite, *Dermatophagoides pteronyssinus* (Trouessart) (Acarina: Pyroglyphidae) in Tasmania. *Journal of the Australian Entomological Society 16:* 281-7

27. Oldham, J.N. and Beresford-Jones, W.A. (1954). Observations on the occurrence of *Cnemidocoptes pilae* in budgerigars and a parakeet (Lavoipierre and Griffiths, 1951). *British Veterinary Journal 110*: 29-30

28. Petrov, D., Milushev, I. and Monov, M. (1976). Acariasis in pigs. *Veterinarna Sbirka 74*: 35-8

29. Rhodes, A.P. (1976). The effect of extensive chorioptic mange of the scrotum on reproductive function of the ram. *Australian Veterinary Journal 52*: 250-7

30. Roberts, I.H., Blachut, K. and Meleney, W.P. (1971). Oversummering location of scab mites, *Psoroptes ovis*, on sheep in New Mexico. *Annals of the Entomological Society of America 64*: 105-8

31. _____ and Meleney, W.P. (1971). Variations among strains of *Psoroptes ovis* (Acarina: Psoroptidae) on sheep and cattle. *Annals of the Entomological Society of America 64*: 109-16

32. Spieksma, F.Th.M. and Spieksma-Boezeman, M.I.A. (1967). The mite fauna of house dust with particular reference to the house-dust mite *Dermatophagoides pteronyssinus* (Trouessart, 1897) (Psoroptidae: Sarcoptiformes). *Acarologia 9*: 226-41

33. Sweatman, G.K. (1957). Life history, non-specificity, and revision of the genus *Chorioptes*, a parasitic mite of herbivores. *Canadian Journal of Zoology 35*: 641-89

34. _____ (1958). Redescription of *Chorioptes texanus*, a parasitic mite from the ears of reindeer in the Canadian arctic. *Canadian Journal of Zoology 36*: 525-8

35. _____ (1958). Biology of *Otodectes cynotis*, the ear canker mite of carnivores. *Canadian Journal of Zoology 36*: 849-62

36. _____ (1958). On the life history and validity of the species in *Psoroptes*, a genus of mange mites. *Canadian Journal of Zoology 36*: 905-29

37. Turner, K.J., Baldo, B.A. and Hilton, J.M.N. (1975). IgE antibodies to *Dermatophagoides pteronyssinus* (house-dust mite), *Aspergillus fumigatus* and β-Lactoglobulin in sudden infant death syndrome. *British Medical Journal 1*: 357-60

38. Voorhorst, R., Spieksma, F.T.M. and Varekamp, H. (1969). *House-dust Atopy and the House-dust Mite Dermatophagoides pteronyssinus* (Trouessart 1897). Stafleu's Scientific Publishing Co., Leiden

39. Wilson, G.I., Blachut, K. and Roberts, I.H. (1977). The infectivity of scabies (mange) mites, *Psoroptes ovis* (Acarina: Psoroptidae), to sheep in naturally contaminated pastures. *Research in Veterinary Science 22*: 292-7

40. Yunker, C. (1973). Mites. pp. 425-92 in R.J. Flynn (ed.), *Parasites of Laboratory Animals*. Iowa State University Press, Ames

21 ACARI — PROSTIGMATA AND GAMASIDA (CHIGGERS, BLOOD-SUCKING MITES)

Prostigmata

The Prostigmata are a large and complex group of mites which vary in size from 100 µm to 10 mm and have equally diverse forms. Most species live by sucking the juices of animals and plants. Predatory prostigmatid mites occur in terrestrial, freshwater and marine habitats, and include the Hydrachnidia or freshwater mites. Plant feeding Prostigmata include the Tetranychidae or spider mites and the Eriophyidae or bud mites, many of which are economically important pests in orchards and in horticulture. Other Prostigmata are parasites of invertebrates including insects, and vertebrates including man. It is the parasitic forms which are of medical and veterinary importance.

The typical prostigmatic mite is weakly sclerotised and, where there is an internal respiratory system, the stigmata open on the gnathosoma or anterior part of the propodosoma. It is this feature that gives rise to the name Prostigmata. The chelicerae are either blade-like as in *Trombicula* or stylettiform as in *Pyemotes*; they are rarely chelate. Specialised sensilla, the trichobothria, are often present on the propodosoma, e.g. *Trombicula* larva. The coxae of the legs may be incorporated into the ventral surface of the body as in *Trombicula*, and may be united with each other as in *Demodex*.

Trombidioidea — Trombiculidae

Trombidioids are generally parasitic in the larval stage and free-living predators in the adult and nymphal stages. The Trombidioidea contain nine families including the Trombidiidae and Trombiculidae. Many species and genera have been described in these two families which, in the adult and nymphal stages, are predators on the eggs and young of other arthropods. The larval stages of both families are parasitic with trombidiids parasitising insects and trombiculids parasitising vertebrates.

More than 1,200 species of trombiculid mites have been described and about 50 of these have been known to attack human beings or livestock. They are widely distributed throughout the world and in many countries cause trombidiosis, a dermatitis due to the feeding of trombiculid larvae. In Europe they are known as harvest bugs, e.g. *Neotrombicula autumnalis*; in the Americas as chiggers, e.g. *Eutrombicula alfreddugesi*; and in Asia and Australia as scrub itch mites, e.g. *Eutrombicula sarcina*. In Japan, southeast Asia and parts of Australia larval trombiculids may also be vectors of *Rickettsia tsutsugamushi*, the causative agent of scrub typhus in man (see

Chapter 25). Two important vectors of scrub typhus are *Leptotrombidium akamushi* and *L. deliense*. Trombiculid mites normally parasitise rodents, insectivores and ground-dwelling birds, but given the opportunity will feed on man, domestic animals and free-ranging poultry.

The female trombiculid deposits its spherical eggs in damp but well drained soil. They give rise to larvae which are about 250 μm long. They ascend grass stems to a height of 60-80 mm to await the passage of a suitable host to which they cling. This habit leads to trombiculid larvae being picked up on the faces and legs of grazing animals. Horses and cattle are most noticeably affected on the face, while *E. sarcina* attacks the legs of sheep in the black soil areas in the central highlands of Queensland.[1]

The larva attaches itself by its chelicerae and feeds on the host's tissues by partially digesting them with saliva, which it pumps to and fro, leading to the formation of a feeding tube or stylostome in the host at the point of larval attachment. The larva feeds for several days before falling from the host and entering a quiescent phase before moulting to the protonymph.

Figure 21.1: Dorsal View of Larva of *Trombicula deliense*

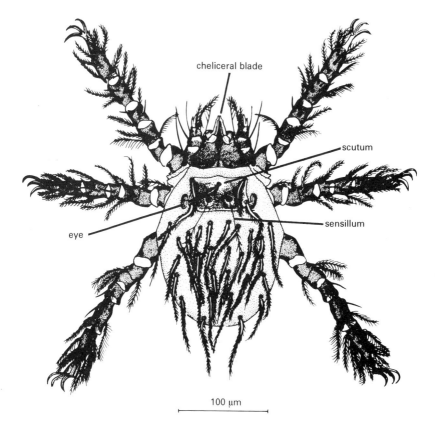

100 μm

There are three nymphal stages but only one, the second, is active. The adult mite is about 1 mm long, and its body is 'waisted' producing a figure-of-eight shape.

In the warmer regions of the world trombiculid mites probably breed continuously throughout the year but in the cooler regions the number of generations per year is limited and infestations with trombiculid mites are seasonal, e.g. larvae of *N. autumnalis* are abundant in late summer and early autumn and hence the popular name 'harvest bug'.

The prominent gnathosoma of the larva bears strong, blade-like chelicerae anteromedially (Figure 21.1). The chelicerae are flanked by stout, segmented palps, the penultimate segment (palpal tibia) of which bears a claw. The terminal segment (palpal tarsus) opposes the claw and bears ciliated setae.[1] There are no true stigmata or tracheae and respiration is cutaneous. Behind the gnathosoma on the dorsal surface, there is a scutum which is very important taxonomically. The scutum bears a pair of sensilla or trichobothria, which are setaceous in many genera but inflated in some, e.g. *Schoengastia*. Typically the scutum also bears five ciliated setae, one at each corner of the more or less rectangular scutum and a single antero-median seta (paired in *Apolonia*). Both the ventral and dorsal body surfaces carry moderately long ciliated setae, the number and distribution of which are specific characters. Nymphal and adult trombiculids and trombidiids are known as velvet mites, a term which refers to the dense covering of pilose setae which cover their legs, body and, to some degree, palps. In these free-living stages the stigmata open at the base of the chelicerae.

Cheyletoidea

The Cheyletoidea are a diverse assemblage of nine families, which are parasitic on arthropods, reptiles, birds and mammals. This superfamily includes: the Demodicidae, a widely distributed family of medical and veterinary importance; the Psorergatidae and Cheyletiellidae of moderate veterinary importance; and the Myobiidae of minor importance.

Psorergates (Psorergatidae)

Two species of *Psorergates* have been recovered from domestic stock. *P. bos* has been found on cattle in the United States where its effect is so slight as to be almost undetectable.[34] A more important parasite is *P. ovis*, which occurs on sheep mainly in the southern hemisphere. It was first described from Australia[38] and has since been found in New Zealand, southern Africa, South America and the USA.[1] A third species, *P. simplex*, occurs on mice in the northern hemisphere. Adult *Psorergates* can be recognised

Figure 21.2: Adult *Psorergates ovis*. A, dorsal view of male with enlargement of penis and genital opening; B, ventral view of male; C, ventral view of female

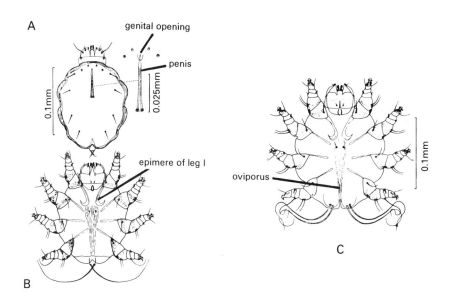

Source: From Fain[13]

by the fact that the legs are radially arranged around a more or less circular body (Figure 21.2).

P. ovis. P. ovis mainly affects merino sheep which respond to the irritation by chewing at the fleece. This results in a condition known as fleece derangement and leads to the wool clip being downgraded.[35] *P. ovis* spreads very slowly through a flock, the reason being that only the adults are motile and they are very sensitive to desiccation, so that they survive for only a short time in the fleece and die within 24-48 h when removed from their host.[27] Consequently the period of transmission from one host to another occurs during a brief period following shearing. Most mites occur under the stratum corneum in the superficial layers of the skin, and infestation with *P. ovis* is confirmed by finding the mites in skin scrapings.

Females lay few eggs during their lifetime. These give rise to larvae with reduced legs. There are three nymphal stages in which the legs become progressively larger until, in the adult stage, the legs are well developed and the mites are motile.[27] Adults of both sexes are very small measuring only 200 μm. The coxae of all the legs are sunk into the body as epimeres. Those of the first pair of legs are relatively broad and reflected laterally to be hook-shaped (Figure 21.2B, C). The female has two pairs of long setae posteriorly, and the oviporus opens posteriorly on the ventral surface. The male is more oval than the rounded female; has only a single pair of long setae on a small posteromedian process; and the genital opening is located anterodorsally (Figure 21.2A, B), behind which the elongated penis may be seen.[13] The complete life cycle of *P. ovis* takes about six weeks.

Demodex (Demodicidae)

Members of the genus *Demodex* are minute, annulate, worm-like (Figure 21.3), parasitic mites which live head down in hair follicles and in the sebaceous and Meibomian glands of the skin. On occasions they may penetrate the epidermis and invade the internal tissues. Demodicid mites occur in man and in a wide range of wild and domestic animals, including bats, insectivores, carnivores, rodents, horses and ruminants. They form a group of sibling species with different species occurring on different hosts, and more than one species may occur on the same host, e.g. *D. folliculorum* and *D. brevis* on man,[9] and the same may be true for other hosts.[28] The relationship between demodicid mites on a host and clinical disease is not simple. They are to be found on both healthy and diseased hosts. The pathological conditions which occur are often the result of secondary infection by bacteria, entry of which is facilitated by the activity of the mites. Demodicid mites cause an itchless mange which is often not noticed until the hides of animals are being prepared for leather.

Demodex in Domestic Animals. Among domestic animals demodectic mange is of greatest importance in dogs and cattle. *D. canis* is part of the normal fauna of the canine skin, but under certain conditions increases and causes demodicosis in which the skin becomes reddened and the hair falls out. Demodicosis occurs almost exclusively in dogs less than a year old with a tendency to be commoner in short-haired breeds. Two clinical conditions are distinguished, a localised and generalised demodicosis.[26] In localised demodicosis a small number of squamous patches develop on the face especially around the eyes and mouth. In most cases the condition cures itself without treatment, and recurrences are rare. Generalised demodicosis begins on the face and spreads to the head, legs and trunk. Secondary infections with bacteria follow and crusted, pyogenic, haemorrhagic lesions develop on much of the body.[26] This condition is difficult to treat and may terminate fatally.

Although in cattle infestation with *D. bovis* is generally benign, resulting in small nodular pustules in the skin,[3] in East Africa it may take a more severe form and end fatally.[5] In pigs the pustules which develop in association with *D. phylloides* may remain inconspicuous and undiagnosed[18] or develop into large abcesses on the chest and belly. Demodectic mange is benign in horses, rare in sheep, and may be severe in goats.[3] Species of

Figure 21.3: Ventral View of *Demodex*

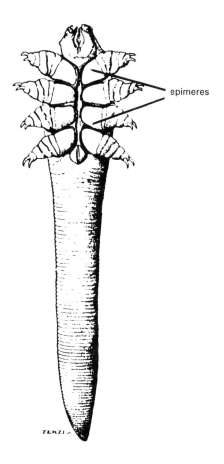

epimeres

Source: From Patton, W.S. and Evans, A.M. (1929). *Insects, Ticks, Mites and Venomous Animals, Part I: Medical.* H.R. Grubb, Croydon

Demodex are host specific and no instance has been documented of interspecific transfer of any *Demodex* species.[29] Transmission of *Demodex* within a host species occurs very early in life while the young are suckling.[15, 26]

Diagnosis of demodectic mange requires the recovery of mites from skin scrapings. They are easily identified as *Demodex* but specific identification is a matter for a specialist. Keys to species of medical and veterinary importance are given by Nutting.[28]

Life Cycle of D. canis. This cycle is representative of all species of *Demodex*. The female lays eggs which give rise to larvae with short legs endings in

Figure 21.4: Stages in Life Cycle of *Demodex*. A, egg; B, larva; C, deutonymph of *D. muscardinus*; D, deutonymph of *D. bovis* containing fully formed adult within (× 350)

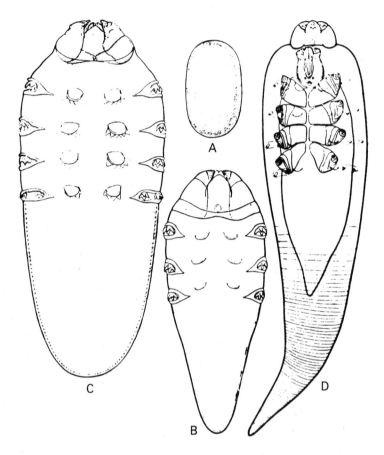

C   B   D

Source: From Hirst, S. (1922). Economic Series no. 13: *Mites Injurious to Domestic Animals*. British Museum (Natural History), London

a single trifid claw (Figure 21.4B). An unusual feature of the life cycle is the production of a second larval form, designated the protonymph by Nutting and Desch.[29] This stage is also hexapod but each leg terminates in a pair of trifid claws. The deutonymph stage which follows is octopod. Both protonymph and deutonymph have a pair of crescent-shaped sternal scutes on the ventral surface between each pair of legs (Figure 21.4C). The deutonymph moults into an adult in which the coxal epimeres are united to form a median longitudinal bar (Figure 21.3). The female genital opening is on the ventral surface just posterior to the fourth pair of legs, while the male genital opening is located dorsally at the level of the second and third pair of legs, as in *Psorergates*. In *Demodex* the legs are closely associated anteriorly so that the striated opisthosoma forms at least half the total body length.

Cheyletiella (Chyletiellidae)

The Cheyletiellidae contains nine genera of mites which are parasitic on birds and small mammals.[36] They are characterised by having stilettiform chelicerae which are used for piercing the host and strong, curved, palpal claws for maintaining the mite in the fur or feathers of its host (Figure 21.5).[4] Species of *Cheyletiella* cause a mild, non-suppurative dermatitis in dogs, cats and rabbits, and a transitory dermatitis in man. Other species have been described from wild animals.[4] *Cheyletiella* is an obligate parasite which lives on the keratin layer of the epidermis,[26] and does not burrow nor is it associated with hair follicles and skin glands.

The mites move about rapidly and this behaviour gives rise to the term 'walking dandruff'. *C. yasguri* causes a highly contagious infection of puppies. This usually begins on the rump from which it may spread over the back to the head. Older dogs may be symptomless carriers with light populations of mites. *C. blakei* causes a mild dermatitis in cats, and *C. parasitivorax* occurs in the scapular region of rabbits. Human infestations with *Cheyletiella* are transitory and the reaction variable. Treatment involves alleviation of the symptoms, and eradication of the mites on the

Figure 21.5: *Cheyletiella parasitivorax* Female (× 140). Leg setae omitted

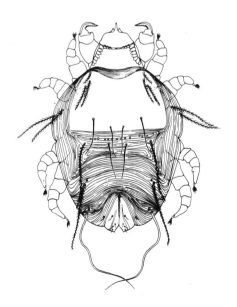

Figure 21.6: *Myobia musculi* (× 125). Minor hairs omitted

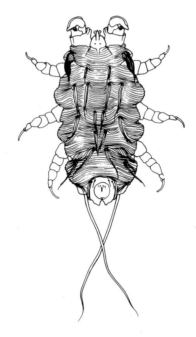

infested pet, the source of the human infestation. *Cheyletiella* dermatitis is diagnosed by finding the mites in the hair of the host. Keys to the three species mentioned are given by van Bronswijk and de Kreek,[4] but identification of species is really a matter for the specialist.

The life cycle is completed on the host. Eggs are attached to the hairs of the host 2 or 3 mm above the skin; the prelarva and larva develop within the eggshell. The larva is hexapod but the prelarva possesses only rudimentary gnathosomal appendages. There are two nymphal stages before the adult stage is reached. Females can survive for approximately ten days in a cool atmosphere, but males and immature stages die within 48 h of removal from the host. Females have been found attached to fleas and louse flies (Hippoboscidae), and phoresy could be an important mode of transfer from host to host.[4] The ready mobility of these mites through the hair of the host makes for rapid spread among hosts which are in close contact.

Myobiidae

The Myobiidae is a cosmopolitan family of ectoparasites which occur on marsupials, rodents, bats and insectivores. In modest numbers they appear to have little effect on the health of the host. Myobiids are readily recognised by the first pair of legs being highly modified for clinging to a single hair (Figure 21.6). *Myobia musculi* causes a mild dermatitis in mice; *Radfordia ensifera* and *R. affinis* infest rats and mice, respectively. They feed at the base of hairs ingesting extracellular tissue fluid and sometimes blood.[21,39]

Pyemotes (Pyemotoidea, Pyemotidae)

Species of *Pyemotes* are predators of insects which attack man and domestic animals that come in contact with infested materials. The grain or hay itch mite is the cause of dermatitis in people in many parts of the world. On susceptible humans a vesicle develops in the centre of an erythematous weal. Rubbing and scratching bursts the vesicle and introduces the possibility of secondary infection. The mites do not establish breeding populations on mammals and, if reinfestation is prevented, the condition subsides in a few days. Infestations of *Pyemotes* are mainly associated with grains, straw, hay and grasses but also occur with pulses and other crops.

For many years the grain itch mite was referred to as *P. ventricosus* but recent work has thrown doubt on that identification, and *P. tritici* is now regarded as the correct name.[25] Species of *Pyemotes* vary in their toxicity to man. *P. tritici* is highly toxic, as is *P. beckeri*,[19] while *P. scolyti* is not toxic.

Figure 21.7: Dorsal View of *Pyemotes triciti* (Female)

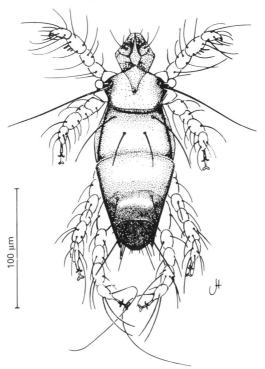

100 μm

Figure 21.8: Lateral View of Gravid *Pyemotes tritici.* All of the swollen area is the opisthosoma

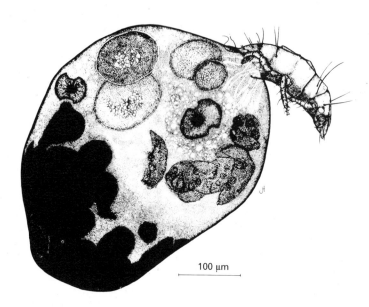

100 μm

The life cycle of *P. tritici* is unusual in that the fertilised female attaches herself to an insect with her chelicerae. The eggs are fertilised within the female, and all the immature stages are spent inside the female's swollen opisthosoma (Figures 21.7 and 21.8). Only adult males and females emerge from the gravid female. The males remain parasitic on the outside of the female opisthosoma, and assist in the birth of virgin females by dragging them through the birth pore. Copulation takes place and the inseminated female moves away to find a host. A fully gravid female will produce 200-300 offspring. The insect hosts of *P. tritici* are larvae of the Angoumois grain moth (*Sititroga cerealella*), the saw-toothed grain beetle (*Oryzaephilus surinamensis*), the cow pea weevil (*Callosobruchus maculatus*) and the rice weevil (*Sitophilus oryzae*).[2, 25]

Parasitiformes

Four suborders are recognised within the Parasitiformes and two of these, the Ixodida and Gamasida, are of medical and veterinary importance. The Ixodida or ticks are also known as the Metastigmata because in many cases (Ixodidae) the stigmata are posterior to the coxae of the fourth pair of legs, but in the Argasidae the stigmata are located above the second or third pair of legs. The Gamasida are also known as the Mesostigmata and their stigmata are located above coxae II to IV. The Ixodida possess a toothed hypostome, no claw on the palps and no forwardly directed peritreme from the stigmata. In the Gamasida the hypostome is rarely toothed, the peritreme is usually well developed, and the last segment of the palp bears a palpal claw or apotele.

Gamasida[11, 12, 20, 21]

Gamasid mites are comparatively large, ranging from 200 μm to more than 2 mm in length. With few exceptions the gamasid mites associated with vertebrates are in the superfamily Dermanyssoidea but most gamasids are predators and are found in a variety of habitats. Some have been used as biocontrol agents, e.g. *Phytoseiulus persimilis* (Phytoseiidae) against red spider mites (Tetranychidae) in glasshouses. *Macrocheles muscaedomesticae* is a ubiquitous inhabitant of dung and is commonly phoretic on houseflies and predacious on their eggs. In Australia *Macrocheles glaber* is phoretic on several species of native Australian dung beetles, e.g. *Onthophagus granulatus* (Scarabaeidae). Experiments in both the field and laboratory have shown that complete control of bushfly (*Musca vetustissima*) breeding can be achieved by as few as 50 *M. glaber* in a litre of dung upon which 300-400 bushfly eggs have been laid.[37]

In connection with the classification of the parasitic Gamasida Radovsky[31] comments that 'The non-specialist must be confused by the currently variable usage, involving recognition of different names and different degrees of lumping or splitting at the subfamily level ... Part of these difficulties result from recognition of the arbitrariness of many traditional criteria, but more important has been the discovery of forms with characteristics intermediate between higher taxa.' The student is reassured when the passage continues 'A fluid condition of the classification does not portend continued confusion, but it does indicate a certain growth in knowledge that has not yet been fully assimilated taxonomically.' Evans and Till[12] would include the external and internal parasites of mammals and birds in a single broadly-based family, the Dermanyssidae. Within that family they recognised a large number of subfamilies. Krantz[21] retains substantially the same format but raises many of the subfamilies to families within the superfamily Dermanyssoidea and this is the classification which will be followed here.

Dermanyssoidea

In the Dermanyssoidea the intermediate gradations between free-living organisms and obligatory parasites are well represented by existing species. In a single genus, e.g. *Haemogamasus*, are to be found non-parasitic, polyphagous nest-dwellers; facultative parasites; and obligatory haematophagous parasites.[31] The early stages of this progression towards parasitism is shown in the family Laelapidae, in which one subfamily, the Hypoaspidinae, does not include any parasites of vertebrates although a number of species in that subfamily are typically found in the nests of small mammals and birds. Two other subfamilies, the Laelapinae and Haemogamasinae, are largely parasitic, but have some polyphagous, nest-dwelling species.[31] The main families of importance to the medical entomologist are the blood-sucking Dermanyssidae and Macronyssidae; the Rhinonyssidae and the subfamily Halarachninae of the Halarachnidae, which infest the respiratory passages of birds and mammals, respectively; and the Raillietiinae, another halarachnid subfamily, which are found in the ears of bovids and goats.

Structure (see Figures 21.9 and 21.10)

In most Dermanyssoidea there is a narrow, elongated, anteriorly directed peritreme associated with each stigma. On the dorsal and ventral surfaces there are a number of sclerotised shields or plates, the arrangement of which is of considerable use in classification. The base of the gnathosoma is known as the basis capituli and bears laterally a pair of palps between

Figure 21.9: Dorsal View of Female *Ornithonyssus bursa*

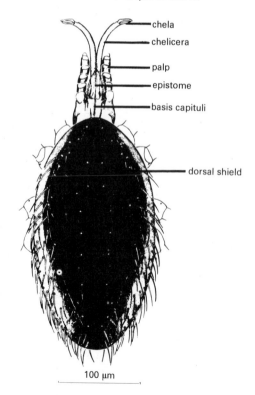

chela

chelicera

palp

epistome

basis capituli

dorsal shield

100 μm

which the hypostome extends anteriorly on the ventral surface. The palps have five free segments, of which the terminal segment, the tarsus, bears at its base a two-tined, claw-like structure, the apotele. The chelicerae are enclosed within the basis capituli inside a system of sheaths from which they can be extruded and into which they can be withdrawn. The chelicerae are 3-segmented and consist of a short, basal segment, followed by a second segment, which may be elongate, and which bears distally the third segment or movable chela (Figure 21.9)

The gnasothoma or capitulum is basically a tube through which fluid is carried to the oesophagus. The roof of the tube is the epistome which covers the chelicerae dorsally. In *Dermanyssus* and other obligate parasites the epistome is continued anteriorly as a forwardly-pointing, triangular or rounded structure. In *Haemogamasus* the lobate epistome is deeply serrated. Ventrally the basis capituli is formed from the fused, expanded coxal segments of the palps. In the midventral line there is the shallow deutosternum, which is marked by several transverse rows of denticles (Figure 21.10B). In parasitic species the number of denticles per row tends to be reduced and often only one is present. Ventrally the hypostome bears on its

Figure 21.10: Ventral View of Female *Ornithonyssus bursa*

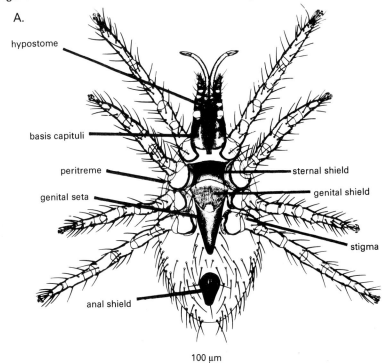

A.

hypostome

basis capituli

peritreme

genital seta

sternal shield

genital shield

stigma

anal shield

100 μm

Figure 21.11: Female *Ornithonyssus bursa* — enlargement of gnathosome area (ventral view)

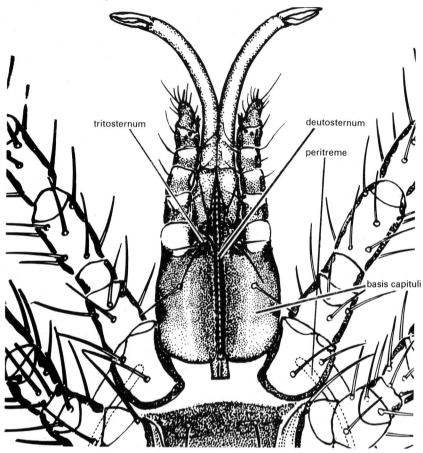

anterior border two pairs of structures, the corniculi and between them the internal malae. In free-living dermanyssoid mites the corniculi form obvious horn-like structures and the internal malae are free, while in obligatory parasites the hypostome is elongated and the corniculi and internal malae, both membranous, form a preoral trough. In the midventral line between the first coxae, is the tritosternum bearing two forwardly directed laciniae, which in life engage with the denticles in the deutosternum. The tritosternum is absent in some reduced dermanyssoids.

There is usually one, large, sclerotised shield on the dorsal surface (Figure 21.9) and a series of smaller shields in the midline on the ventral surface. The main unpaired shields are: the sternal shield at the level of the second and third pairs of legs; an epigynial or genital shield, the anterior border of which covers the genital opening; a ventral shield; and a shield surrounding the anus (Figure 21.10). The ventral shield is usually fused with either the genital or anal shields, and in males the shields on the ventral surface may merge to form a single holoventral shield.

The chaetotaxy, i.e. distribution of setae on the body, is useful in identification. Full details are given in Hughes,[20] Krantz[21] and in Evans and Till.[11] On the ventral surface there are three pairs of setae on the hypostome; one pair on the basis capituli; three pairs on the sternal shield; usually one pair posterior to the sternal shield; often one pair on the genital shield; and usually three setae on the anal shield, one on each side of the anus and a single seta posterior to the anus.

The pretarsus bears the ambulacral apparatus consisting of a pulvillus, often deeply incised, and a pair of well-developed claws. The anterior legs are not wholly used for walking but serve as sensory organs and are often different from the other walking legs.

Biology and Medical Importance

Dermanyssoids have evolved a complicated process for the transfer of sperm to the female. Sperm are passed to the chelicerae from the male genital opening and move into the hollow spermadactyl which is a specialised genital opening and move into the hollow spermadactyl which is a specialised structure on the movable digit of the male chelicera. Sperm are then transferred to special sperm induction pores on the third or fourth coxae of the female. This phenomenon is referred to as podospermy. These pores lead by a complicated route to the spermatheca which connects through a minute lumen with the ovary. In both sexes the genital openings are on the ventral surface about one third of the way back from the anterior end. In the female the opening is a slit posterior to the sternal plate and covered by the flexible epigynial plate. In the male the genital opening is at the anterior edge of the sterno-genital shield.

The life cycles of the internal parasitic Dermanyssoids are imperfectly known. In the external parasitic, haematophagous dermanyssoids the female lays a few, large, heavily yolked eggs after each blood meal. In her lifetime an individual female will lay several, about six, batches of eggs totalling less than 100 eggs. These hatch into larvae which are followed by two nymphal stages before moulting to the adult mite. One or more of the immature stages may be inactive and non-feeding. One feature which is common to the haematophagous dermanyssoids is the speed with which the life cycle can be completed. Under optimal conditions development from egg to adult may take as little as seven days and always less than a month. As a result, populations of these mites can build up to astronomical levels in a very short space of time.

Most of the damage caused by haematophagous dermanyssoids results from the direct effect of large numbers feeding on the host rather than from their transmitting pathogens. Various pathogens have been recovered from dermanyssoids in the field and some have been transmitted under experimental conditions in the laboratory. The results are inconclusive and it is generally considered that, with the exception of *Rickettsia akari,* bloodsucking dermanyssoids play little part in the epidemiology of blooddwelling pathogens.

Blood-sucking dermanyssoids may be host specific or parasitise a range of related hosts, but in certain circumstances, e.g. when birds desert an infested nest, they will attack unusual hosts. Attacks on man are in the last category. There is no blood-sucking mite for which man is the main host. The common hosts are birds and rodents. It is this ability to feed opportunisitically on other hosts which accounts for *Liponyssoides sanguineus* (also known as *Allodermanyssus sanguineus*) acting as a vector of *R. akari* to man from rodents. Infestations of mites have to be dealt with postively. Merely vacating infested premises for a short period will not eliminate an infestation because adult mites are able to survive for several months in the unfed state, e.g. *Dermanyssus gallinae* can survive four to five months, and *L. sanguineus* two months.[1]

Dermanyssidae[1, 11, 12, 39]

Dermanyssid mites are haematophagous ectoparasites of birds and mammals. The adults are 750-1000 µm long, and in the unfed state are greyishwhite becoming bright red after feeding and darker as the meal is digested. The chelicerae are chelate and the digits are minute and weakly dentate. In the nymphs and female the chelicerae are elongate and stylet-like with the second segment considerably lengthened. In the male the second segment is of normal length and a long, grooved spermadactyl is fused with the movable digit which is considerably longer than the fixed digit. The corniculi are membranous and there are nine or more deutosternal denticles in a single file. In the life cycle the larva is non-feeding while both the protonymph and deutonymph are actively feeding stages. Two species are of medical and veterinary importance — *Dermanyssus gallinae* and *Liponyssoides sanguineus.*

Dermanyssus gallinae

D. gallinae is a cosmopolitan species which is ectoparasitic on poultry and a range of wild birds including pigeons, sparrows and starlings, and will attack mammals when other hosts are not available.[12] Unfed *D. gallinae* are approximately 700 µm long × 400 µm wide but increase to more than 1 mm long when engorged. In the female the second segment of the chelicera measures about 275 µm compared with a first segment of 45 µm. In the male the corresponding lengths are 84 and 54 µm and the spermadactyl is 105 µm long. The female has a single large dorsal shield which is truncate posteriorly. The setae on the dorsal shield are shorter than those on the adjacent body surface. There are only two pairs of setae on the sternal plate, the posterior pair being remote from the plate. There are also two pairs of pores on the sternal plate. The genito-ventral plate is rounded posteriorly and bears one pair of setae. The anal plate is large and bears three setae. In the male there is a single holoventral shield.

Very large populations of *D. gallinae* can rapidly build up in poultry houses and bird nests. The mites are nocturnal, feeding on roosting birds and by day hide away in cracks and crevices. Under optimal conditions the life cycle can be completed very rapidly in the presence of hosts. The eggs hatch in two to three days, both nymphal stages moult one to two days after a blood meal, and adult females are ready to oviposit 12 to 24 hours after feeding. Fed adults can survive four to five months without feeding, making it difficult to eliminate infestations by removing the domestic hosts.[1]

Large populations of *D. gallinae* have a serious effect on domestic poultry. Egg production is reduced, hens may leave eggs that they are incubating and death may occur from exsanguination. A number of pathogens have been recorded from *D. gallinae* and it has been shown to transmit some of these experimentally, but its role in the epidemiology of these pathogens and their diseases is not known.

Liponyssoides sanguineus

L. sanguineus is an ectoparasite of small rodents. It was originally described from Egypt where it was found on rats and has since been identified in the United States. *L. sanguineus* is very similar to *D. gallinae* but differs by having two dorsal shields, a larger tapering anterior shield and a very small posterior one, bearing one pair of setae. The sternal plate has three pairs of setae and two pairs of pores. The genital plate is slender and tapering and there is a small anal plate. Development of *L. sanguineus* is slower than that of *D. gallinae* with the life cycle from egg to adult taking 18-23 days,[1] compared with seven days for *D. gallinae*. *L. sanguineus* is of medical importance because it is the vector of *Rickettsia akari*, the agent which causes rickettsial pox in man. *L. sanguineus* is normally a nest dweller, only occurring on the host when it is feeding.

Macronyssidae

Members of the Macronyssidae are haematophagous ectoparasites of mammals, birds and reptiles. It is believed that they evolved primarily on bats and secondarily have transferred to other mammals, birds and reptiles.[31] In the feeding protonymph and female the chelicerae are chelate and edentate, and in the inactive, non-feeding larva and deutonymph the cheliceral digits are rudimentary. In the male the grooved spermadactyl is relatively short and incompletely fused to the movable digit and is rarely longer than the fixed digit. The deutosternal denticles are arranged in a single file.

Two genera are of interest, *Ornithonyssus*, which occurs on birds and mammals, and *Ophionyssus*, an ectoparasite of reptiles. The characters given here to separate the two genera apply to the four species dealt with (*Ornithonyssus bacoti, O. sylviarum, O. bursa* and *Ophionyssus natricis*), but are not necessarily applicable to all species in these genera. Female *Ornithonyssus* have the genital setae inserted on the genital shield and there is only a single dorsal shield, while in *Ophionyssus* there are two dorsal shields and the genital setae are inserted on the integument adjoining the genital shield. In male *Ornithonyssus* the anal shield is fused with the other ventral shields while in male *Ophionyssus* the anal shield is discrete.

In female *Ornithonyssus* the dorsal shield tapers posteriorly, and in the male it is more extensive. On the ventral surface there are three separate shields. The sternal shield bears three pairs of setae (two pairs in *O. sylviarum*); the genital shield, which tapers posteriorly, bears one pair of setae; and the anal shield is of the usual type being oval, tapering posteriorly and bearing three setae.

Ornithonyssus bacoti

Although *Ornithonyssus bacoti* is referred to as the tropical rat mite it is cosmopolitan, occurring in both tropical and temperate areas of the world, especially in sea ports. *O. bacoti* is a pest of mice, rats, hamsters and small marsupials. It is distinguished by the setae on the dorsal shield being of similar length to those on the adjoining integument, and there being three pairs of setae on the sternal shield.

The life cycle is completed rapidly under optimal conditions with the cycle from egg to adult being completed in 11 to 16 days. As with other haematophagous gamasid mites high populations can cause the death of their host by exsanguination. *O. bacoti* is the vector of the filarial worm *Litomosoides carinii* to rodents. A number of other pathogens have been transmitted experimentally using *O. bacoti* but their role in nature is not considered to be important.

Ornithonyssus sylviarum

O. sylviarum is a serious pest of poultry and wild birds throughout the northern temperate region of Europe and North America, and is common in southern Australia. It has also been recorded from wild birds in South Africa. The setae on the dorsal shield are shorter than those on the adjoining integument, and there are only two pairs of setae on the sternal plate, the third pair being on the integument.

An unusual feature of the life cycle of *O. sylviarum* is that the adults remain on the host giving heavily infested birds a greyish to blackish appearance. Oviposition occurs on the host and egg development is completed in one to two days. The protonymph requires at least two feeds before moulting to the non-feeding deutonymph. The entire life cycle can be completed in a week.[1] This enables populations of *O. sylviarum* to build up rapidly. Heavily infested poultry suffer losses of weight, decreased egg production and even death from exsanguination.

Ornithonyssus bursa (see Figures 21.9 and 21.10)

O. bursa is the tropical poultry mite, which occurs also on pigeons, sparrows and mynah birds as well as attacking man on occasions. Its effect on man is irritating but temporary because *O. bursa* is unable to survive for long away from its bird hosts. In this species, as in *O. sylviarum*, the setae on the dorsal shield are shorter than those on the integument, but it differs from the latter by having three pairs of setae on the sternal plate. *O. bursa* occurs either on the bird or in its nest. Attacks on man in Queensland frequently result from the dispersal of mites from infested nests when the breeding birds and their nestlings have deserted them.

Ophionyssus natricis[7]

Ophionyssus natricis is an ectoparasite of reptiles which is rare in the wild but troublesome in zoos. This species has two dorsal plates, an anterior lemon-shaped plate on the podosoma and a posterior plate which is immediately dorsal to the anal plate but considerably smaller. The posterior plate bears no setae. There are two pairs of setae and two pairs of pores on the sternal plate with the third pair of each located behind the plate on the integument. The anal plate bears the usual three setae.

The adult mite feeds under the scales on the snake and then leaves its host to oviposit in dark, moist crevices. Where there is no shortage of hosts the life cycle can be completed in two to three weeks and in their absence some females can survive unfed for five to six weeks. Heavy infestations seriously affect the health of snakes causing a severe anaemia, which may lead to the snake's death. *O. natricis* is believed to be a mechanical vector of a haemorrhagic septicaemia of snakes caused by *Aeromonas hydrophila hydrophila* (=*Proteus hydrophilus*), a motile, facultatively anaerobic bacillus.[6] Infestations of snakes in captivity can be reduced by providing the snakes with water in which they may immerse themselves.

Halarachnidae

Two subfamilies are recognised within the Halarachnidae.[31] They are the Halarachninae which are obligatory parasites of the respiratory tract of

Figure 21.12: Female *Pneumonyssus caninum.* A, dorsal view; B, ventral view; C, detail of tarsus, typical of legs II, III and IV; D, tarsus of leg I

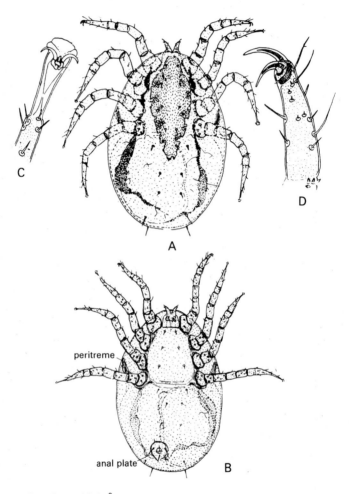

Source: From Chandler and Ruhe[8]

mammals, and the Raillietiinae which are obligatory parasites occurring in the external ear of mammals. As adaptations to an internal parasitic mode of life the dorsal and ventral shields in the Halarachninae are delicate and reduced and the genital plate is much reduced. In addition the tritosternum is reduced or absent and the peritremes, associated with the stigmata, are reduced or vestigal. These mites are active within the respiratory system and consequently the ambulacral apparatus at the ends of the legs is well developed. In the Raillietiinae the genital shield is well developed, a bifid tritosternum is present and the peritremes are elongate and well developed.[16] In both subfamilies the life cycle is compressed. The protonymph and deutonymph are non-feeding, non-motile, ephemeral stages with rudimentary claws. The female is ovoviviparous and the hexapod larva is active.

Halarachninae

Species of the Halarachninae parasitise a wide range of mammals, seals being the classic example, but also including primates, suids, carnivores and rodents. Halarachnine mites appear to transfer easily from one host species to another. An Asiatic macaque, which had been kept in a zoo where numerous African monkeys were present, was found to be infected with three species of lung mites, normally parasites of African monkeys. This may help to explain the wide distribution among mammals of mite species of the same genus. For example the 14 species in the genus *Pneumonyssus* are mainly found on Old World simians but species also occur on hyraxes and on a marsupial, the cuscus (*Phalanger maculatus*). Similarly the four species of *Pneumonyssoides* occur on pigs, the dog and New World monkeys.[16] Two species are of veterinary importance, the dog parasite *Pneumonyssoides caninum* and the monkey parasite *Pneumonyssus simicola*.

Pneumonyssoides caninum. *P. caninum* occurs in the sinuses and nasal passages of dogs in Australia, South Africa and the USA. Infections with *P. caninum* run a mild course and are relatively free from marked symptoms.[8, 39] However, in some cases, the mites penetrate tissues and migrate throughout the body. They have been found in the bronchi, the renal fat and the liver.[17]

Adult *P. caninum* are pale yellow, oval mites with few body setae (Figure 21.12). The chelicerae are well developed with opposable digits. The dorsal plate is small, irregular in shape and covered with microscopic spines. The first pair of legs is equipped with a pair of heavily sclerotised brown claws, while the other three pairs are tipped with a long, stalked pulvillus and two slender claws.

Pneumonyssus simicola. *P. simicola* is an extremely common parasite of the lungs of the rhesus monkey (*Macaca mulatta*) in which 100 per cent infestation may occur. This species also occurs, but less commonly, in a range of Old World primates. Furman[16] considers *Pneumonyssus* to be the most specialised genus on the grounds that its palps are reduced both in size and number of segments, and the denticles in the deutosternal groove are reduced to a single file. *P. simicola* is similar to *P. caninum* but smaller. The mites live and feed in the lung where they may be grouped in nodules superficially resembling tubercles. The nodules contain a characteristic golden brown to black pigment which may be faecal material resulting from

Figure 21.13: Female *Raillietia auris* (× 40). A, dorsal view; B, ventral view

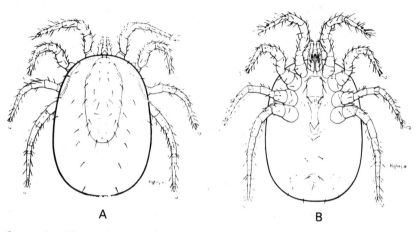

Source: From Hirst, S. (1922). Economic Series no. 13: *Mites Injurious to Domestic Animals.*
British Museum (Natural History), London

the mite feeding on blood. Clinical signs are usually absent. The mite
spreads readily through susceptible animals by coughing and sneezing.
Rhesus monkeys taken from their mothers at birth and reared in isolation
are free from infection.

Raillietiinae

Only five species of Raillietiinae have been described and they are all
assigned to the genus *Raillietia.* Two occur in the ears of East African
antelopes of the genus *Kobus*,[30] one species in the common Australian
wombat (*Vombatus ursinus*),[10] *R. caprae* in goats and *R. auris* in domestic
bovids. *R. auris* occurs in the ears of cattle in North America, Europe and
Australia, and of sheep in Iran.[32] The mite is considered to feed on epidermal cells and wax but not on blood. Infestations are usually benign, lacking
obvious symptoms, but in northern Queensland *R. auris* has been associated with otitis media.[22] *R. auris* is an oval mite about 1 mm long with a
small oval dorsal plate (Figure 21.13). The second pair of legs in the male
are modified for grasping the female. The movable digit of the chelicera is
entirely fused with the hypertrophied spermadactyl which collects sperm
from the male genital opening and deposits them into the sperm induction
pores of the female.

Rhynonyssidae

Most members of the Rhynonyssidae are parasites of the naso-pharynx of birds. They share a number of characters with the Halarachnidae but these features may be common adaptations to an endoparasitic mode of life. Rhinonyssids are weakly sclerotised, elongate mites with well-developed legs; peritreme reduced or absent; and the tritosternum usually absent. Little is known about the life cycle but the female may be ovoviviparous.[1] One species of minor veterinary importance is the canary lung mite *Sternostoma tracheacolum.*

Sternostoma tracheacolum

S. tracheacolum has been recorded from a range of domestic and wild birds, including canaries and budgerigars.[14, 23, 24] The species is widely distributed throughout the world, occurring in Africa, North and South America, Europe, Australia and New Zealand. *S. tracheacolum* is a yellowish brown mite about 0.5 mm long with two dorsal plates, a pentagonal anterior plate and a narrower, posterior one (Figure 21.14); distinct sternal and genital plates, and a reduced anal plate; strong, thick-set palps; large, mobile and chelate chelicerae. On legs II to IV the ambulacral apparatus consists of paired claws and a pulvillus, but on leg I it is much modified (Figure 21.14A).

Figure 21.14: Female *Sternostoma tracheacolum.* A, dorsal view; B, ventral view

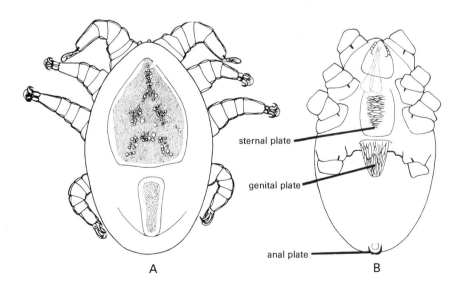

sternal plate

genital plate

anal plate

A   B

Source: From Lawrence[23]

S. tracheacolum has been found in the tracheae, air sacs, bronchi, parenchyma of the lung and also on the surface of the liver,[1] but rarely in the
nasal cavities.[14] In canaries the mites were firmly attached to the inner walls
of the tracheae from which they were imbibing blood.[23] In Gouldian
finches the mites were found in the lungs as well as the tracheae and air
sacs, and a wasting disease developed from which the birds died.[33]

References

1. Baker, E.W., Evans, T.M., Gould, D.J., Hull, W.B. and Keegan, H.L. (1956). *A Manual of Parasitic Mites of Medical or Economic Importance.* National Pest Control Association, New York
2. _____ and Wharton, G.W. (1959). *An Introduction to Acarology.* Macmillan, New York
3. Blood, D.C., Henderson, J.A. and Radostits, O.M. (1979). *Veterinary Medicine — a Textbook of the Diseases of Cattle, Sheep, Pigs and Horses.* Baillière Tindall, London
4. Bronswijk, J.E.M.H. van and Kreek, E.J. de (1976). *Cheyletiella* (Acari: Cheyletiellidae) of dog, cat and domesticated rabbit, a review. *Journal of Medical Entomology 13*: 315-27
5. Bwangamoi, O. (1970). The pathogenesis of demodicosis in cattle in East Africa. *British Veterinary Journal 127*: 30-3
6. Camin, J.H. (1948). Mite transmission of a hemorrhagic septicemia in snakes. *Journal of Parasitology 34*: 345-54
7. _____ (1953). Observations on the life history and sensory behaviour of the snake mite, *Ophionyssus natricis* (Gervais) (Acarina: Macronyssidae). *Chicago Academy of Sciences Special Publication No. 10*: 1-75
8. Chandler, W.L. and Ruhe, D.S. (1940). *Pneumonyssus caninum* n.sp., a mite from the frontal sinus of the dog. *Journal of Parasitology 26*: 59-70
9. Desch, C.E. and Nutting, W.B. (1972). *Demodex folliculorum* (Simon) and *D. brevis* Akbulatova of man: redescription and reevaluation. *Journal of Parasitology 58*: 169-77
10. Domrow, R. (1961). New and little known Laelaptidae, Trombiculidae and Listrophoridae (Acarina) from Australian mammals. *Proceedings of the Linnean Society of New South Wales 86*: 60-95
11. Evans, G.O. and Till, W.M. (1965). Studies on the British Dermanyssidae (Acari: Mesostigmata). Part I. External morphology. *Bulletin of the British Museum of Natural History (Zoology) 13*: 247-94
12. _____ and Till, W.M. (1966). Studies on the British Dermanyssidae (Acari: Mesostigmata). Part II. Classification. *Bulletin of the British Museum of Natural History (Zoology) 14*: 107-370
13. Fain, A. (1961). Notes sur le genre *Psorergates* Tyrrell. Description de *Psorergates ovis* Womersley et d'une espèce nouvelle. *Acarologia 3*: 60-71
14. _____ and Hyland, K.E. (1962). The mite parasitic in the lungs of birds. The variability of *Sternostoma tracheacolum* Lawrence, 1948, in domestic and wild birds. *Parasitology 52*:401-24
15. Fisher, W.F. (1973). Natural transmission of *Demodex bovis* Stiles in cattle. *Journal of Parasitology 59*: 223-4
16. Furman, D.P. (1979). Specificity, adaptation and parallel evolution in the endoparasitic Mesostigmata of mammals. pp. 329-37 in volume II, *Recent Advances in Acarology*, J.G. Rodriguez (ed.), Academic Press, New York
17. Garlick, N.L. (1977). Canine pulmonary acariasis. *Canine Practice 4* (4): 42-7
18. Harland, E.C., Simpson, C.F. and Neal, F.C. (1971). Demodectic mange of swine. *Journal of the American Veterinary Medical Association 159*: 1752-4
19. Hewitt, M., Barrow, G.I., Miller, D.C. and Turk, S.M. (1976). A case of *Pyemotes*

dermatitis with a note on the role of these mites in skin disease. *British Journal of Dermatology 94*: 423-30

20. Hughes, A.M. (1976). *The Mites of Stored Food and Houses.* Ministry of Agriculture, Fisheries and Food, Technical Bulletin No. 9, HMSO, London

21. Krantz, G.W. (1978). *A Manual of Acarology.* Oregon State University Book Stores, Corvallis, Oregon

22. Ladds, P.W., Copeman, D.B., Daniels, P. and Trueman, K.F. (1972). *Raillietia auris* and otitis media in cattle in northern Queensland. *Australian Veterinary Journal 48*: 532-3

23. Lawrence, R.F. (1948). Studies on some parasitic mites from Canada and South Africa. *Journal of Parasitology 34*: 364-79

24. Mathey, W.J. (1967). Respiratory acariasis due to *Sternostoma tracheacolum* in the budgerigar. *Journal of the American Veterinary Medical Association 150*: 777-80

25. Moser, J.c. (1975). Biosystematics of the straw itch mite with special reference to nomenclature and dermatology. *Transactions of the Royal Entomological Society of London 127*: 185-91

26. Muller, G.H. and Kirk, R.W. (1976). *Small Animal Dermatology.* W.B. Saunders, Philadelphia

27. Murray, M.D. (1961). The life cycle of *Psorergates ovis* Womersley, the itch mite of sheep. *Australian Journal of Agricultural Research 12*: 965-73

28. Nutting, W.B. (1976). Hair follicle mites (*Demodex* spp.) of medical and veterinary concern. *Cornell Veterinarian 66*: 214-31

29. _____ and Desch, C.E. (1978). *Demodex canis* redescription and reevaluation. *Cornell Veterinarian 68*: 139-49

30. Potter, D.A. and Johnston, D.E. (1978). *Raillietia whartoni* sp.n. (Acari — Mesostigmata) from the Uganda kob. *Journal of Parasitology 64*: 139-42

31. Radovsky, F.J. (1969). Adaptive radiation in the parasitic Mesostigmata. *Acarologia 11*: 450-78

32. Rak, H. and Naghshineh, R. (1973). First report and redescription of *Raillietia auris* (Trouessart, 1902) (Acar., Gamasidae). *Entomologist's Monthly Magazine 109*: 59

33. Riffkin, G.G. and McCausland, I.P. (1972). Respiratory acariasis caused by *Sternostoma tracheacolum* in aviary finches. *New Zealand Veterinary Journal 20*: 109-12

34. Roberts, I.H. and Meleney, W.P. (1965). Psorergatic acariasis in cattle. *Journal of the American Veterinary Medical Association 146*: 17-23

35. Sinclair, A.N. (1976). Fleece derangement of merino sheep infested by the itch mite *Psorergates ovis. New Zealand Veterinary Journal 24*: 149-52

36. Smiley, R.L. (1978). Further studies on the family Cheyletiellidae (Acarina). *Acarologia 19*: 225-41

37. Wallace, M.M.H., Tyndale-Biscoe, M. and Holm, E. (1979). The influence of *Macrocheles glaber* on the breeding of the Australian bushfly, *Musca vetustissima* in cow dung. pp. 217-22 in volume II, *Recent Advances in Acarology*, J.G. Rodriguez (ed.), Academic Press, New York

38. Womersley, H. (1941). Notes on the Cheyletidae (Acarina, Trombidoidea) of Australia and New Zealand with descriptions of new species. *Records of the South Australian Museum 7*: 51-64

39. Yunker, C. (1973). Mites. pp. 425-92 in R.J. Flynn (ed.), *Parasites of Laboratory Animals*, Iowa State University Press, Ames

22 IXODIDA — ARGASIDAE (SOFT TICKS)

The Ixodida or ticks are relatively large acarines, which are blood-sucking ectoparasites of vertebrates. The movable capitulum consists of the basis capituli, paired 4-segmented palps, paired chelicerae and ventrally a median hypostome (Figures 22.1C, D and 22.6C, D). The hypostome is armed with rows of backwardly-directed teeth which securely attach the tick to its host. The genital opening and anus are both located ventrally, the genital opening being at the level of the second pair of legs, and the anus a little posterior to the fourth pair of legs (Figure 22.3). Haller's organ, which is used in host seeking, is located on the tarsus of the first pair of legs (Figure 22.6E).

About 800 species are included in the Ixodida and they are classified into three families with the largest, the Ixodidae (hard ticks), having 650 species in 13 genera, the Argasidae (soft ticks) with 150 species in five genera, and the Nuttalliellidae with one genus and species.[14] The terms hard and soft refer to the possession of a dorsal scutum in the Ixodidae (Figure 23.2), which is absent in the Argasidae. In a short article Hoogstraal[14] gives a fascinating picture of the evolution of ticks over the last 200 million years as they adapt from reptiles to the newly evolving free-ranging warm-blooded birds and mammals.

Argasids are tough, leathery ticks in which there is little differentiation between the sexes. In nymphs and adults the capitulum is not visible from the dorsal view, being located ventrally in a recess, the camerostome (Figures 22.3 and 22.5). The fourth segment of the palp is similar in size to the other three (Figure 22.1D). When eyes are present they are lateral in position in folds above the legs (Figure 22.4). The stigmata are small and placed anterior to the coxa of the fourth pair of legs. The pad-like pulvillus between the claws is either absent or rudimentary.

In the Ixodidae sexual dimorphism is well developed, the dorsal scutum being small in the female and almost covering the whole of the dorsal surface in the male (Figure 23.2). The capitulum is terminal and always visible when the tick is viewed from above. When eyes are present they are located dorsally at the sides of the scutum (Figure 23.5). The fourth segment of the palp is reduced and recessed on the ventral surface of the third segment (Figure 23.1). The stigmata are large and posterior to the coxae of the fourth pair of legs (Figure 23.1). The pulvillus is well developed.

The two families differ in many aspects of their biology. In the Ixodidae there is a single nymphal stage. The adult female engorges, develops a very large batch of eggs, which she lays and then dies. In the Argasidae there are several nymphal stages, and the female feeds several times during her lifetime and lays several batches of eggs. Ixodid ticks feed on the host for a number of days. Argasids, with some exceptions, are nocturnal and visit the host to feed for a period of minutes.

The Argasidae will be considered in this chapter and the Ixodidae in the next.

Figure 22.1: *Otobius megnini.* A, B, dorsal and ventral views of larva; C, D, dorsal and ventral views of larval capitulum

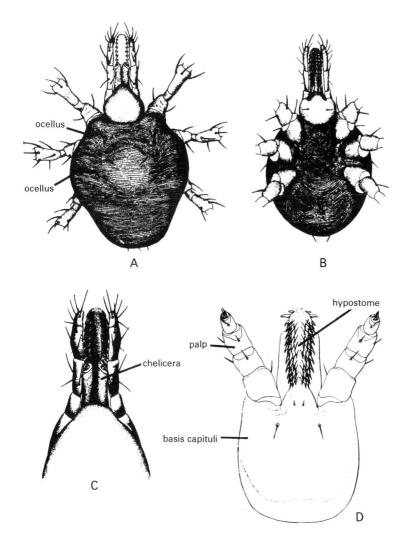

Source: From Cooley and Kohls[7]

Argasidae

Three genera of argasids, *Argas, Ornithodoros* and *Otobius,* contain species of medical and/or veterinary importance, and a fourth genus, *Antricola,* parasitises bats.[7] The name of the second genus is sometimes spelt differently as *Ornithodorus.* This arises because Koch used the 'os' ending in his original description in 1844, and this was emended to 'us' by Erickson the next year. The 'os' ending has priority and should be used.

In *Argas* the margin of the body is distinctly flattened and usually structurally different from the dorsal surface (Figure 22.5C). The flattened margin remains distinct even when the tick is fully fed. There is usually a lateral sutural line present (Figure 22.5D). Eyes are absent. All stages of *Argas* are found in the resting places of birds and bats which they parasitise.

In *Ornithodoros* and *Otobius* there is no lateral sutural line and no distinct margin to the body. In *Ornithodoros* the integument bears mammillae (Figure 22.3), and in *Otobius* the integument is spiny in the nymph (Figure 22.2) and granulated in the adult. The main species of medical importance is *Ornithodoros moubata,* and of veterinary importance *Otobius megnini* and species of *Persicargas* a subgenus of *Argas.*

Two species of *Otobius* have been described, *O. megnini* from cattle, and *O. lagophilus* from cottontail and jack rabbits.[7]

Figure 22.2: *Otobius megnini.* A, dorsal and B, ventral views of partially fed nymph

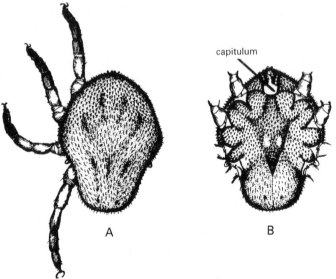

A   B

Otobius megnini (see Figures 22.1 and 22.2)

O. megnini, the spinose ear tick, originated in the Americas from where it has been introduced into southern Africa and India. It is mainly a parasite of cattle and horses but has been recorded from a range of hosts in North America including donkeys, sheep, goats, dogs, cats, deer and rabbits.[7] In India it has been recorded from cattle, sheep and man.[5, 6] This tick is associated with stables and animal shelters and this may explain why it 'has apparently not spread to wild animals' in southern Africa.[34] The female tick lays her eggs in cracks and crevices several feet above the ground in the walls of animal shelters. This behaviour ensures that the emerging larva is at a height to transfer easily to the bodies of large, stabled domestic animals.

Life Cycle. The eggs hatch in 11 days in summer,[29] but can take three to eight weeks under cooler conditions.[3] The eggs are small, oval and reddish in colour. A hexapod larva just over 0.5 mm in length emerges from the egg (Figure 22.1A, B). The capitulum is very long, accounting for more than one third of the length of the unfed larva, and is terminal. There are two pairs of ocellus-like eyes present dorsally.[7] The larva enters an ear of its host where it engorges and may attain a length of 4 mm.[29] Engorgement which takes five to ten days is followed by a quiescent period before the larva moults to become an octopod nymph.

There are two nymphal stages and both are characterised by having the capitulum on the ventral surface, and a spiny integument, from which the tick acquires the common name, spinose ear tick (Figure 22.2). The nymphs reattach to the skin lining the ear, suck blood and remain in the ear for an unusually long time. Most nymphs leave the host within five weeks but they may remain for several months.[3] The fully-fed nymph measures up to 8 mm. Nymphs drop from the host and 'creep into cracks and crevices in walls and woodwork, under stones or under the bark of trees, usually low down, where they develop into adults'.[34] The second stage nymph moults to an adult one to four weeks later.

The body of the adult is fiddle-shaped, being constricted posterior to the fourth pair of legs. The adult does not feed, and its hypostome is poorly developed and without teeth.

Bionomics. The female can wait up to 18 months to be impregnated and then 'lays up to 1,500 eggs in small batches over a period of a few weeks to several months'.[34] This species has considerable powers of survival in the absence of hosts and it can persist in empty cattle sheds and stables for more than two years.[34] Unfed larvae usually survive for less than a month but under favourable circumstances can survive for as long as four months. Infestations of *O. megnini* cannot be eradicated by vacating premises except for excessively long periods.

O. megnini favours hot, arid areas and is not present in wet areas. In South America it has been found up to 2,600 m.[4] At this altitude in Bolivia nymphs of *O. megnini* were present all the year round in the ears of dairy cattle, and during the rainy season clusters of 150 nymphs and larvae could be found under the tails of a small percentage ($<$ 15 per cent) of cattle.[4] These ticks do not transmit pathogens but do considerable damage to the ears, ear drums and auricular nerves by their feeding. The ear can be choked with ticks, wax and other debris, and the ear drum be ruptured favouring secondary infections. Badly infested calves, sheep and goats may die and loss of condition in infested beasts is common.[3]

Ornithodoros

Two species of *Ornithodoros, O. moubata* and *O. savignyi,* have become associated with man and/or his domestic animals. The taxonomic position of the two or more strains of *O. moubata* is not satisfactorily resolved and the term *O. moubata* will be used to cover both the hut-dwelling strain feeding on man and chickens, and a strain living in burrows and feeding on the occupants — warthogs, antbears and porcupines. A note on this taxonomic difficulty is given in Chapter 26.

Ornithodoros moubata (see Figure 22.3)

O. moubata is widely distributed throughout East Africa and northern

Figure 22.3: *Ornithodoros moubata.* A, dorsal and B, ventral views of female

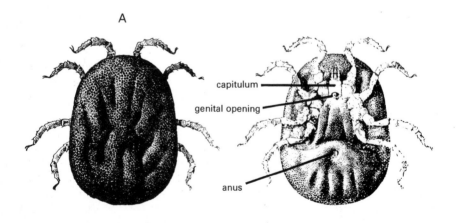

Source: From Castellani, A. and Chalmers, A.J. (1913). *A Manual of Tropical Medicine.* Baillière Tindall, London

South Africa, extending into the drier parts of central Africa.[13] It lives in cracks in walls and in the earth floors of huts. During the day it hides away in dark locations including the possessions of the occupants. Consequently *O. moubata* has been spread by man with his goods and chattels as he moves from one area to another.

Oviposition. Over a considerable period of time a female will lay several batches of comparatively large, spherical (0.9 mm in diameter), glistening golden yellow eggs.[29] During oviposition the tick bends its head towards the genital opening and extrudes Gene's organ from the base of the capitulum. Each egg is 'handled' by Gene's organ which coats the egg with a waxy waterproof layer. Eggs which do not get this treatment quickly shrivel and die. The wax on the eggs has a lower melting point (50-54°C) than the crystalline cuticular wax which has a melting point of 65°C. The function of both waxes is to waterproof the organism, an essential requirement for survival in its arid natural environment.[26]

Life Cycle. The eggs hatch in about eight days at 30°C and give rise to larvae which do not feed but remain motionless until they moult into nymphs four days later.[17] The nymphs feed on blood taking 20-25 min to acquire a full meal. After an interval the first nymphal stage moults into the second stage which feeds and repeats the process. The number of nymphal stages is variable with adult males being produced after four nymphal stages and females after five.[17] Mating occurs after the female has fed, and stimulates egg development with oviposition occurring 10 to 15 days later. Full digestion of the blood meal and egg development can be delayed for many months if the female is not mated. Virgin females mated 150-200 days after a blood meal produce eggs in the normal preoviposition period of 10 to 15 days.[2]

Feeding. When the tick feeds, the tips of the chelicerae press against the skin and cut it by alternate movements. The hypostome enters the host passively with the chelicerae. Feeding involves periods of active suction in which blood is stored in the midgut and its diverticula, and periods of rest when saliva is introduced into the host.[21]

There is no open connection between the midgut and the rectum and no faeces are passed. The malpighian tubules open into the hindgut and their excretory products are deposited. The tick excretes a great deal of the watery component of blood via the coxal apparatus which opens just behind the coxae of the first pair of legs. Excretion of coxal fluid begins about 15 min after the start of feeding, continues during feeding and for about an hour afterwards.[24] The coxal apparatus can excrete 30 times its own volume in 20 minutes.[24]

Effect of Host on Fecundity. The source of the blood meal can have a considerable effect on the fecundity of the female. Thus a laboratory strain of *O. moubata* produced nearly twice as many eggs (147 cf. 80) when fed on porcine compared with bovine blood. In both cases the ticks took up similar amounts of blood, increasing their bodyweight from 45 mg to 175 mg, i.e. taking up three times their bodyweight of blood.[27] Nymphs reared on porcine blood developed more quickly and reached the adult stage in fewer instars than nymphs fed on bovine blood. Some nymphs fed on porcine blood became adults after four instars and 62 per cent were adult within six instars, whereas only 13 per cent became adult within six instars when fed on bovine blood and none took less than five instars.[27]

In the laboratory vigorous colonies of *O. moubata* have been maintained on rabbits, a host that this tick will not have encountered in nature. So well has it become adapted that its fecundity per unit weight of blood is 30 per cent higher than when the colony is fed on porcine blood.[27] The same colony of *O. moubata* fed equally readily on rabbit, chicken and guinea pig (84-92 per cent), but 'showed considerable reluctance to feed on rat, mouse or hamster'.[9] The blood meals taken from different hosts were comparable in size (118-125 mg), with a smaller meal (100 mg) being taken from a mouse and a larger meal (147 mg) from a guinea pig; yet the fecundity of females fed on mouse or guinea pig were similar, and the highest fecundity was recorded on rabbit and chicken.[9] The last observation is of interest because this colony has been derived from ticks collected from a warthog burrow and reared for many generations on rabbits, and yet gave high fecundity when fed on chickens. In contrast *O. tholozani* fed equally readily on all six hosts, and produced similar numbers of eggs.[9]

Mating. Aggregations of *O. moubata* develop in response to pheromones emitted by both sexes. Males respond more readily to the female pheromone than do females to the male pheromone. The receptors are located on the fourth segment of the palps. The function of the pheromone is to bring the sexes together for mating and for food location, and hence starved ticks show an enhanced response to pheromones.[22] The pheromones are not species specific and *O. moubata* is attracted to *O. tholozani* and *A. persicus.*[22]

In mating the male crawls beneath the female so that their ventral surfaces are in contact and the male uses its mouthparts to dilate the female genital opening. A bulb-shaped spermatophore appears at the genital opening of the male and is introduced into the female opening by the mouthparts of the male. The outer exospermatophore remains attached externally and the endospermatophore evaginates, entering the female genital tract and depositing developing sperm in paired capsules. Later when the sperm are mature the capsule ruptures and they are released into the uterus.[8, 13, 32] A female may mate more than once and 80 capsules have been found in the uterus of a single female in a laboratory colony, indicating that 40 successive matings have taken place.[1]

Mating and Fecundity. A female may produce up to eight egg batches but the number of eggs in each batch steadily declines from about 140 in the first batch to 33 in the seventh batch.[1] In the absence of repeated mating the percentage of females ovipositing declines rapidly after the third batch of eggs to less than 30 per cent. When females were mated after every blood meal, the proportion which oviposited remained very high for the first four batches and was about 70 per cent of the surviving females in the seventh batch.[1] On average a female will lay about 500 eggs in her lifetime. Even where the female is mated after every blood meal there is a steady decline in fertility from 93 per cent in the first batch to 73 per cent in the seventh batch. Mating after each blood meal ensured high fertility in the eggs subsequently laid but shortened the life of the female.[1]

Bionomics. In common with other argasid ticks *O. moubata* has considerable powers of survival against starvation and desiccation. The crystalline cuticular wax coating over the body is protected by a cement layer and prevents water loss through the cuticle.[25] It is extremely effective, and the cuticle of *O. moubata* has a very high vapour diffusion resistance, being fourth highest out of 18 terrestrial organisms, which included vertebrates, arthropods and plants.[28]

Unmated and unfed adult female *O. moubata* have survived for more than three months when kept at 32°C over concentrated sulphuric acid in an atmosphere of 0 per cent RH.[35] When fed once before being starved and maintained under a more favourable humidity (85 per cent RH) there were differences in survival between different strains of *O. moubata*. In three different populations 40 per cent mortality (60 per cent survival) occurred after nine, 18 and 56 months, respectively.[35] Survival is favoured by the fact that *O. moubata* is able to take up water through the spiracles when exposed to humid air (95 per cent RH).[23]

Peirce[30] studied the distribution of *O. m.porcinus* in animal burrows in East Africa and found over 40 per cent of them infested. The estimated numbers of ticks ranged from a few up to 250,000 with a predominance of second- and third-stage nymphs accounting for more than 70 per cent of the population. Adults formed only 6 per cent of the population, and they and the larger nymphs were suspected of being subject to predation by insectivorous carnivores, rodents and reduviid bugs. The ticks were found on and in the soil to a depth of 5 cm and on the roof of the burrow, which was interpreted as being a response to hunger.

The most important environmental conditions for the tick are a neutral soil, high pH and a favourable temperature with an optimum at 24°C. Vegetation around the burrow conceals the occupants from predators and favours the presence of suitable hosts for the tick. The optimum altitude for *O. m.porcinus* is 900-1500 m and the tick has not been found above 1900 m.[30] In the absence of hosts the tick is able to survive for long periods, even up to five years under suitable conditions of humidity.[35] Such resistance to starvation enables foci of *O. moubata* to persist in the absence of hosts for a long period. Coupled with the ability to feed on alternate hosts, foci can be regarded for practical purposes as permanent.

Medical and Veterinary Importance. The population of *O. moubata* which lives in human habitations is of medical importance as the vector of endemic relapsing fever caused by *Borrelia duttoni* and is considered in Chapter 26. Wild suids are considered to act as reservoirs of African swine fever, and the virus has been isolated from *O. m. porcinus* taken from warthog burrows. Experimentally the virus passes from one generation to another by transovarian transmission but there is a problem with regard to warthogs being reservoirs of the virus for ticks. The level of viraemia needed to infect the tick has never been detected in warthogs, which raises the possibility of another host being involved or of special conditions under which warthogs produce a sufficiently intense viraemia.[31]

Ornithodoros savignyi (see Figure 22.4)

O. savignyi is known as the eyed tampan in contrast to *O. moubata*, the eyeless tampan, on account of its possession of two pairs of simple eyes (Figure 22.4) in the folds above coxa I and between coxae III and IV.[29] It is also known as the sand tampan because it buries itself in sandy and loose clayey soils, under trees, near wells and shady spots frequented by domestic stock — particularly camels, cattle, mules — and man, on which it feeds.[13,34] It does not occur in huts. On standing cattle it feeds on the legs just above the hooves. The numbers of *O. savignyi* in infested localities reach plague proportions. Their behaviour has been graphically described by Hoogstraal (p. 197):[13]

> At the Khartoum quarantine one may see a long, seething line of thousands of hungry tampans helplessly confined to the shade of a row of acacia trees. A few yards away, separated only by the hot, 9 o'clock sun, newly arrived cattle tied to a post fence tempt the tampans to cross the glaring strip. The next morning, in the coolness of 7 o'clock, those tampans under the trees are all blood bloated and resting comfortably in the sand, others are dragging back from their hosts across the now non-existent barrier and the legs of the cattle are beaded with yet other pod-shaped ticks taking their fill of blood in a regular line just above the hoof.

The biology and life cycle of *O. savignyi* is very similar to that of *O.*

moubata, but it has a much wider geographical distribution occurring in the arid parts of Africa, the Near East, India and Ceylon.[13] *O. savignyi* is not known to transmit any pathogen but 'camels and cattle suffer greatly and may even be killed by the volume of blood lost'.[13]

Argas (see Figures 22.5 and 22.6)

Fifty-six species have now been described in the genus *Argas* and they are allocated to seven subgenera which are structurally and biologically distinct. Two subgenera, *Argas* and *Persicargas*, parasitise birds; other subgenera are associated with bats and a small number of other mammals; and one monotypic subgenus occurs on the Galapagos giant tortoise.[15] All species of *Argas* are nocturnal except one, and with one exception all are restricted to arid habitats with long dry seasons. Where birds are present all year round enormous populations of ticks can build up and this applies to domestic poultry. These ticks have a strongly developed positive thigmotactic response and penetrate deeply into crevices in wood or stone to a situation where both surfaces of their body are in contact with the substrate.[15]

Until 1964 *A. persicus* was regarded as being a widespread species parasitising domestic chickens and a range of wild birds. Following the creation of the subgenus *Persicargas* and the recognition that the species parasitising the cattle egret in Egypt was a separate species, *A. (P). arboreus*, several

Figure 22.4: *Ornithodoros savignyi*. Lateral view

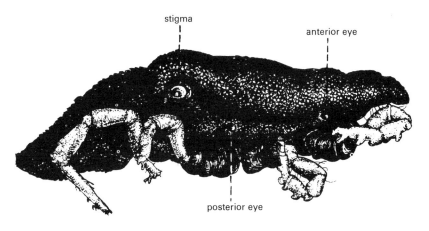

Source: From Patton, W.S. and Evans, A.M. (1929). *Insects, Ticks, Mites and Venomous Animals, Part 1: Medical*. H.R. Grubb, Croydon

Figure 22.5: *Argas (Persicargas) walkerae.* A, dorsal and B, ventral views of female; C, female dorsal integument (posterior quadrant); D, lateral integument in the same area

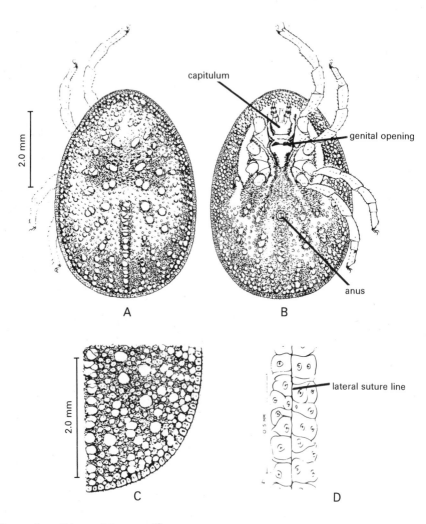

Source: From Kaiser and Hoogstraal[18]

other closely related species have been identified.[15, 19] *A. (P). persicus,* as now defined, is regarded as originating in the Palaearctic region where it occurs on domestic poultry and wild birds. It has been introduced by man with chickens into all other zoogeographical regions of the world, with the possible exception of the Neotropical region.[15] It has recently been reported from a galah's nest in Australia.[16]

In southern Africa the main argasid parasitising poultry is *A. (P). wal-kerae,*[18] *A. (P). robertsi* parasitises Ciconiformes (herons, egrets, storks, ibises) in the Australian and Oriental regions, filling the niche occupied by *A. (P). arboreus* in the Afrotropical region. In Queensland, Australia, *A. (P.) robertsi* also parasitises chickens, and may do so elsewhere in the region, but the commoner chicken argasid in the region is *A. (P.) persicus.*[16] The validity of three of these four closely related species has been confirmed by cross-breeding in the laboratory. Few eggs and no progeny are produced when *A. (P.) arboreus, A. (P.) walkerae* and *A. (P.) persicus* are cross-mated, proving that these three species are reproductively isolated.[11]

A. (P.) persicus

A. persicus is of considerable veterinary importance as the most widespread argasid tick feeding on poultry. The unfed adult tick is pale yellow in colour, becoming darker when fed. In outline the body is oval to pear shaped being broadest behind the legs at about the level of the anus. Females measure 7-10 mm × 5-6 mm and males are slightly smaller measuring 4-5 mm × 2.5-3 mm.[29] As in all species of *Persicargas* the quadrangular cells at the body margin are not striated (Figure 22.5C, D), a point which distinguishes this subgenus from the subgenus *Argas.*[19] The life cycle is similar to that of *O. moubata* with two major differences: there are fewer nymphal stages and the larva feeds on the host for several days.

Life Cycle. Females deposit yellowish-brown, spherical eggs in cracks and crevices of poultry houses where they hatch to produce a larva (Figure 22.6), which has a more or less circular outline, subterminal mouthparts visible from above, and no stigmata. The larva attaches itself to its host, particularly under the wings, where it feeds for about a week. It then falls off the host and has a period of relative inactivity before moulting to become a nymph. There are two to four nymphal stages before the adult.

Mating. The adults produce an aggregation pheromone which brings the sexes together for mating, and males of *A. persicus* were the most responsive not only to their own females, but to the pheromones produced by other species of *Argas* and *Ornithodoros.*[22] Usually the female feeds before mating and the coxal fluid is excreted after the tick has fed and not during feeding as in *O. moubata.* During mating the male inserts a spermatophore into the female genital opening. Eggs are matured and laid over a period of several days after a blood meal and not in a single batch.[13]

Quantitative Studies. Quantitative studies on the life cycle of *A. persicus* have been made by Gothe and Koop[10] and Khalil.[20] Both sets of observations were made on material originating from a colony maintained by Dr Hoogstraal's unit in Cairo. The environmental conditions were similar: 28-

Figure 22.6: *Argas (Persicargas) walkerae*. A, dorsal and B, ventral views of larvae; C, dorsal and D, ventral views of larval capitulum; E, dorsal view of tarsus I

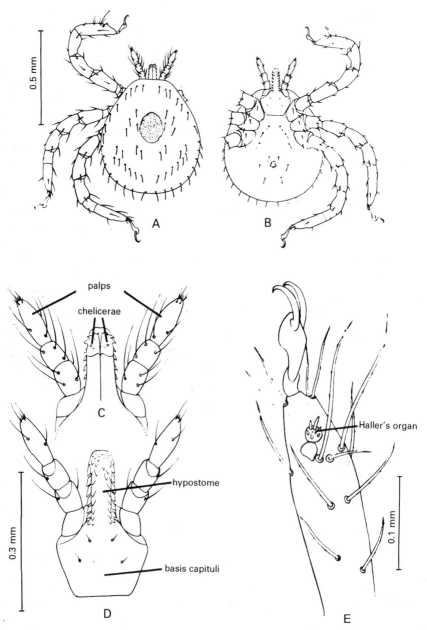

Source: From Kaiser and Hoogstraal[18]

29°C and 75 per cent RH[20] and 27°C and 90-95 per cent RH.[10] Khalil fed her ticks on domestic pigeons and Gothe and Koop fed theirs on chickens. This may explain the differences between the two sets of results. In Khalil's study[20] the range of variation was greater, the average time taken for each stage longer, and an extra nymphal stage occurred.

It is known that there is an interaction between host and tick. Tatchell *et al.*[33] found that when *A. persicus* was fed on pigeons it took in only two-thirds of the amount of blood it would imbibe from poultry. The reverse was true for *A. (P.) arboreus.*[33] Galun *et al.*[9] obtained a different result and found *A. persicus* taking a considerably larger (× 1.5) meal from pigeons compared with chickens. However, in terms of egg production, pigeon blood was less productive (× 0.75) than chicken blood. This may explain the differences between the results, and since chickens are the more important host economically, the results of Gothe and Koop will be considered first, and then additional results from Khalil be presented.

Larvae of *A. persicus* attached to chickens for four to seven days with the majority falling off after five days' attachment. There followed a pre-moult period of eight days (6-10 days) before moulting to the first nymph. Following a blood meal the nymph moulted to a second nymphal stage in 12 days (10-17 days). After the first blood meal most second-stage nymphs moulted to the adult stage in 14 days (11-20 days) with only a small proportion (6 per cent) becoming third-stage nymphs. After these had fed they moulted to the adult in 15 days and there was no fourth nymphal stage.

When the female had fed and mated there followed a preoviposition period of eight days, before an oviposition period of eleven days during which the female deposited on average about 140 eggs but there was considerable variation between individual females with a standard deviation of 38. Eggs were deposited at a rate of 12-18 per day from the second to ninth day of oviposition inclusively. Larval emergence took place two weeks after the first egg was laid and just over three weeks from the blood meal. Just over 60 per cent of the nymphs become adults.[10]

In view of the large variation in individual results it is preferable to present Khalil's data as median values representing the point at which 50 per cent of the population had completed the stage. The ability of larval *A. persicus* to attach successfully was a function of age and was highest when larvae were six to 14 days old, when 60 per cent of the larvae attached. Nymphs fed for varying periods up to an hour, and after each moult there was a pre-feeding period of one to four days in all stages. Adults fed for a longer period up to two to three hours. In all cases the coxal fluid was excreted after detaching from the host. Rather less than half the individuals required three or more nymphal stages to become adult, and 10 per cent required four nymphal stages. All adults produced from the fourth stage were females. Females had four to six periods of oviposition following blood meals, and the number of eggs produced in the first and second ovipositions were similar (63 and 74), but only about half the number (142) reported by Gothe and Koop[10] for the same species after a single blood meal.

Bionomics. The median time for survival of unfed larvae of *A. persicus* was 20 days. Nymphs survived considerably longer, especially the first nymphal stage which had a median survival period of nearly four months compared with eight weeks for the second to fourth nymphal stages. The latter value was closer to the survival ability of the adult which was nine weeks for males and ten weeks for females. Depending upon the availability of hosts Khalil[20] suggests that there could be up to ten generations a year and the life cycle could extend to two years where hosts were only available infrequently.

Desiccation is a major threat to the survival of unfed ticks. Experiments with *A. (P.) arboreus* shows that this species has considerable resistance to desiccation. More than 50 per cent of adults survived unfed for 105 days when kept over concentrated sulphuric acid at 0 per cent RH. During that time they lost about half their initial bodyweight, mostly due to loss of water. At 96 per cent RH survival is almost 100 per cent and the loss of weight a mere 4-5 per cent after 105 days. Indeed, in the early stages the ticks actually took up water and increased their weight by 7 per cent.[12]

Economic Importance. A. persicus, and probably the other related chicken-feeding species, transmits two important pathogens to poultry, *Borrelia anserina* and *Aegyptianella pullorum,* which are dealt with in Chapters 25 and 26. In addition by their feeding they can cause a condition known as fowl paralysis. A similar phenomenon is caused by ixodid ticks on mammals and will be considered in the next chapter. Populations of *A. persicus* can be very high and cause the death of poultry from exsanguination.[13]

References

1. Aeschlimann, A. and Grandjean, O. (1973). Observations on fecundity in *Ornithodorus moubata,* Murray (Ixodoidea: Argasidae). *Acarologia 15*: 206-17
2. _____ and Grandjean, O. (1973). Influence of natural and 'artificial' mating on feeding, digestion, vitellogenesis and oviposition in ticks (Ixodoidea). *Folia Parasitologia 20*: 67-74
3. Bedford, G.A.H. (1925). The spinose ear-tick (*Ornithodorus megnini* Dugès). *Journal of the Department of Agriculture, Union of South Africa 10*: 147-53
4. Bulman, G.M. and Walker, J.B. (1979). A previously unrecorded feeding site on cattle for the immature stages of the spinose ear tick, *Otobius megnini* (Dugès, 1844). *Journal of the South African Veterinary Association 50*: 107-8
5. Chellappa, D.J. (1973). Notes on spinose ear tick infestations in man and domestic animals in India and its control. *Review of Applied Entomology B 63*: 2902
6. _____ and Alwar, V.S. (1972). On the incidence of *Otobius megnini* (Dugès, 1883) on sheep in India. *Review of Applied Entomology B 62*: 1459

7. Cooley, R.A. and Kohls, G.M. (1944). *The Argasidae of North America, Central America and Cuba.* American Midland Naturalist Monograph No. 1, University Press, Notre Dame

8. Feldman-Muhsam, B. (1967). Spermatophore formation and sperm transfer in *Ornithodoros* ticks. *Science 156*: 1252-3

9. Galun, R., Sternberg, S. and Mango, C. (1978). Effects of host species on feeding behaviour and reproduction of soft ticks (Acari: Argasidae). *Bulletin of Entomological Research 68*: 153-7

10. Gothe, R. and Koop, E. (1974). Zur biologischer Bewertung der Validität von *Argas (Persicargas) persicus* (Oken, 1818), *Argas (Persicargas) arboreus* Kaiser, Hoogstraal und Kohls, 1964 and *Argas (Persicargas) walkerae* Kaiser und Hoogstraal, 1969. I. Untersuchungen zur Entwicklungsbiologie. *Zeitschrift für Parasitenkunde 44*: 299-317

11. _____ Koop, E. (1974). Zur biologischen Bewertung der Validität von *Argas (Persicargas) persicus* (Oken, 1818), *Argas (Persicargas) arboreus* Kaiser, Hoogstraal und Kohls, 1964 und *Argas (Persicargas) walkerae* Kaiser und Hoogstraal, 1969. II. Kreuzungsversuche. *Zeitschrift für Parasitenkunde 44*: 319-28

12. Hefnawy, T., Bishara, S.I. and Bassal, T.T.M. (1975). Biochemical and physiological studies of certain ticks (Ixodoidea): effects of relative humidity and starvation on the water balance and behaviour of adult *Argas (Persicargas) arboreus* (Argasidae). *Experimental Parasitology 38*: 14-19

13. Hoogstraal, H. (1956). *African Ixodoidea. I. Ticks of the Sudan (with special reference to Equatoria Province and with Preliminary Reviews of the Genera Boophilus, Margaropus* and *Hyalomma).* Research Report NM 005 050.29.07, Bureau of Medicine and Surgery, Department of Navy, Washington

14. _____ (1978). Biology of ticks. pp. 3-14 in *Tick-borne Diseases and their Vectors,* J.K.H. Wilde (ed.), Centre of Tropical Veterinary Medicine, University of Edinburgh

15. _____ Clifford, C.M., Keirans, J.E. and Wassef, H.Y. (1979). Recent developments in biomedical knowledge of *Argas* ticks (Ixodoidea: Argasidae). pp. 269-78 in volume II, *Recent Advances in Acarology,* J.G. Rodriguez (ed.), Academic Press, New York

16. _____ Kaiser, M.N. and McClure, H.E. (1975). The subgenus *Persicargas* (Ixodoidea: Argasidae: *Argas*). 20. *A. (P.) robertsi* parasitizing nesting wading birds and domestic chickens in the Australian and Oriental regions, viral infections and host migration. *Journal of Medical Entomology 11*: 513-24.

17. Jobling, B. (1925). A contribution to the biology of *Ornithodorus moubata* Murray. *Bulletin of Entomological Research 15*: 271-9

18. Kaiser, M.N. and Hoogstraal, H. (1969). The subgenus *Persicargas* (Ixodoidea: Argasidae: *Argas*). 7. *A. (P.) walkerae*, new species, a parasite of domestic fowl in southern Africa. *Annals of the Entomological Society of America 62*: 885-90

19. _____ Hoogstraal, H. and Kohls, G.M. (1964). The subgenus *Persicargas*, new subgenus (Ixodoidea: Argasidae: *Argas*). 1. *A. (P.) arboreus*, new species, an Egyptian *Persicus*-like parasite of wild birds, with a redefinition of the genus *Argus. Annals of the Entomological Society of America 57*: 60-9

20. Khalil, G.M. (1979). The subgenus *Persicargas* (Ixodoidea; Argasidae: *Argas*). 31. The life cycle of *A. (P.) persicus* in the laboratory. *Journal of Medical Entomology 16*: 200-6

21. Lavoipierre, M.M.J. and Riek, R.F. (1955). Observations on the feeding habits of argasid ticks and on the effect of their bites on laboratory animals, together with a note on the production of coxal fluid by several of the species studied. *Annals of Tropical Medicine and Parasitology 49*: 96-113

22. Leahy, M.G. (1979). Pheromones of argasid ticks. pp. 297-308 in volume II, *Recent Advances in Acarology,* J.G. Rodriguez (ed.), Academic Press, New York

23. Lees, A.D. (1946). The water balance in *Ixodes ricinus* L. and certain other species of ticks. *Parasitology 37*: 1-20

24. _____ (1946) Chloride regulation and the function of the coxal glands in ticks. *Parasitology 37*: 379-410

25. _____ (1947). Transpiration and the structure of the epicuticle in ticks. *Journal of Experimental Biology 23*: 379-410

26. _____ and Beament, J.W.L. (1948). An egg-waxing organ in ticks. *Quarterly Journal of Microscopical Science 89*: 291-332

27. Mango, C.K.A. and Galun, R. (1977). *Ornithodoros moubata*: breeding *in vitro*. *Experimental Parasitology 42*: 282-8
28. Monteith, J.L. and Campbell, G.S. (1980). Diffusion of water vapour through integuments — potential confusion. *Journal of Thermal Biology 5*: 7-9
29. Nuttall, G.H.F., Warburton, C., Cooper, W.F. and Robinson, L.E. (1908). *Ticks: A Monograph of the Ixodoidea. Part I. The Argasidae.* Cambridge University Press, Cambridge
30. Peirce, M.A. (1974). Distribution and ecology of *Ornithodoros moubata porcinus* Walton (Acarina) in animal burrows in East Africa. *Bulletin of Entomological Research 64*: 605-19
31. Pini, A. and Hurter, L.R. (1975). African swine fever: an epizootiological review with special reference to the South African situation. *Journal of the South African Veterinary Association 46*: 227-32
32. Robinson, G.G. (1942). The mechanism of insemination in the argasid tick, *Ornithodorus moubata* Murray. *Parasitology 34*: 195-8
33. Tatchell, R.J., Kerr, J.D. and Boctor, F.N. (1973). Biochemical and physiological studies of certain ticks (Ixodoidea). Haemolysis rate and meal size in the interactions between *Argas (Persicargas) arboreus* Kaiser, Hoogstraal and Kohls, *A. (P.) persicus* (Oken) (Argasidae) and some avian hosts. *Parasitology 67*: 41-51
34. Walker, J.B., Mehlitz, D. and Jones, G.E. (1978). *Notes on the Ticks of Botswana.* German Agency for Technical Cooperation, Eschborn, West Germany
35. Walton, G.A. (1960). The reaction of some variants of *Ornithodoros moubata* Murray (Argasidae, Ixodoidea) to desiccation. *Parasitology 50*: 81-8

23 IXODIDA — IXODIDAE (HARD TICKS)

The Ixodidae are large, blood-sucking Acarina with terminal capitulum in all stages; a dorsal shield or scutum showing sexual dimorphism, being small in the female and almost covering the dorsal surface in the male (Figure 23.1A and C); reduced fourth palpal segment inserted on the ventral side of the third (Plate 23.1); and the stigmata located behind the

Figure 23.1: Diagnostic Features of *Ixodes* Ticks. A, dorsal and B, ventral views of female; C, dorsal and D, ventral views of male

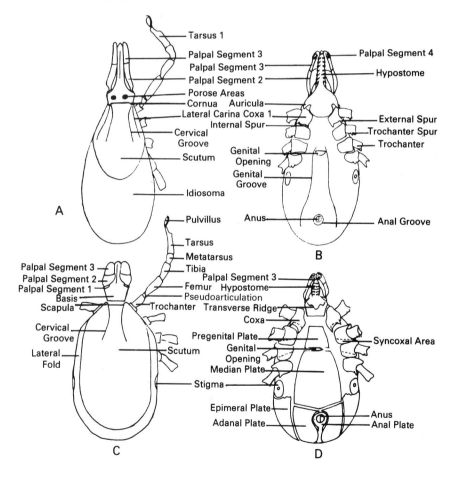

Source: From Arthur[2]

fourth pair of legs. There is only one nymphal stage in the life cycle. Thirteen genera are recognised of which seven contain species of major veterinary importance, and some are of minor medical importance.

Genera of Veterinary Importance

Ixodes (see Figure 23.1)

Ixodes are small, inornate ticks, easily overlooked when searching a host. The capitulum of the female is considerably longer than that of the male. Often the second segment of the palp is constricted at the base, creating a gap between the palp and the mouthparts. There are no eyes (Figure 23.3) or festoons (Figure 23.2). The anal groove passes anteriorly to the anus and *Ixodes* is said to be prostriate. In the other genera the anal groove is

Figure 23.2: *Haemaphysalis longicornis.* A, dorsal and B, ventral views of male; C, dorsal and D, ventral views of female

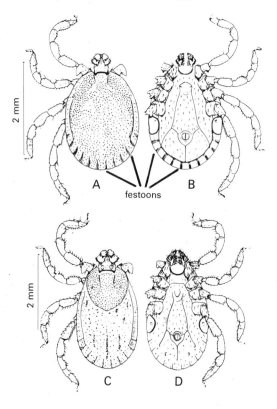

either posterior to the anus or obsolete and they are referred to as meta-striate. In the male there are seven ventral plates including a median row of three — pregenital, median, anal — a pair of adanals and a pair of epi-merals. The margins of the epimerals, which are placed posterolaterally, are often indistinct.[2] Ixodes ticks are highly specialised in their habits with some species occurring on bats and even on sea birds. Important species in this genus are the European sheep tick (*I. ricinus*) and two species which cause paralysis in mammals, *I. rubicundus* in southern Africa and *I. holocyclus* in Australia.

Haemaphysalis (see Figure 23.2 and 23.9)

These are small, inornate ticks with short mouthparts, i.e. brevirostrate. The basis capituli is rectangular and the base of the second palpal segment is expanded, projecting laterally beyond the basis capituli. The second and third palpal segments taper anteriorly so that the capitulum anterior to the basis capituli appears to be triangular. There are no eyes in either sex and no ventral plates in the male. Festoons are present. These are uniform, rectangular areas along the posterior margin of the body, separated by grooves. They are best seen in unfed specimens, and are lost in engorged females. This genus reaches its maximum development in the Oriental region where *H. spinigera* is the vector of the arbovirus causing Kyasanur

Figure 23.3: A, Dorsal and B, Ventral Views of Male *Boophilus microplus*

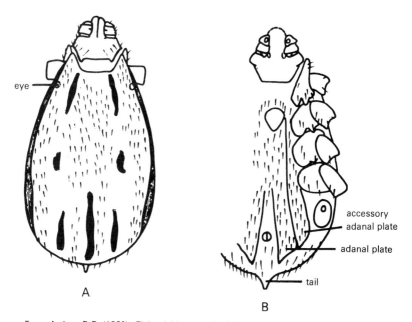

Source: From Arthur, D.R. (1960). *Ticks: A Monograph of the Ixodoidea, Part V*, p. 209. Cambridge University Press

Forest Disease (see Chapter 24). The yellow dog tick *H. leachi leachi* is widespread in the tropics and subtropics. *H. punctata* is a parasite of cattle in the Palaearctic region, as is *H. longicornis* in the Australian and Oriental regions.[15] *H. longicornis* is the only cattle tick in New Zealand.

Boophilus (see Figure 23.3)

Boophilids are small, inornate, brevirostrate ticks in which the anal groove is obsolete. The basis capituli is hexagonal dorsally, and there are simple eyes laterally on the scutum. Ventrally coxa I is bifid, and there are paired adanal and accessory adanal plates flanking the anus posteriorly. In some

Plate 23.1: Scanning Electron Micrograph of Ventral Surface of Mouthparts and Palps of Female *Boophilus microplus*. Note: lateral palps with 4th segment located on ventral surface of 3rd segment; median toothed hypostome; and, at the top, the chelicerae protruding from the cheliceral sheaths

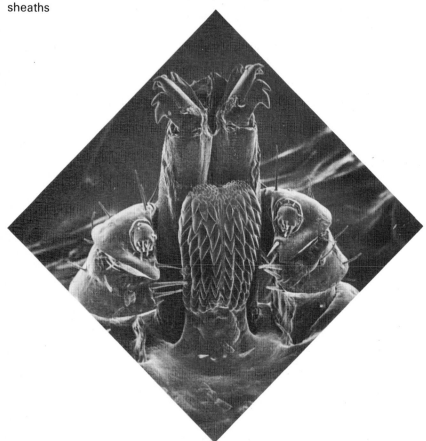

Courtesy of J.V. Hardy, M.J. Rice and S.M. Waladde

species the replete male develops a median tail. They are one-host ticks (see below) which parasitise large mammals, especially cattle, and are important vectors of disease to livestock. Important species are *B. microplus*, the pantropical cattle tick, which occurs in the Neotropical, Afrotropical and Australian regions, *B. decoloratus* in tropical Africa, and *B. annulatus* in North America.

Rhipicephalus (see Figure 23.4)

These are small metastriate, brevirostrate, reddish or blackish-brown ticks which are mostly inornate. The basis capituli is hexagonal dorsally and eyes and festoons are present. Coxa I is bifid in both sexes. The male has adanal

Figure 23.4: Above, Dorsal and Below, Ventral Views of Male *Rhipicephalus sanguineus*

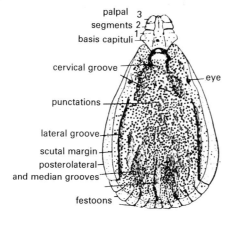

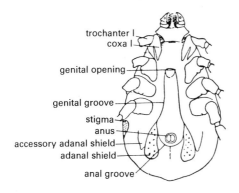

Source: From Nuttall, G.H.F. (1911). *Ticks: A Monograph of the Ixodoidea, Part II*, p. 122. Cambridge University Press

and accessory adanal plates on the ventral surface and when replete has a tail. The genus reaches its greatest development in the Afrotropical region where *R. appendiculatus*, the brown ear tick, is the main vector of *Theileria parva*, the causative agent of east coast fever in cattle in eastern Africa. Other important species on domestic animals are *R. eversti* and *R. simus.* The red dog tick, *R. sanguineus*, is now the most widespread of any ixodid species but is commoner in the warmer parts of the world.

Figure 23.5: *Dermacentor andersoni.* A, dorsal view of female. B, dorsal view of male

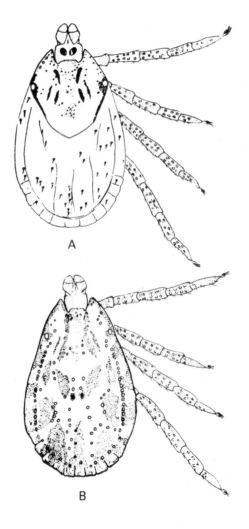

Source: From Arthur[1]

Figure 23.6: A, Dorsal and B, Ventral Views of Male *Dermacentor reticulatus*

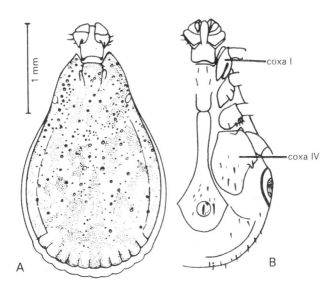

Source: From Arthur, D.R. (1963). *British Ticks*. Butterworth, London

Dermacentor (see Figures 23.5 and 23.6)

These are larger, usually ornate, metastriate, brevirostrate ticks. The basis capituli is rectangular dorsally and eyes and festoons are present. Coxa I is bifid in both sexes and coxa IV is greatly enlarged in the male which has no ventral plates (Figure 23.6B). This genus has its greatest development in the New World, and includes the wood tick *D. andersoni* (Figure 23.5), which causes tick paralysis, and is the vector of Rocky Mountain spotted fever and tularaemia. *D. reticulatus* (Figure 23.6) parasitises cattle and horses in the Palaearctic region.

Hyalomma (see Figure 23.7)

These are medium sized metastriate ticks with long mouthparts, i.e. longirostrate. The basis capituli is subtriangular dorsally (Figure 23.7E) and eyes are present. Festoons and ornamentation of the scutum are variable characters which may be present or absent. The male has one pair of adanal plates and accessory adanal plates may or may not be present. Coxa I is bifid. Hyalommas are tough, hardy ticks which survive where humidity is low, climatic conditions extreme, hosts rare and hiding places sparse.[13] They probably originated in the desert regions of the southern Soviet Union and Iran in the Palaearctic region.[13] *H. anatolicum anatolicum* and species of the *H. marginatum* complex play a major part in the

Figure 23.7: A, Dorsal and B, Ventral Views of Female *Hyalomma excavatum*; C, Dorsal and D, Ventral Views of Male *H. excavatum*; E, Dorsal and F, Ventral Views of Capitulum of Female *H. aegyptium*

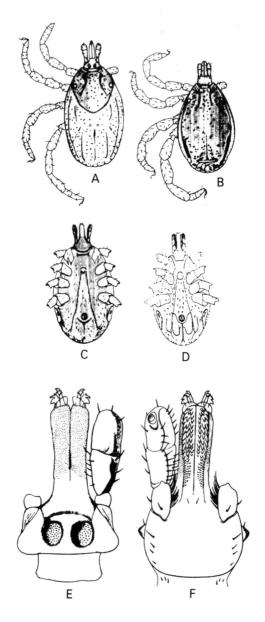

Sources: A, B, C, D from Arthur.[1] E and F from Nuttall, G.H.F. (1911). *Ticks: A Monograph of the Ixodoidea, Part II*, p. 122. Cambridge University Press

transmission of the arbovirus causing Crimean-Congo haemorrhagic fever (see Chapter 24).

Amblyomma (see Figure 23.8)

These are large ornate metastriate longirostrate ticks with eyes and festoons but no adanal plates in the male. The genus is particularly well represented in the New World. In the Afrotropical region *A. hebraeum* (Figure 23.8) and *A. variegatum* are important parasites of cattle. The feeding of numbers of large longirostrate ticks can cause extensive damage to hides and skins, and their lesions provide a route for the invasion of pathogens.[53]

Figure 23.8: A, Dorsal View of Female, and B, Dorsal View of Male *Amblyomma hebraeum*

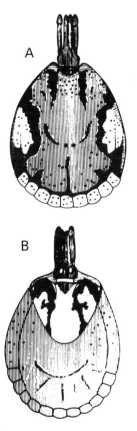

Source: From Arthur[1]

Life Cycle

Oviposition

There are four stages in the life cycle: egg, larva, nymph and adult. The female drops off its vertebrate host and seeks a sheltered situation in which to develop and lay a single large batch of eggs, after which she dies. Typically a batch contains several thousand brown globular eggs, and oviposition continues for many days. *I. ricinus* has been recorded as depositing an egg every three to twelve minutes.[20] During oviposition the

Figure 23.9: *Haemaphysalis longicornis.* A, dorsal and B, ventral views of nymph. C, dorsal and D, ventral views of larva

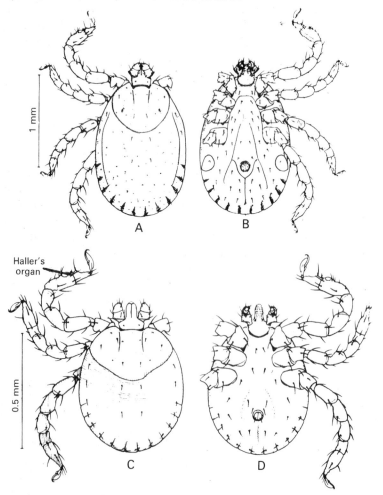

Source: From Hoogstraal, Roberts, Kohls and Tipron[15]

tick bends its capitulum in an arc ventrally until it is tightly oppressed to the ventral surface and the tip of the capitulum is near the genital opening. Gene's organ is everted between the scutum and the basis capituli. This structure has a swollen base and two short horns. During the extrusion of an egg the lining of the vagina prolapses through the genital opening holding the egg which is deposited between the horns of Gene's organ. The prolapse is then retracted.

The function of Gene's organ is to apply a waterproofing wax to the egg after which the organ is withdrawn and the egg is left on the hypostome. When the capitulum returns to its normal forwardly directed position the egg is deposited above the female. Consequently the egg batch is to be found above the shrivelled body of the female. If the eggs do not receive a wax coat they shrivel and die. In *I. ricinus* an incomplete waterproof layer is added during the egg's passage down the vagina, and this proofing is completed by the application of the secretion of Gene's organ which, in this species, is an easily spreading and penetrating soft wax. In the first few days of incubation the wax penetrates the outer layers of the egg to reach the inner membrane. The critical temperature at which the wax ceases to waterproof the egg is 35°C in *I. ricinus*, and 44°C in *Hyalomma savignyi*.[20]

Larva (see Figure 23.9C, D)

Depending upon climatic conditions eggs hatch in two weeks to several months,[13] giving rise to a hexapod larva which seeks a host by climbing vegetation. Larvae accumulate near the tips of grasses and similar vegetation. When a host approaches the larvae quest for it by waving their first pair of legs in the air. Larvae of *B. microplus* quest in response to odours, vibrations, air currents, warmth, moisture and interrupted illumination.[47] Haller's organ on the dorsal surface of the tarsus of the first pair of legs houses receptors for many of these stimuli (Figure 23.9C). Larvae have neither spiracles nor tracheal system and therefore water loss is solely through the cuticle. When a larva succeeds in getting on to a host it attaches and feeds for several days before dropping off engorged. All larvae are not successful in finding a host and larvae of *I. ricinus* move down to the more humid layers near the ground where, at suitable humidities, they are able to take up water from the atmosphere.[1] In this way larvae can survive for considerable periods unfed.

Nymph and Adult

The larva digests its blood meal and moults to an octopod nymph (Figure 23.9A, B) which repeats the larval pattern of behaviour to find a host. The nymph has spiracles and a tracheal system which makes it more susceptible to desiccation. The nymph feeds for four to eight days on the host, engorging more rapidly towards the end of the period before dropping off to find a suitable location in which to digest its meal and moult to the adult stage.

The adults repeat the process of host finding. The female attaches but does not engorge until mating has taken place. The male feeds but does not engorge. The engorged female drops off the host and hides away in a suitable location to digest the blood meal and lay her egg batch.

Variations on Life Cycle

The majority of ixodid ticks have the type of life cycle just described and are referred to as three-host ticks, but two genera *Boophilus* and *Margaropus* are one-host ticks in which engorged larvae and nymphs do not drop off the host but remain attached and moult *in situ*, and the subsequent stage re-attaches on the same individual host. The genus *Margaropus* contains three species, two of which are parasites of giraffe, and *M. winthemi*, the winter horse tick of the high veld of southern Africa.[14]

A few species in other genera are one-host ticks, including *D. (Anocentor) nitens*, a Neotropical ear-tick of horses; *D. albipictus*, the North American moose tick; and *Hy. scupense* in the Palaearctic region.[14] A few species have adopted a two-host cycle in which the larva and nymph occur on the same individual host, the nymph then dropping off and the adult parasitising a different individual of the same or another host species. Included in the two-host ticks, which parasite domestic animals, are: *R. evertsi* of the Afrotropical region, and *R. bursa*, *Hy. marginatum* and *Hy. detritum* of the Palaearctic region.[14]

Although ixodid ticks are not host specific they are not indiscriminate in the hosts they parasitise. A few show an extremely wide range and these are often of economic importance, but most occur on a limited range of hosts which they parasitise with varying intensities. Some hosts are commonly and heavily infested and others infrequently and lightly. Each species is adapted to its hosts, concentrating on particular parts of the host's body and adjusting its seasonal and daily activity cycles to the host's behaviour and availability.[14] To overcome adverse conditions or times when the host is not present diapause may occur at any stage of the life cycle and both pre- and post-feeding. There may be several generations in a year, e.g. *B. microplus*, or the life cycle may extend over three to four or even seven years in cold subarctic latitudes.[14]

Biology and Behaviour

Feeding and Water Elimination

The ixodid tick pierces the skin of its host with its chelicerae and inserts the barbed hypostome to secure it to the host initially. In brevirostrate ticks cement is secreted during the first 24 h which spreads over the skin firmly anchoring the tick to its host. Extra cement is secreted up to 96 h to secure the tick more firmly by penetrating the keratinised layers of the stratum corneum and filling the lesion.[23] In longirostrate ticks there is less need of cement which is reduced to form a sheath around the mouthparts within the host.[4] In *I. holocyclus* the female is longirostrate and secretes no cement.[4]

During engorgement the bodyweight of a tick increases by about × 200.[4] An unfed female *I. ricinus* weighs about 2 mg and takes in 600 mg of blood while feeding, but a half to two thirds of the water contained in the ingested blood is eliminated before feeding ceases and the final weight of the engorged tick is about 240 mg.[18] In argasid ticks excess water is eliminated via the coxal apparatus but no such structure is present in ixodid ticks.[16] Little urine is produced by the malpighian tubules and excess fluid is eliminated by salivation, the voluminous saliva being passed back into the host.

Mammalian blood is hyposmotic to tick tissues. When *I. ricinus* feeds on its main host the sheep, which has a blood chloride concentration of 0.5 per cent, the chloride content of its haemolymph rises from 0.72 per cent in the unfed tick to 0.88 per cent in the fed tick.[17] This can only be achieved by the secretion of hyposmotic saliva.[16] The saliva contains many compounds some originating in the salivary glands and others being derived from the haemolymph. Some compounds could play important roles in the feeding process but other explanations for their presence can be advanced. The position can be summarised by quoting Binnington and Kemp:[4] 'The accumulated evidence outlined above suggests that secretion of anti-coagulants, weak hydrolytic enzymes, and pharmacological agents coupled with capillary blood pressure and some tissue damage by cheliceral teeth, can liberate enough host blood for tick engorgement'. The question of toxins in the saliva is considered below under Tick Paralysis.

Water Balance

In ixodid ticks the cuticle is impermeable to water due to the presence of an outer wax layer which is not protected by a cement layer as in the Argasidae. The critical temperature of the wax layer varies being low in *I. ricinus* (32°C) and high in *Hyalomma savignyi* (45°C), but not as high as in argasids.[19] *I. ricinus* is associated with a moist microclimate, and when kept at 0 per cent RH and 25°C unfed females lost 17 per cent of their body weight in 24 hours, compared with the loss of 0.8 per cent under the same conditions by *Hy. savignyi*, an inhabitant of arid regions.[19] Loss of water also occurs through the spiracles, and in an atmosphere of high CO_2 when the spiracles were kept open, female *A. variegatum* lost 17 times as much water at 0 per cent RH compared to 93 per cent RH. Larvae of the same species have no spiracles and their water loss remained unchanged in the presence of high concentrations of carbon dioxide.[34]

Opening of the spiracles and loss of water will depend upon the activity of the individual tick. Ticks can compensate for water loss by absorbing water from an unsaturated atmosphere. Such absorption has been demonstrated in 30 species; the most efficient can absorb water in an atmosphere of 75 per cent RH and the least efficient at 94 per cent RH. The rate of absorption depends upon the humidity, being seven times as high in *A. variegatum* exposed to 93 per cent RH, compared with 85 per cent RH.[34] The mechanism is believed to involve secretion of a hygroscopic saliva which extracts water from the atmosphere and is then imbibed. It is of some interest that stages in the life cycle of 1- or 2-host ticks which are not required to search for a host do not have this ability to absorb water. Unfed nymphs and adults of *B. annulatus* when removed from the host survive for only 14 days at 25°C even though maintained at 90 per cent RH.[34]

Pheromones, Aggregation and Mating

Three different types of pheromones have been detected among ixodid ticks: aggregation pheromones produced off the host, and different pheromones produced by males and females on the host. Receptors for pheromones are located on Haller's organ.[11] Aggregation pheromones have been demonstrated in *I. holocyclus*, a paralysis tick, and *Aponomma concolor*, which parasitises echidnas, monotreme mammals.[45] Female *I. ricinus* produce a pheromone which strongly attracts males and also attracts females but more weakly. *Ixodes* species are said to mate both on and off their hosts,[28] and pheromones will serve to bring the sexes together. The pheromone produced by female *I. ricinus* is water soluble and different from the phenolic compounds produced by female metastriate ticks. One such pheromone, 2, 6 dichlorphenol, is found in at least four genera of ticks: *Amblyomma*, *Rhipicephalus*, *Dermacentor* and *Hyalomma*.[38]

In *D. andersoni* the pheromone is synthesised early in adult life by the foveal gland but it is not released until the female is feeding. In *R. appendiculatus* both synthesis and release of the pheromone are associated with feeding.[38] In response to the pheromone the male detaches and orientates to the female. In *D. variabilis* males may migrate as far as 43 cm to reach females on the opposite side of the host, a dog.[38] Males of five species of *Amblyomma* secrete a pheromone which attracts both adults and nymphs, but which is not secreted until the male has been feeding for five days reaching a peak after six to eight days. A similar period is required to complete spermatogenesis. This pheromone is species specific and in the absence of fed males, female *A. hebraeum* and *A. variegatum* do not readily attach.[32] Another pheromone which is not specific accelerates attachment and both sexes attach near feeding males.[32]

Metastriate ticks mate on the host and, as in the Argasidae, the mouthparts are used to dilate the female genital opening, then a spermatophore is produced by the male and introduced into the vagina, but there is uncertainty with regard to the role of the mouthparts in effecting transference of the spermatophore.[28] In *D. occidentalis* and *Ha. leporispalustris* the endospermatophore contains only one capsule compared with the two present in argasids. A maximum of five capsules have been found in a single female *D. occidentalis* indicating that it had mated five times.[28] *Ha. longicornis* is unusual in that it has sexual reproduction in the greater part of its range but in the cold northern part of the range the species is parthenogenetic.[14]

Two ticks of economic importance will be considered in more detail. They are the 3-host *Rhipicephalus appendiculatus* and the 1-host *Boophilus microplus*. Both are vectors of important protozoal diseases to cattle.

Rhipicephalus appendiculatus

Distribution

R. appendiculatus occurs mainly in the eastern and southern parts of Africa, south of the equator. It does not occur in West Africa.[13] It ranges from sea level at the coast up to 2,100 m inland but is absent from deserts and areas lacking shrub cover.[13,53] It is commoner in areas of tall grass rather than short grass, and in areas of moderate or higher rainfall, which is often defined as more than 750 mm per annum.[3] In Tanzania, Yeoman and Walker[53] found it rare in areas where the rainfall was less than 500 mm, and widely distributed in the 500-1,000 mm rainfall zone, but not ubiquitous on cattle within that zone. In areas where the rainfall exceeded 1,000 mm heavy infestations of *R. appendiculatus* could be expected wherever cattle were present in any number. The distribution of *R. appendiculatus* is the result of a complex interaction between climate, vegetation and cattle. Yeoman and Walker do not believe that *R. appendiculatus* is present in undisturbed habitats but that it is introduced with cattle during settlement.[53]

Biology

Daily Activity. There is a rhythm in the host-seeking behaviour of *R. appendiculatus* with activity being greater by day with bimodal diurnal periodicity. In the cooler months one peak occurred before midday and the other before sunset while in the warmer months the morning peak was earlier (08.00 h), and the afternoon peak reduced. Under shade conditions peak activity occurred in the late afternoon.[30]

Hosts. R. appendiculatus is primarily a parasite of cattle but also occurs on sheep and goats and to a very limited extent on wild animals.[53] Infestations of up to nearly 2,000 adult *R. appendiculatus* have been found on a single beast but infestations are usually considerably smaller.[53] Yeoman and Walker[53] consider that in the absence of cattle *R. appendiculatus* is not able to sustain itself on other domestic or wild animals. Smaller wild animals tend to be infested with nymphs but only in the presence of cattle.

Distribution on Host. The site most frequented by adult *R. appendiculatus* is inside the ear flap which can support a maximum population of about 250 adults.[53] Larvae and nymphs of the 2-host tick, *R. eversti,* which occur on the same individual host are present deep inside the ear, and the adults almost exclusively in the perianal region,[25, 53] whereas 87 per cent of adult *R. appendiculatus* occur on the ears and only 2 per cent in the perianal region.[25] Adults of *R. kochi,* which also parasitises cattle, occur mainly elsewhere on the body with only small numbers on the ear or in the perianal region.[25] Larvae and nymphs of the blue tick *B. decolaratus* are often found on the ears of cattle in a similar position to the immature stages of *R. appendiculatus.*[53] Where low infestations of *R. appendiculatus* are present the ticks will be confined to the ear, but in heavier infestations they will occur elsewhere on the head, spreading to the neck and body.

Length of Life Cycle. Branagan[5] studied in the laboratory the effect of temperature and humidity on the duration of those stages in the life cycle of *R. appendiculatus* which occur off the host. He found that at 25°C these stages took nine weeks (Table 23.1), and at 18°C six months. Assuming that hosts are readily available and that the total time spent by the three feeding stages on the host is three to four weeks, then the minimum time in which the life cycle could be completed at 25°C would be three months, and at 18°C seven months. Over the range 18 to 85 per cent RH, humidity had no effect on the speed of development.

These are minimum times. At 25°C 40 per cent of the egg batch is laid in the first four days of oviposition and 90 per cent within 12 days, but at 18°C the respective percentages are 29 and 46. At 25°C hatching of the

Table 23.1: Duration of Various Stages in Life Cycle of *Rhipicephalus appendiculatus*

Stage in life cycle	25°C	18°C
Pre-oviposition	6.2	12.8
Pre-eclosion	29.3	71.8
Engorged larva to nymph	11.9	34.3
Engorged nymph to female (male)	16.5 (18.2)	56.5 (64.2)
Total	63.9	175.4

Notes: Average duration in days. Pre-oviposition = time to deposition of first egg. Pre-eclosion = time to emergence of first larva from eggs

Source: From Branagan[5]

eggs is spread over two weeks with 50 per cent of the larval emergence being reached by day five, and at 18°C hatching is prolonged to nearly four weeks with 50 per cent emergence by day eight.[5]

Seasonal Abundance

In southern Africa there is a definite seasonal cycle with one generation per year. In the eastern Cape, which has summer rainfall, adult *R. appendiculatus* appear in November, reach a peak in January-February and then decrease in the autumn.[31] Peak numbers of larvae on cattle occur in the autumn (April-May), and of nymphs in late winter in August-September. The activity of adult *R. appendiculatus* is regulated by day length which controls the timing of the annual cycle, but the activity of larvae and nymphs is independent of day length. The size of the *R. appendiculatus* population is dependent upon the rainfall distribution.[31]

A similar cycle has been recorded on the highveld of Zimbabwe with peak adult activity coinciding with the rainy season, and larval and nymphal activity with the dry season.[36] Here, too, adult activity was controlled by day length, temperature and humidity, and there was evidence to suggest that adult *R. appendiculatus* had a quiescent period when they were present on the vegetation but not actively seeking a host.[36]

Under optimal conditions the life cycle of *R. appendiculatus* can be completed in about four months in Malawi,[51] but it was found that females only engorged and oviposited in the rainy season, when the relative humidity was above 75 per cent.[50] Branagan[5] points out that this is a description of actual events, but that on his experimental findings humidity itself would not limit female engorgement and oviposition. Unengorged larvae fail to survive the cold, dry months,[51] and Branagan[5] considers that *R. appendiculatus* survives the winter as engorged nymphs.

At Mwanza on Lake Victoria in Tanzania McCulloch *et al.*[22] estimated, on field data, the duration of the off-the-host stages to be 90 days. Allowing a month for the three feeding stages to find a host and engorge it would be possible to have two or three cycles completed in a year, but optimal conditions are not continuously present, and the number of cycles is dependent on local conditions. At Mwanza adult *R. appendiculatus* were present all the year round, and there were smaller fluctuations in the numbers of adults than there were in the immature stages, in which cycles of abundance were more apparent.[22] There were two generations per annum with peaks of larvae and nymphs in the dry interlude in the wet season early in the year, and a second peak following the rains in the middle of the year. In the drier zone of Sukumaland, east of Lake Victoria, the seasonal pattern of *R. appendiculatus* was closer to that of southern Africa with a single generation per annum with peak adult activity during the rains.[52]

At a similar latitude on the Kenya coast adult *R. appendiculatus* were present all the year round, but the annual cycle was bimodal with a small peak in April at the start of the rains, and a larger second peak in September-October, when dry conditions were likely to prevail. It is suspected that much of the second generation is lost.[25]

Survival of *R. appendiculatus* depends on temperature, humidity and activity. Exposure to 4°C continuously for two to three days was fatal to all engorged stages.[5] In the dry season at Kedong in the Rift Valley desiccation of egg batches frequently prevented any emergence of larvae.[6] Larvae that do emerge prolong survival by resting on grasses where transpiration is taking place, creating a humid microclimate.[6] The survival of adult *R. appendiculatus* is inversely related to their activity. Regular activation reduced survival from more than four months to less than three months.[29]

Veterinary Importance

R. appendiculatus is the main vector of *Theileria parva,* a virulent pathogen causing east coast fever of cattle in eastern and central Africa. It is also a vector of *Babesia bigemina,* the cause of redwater in cattle, but not the most important vector of this disease.[13, 53] These pathogens are dealt with in Chapter 28.

Boophilus microplus

Distribution and Hosts

B. microplus is widely distributed in, but not limited to, the southern hemisphere. It occurs in Central and South America, southern Florida and Mexico, from which it may extend into Texas. It is present in the Oriental region from which it has been introduced into northern Australia, where it now extends down the eastern coast into northern New South Wales. From the Oriental region *B. microplus* was introduced into Madagascar and from there into eastern, central and southern Africa.[12, 13, 35]

In all regions *B. microplus* is primarily a parasite of cattle, but heavy infestations can develop on horses and sheep; goats and deer can also be infested. Indeed, in southern Florida *B. microplus* survives on white-tailed deer (*Odocoileus virginianus*).[12] In Tanzania only light infestations occurred on sheep and goats,[53] and in Australia the sheep-rearing areas are too arid for *B. microplus.*[35]

Life Cycle

The female *B. microplus* deposits 2,000-3,000 shiny, dark yellow-brown eggs, almost spherical measuring 0.5 mm × 0.4 mm. Providing the humidity remains above 70 per cent, they hatch in summer in about two weeks.[33] Larvae show positive phototaxis and ascend grass stems, occurring in groups of 20 or more on the tips of grasses. They do not show the ascending-descending pattern of activity described for *I. ricinus* but remain on the upper parts of the grass, avoiding direct sunlight, and aggregating on the tips of the grass particularly in the early morning.[47] Larvae show a strong response to odours, breath and contact in their search for a host.[47]

On the host larvae attach themselves and feed for about four days after which there is a quiescent period of about two days before the larva moults to a nymph while still on the host. The nymph may wander around on the host for a while before attaching, when it feeds for nearly a week followed by a short quiescent period, and then it moults to the adult. The female attaches particularly on the neck, brisket, flank, inguinal region and escutcheon.[33] The female feeds slowly at first and then after mating engorges rapidly and drops from the host about three weeks after attachment of the larva. Most female ticks drop from their hosts in the early morning (06.00-10.00 h).[35] After a minimum preoviposition period of two days the female commences to lay eggs over a period of ten or more days. The minimum time to complete the life cycle is therefore five weeks, and under less favourable conditions will extend to several months.[33]

Seasonal Abundance

B. microplus is a high rainfall species (750 mm or more)[53] and does not persist in dry areas with low humidities.[35] In parts of the tropics where rainfall and humidity are high, *B. microplus* reproduces continuously throughout the year.[46] In subtropical regions such as south eastern Queensland, the tick has a pronounced seasonal cycle. The spring rise of larvae results in a first generation of adults in November-December, and the population steadily increases reaching a peak in the fourth generation at the end of the autumn (June), followed by a population crash in the winter.[46] The rapid decline in the numbers of ticks on cattle in the winter results from the fact that female ticks which drop in April until mid-July produce virtually no progeny.[37] Ticks dropping from late July onwards do produce progeny. The tick 'overwinters' through larvae hatching from eggs laid by females that dropped from cattle in March or early April. These are the source of the spring rise.[46] Continuation of the species in a locality depends upon larval survival which is of the order of three to four months in summer and five to six months in winter but larvae, like eggs, are susceptible to low temperatures and humidities.[35]

Population Dynamics and Modelling

Models have been constructed which relate the population of *B. microplus* to its host and the time of year.[42] Such a model is a valuable tool in evaluating the effect of various management decisions, e.g. when and how frequently to dip. Models require more elaborate data than that given above and indeed the components of the model have different values depending on the season. Thus egg production is constant over the range

16-33°C which equates to the period September to April, when a reasonable figure is 2,000 eggs per female. In May, the second half of July and August it is half that, but in June and the first half of July egg production drops to about 200 eggs per female.[42]

Egg development is prolonged at lower temperatures and survival of eggs laid from mid-April through to mid-July is virtually zero. Eggs laid in late July and later which contribute to the first generation have about 20 per cent survival. Larvae of the spring rise and the following second generation (10 per cent survival) can survive unfed for four to six weeks; this is slightly longer in the third generation and is seven to eleven weeks in the fourth generation (April-September).

The obverse to larval survival is host finding and this is a function of density of hosts; having found a host, survival is a function of tick density on the host. Experiments conducted during the major active period of larvae of *B. microplus*, i.e. from the end of October until mid-April, showed that at a density of two beasts per hectare 30-70 per cent of the larvae were picked up per week, and at five beasts per hectare that rate had increased to 50-85 per cent.[41] This is equivalent to each beast picking up all ticks from 0.022-0.75 hectares per day with the lower values being associated with lower temperatures.[41]

Survival of larvae that have found a host depends upon a number of factors including the breed of host and time of year. All breeds have lower resistance to ticks in winter and Zebu are more resistant than Hereford cattle. This relationship can be represented by the expression:

$$M = aL^c$$

where M = number of females dropped, L = number of larvae and a and c are constants.[44] The percentage survival will depend upon the values of c and L. When L equalled 20,000, 28 per cent were found to survive in winter on Hereford cattle compared with 9 per cent on Zebu crossbreds, but the same level of initial infestation had only 1.3 per cent survival in spring on Zebu crossbreds.[44]

Principles of control

Use of Acaricides. In theory it would appear to be easy to control boophilids. They are the most species specific of the ixodid ticks with the bulk of the population occurring on domestic animals which can be mustered and treated. In addition it is a 1-host tick spending a minimum of three weeks on the host, and therefore dipping of all the hosts in an area at three weekly intervals with an effective acaricide, for a period to exceed that for which unfed larvae can survive, should eradicate the tick. Application of a rigorous, well organised programme of eradication in the United States was highly successful against *B. annulatus*. By 1940, using arsenic as the only acaricide, *B. annulatus* had been eradicated from the USA, except for border areas in Texas; and in the south of Florida *B. microplus* persisted. Elimination of the Florida population was completed by 1943, and although there were limited subsequent outbreaks no *Boophilus* has been found in Florida since 1960.[12] During this campaign no evidence of resistance to acaricides in either *B. annulatus* or *B. microplus* was detected.

Acaricidal Resistance. In other parts of the world similar programmes have been thwarted by the development of resistance in *B. microplus.* Resistance to arsenic appeared before 1940 in Australia; to DDT and other chlorinated hydrocarbons in the early 1950s; and to organophosphorus acaricides and carbamates in the late 1960s.[46] The range of potential acaricides available was further reduced by the withdrawal of chlordimeform and the finding that in a tick population containing a small percentage of DDT-resistant ticks, specific pyrethroid resistance developed very rapidly.[26] Clearly it was time to look at alternative methods of control.

Controlled Dipping. Dipping can be made more efficient and less frequent, which should slow down the appearance of resistance, by concentrating attack on the ticks at the most vulnerable points in their life system. These are during the spring rise of larvae, in the autumn to kill the females that will produce the overwintering larvae, and in late winter when those overwintering larvae will be on the host.[27,46]

Pasture Spelling. Since unfed larvae can only survive for three to four months in pasture, a high degree of control can be obtained by pasture spelling which involves grazing cattle on alternate paddocks with intervals of three to four months in each paddock alternately. This can be highly effective.[46, 48] It does, however, produce problems in farm management and is not always practical.

Tick-Resistant Hosts. Reference has already been made to the fact that cattle vary in their resistance to ticks. All cattle are equally susceptible initially but some develop resistance on challenge.[46] Brahman cattle, for example, are 99 per cent resistant, i.e. only 1 per cent of the larvae survive to give engorged females.[46] In general, European breeds, e.g. Friesian and Hereford, have very low resistance (15 per cent survival) but Jersey cattle are unexpectedly resistant (2 per cent).[46] Programmes of breeding are being undertaken to combine tick resistance with the other qualities which are involved in good dairy and beef cattle.

Development of resistance to ticks by the host is not universal. Dogs do not become immune to *R. sanguineus* nor do sheep to *A. hebraeum*.[49] A variety of immunological responses are involved. The saliva of ixodid ticks contains a range of compounds with varying functions either within the tick or on its host, and it is likely that many of these will be important antigens.[49] Sutherst and Utech[43] have studied the ways of measuring resistance and increasing its expression by appropriate culling of susceptible animals.

Economic Importance

Two separate issues are involved in controlling *B. microplus*. There is the direct damage caused by the presence of large numbers of ticks, the so-called tick burden, and the indirect effect of the tick as a vector of babesiosis in cattle. Eradication, if it can be achieved, would be the ideal answer in both cases, but elimination of the vector tick followed by its reintroduction can be more damaging because the cattle will have lost their immunity. Cattle infected early in life develop immunity without developing clinical disease and maintain their immunity throughout adult life. Non-immune adult cattle develop clinical disease. The aim should be to maintain tick infestation at a level which confers immunity on the young beasts so that there is no clinical disease and at the same time infestation is not heavy enough to cause direct damage. In Australia this result can be achieved by limiting numbers of engorged female *B. microplus* to about 10 per beast per day.[46]

Economic Importance of Ixodid Ticks

In 1906 economic loss due to *B. annulatus* in the USA was estimated at 130 million dollars per annum which in 1976 terms would be of the order of a billion dollars.[12] Even when *B. annulatus* and *B. microplus* had been eradicated, tick losses in the cattle and sheep industries were estimated to be 65 million dollars in 1965.[39] In Australia the cost to the cattle industry of tick control in 1975 was estimated at 40 million dollars, of which one third was the cost of control and two thirds loss in production.[42] Heavy tick infestations damage hides, and cause a loss in live-weight gain which has been estimated at 1 kg per beast per year for every 1,400 tick-years, or the equivalent of four female ticks dropping per day over a year.[42] Heavy infestations of *Haemaphysalis hoodi* can cause the death of poultry.[21]

The more important role of ixodid ticks is as vectors of a wide range of pathogens of man and domestic animals. These include the agents of theileriasis and babesiosis of cattle, which are dealt with in Chapter 28. Ixodid ticks transmit tick typhus (*Rickettsia* spp) to man, and other rickettsial diseases and anaplasmosis to domestic animals (see Chapter 25). They are also involved in the transmission of arboviruses to man, including Crimean-Congo haemorrhagic fever and Kyasanur Forest disease, and other arboviruses to domestic animals (see Chapter 24). Ixodid ticks are also involved in the transmission of tularaemia, a disease which affects man and sheep (see Chapter 26). Recently in Australia and the USA ticks of the genus *Ixodes* have been associated with Lyme arthritis, the aetiological agent of which is not known for certain.[7]

Tick Paralysis

Paralysis in man caused by ticks has been known since 1843 in Australia, and 1912, possibly earlier, in the United States.[24] At the onset, paralysis affects the lower limbs ascending to the torso, upper limbs and head regions within a few hours. Typically it is an ascending, symmetrical paralysis involving all limbs.[9] Forty-three different species of ticks belonging to ten genera have been associated with this condition in man and/or animals but the connection is not necessarily proven in all these species.[9] From the human standpoint the most important paralysis-causing ticks are *Ixodes holocyclus* in Australia, *Dermacentor andersoni* in western North America and *D. variabilis* in eastern North America.[9, 24]

Paralysis is associated with the feeding of a female tick and first symptoms occur five to seven days after attachment and 'a single female tick suffices to completely paralyse and kill an adult human'.[9] The toxin involved is not the same in the different species. 'Removal of *D. andersoni* usually leads to an immediate improvement whereas this does not necessarily occur in *I. holocyclus* and the animal (or man) may subsequently die.'[40] In the case of *I. holocyclus* an effective hyperimmune serum has been developed for the treatment of animals and man. This serum is ineffective against *D. andersoni*.

I. holocyclus is present in the moist, densely vegetated areas of eastern coastal Australia. It was originally a parasite of the native monotreme and marsupial fauna, but now parasitises introduced cattle, dogs and cats, frequently causing paralysis in the first two.[35] Animals that have been attacked develop immunity to further paralysis. In South Africa tick paralysis was recognised in sheep in 1890. The species involved are *I. ribicundus* and *R. eversti eversti.*[9]

Argasid ticks of the subgenus *Persicargas* can cause paralysis among poultry through the feeding of their larvae, which attach and feed for days as do ixodid ticks.

Two reviews of tick paralysis have recently appeared. One by Murnaghan and O'Rourke[24] gives a broad coverage of the topic and the other by Gothe *et al.*[9] gives a detailed account of the mechanisms of pathogenicity in *Dermacentor, I. holocyclus* and *A.(P.) walkerae.* In a comparative study of three species of *Argas (Persicargas)* it was found that there was 'nearly direct proportional relation between the intensity of infestation and the clinical manifestation',[10] and in order of pathogenicity the species could

446 *Ixodida — Ixodidae (Hard ticks)*

be arranged in descending order as *A.(P.) arboreus, A.(P.) walkerae* and *A.(P.) persicus.*[10] In a further set of experiments involving two other species of *Argas (Persicargas)* similar results were obtained, and the order of pathogenicity was *A.(P.) radiatus, A.(P.) persicus* and *A.(P.) sanchezi.*[8]

Binnington and Kemp[4] have pointed out that there is no apparent advantage to the tick to cause paralysis of its host, and put forward the suggestion that the toxic substance may have an important function in tick feeding. Bandicoots, which are natural hosts of *I. holocyclus,* do not develop paralysis unless they have been reared tick-free, and it is considered that exposure to larvae and nymphs of *I. holocyclus* throughout much of the year could stimulate the bandicoots' immunity to the toxin.[40]

References

1. Arthur, D. R. (1962). *Ticks and Disease.* Pergamon Press, Oxford
2. _____ (1965). Ticks of the genus *Ixodes* in Africa. Athlone Press, London
3. _____ (1966). The ecology of ticks with reference to the transmission of protozoa. pp. 61-84 in *Biology of Parasites,* E.J.L. Soulsby (ed.), Academic Press, London
4. Binnington, K.C. and Kemp, D. H. (1980). Role of tick salivary glands in feeding and disease transmission. *Advances in Parasitology 18:* 315-39
5. Branagan, D. (1973). The developmental periods of the ixodid tick *Rhipicephalus appendiculatus* Neum. under laboratory conditions. *Bulletin of Entomological Research 63:* 155-68
6. _____ (1973) Observations on the development and survival of the ixodid tick *Rhipicephalus appendiculatus* Neumann, 1901 under quasi-natural conditions in Kenya. *Tropical Animal Health and Production 5:* 153-65
7. Fraser, J.R. E. (1982). Lyme disease challenges Australian clinicians. *Medical Journal of Australia, February 6:* 101-2
8. Gothe, R. and Englert, R. (1978). Quantitative Untersuchungen zur Toxinwirkung von Larven neoarktischer *Persicargas* spp. bei Hühnern. *Zentralblatt für Veterinärmedizin Reihe B 25:* 122-33
9. _____ Kunze, K. and Hoogstraal, H. (1979). The mechanism of pathogenicity in the tick paralyses. *Journal of Medical Entomology 16:* 357-69
10. _____ and Verhalen, K.H. (1975). Zur Paralyse-induzierenden Kapizität verschiedener *Persicargas*-Arten und -Populationen bei Hühnern. *Zentralblatt für Veterinärmedizin Reihe B 22:* 98-112
11. Graf. J.F. (1975). Écologie et Éthologie d'*Ixodes ricinus* L. en Suisse (Ixodoidea; Ixodidae). Cinquième note: mise en évidence d'une phéromone sexualle chez *Ixodes ricinus. Acarologia 17:* 436-41
12. Graham, O.H. and Hourrigan, J.L. (1977). Eradication programs for the arthropod parasites of livestock. *Journal of Medical Entomology 13:* 629-58
13. Hoogstraal, H. (1956). *African Ixodoidea. I. Ticks of the Sudan (with special reference to Equatoria Province and with Preliminary Reviews of the Genera Boophilus, Margaropus and Hyalomma).* Research Report NM 005 050.29.07, Bureau of Medicine and Surgery, Department of Navy, Washington
14. _____ (1978). Biology of ticks. pp. 3-14 in *Tick-borne Diseases and their Vectors,* J.K.H. Wilde (ed.), Centre for Tropical Veterinary Medicine, University of Edinburgh
15. _____ Roberts, F.H.S., Kohls, G.M. and Tipton, V.J. (1968). Review of *Haemaphysalis (Kaiseriana) longicornis* Neumann (resurrected) of Australia, New Zealand, New Caledonia, Fiji, Japan, Korea and north-eastern China and USSR, and its parthenogenetic and bisexual populations (Ixodoidea, Ixodidae). *Journal of Parasitology 54:* 1197-1213
16. Kaufman, W.R. (1979). Control of salivary fluid secretion in ixodid ticks. pp. 357-63 in

volume I, *Recent Advances in Acarology*, J.G. Rodriguez (ed.), Academic Press, New York

17. Lees, A.D. (1946). Chloride regulation and the function of the coxal glands in ticks. *Parasitology 37*: 172-84

18. _____ (1946). The water balance in *Ixodes ricinus* L. and certain other species of ticks. *Parasitology 37*: 1-20

19. _____ (1947). Transpiration and the structure of the epicuticle in ticks. *Journal of Experimental Biology 23*: 379-410

20. _____ Beament, J.W.L. (1948). An egg-waxing organ in ticks. *Quarterly Journal of Microscopical Science 89*: 291-332

21. Lucas, J.M.S. (1954). Fatal anaemia in poultry caused by heavy tick infestation. *Veterinary Record 66*: 573-4

22. McCulloch, B., Kalaye, W.J., Tungaraza, R., Suda, B'Q.J. and Mbasha, E.M.S. (1968). A study of the life history of the tick *Rhipicephalus appendiculatus* — the main vector of east coast fever — with reference to its behaviour under field conditions and with regard to its control in Sukumaland, Tanzania. *Bulletin of Epizootic Diseases of Africa 16*: 477-500

23. Moorhouse, D.E. (1969). The attachment of some ixodid ticks to their natural hosts. *Proceedings of the 2nd International Congress of Acarology*: 319-27

24. Murnaghan, M.F. and O'Rourke, F.J. (1978). Tick paralysis. pp. 419-64 in *Arthropod Venoms*, S. Bettini (ed.), Springer-Verlag, New York

25. Newson, R.M. (1978). The life cycle of *Rhipicephalus appendiculatus* on the Kenyan coast. pp. 46-50 in *Tick-borne Diseases and their Vectors*. J.K.H. Wilde (ed.), Centre for Tropical Veterinary Medicine, University of Edinburgh

26. Nolan, J., Roulston, W.J. and Schnitzerling, H.J. (1979). The potential of some synthetic pyrethroids for control of the cattle tick (*Boophilus microplus*). *Australian Veterinary Journal 55*: 463-6

27. Norris, K.R. (1957). Strategic dipping for control of the cattle tick, *Boophilus microplus* (Canestrini), in south Queensland. *Australian Journal of Agricultural Research 8*: 768-87

28. Oliver, J.H., Al-Ahmadi, Z. and Osburn, R.L. (1974). Reproduction in ticks (Acari: Ixodoidea). 3. Copulation in *Dermacentor occidentalis* Marx and *Haemaphysalis leporispalustris* (Packard) (Ixodidae). *Journal of Parasitology 60*: 499-506

29. Payne, R.C. and Purnell, R.E. (1975). The effect of induced activity on the survival of the brown ear tick, *Rhipicephalus appendiculatus*, under laboratory conditions. *Bulletin of Animal Health and Production in Africa 23*: 297-301

30. Punyua, D.K. and Newson, R.M. (1979). Diurnal activity behaviour of *Rhipicephalus appendiculatus* in the field. pp. 441-5 in volume I, *Recent Advances in Acarology*, J.G. Rodriguez (ed.), Academic Press, New York

31. Rechav. Y, (1981). Ecological factors affecting the seasonal activity of the brown ear tick *Rhipicephalus appendiculatus*. pp. 187-91 in *Tick Biology and Control*, G.B. Whitehead and J.D. Gibson (eds.), Tick Research Unit, Rhodes University, Grahamstown

32. _____ and Whitehead, G.B. (1979). Male produced pheromones of Ixodidae. pp. 291-5 in volume II, *Recent Advances in Acarology*, J.G. Rodriguez (ed.), Academic Press, New York

33. Roberts, F.H.S. (1952). *Insects Affecting Livestock*. Angus and Robertson, Sydney

34. Rudolph, D. and Knulle, W. (1979). Mechanisms contributing to water balance in nonfeeding ticks and their ecological implications. pp. 375-83 in volume I, *Recent Advances in Acarology*, J.G. Rodriguez (ed.), Academic Press, New York

35. Seddon, H.R. and Albiston, H.E. (1968). *Diseases of Domestic Animals in Australia. Part 3 Arthropod Infestations (Ticks and Mites)*. Department of Health, Commonwealth of Australia.

36. Short, N.J. and Norval, R.A.I. (1981). The seasonal activity of *Rhipicephalus appendiculatus* Neumann 1901 (Acarina: Ixodidae) in the highveld of Zimbabwe Rhodesia. *Journal of Parasitology 67*: 77-84

37. Snowball, G.J. (1957). Ecological observations on the cattle tick, *Boophilus microplus* (Canestrini). *Australian Journal of Agricultural Research 8*: 394-413

38. Sonenshine, D.E., Silverstein, R.M. and Homsher, P.J. (1979). Female produced

pheromones of Ixodidae. pp. 281-90 in volume II, *Recent Advances in Acarology*, J.G. Rodriguez (ed.), Academic Press, New York

39. Steelman, C.D. (1976). Effects of external and internal arthropod parasites on domestic livestock production. *Annual Review of Entomology 21*: 155-78
40. Stone, B.F., Doube, B.M., Binnington, K.C. and Goodger, B.V. (1979). Toxins of the Australian paralysis tick *Ixodes holocyclus*. pp. 347-56 in volume I, *Recent Advances in Acarology*, J.G. Rodriguez (ed.), Academic Press, New York
41. Sutherst, R.W., Dallwitz, M.J., Utech, K.B.W. and Kerr, J.D. (1978). Aspects of host finding by the cattle tick, *Boophilus microplus*. *Australian Journal of Zoology 26*: 159-74
42. _____ Norton, G.A., Barlow, N.D., Conway, G.R., Birley, M. and Comins, H.N. (1979). An analysis of management strategies for cattle tick (*Boophilus microplus*) control in Australia. *Journal of Applied Ecology 16*: 359-82
43. _____ and Utech, K.B.W. (1981). Controlling livestock parasites with host resistance. pp. 385-407 in volume II, *CRC Handbook of Pest Management in Agriculture*, CRC Press, Boca Raton, Florida
44. _____ Utech, K.B.W., Kerr, J.D. and Wharton, R.H. (1979). Density dependent mortality of the tick, *Boophilus microplus*, on cattle — further observations. *Journal of Applied Ecology 16*: 397-403
45. Treverrow, N.L., Stone, B.F. and Cowie, M. (1977). Aggregation pheromones in two Australian hard ticks, *Ixodes holocyclus* and *Aponomma concolor*. *Experentia 33*: 680-2
46. Wharton, R.H. and Norris, K.R. (1980). Control of parasitic arthropods. *Veterinary Parasitology 6*: 135-64
47. Wilkinson, P.R. (1953). Observations on the sensory physiology and behaviour of larvae of the cattle tick, *Boophilus microplus* (Can.) (Ixodidae). *Australian Journal of Zoology 1*: 345-56
48. _____ (1957). The spelling of pasture in cattle tick control. *Australian Journal of Agricultural Research 8*: 414-23
49. Willadsen, P. (1980). Immunity to ticks. *Advances in Parasitology 18*: 293-313
50. Wilson, S.G. (1946). Seasonal occurrence of Ixodidae on cattle in Northern Province, Nyasaland. *Parasitology 37*: 118-25
51. _____ (1950). A check-list and host-list of Ixodoidea found in Nyasaland, with descriptions and biological notes on some of the rhipicephalids. *Bulletin of Entomological Research 41*: 415-28
52. Yeoman, G.H. (1966). Field vector studies of epizootic east coast fever. II. Seasonal studies of *R.appendiculatus* on bovine and non-bovine hosts in east coast fever enzootic, epizootic and free areas. *Bulletin of Epizootic Diseases of Africa 14*: 113-40
53. _____ and Walker, J.B. (1967). *The Ixodid Ticks of Tanzania*. Commonwealth Institute of Entomology, London

PART III:
DISEASES OF WHICH THE PATHOGENS ARE TRANSMITTED
BY INSECTS OR ACARINES

24 ARBOVIRUSES

Viruses transmitted to vertebrates by insects and acarines are known as arboviruses. The term simply means arthropod (ar) borne (bo) viruses. Originally the term was arborviruses but this suggested associations with trees and the second 'r' was omitted. Arboviruses are defined as viruses which multiply in both their vertebrate and invertebrate hosts, and the term is therefore restricted to viruses which are transmitted biologically. It excludes viruses which are transmitted mechanically, such as the virus of myxomatosis which is spread among rabbits in England by the rabbit flea (*Spilopsyllus cuniculi*) and in Australia by mosquitoes; and the viruses of hog cholera and equine infectious anaemia which are transmitted mechanically by tabanids.[30,76]

In the 1950s about 30 arboviruses were recognised but in the 1960s and 1970s improved techniques led to a rapid increase in their recognition, and at the end of 1978 the total stood at 388.[43] The classification used here is that of Matthews.[48] The criteria for a virus being an arbovirus is based on its biology and ecology and not on its morphology, consequently arboviruses are found in several families of viruses including the Togaviridae, Bunyaviridae, Rhabdoviridae and Reoviridae. The greatest number of important viruses is in the Togaviridae.

The account given here of arboviruses and the diseases they cause will have an entomological bias. The medical aspects are to be found in Manson-Bahr and Apted[47] and Woodruff,[81] and the veterinary aspects in Blood *et al.*[7] Details of virus structure and taxonomy are dealt with in Matthews,[48] Andrewes *et al.*[2] and Theiler and Downs.[75]

In common with other pathogens there is interest in how arboviruses survive from season to season and spread from endemic areas to areas previously free from infection. It used to be considered that arbovirus infections were restricted to the adult insect vector and did not pass to the next generation, while infections in acarines often passed from one generation to another by transovarian transmission. This view was first queried with regard to the virus of sandfly fever, where there was epidemiological evidence for transovarian transmission in *Phlebotomus papatasi*. It was then undermined by it being demonstrated that La Crosse virus overwintered in larvae of *Aedes triseriatus*.[78] More recently the original view has been seriously questioned as a result of experiments showing that the viruses of yellow fever, Japanese encephalitis and St Louis encephalitis, can be passed transovarially to the progeny of *Ae aegypti*, *Cx tritaeniorhynchus* and *Cx tarsalis*, respectively.[6,59,63] The epidemiological significance of these findings is still being assessed.

Some arboviruses, such as bluetongue and African horsesickness, have spread widely in the last 30 years. These diseases could have been introduced into new areas by the introduction of infected hosts but there is evidence accumulating that the wind-borne carriage of infected vectors may be an important alternative route for arbovirus dissemination.[66]

Togaviridae

In this family the virus particles or virions are spherical in shape with a diameter of 40-70 nm. The genetic material or genome is a single molecule of a single-stranded RNA with a molecular weight of 4×10^6, and forms about 4-8 per cent of the molecular weight of the virion. The virion is bounded by a lipoprotein envelope which makes the particles sensitive to ether and other lipid solvents, providing a valuable tool in the first-level separation of viruses.

Two genera of arboviruses, *Alphavirus* and *Flavivirus*, are recognised in the Togaviridae. The species within each genus are serologically related but quite distinct from species in other genera. The two genera differ in their methods of replication, and in the conditions under which they can be grown in cell culture.[79] Entomologically the most important feature is that all species of *Alphavirus* are transmitted by mosquitoes while only some species of *Flavivirus* are transmitted by mosquitoes, others being transmitted by acarines, and for some the method of transmission is not known.

Alphaviruses were previously known as group A viruses and hence the generic name *Alphavirus*. They include such viruses as Sindbis, the type species; Ross River; O'Nyong-nyong; and three equine encephalitis viruses — eastern, western and Venezuelan.[47] Species of *Flavivirus* were previously known as group B viruses. The type species is the yellow fever virus, which explains the generic name *Flavivirus* when Betavirus might have been expected. Some other members of the genus are the dengue virus and several encephalitis viruses including Murray Valley, Japanese (formerly known as Japanese B), and St Louis. These viruses are mosquito-borne, while Kyasanur Forest disease, louping ill and Russian spring-summer encephalitis viruses are tick-borne.

The isolation and propagation of some arboviruses, e.g. dengue, have been aided by intrathoracic inoculation of material into adult *Aedes aegypti* and *Ae albopictus*. The usefulness of this technique is limited by the small size of these mosquitoes, and the danger posed by infected female mosquitoes. Rosen[61] has shown that both sexes of the large, non-blood-feeding *Toxorhynchites* mosquitoes were highly suitable for the detection and propagation of dengue virus, of which hundreds of strains had been isolated using *Tx amboinensis*. In addition the viruses of St Louis encephalitis and Japanese encephalitis replicated to very high titres in the same mosquito. Other arboviruses which also replicated in *Tx amboinensis* included some other flaviviruses; Ross River, an alphavirus; and some bunyaviruses and rhabdoviruses.[61]

Yellow Fever

Yellow fever is a disease which has had a considerable impact on man's social development. It was yellow fever which caused de Lesseps to abandon the first attempt to build the Panama Canal.[69] It was greatly feared by the inhabitants of Western Europe and was one of three diseases (cholera, plague, yellow fever) for which ships entering British waters, had to fly the special yellow and black quarantine flag, the Yellow Jack.[3] Even in the present day travellers from areas where yellow fever is endemic have to carry international certificates of vaccination against the disease. Fortunately, a fully effective vaccine is available, which probably protects for life and is currently valid for ten years.

Classically the disease in an individual followed a rapid course which often terminated fatally within a week. Epidemics occurred regularly in urban areas of tropical and subtropical America during the seventeenth, eighteenth and nineteenth centuries.[69] In recent years there have been epidemics of yellow fever in Central America (1948-57),[24] Sudan (1959),[65] Ethiopia (1959-66),[68] Senegal (1965),[11] Gambia (1978)[58] and in Ghana (1979-80).[5] Yellow fever was regarded as of such importance that in the early part of the twentieth century the Rockefeller Foundation concentrated a great deal of its funding and activity on overcoming this disease, establishing laboratories and research workers in endemic areas.[69]

Yellow fever is endemic in Africa, particularly West Africa, and in tropical Central and South America, from which it may spread into other areas. Two extreme patterns of disease are recognisable, urban epidemics involving thousands of cases and sylvan endemics involving sporadic individual cases. Walter Reed, whose name has been commemorated by the US military forces in the Walter Reed Army Institute of Research and the Walter Reed Army General Hospital, was the first to link yellow fever transmission with the mosquito *Aedes aegypti*. By instituting strict measures for the control of this mosquito General Gorgas stopped yellow fever transmission in Cuba in 1901 and then applied the same techniques successfully in Panama in 1903, enabling the Panama Canal to be completed.

Aedes aegypti becomes infected with the virus of yellow fever when it feeds on an infected man in the early stages of his disease. An infected person is infective to the mosquito from about six hours before the onset of clinical signs to about four days later. The virus undergoes a cycle in the mosquito which takes about 12 days. When that is completed the virus appears in the saliva of the mosquito, which remains infective for the rest of its life. Every time an infective mosquito feeds it passes virus into its host together with saliva. In a susceptible individual the virus will be incubated for three to six days before the onset of clinical symptoms of disease.

The reservoir of yellow fever is not to be found in urban areas experiencing a dramatic epidemic but in the sylvan setting where the disease is endemic. The virus is maintained in the forest primates of Africa and South America. In Africa one of the main vectors among the primate population is *Aedes africanus*,[27] and among South American monkeys, *Sabethes chloropterus* and *Haemagogus spegazzini*.[24] The mosquito genera *Sabethes* and *Haemagogus* are solely Neotropical in distribution.

African monkeys show no recognisable signs of disease when infected with yellow fever but some American monkeys develop disease and die. This suggests that yellow fever is a relatively recent introduction into the Neotropical region from Africa, possibly with the slave trade when there was a great deal of movement of ships across the Atlantic from Africa to the New World. Water storage containers on board would be ideal breeding sites for *Aedes aegypti* which may have been introduced into the Americas at the same time.

The dispersal of yellow fever by shipping can be demonstrated by the history of the disease in Jamaica. During the Napoleonic wars at the start of the nineteenth century yellow fever took a heavy toll of army and navy personnel stationed on the island. In an attempt to reduce the incidence of the disease the main army and naval barracks were built in the Blue Mountains 1,200 m above sea level, not the obvious place to build naval headquarters, and represented an act of desperation. Plaques in the garrison church in Port Royal at the foot of the Blue Mountains bear ample testimony to the destruction yellow fever wrought among the young servicemen.

Yellow fever disappeared from Jamaica about 1870 following cessation of the coastal schooner trade between South America and Trinidad, and the islands of the Greater and Lesser Antilles. When the schooner trade stopped, yellow fever stopped in Jamaica because of the absence of reservoir hosts on the island, but in Trinidad yellow fever continued because there monkeys are indigenous. A schooner with *Aedes aegypti* breeding in its water containers, a susceptible crew and virus present either in the mosquito or a crew member, could disseminate yellow fever at every port at which it called on its voyage.

One of the puzzles with regard to the distribution of yellow fever throughout the world is its absence from the Oriental region. There are monkeys in the Indian subcontinent which are susceptible to yellow fever and could act as reservoir hosts. *Ae aegypti* is well established in India yet yellow fever does not exist there. There is no simple answer. If the South American schooner trade could introduce yellow fever into Jamaica, Arab dhows, which sailed the coasts of the Indian Ocean, could similarly have introduced yellow fever into India. Several reasons can be put forward, none of which is entirely satisfactory.

Firstly, yellow fever is not prevalent in the coastal areas of East Africa. The coastal fringe and the main port of Mombasa are separated from the main forested area of tropical Africa by a broad belt of desert. Secondly, Arab dhows would take considerably longer to make their journey to India than those travelling in the Caribbean. In this long journey an epidemic on board an infected vessel could burn itself out with the survivors becoming immune. Lastly, there may be a maximum number of viruses offering cross-immunity, as do those of the *Flavivirus* group, which are able to sustain themselves in a given ecosystem. The Oriental region already has several members of the *Flavivirus* genus, including dengue, Japanese encephalitis and Kyasanur Forest disease.

Yellow fever circulates among the monkeys of the forest and man becomes involved when he enters the enzootic area and is bitten by an infected mosquito. The man, incubating yellow fever virus, returns to the human ecosystem where he is in contact with *Ae aegypti* and the scene is then set for an outbreak of urban yellow fever. Interchange between the two ecosystems can also be achieved by monkeys entering the human ecosystem.

In western Uganda yellow fever circulates among the forest monkeys through *Ae africanus.* Monkeys are attracted into groves of bananas planted by man. While there the monkeys are exposed to attack by day-biting *Ae simpsoni* which breeds in water accumulating in the axils of plants including bananas. *Ae simpsoni* is susceptible to infection with yellow fever virus and readily bites both monkeys and man, making it potentially a very important vector.[27] Indeed, it is considered that *Ae simpsoni* was the main vector of yellow fever during the Ethiopian epidemic of the early 1960s, which was a rural rather than an urban epidemic.[53, 68]

In the Sudan epidemic of 1959 *Ae vittatus,* a rock hole breeding species, was considered to be the vector between monkeys and man, and together with *Ae aegypti* transmitted yellow fever virus among the human population.[65] All the *Aedes* species mentioned so far — *Ae aegypti, Ae simpsoni, Ae africanus, Ae vittatus* — are members of the subgenus *Stegomyia,* a group of black mosquitoes with silvery markings. In The Gambia, species of the subgenus *Diceromyia* belonging to the *Ae furcifer/taylori* complex were considered to be involved in transmission of yellow fever but their precise role was not resolved.[58]

Dengue Virus[47,81]

Dengue or break-bone fever is widely distributed throughout the tropics and subtropics (Figure 24.1). It probably originated as a rural infection in tropical Asia,[81] but has spread with *Ae aegypti* to other parts of the tropics and subtropics and is now endemic in south-east Asia, the Pacific area,

Figure 24.1: World Distribution of Dengue Infections Based on Virus Isolation from Man Within the Past Decade, or Areas Considered Permissive to Dengue Because of the Prevalence of Urban *Aedes aegypti*

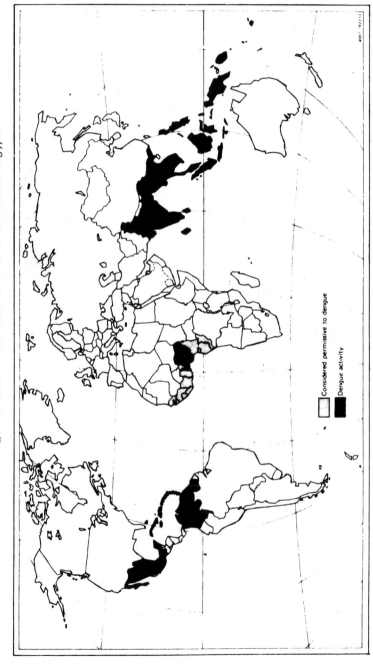

Source: from Halstead (1980)[28]

Africa and the Americas (Figure 24.1).[46] The vectors of dengue to man are species of the subgenus *Stegomyia* of *Aedes*, particularly *Ae aegypti*, *Ae albopictus*, *Ae scutellaris* and *Ae polynesiensis*. Until recently there had been no convincing evidence for a reservoir host other than man himself, although monkeys were suspected of being maintenance hosts. In Malaysia a forest cycle of dengue, similar to that of yellow fever, has been shown to exist among canopy-dwelling primates with the vectors being members of the *Ae (Finlaya) niveus* group.[64]

The incubation period for dengue fever is five to eight days and attacks last five to six days, often being composed of two feverish periods. There is no mortality. Recovery is complete but convalescence may be prolonged with weakness and depression lasting several weeks. Epidemics of dengue are noted for affecting a large proportion of urban communities and can seriously disrupt social organisation. An epidemic of dengue fever in Ajmer City, Rajasthan, in India in 1969 affected 34 per cent of the population.[42] The cost of an outbreak of dengue fever in Puerto Rico in 1977 was calculated to be $6.0-15.6 million in direct costs and indirect losses to the economy.[1]

There are four different serological types of dengue virus which offer only cross-immunity of short duration. Two epidemics of dengue in north Queensland were caused by Types 1 and 2 in 1942-44 and by Type 3 in 1953-55, with a significant number of people being affected in both epidemics. Three of the four known types of dengue virus have been isolated from sentinel monkeys, maintained in high canopy forest in Malaysia.[64]

Dengue Haemorrhagic Fever[28]

Dengue haemorrhagic fever (DHF) and the associated dengue shock syndrome (DSS) were confined originally to south-east Asia, but in 1981 DHF/DSS was reported from Cuba.[4] According to Manson-Bahr and Apted[47] this disease was first recognised in Manila in 1953, spreading to Thailand where it caused 150,000 to 200,000 cases. Halstead[28] calculates that since 1956 (his article appeared in 1980) over 350,000 patients have been hospitalised and nearly 12,000 deaths have been reported from DHF/DSS.

DHF has been associated with all four types of dengue virus. It differs from classical dengue fever by being largely restricted to young children under 15 years of age, and by being a much more severe disease, terminating fatally in a small percentage of cases. When the condition passes to DSS mortalities are much higher, occurring in 10 to 40 per cent of cases.[29]

Encephalitides[7,47,81]

Six viruses of the Togaviridae can be grouped together on the grounds that they have a number of features in common and cause encephalitis in man and some other mammals. Three of these viruses — eastern equine, Venezuelan equine and western equine — are species of *Alphavirus* and three — Japanese, Murray Valley and St Louis — are species of *Flavivirus*. They are all primarily viruses of wild hosts, often birds, and are transmitted by mosquitoes. From the human point of view three cycles of the virus may be distinguished. There is a maintenance cycle in a wild host, an amplifying cycle in a susceptible domestic or wild host, and a possible cycle in the human population. In some cases the viraemia in man is inadequate to infect the vector.

Horses are particularly susceptible to these viruses and hence some of the diseases are known as equine encephalitis. Other domestic hosts may also act as amplifiers, e.g. pigs for Japanese encephalitides, and dogs and chickens for Murray Valley encephalitis. A common feature of infections in the human population is that only a small percentage of human beings that become infected with the virus actually develop clinical disease. In Murray Valley encephalitis it has been estimated that for every individual who becomes clinically ill, 700-1,000 people develop antibodies to the virus without any clinical symptoms. In almost all clinical cases encephalitis viruses do irreparable damage to the brain.

Murray Valley Encephalitis[17]

Murray Valley encephalitis (MVE) has caused epidemics in south-eastern Australia, especially in the Murray-Darling Basin, but it also occurs widely throughout Australia. Outbreaks occur at infrequent intervals and the number of cases, although small in absolute terms, is significant compared to the population at risk. The vector is *Culex annulirostris* which breeds in temporary breeding sites created by rainfall or flooding. Attempts to relate outbreaks of MVE with climatic conditions, particularly rainfall in the catchment areas, have not been particularly successful. In part, this may be due to the fact that by far the greater number of infections remain sub-clinical. Horses, dogs and chickens develop high levels of viraemia and chickens have been used as sentinel hosts to give warning of active transmission. Chickens are convenient sentinel hosts but not the most satisfactory because *Cx annulirostris* does not readily feed on birds.

Japanese Encephalitis

Japanese encephalitis is widespread in Asia causing large-scale epidemics. In Japan in the spring there is intense virus transmission among young herons by *Culex tritaeniorhynchus*. This may be regarded as an amplifying cycle among the susceptible young of the maintenance hosts. The virus then spreads to pigs, in which it causes abortion, and to horses which develop encephalitis. These are the main amplifier hosts from which the virus is transmitted to man. Mortality varies with the age group but it is always considerable and may reach nearly 40 per cent in a susceptible age class.[81]

St Louis Encephalitis (SLE)

St Louis encephalitis is restricted to the New World and is the most important mosquito-borne encephalitis in the USA.[81] It also occurs in the Caribbean and tropical South America. In the western United States the vector is *Culex tarsalis,* and the *Culex pipiens* complex which is abundant is at best a secondary vector.[59] In other parts of the country the *Cx pipiens* complex is the primary vector during epidemics. Part of the explanation for this difference is that in more eastern parts of the United States the strains of SLE virus produce higher viraemias in birds than the strains present in the western USA, and *Cx tarsalis* is more readily infected at low viraemias than is the *Cx pipiens* complex.[59] In Florida and Jamaica the vector of SLE is probably *Aedes nigripalpus.*[81]

Equine Encephalitides

Three arboviruses, which occur only in the New World, cause disease in man and horses, and are given the appellation 'equine encephalitis'. They are western, eastern and Venezuelan encephalitides.

Western Equine Encephalitis (WEE). In the western and central areas of the United States the primary vector of WEE is *Cx tarsalis.*[31] Populations of this species show considerable variation in their ability to transmit WEE.[59] *Culiseta melanura,* which is mainly an ornithophilic species, is the primary vector of WEE among the avian reservoir hosts.[31] It breeds in wooded fresh water swamps and this habitat restriction combined with its avian feeding preferences contributes to WEE not being a public or veterinary health problem in the eastern USA.[31] WEE has caused large epidemics in North America and human disease in Brazil.[81]

Eastern Equine Encephalitis (EEE). Eastern equine encephalitis virus has been recorded from the USA to the Argentine, with small outbreaks occurring in the USA, the Dominican Republic (1948-9) and Jamaica (1962).[81] The primary vector of EEE among the wild avian reservoir hosts is *Cs melanura,* and in the eastern USA *Aedes sollicitans* and *Ae vexans* are suspected of being the vectors to horses and man, as is *Ae canadensis* in New York State.[31] During outbreaks of EEE epizootics have occurred among pheasants.[81]

Venezuelan Equine Encephalitis (VEE). Venezuelan equine encephalitis is more tropical in distribution being recorded from tropical South America, Trinidad and Mexico.[81] In the 1962-3 epidemic in Venezuela and Columbia the death rate was low with about 200 deaths resulting from an estimated 30,000 cases.[81] In Panama *Culex aikenii* is both an efficient natural vector and the principal vector of VEE.[23]

Some Other Mosquito-borne Arboviruses of the Togaviridae

Ross River. Ross River virus is an alphavirus which causes a syndrome with polyarthralgia, i.e. painful joints, and rash in man in Australia, New Guinea and the Solomon Islands. The condition is often referred to as polyarthritis, i.e. inflamed joints. Fever is rarely an important symptom of the disease, but the arthralgia may last for a month, and in extreme cases for up to eight months.[81] In Australia the virus occurs commonly in large mammals such as cattle, horses, kangaroos and wallabies.[18] The vectors of Ross River virus in Australia are *Aedes vigilax* and *Culex annulirostris*, the former being restricted to coastal areas.[17] They are probably vectors of the virus elsewhere in their range.

In 1979 and 1980 Ross River virus spread eastwards in the Pacific, occurring in epidemic form in Fiji in the first half of 1979, in American Samoa in the second half of 1979, and in Rarotonga, an island of the Cook group, early in 1980.[62] The vector in Rarotonga was *Aedes polynesiensis*, from which six isolations of the virus were made, and virus transmission by bite was successfully achieved in the laboratory.[62] For the first time many isolations of virus were made from patients by inoculating undiluted human sera into intact *Tx amboinensis* mosquitoes.[62]

O'Nyong-nyong. O'Nyong-nyong virus is an alphavirus which caused an epidemic in Uganda in 1959, one unusual feature of which was that the vectors were *Anopheles gambiae* and *An funestus*, the main vectors of malaria in tropical Africa, and consequently outbreaks of O'Nyong-nyong coincided with outbreaks of malaria. Cases of O'Nyong-nyong were detected early in the epidemic, and the staff of the East African Virus Research Institute were able to follow the course of the virus as it spread eastwards from Uganda across East Africa to the Indian Ocean. There were no sequelae or deaths due directly to the disease.[81]

Chikungunya. Chikungunya virus is an alphavirus which is distributed in Africa and the Oriental region. It is frequently associated with dengue haemorrhagic fever and causes a similar disease in man but without shock. Like dengue fever Chikungunya is not a life-threatening disease and the death rate is very low. Large urban epidemics of Chikungunya virus have occurred in the Oriental region where the vector is *Ae aegypti*. In a rural epidemic of Chikungunya in the wooded savannah of the eastern Transvaal, South Africa, the vector was *Ae furcifer/taylori* which was transmitting the virus among baboons and man. Baboons were regarded as the primary vertebrate host from which the virus extended into the human population.[49]

Sindbis and West Nile. Sindbis, an alphavirus, and West Nile, a flavivirus, cause mild disease in man which, in many cases, goes undetected. Sindbis virus occurs in Africa, India, Malaysia, the Philippines and Australia, and causes a fairly rare febrile illness with vesicular rash.[81] In Australia there have been several recoveries of Sindbis virus from *Cx annulirostris*.[17] West Nile virus has been isolated in Egypt, Uganda, Congo, South Africa, India, Borneo, France, and has been epidemic in Israel.[81] In France, West Nile virus affects man and horses in which it causes encephalitis.[81] The avian hosts are pigeons and crows and the vectors species of *Culex*, including *Cx modestus*, a Palaearctic species, and *Cx antennatus* which occurs in Egypt, and East and West Africa.[47]

In an epidemic in an arid region of South Africa in 1974, 55 per cent of the human population had been infected by West Nile virus and 16 per cent by Sindbis virus. Isolations of both viruses were made from *Culex univittatus* and *Cx theileri*. The major vector was *Cx univittatus*, a species which is usually ornithophilic but which also feeds on man. It is believed that an epizootic occurred among wild birds at the same time and that these were the source of infection to *Cx univittatus* and man.[50]

Some Tick-borne Flaviviruses [32,34]

Kyasanur Forest Disease. Kyasanur Forest disease virus (KFD) was detected in India in 1957 when an epidemic in the human population was associated with an epizootic in monkeys, with deaths occurring in both humans and monkeys. The mortality among human cases is of the order of 2-5 per cent. Isolations of virus have been made from seven species of *Haemaphysalis* ticks of which the most important is *H. spinigera* in which transstadial transmission but not transovarian transmission occurs. KFD virus has been recovered from a variety of small rodents, squirrels and shrews which are probably the maintenance hosts of KFD with monkeys acting as amplifying hosts. The emergence of KFD as a human disease resulted from a rapidly increasing human population having increased contact with the forest. Cattle were grazed in and beside the forest, providing additional hosts for *H. spinigera*, and greater numbers of people visited the forest to collect firewood and other forest products.

Russian Spring-Summer Encephalitis and Tick-borne Encephalitis. The viruses causing Russian spring-summer encephalitis (RSSE) and tick-borne encephalitis (TBE) were regarded as subtypes of the same virus[48] which caused different diseases and had different geographical distributions. Hoogstraal[34] is of the opinion that two different viruses are involved with separate epidemiologies: RSSE occurring in the eastern Palaearctic region in Siberia, southern USSR and north-eastern China; while TBE occurs in Europe including the European part of the USSR.

The vectors of both viruses are species of *Ixodes* ticks. *I. persulcatus* is the main vector of RSSE, and *I. ricinus* of TBE. Both viruses survive in the ticks by transstadial and transovarial transmission. RSSE was classified as an occupational disease of forest workers but in the last 20 years has affected urban residents of Soviet Siberian towns, who become infected when relaxing in the adjoining countryside. In the 1960s, 65-80 per cent of RSSE cases were contracted within 3-8 km of towns.[34] A large range of small forest mammals and birds circulate RSSE virus and provide hosts for larvae and nymphs of *I. persulcatus*. Adult *I. persulcatus* parasitise larger wild and domestic mammals.[32]

TBE has been reported in Europe from France to the Urals but not from the Benelux countries or the Iberian peninsula. Outbreaks have occurred recently in Germany and central Europe among visitors to forests or rural regions. Transmission of TBE can also occur through consuming fresh milk or cheese from infected goats or sheep.[34]

Omsk Haemorrhagic Fever. The virus of Omsk haemorrhagic fever (OHF) was first isolated in 1947 from human cases occurring in south-western Siberia.[32] It was considered to be an arbovirus transmitted by ixodid ticks. Virus was recovered from *Dermacentor pictus*, which could transmit the virus to laboratory animals during feeding.[32] 'Recent studies show that OHF virus spreads chiefly by contact with, or drinking, water containing infected urine and faeces of water-frequenting rodents and muskrats',[34] or from handling infected muskrat carcases. Ticks do not appear at present to be important vectors of OHF.

Louping Ill. Louping ill virus causes an acute encephalolyemitis in sheep and occasionally in other animals and man. It is recorded only from Scotland, the border counties of England, and Ireland.[7] In enzootic areas morbidity is low in adult sheep (1-4 per cent), but may be as high as 60 per cent in lambs. The mortality rate is of the order of 10 to 15 per cent.[7] The main vector is the sheep tick, *I. ricinus*, in which transstadial but not transovarian transmission occurs. The virus or antibodies to it have been demonstrated in a range of wild birds and mammals and it possible that other ixodid ticks may maintain the virus among these vertebrates.[32]

Bunyaviridae

Viruses of the Bunyaviridae have spherical virions, 90-100 nm diameter, surrounded by a lipid envelope with glycoprotein projections. The lipids form about one third of the weight of the virus particle. The genome consists of three molecules of single-stranded RNA with a total molecular weight of $5\text{-}6 \times 10^6$. They multiply in the cytoplasm and mature by budding.[48] The Bunyaviridae includes agents such as Phlebotomus fever;

Crimean-Congo haemorrhagic fever; Oropouche and La Crosse viruses which cause disease in man; and Akabane, Rift Valley fever and Nairobi sheep disease, which are solely or mainly of concern as agents of disease in livestock.

Phlebotomus Fever and La Crosse Viruses

More than 27 viruses are included in the Phlebotomus fever group of which the Sicilian and Naples strains of sandfly fever are the most important.[47, 48] They cause a short, sharp, non-fatal fever in man. Sandfly fever occurs in the Mediterranean region from Italy eastwards through the desert regions of the Middle East and Central Asia to Pakistan.[75] The vector is *Phlebotomus papatasi* and the fever is also known as papatasi fever. Man is the only known host of sandfly fever and it has been suspected that the virus overwinters in the *Phlebotomus* population, passing from one generation to another by transovarian transmission. This has not been proved conclusively but weight is given to this proposition by the demonstration that La Crosse virus, another member of the Bunyaviridae, is transmitted transovarially in *Aedes triseriatus*.[78] La Crosse virus is a Nearctic species which circulates in chipmunks, rabbits and squirrels, and is one cause of California encephalitis in man. *Ae triseriatus* is a tree-hole breeder, which overwinters in the larval stage. These larvae may be infected with the virus and give rise to adults which are capable of transmitting it at their first feed. Therefore cases are likely to occur in the spring.

Oropouche Virus[22,55,56]

Oropouche virus (ORO) was first isolated in 1955 in Trinidad, and since then has caused several epidemics in Brazil. Between 1961 and 1979 there have been eight outbreaks of ORO in Para State, Brazil, in small and large urban communities. Infection with ORO causes an acute febrile illness with general aches and pains, which usually lasts for two to five days. No deaths have been reported, although a proportion of patients become severely ill. In the 1967 outbreak in Bragança and in 1975 in Santarém over 30,000 people became infected.

ORO virus has been isolated from *Culex quinquefasciatus* and *Culicoides paraensis*, the latter proving to be the more efficient vector in the laboratory with transmission rates varying from 25 to 83 per cent for *C. paraensis* and less than 5 per cent for *Cx quinquefasciatus* under the same conditions. *C. paraensis* is capable of transmitting ORO four to nine days after feeding on a viraemic hamster.[55] The maximum duration of the urban cycle is apparently only six months and it is likely that there is a sylvatic cycle. Isolations of virus have been made from the three-toed sloth (*Bradypus tridactylus*), and antibodies against ORO have been found in several genera of monkeys. *C. paraensis* is active during the daytime reaching peak activity just before sunset, and feeds on humans both inside and outside houses.[60]

Crimean-Congo Haemorrhagic Fever[33]

The epidemiology of Crimean-Congo haemorrhagic fever (CCHF) has recently been reviewed by Hoogstraal.[33] CCHF virus is enzootic in the Palaearctic, Oriental and Afrotropical regions, chiefly in steppe, savanna, semi-desert and foothill biotopes where one or two *Hyalomma* species are the predominant ticks parasitising domestic and wild animals. Human infections may be clinically inapparent but among CCHF patients mortality rates have ranged from 15-40 per cent or higher. Infection occurs through the bite of the infected tick or by crushing infected ticks in contact with the skin or from shearing tick-infested sheep.

CCHF virus survives transstadially and interseasonally in several tick species and is transmitted transovarially in members of the *Hyalomma marginatum* complex. Twenty-seven tick species and subspecies have been reported to be CCHF reservoirs or vectors. These include one-host ticks of the genus *Boophilus*, two-host ticks of the genus *Hyalomma*, including the *H. marginatum* complex, *H. anatolicum anatolicum* and *Rhipicephalus bursa.* Three-host ticks of the genera *Haemaphysalis, Amblyomma, Dermacentor, Hyalomma* and *Rhipicephalus* serve chiefly to maintain enzootic foci of CCHF virus circulation between ticks and wild and domestic animals.

Ticks of the *H. marginatum* complex and *H. anatolicum* are especially important in causing epidemics and outbreaks of CCHF on account of their great numbers and their aggressiveness in seeking human hosts. Epidemics of CCHF occur under a combination of favourable conditions and environmental changes which favour the survival of large numbers of hyalommas and of their hosts. Unusually severe winter-spring weather results in a reduction of the *Hyalomma* populations and is responsible for virus circulation reverting from epizootic (epidemic) to enzootic intensity.

Rift Valley Fever

Rift Valley fever (RVF) occurs only in Africa, where it causes an acute, febrile disease of cattle, sheep and man, characterised by high mortality in lambs and calves, and abortion in adult sheep and cattle.[7] In 1951 a very severe epidemic of RVF occurred in South Africa with more than 100,000 deaths in sheep and cattle, and an estimated 20,000 human cases.[75] In 1975 there was another extensive outbreak of RVF in South Africa in which thousands of livestock died, and there were many human cases with seven deaths.[25] RVF is mosquito-borne with the major vectors in South Africa being *Aedes caballus* and *Culex theileri,* and in Uganda *Eretmopodites chrysogaster.*[25,70] Human infections may result from being bitten by infected mosquitoes but in six of the seven fatalities previously referred to, infection was considered to have occurred from contact with infected animal tissues.[25]

In 1977-8 there was a widespread epizootic in Egypt and an epidemic which involved an estimated 18,000 cases and 598 deaths.[39] The most ubiquitous and prevalent species in the Nile Valley and Delta was the *Cx pipiens* complex, and RVF was isolated from unengorged mosquitoes. Laboratory transmission of RVF by *Cx pipiens* implicated it as the chief vector in Egypt.[35] Human infections occurred through handling infected carcases and by inhaling natural virus aerosols.[35]

Nairobi Sheep Disease[14,15]

Nairobi sheep disease (NSD) is a severe disease of sheep and goats in which mortality may reach 90 per cent. The vector is the three-host tick *Rhipicephalus appendiculatus* in which transovarian transmission occurs. No virus or antibodies to NSD have been found in wild ruminants or rodents, and the virus appears to be restricted to sheep, goats and *R. appendiculatus*. Human infections with NSD occur rarely and the disease is mild.[81]

Akabane Virus

Akabane virus occurs in cattle in Australia and Japan. In both countries Akabane virus has been incriminated in the production of teratogenic effects on calves *in utero*. Infection with Akabane virus at certain stages of pregnancy results in the cow producing a calf with deformities involving the brain (hydranencephaly) and the limbs (arthrogryposis).[12] The suspected vector of Akabane virus is *Culicoides brevitarsis* from which virus has been recovered in the field. *C. brevitarsis* is well adapted to being a vector of pathogens among cattle because its whole mode of life is dependent on cattle.[44] Female *C. brevitarsis* feed readily on them and oviposit only in naturally-lying cattle dung, in which the larvae and pupae complete their development. Male *C. brevitarsis* form swarms, which probably play a role in mating and, although male *C. brevitarsis* do not feed on blood, the arrangement and structure of their swarms are modified in the presence of cattle.

Rhabdoviridae

In the members of the Rhabdoviridae the virions are either bullet-shaped, with one convex and one truncated end, or bacilliform, with both ends convex. The virions measure 130-380 nm × 50-95 nm and are surrounded by a lipoprotein envelope with surface projections. The genome is a single molecule of single-stranded RNA with a molecular weight of $3\text{-}5 \times 10^6$ and forming 1-2 per cent of the molecular weight of the virion. This family includes members which multiply in arthropods as well as in vertebrates and some which multiply in higher plants. Two members of this family, vesicular stomatitis virus and bovine ephemeral fever virus, are arboviruses.[48]

Vesicular Stomatitis

Vesicular stomatitis is primarily a disease of horses but is assuming increasing importance as a pathogen of cattle and pigs.[7] This virus (VSV) is enzootic in the Nearctic and Neotropical regions. The morbidity rate in herds is usually low and there is no mortality. This condition has achieved some notoriety because the symptoms it produces superficially resemble foot and mouth disease, a much more serious disease.[7] VSV multiplies in *Lutzomyia trapidoi*, a phlebotomine sandfly, in which transovarian transmission occurs. The infection rate obtained in the F1 generation was 20 to 27 per cent, and infected females transmitted VSV by bite and to the F2 generation transovarially. Infection with VSV appeared to have no effect on fecundity or survival to the adult stage, although the virus multiplied during the development of the sandfly from egg to adult. Transovarian transmission also occurred in *L. ylephilator* but not in *L. sanguinaria* or *L. gomezi.*[74]

Bovine Ephemeral Fever

Bovine ephemeral fever or 3-day sickness is a disease of cattle, which is enzootic in Africa and the Oriental region and causes epizootics in Australia. In highly susceptible populations morbidity in an epizootic area may reach 100 per cent while in enzootic areas infection rates of 5-10 per cent are more common. Usually there is no mortality but when the central nervous system is involved free-ranging animals may be unable to reach water and die from dehydration. The main adverse effect of infection with bovine ephemeral fever is seen in dairy herds where milk yields will be dramatically reduced and conception of the next calf abnormally delayed.[7]

The vector is not known for certain but the virus has been recovered from *Culicoides,*[16] which are generally considered to be the most likely vectors. Bovine ephemeral fever virus has been recovered from mosquitoes in Australia but seasonal and geographical distributions of the species of mosquitoes from which the virus was recovered make it unlikely that they were important vectors.[73] The likelihood of the disease being transmitted by an insect vector is increased by the finding that the disease spreads sequentially across Australia from north to south in the direction of the prevailing winds, which are considered to disperse the insect vector population.[52]

Reoviridae

In members of this family the virion is an icosahedral particle measuring

60-80 nm. The virion has no lipoprotein envelope and indeed contains no lipid but it has two protein coats. Replication occurs in the cytoplasm. Four groups can be distinguished within this family on the basis of their hosts. Some are restricted solely to vertebrates, others to plants or insects and members of the genus *Orbivirus* to both insects and vertebrates. In species of *Orbivirus* the virion has both an inner and an outer protein shell. The genome consists of ten pieces of double-stranded RNA with a total molecular weight of 12×10^6, which is about 20 per cent of the molecular weight of the virion. Orbiviruses are sensitive to acidity with infectivity being lost at pH 3, and show reduced infectivity (ten-fold) after exposure to lipid solvents.[48] Four species of *Orbivirus* will be considered — bluetongue virus, African horsesickness virus, epizootic haemorrhagic disease of deer virus and Colorado tick virus.

Bluetongue Virus

Bluetongue virus (BTV) causes severe disease in sheep involving fever, ulceration of the tongue, enteritis and foot lesions causing lameness. In cattle most infections are inapparent although a few animals may become severely affected.[7] Originally BTV was enzootic in Africa but in the last 40 years it has become widely distributed throughout the world and is now present in all zoogeographical regions. BTV was recognised in Cyprus in 1943, but had probably been present since 1924. It appeared in Turkey in 1944, and in the United States in Texas in 1948 and in California in 1952.[38] Since then the virus has spread widely in the United States and has been isolated from ruminants in all states except North Dakota and the northern New England states.[54] In a serological survey in 1977-78 there was high prevalence of BTV antibody throughout the south-western US from California to Texas; from Nevada to western Missouri; and in north-eastern Georgia, south-western South Carolina, Florida and Puerto Rico.[51]

In 1956 BTV appeared in the Iberian peninsula where, in the first four months of the epizootic, the disease caused the death of 179,000 sheep, representing a mortality of 75 per cent among infected animals.[38] A most unusual feature of this epizootic was the disappearance of BTV from the area within four years and the absence of subsequent clinical cases.[38] By 1951 bluetongue had spread to West Pakistan, and appeared in cattle in Japan. In 1977 BTV was identified from cattle in Australia.[26]

BTV can cause very high morbidities (75 per cent) and mortalities (20-50 per cent) in susceptible sheep.[7] Control of the disease is complicated by the existence of 20 different serotypes which necessitate production of polyvalent vaccines. Four serotypes are present in the USA,[54] and three in Australia.[26] Losses from BTV infection are both direct, i.e. mortality, and indirect through abortion of pregnant ewes and reduction in quality and quantity of the fleece.[7]

Du Toit[19] was the first to implicate *Culicoides* in the transmission of

BTV, and his findings have been thoroughly confirmed by American workers, using a laboratory colony of *Culicoides variipennis*. In a series of experiments they transmitted BTV by the bite of *C. variipennis* from sheep to sheep, from sheep to cattle, from cattle to sheep and from cattle to cattle.[45] Their work included the first EM photographs of an arbovirus multiplying in an insect vector.[10]

After an infected blood meal there was a great increase in virus titre four days after the meal and a second marked increase between 10 to 14 days, after which the virus titre remained steady until the experiment was terminated after five weeks.[21] The parent colony used by the American workers had a susceptibility rate to infection with BTV of 30 per cent. By selected breeding from this parent colony Jones and Foster[40] were able to develop lines of *variipennis* which were fully susceptible or highly resistant. The possibility of the existence of resistance and susceptible strains of vector species greatly complicates the identification of insect vectors of pathogens.

Culicoides variipennis was used for laboratory experiments because it was large, for a *Culicoides* species, with a wing length of 2 mm; was relatively easily colonised; and in the field fed on cattle and sheep. However, *C. variipennis* belongs to the subgenus *Monoculicoides* which is absent from Australia and represented by only one species, *C. cornutus*, in East Africa. Other species of *Culicoides*, particularly those of the subgenus *Avaritia*, appear to be important vectors of BTV.

Du Toit's original observation was made on *C. (Avaritia) imicola* (= *pallidipennis*).[19] In Australia field and laboratory work has shown that three species of the subgenus *Avaritia* are the most likely vectors of BTV.[71,72] The possibility of the spread of disease by wind-borne dispersal of infected vectors has been proposed for BTV[67] as it has for ephemeral fever, of which *Culicoides* are also strongly suspected of being vectors. In the temperate regions bluetongue is a summer disease, a time when insect vectors will be active. In the tropics outbreaks of the disease have been associated with the rainy season when breeding sites of *Culicoides* would be more widespread. However, the association between rainfall, vector density and BTV transmission is much more complicated and the correlation between the three factors is low.[13,77]

A problem arises as to how the virus is maintained during the period when there is no active transmission. A number of wild ruminants are susceptible to infection with BTV but present information is to the effect that viraemia is comparatively short lived, i.e. 35 days.[36] Sheep that recover from infection normally develop a solid immunity to the strain with which they have been infected. However, virus has been isolated from sheep four months after an attack, and in some cases after longer periods.[7] In addition, cattle do not develop a significant immunity and could, in theory, sustain the virus over winter. Latent virus in cattle has been demonstrated by recovering virus from *C. variipennis* which had fed on cattle, and then been maintained for a period to allow viral multiplication.[46] There is no evidence for transovarian transmission in *C. variipennis.*

African Horsesickness Virus[7,37]

African horsesickness (AHS) is an acute or subacute, highly fatal disease of equines which is enzootic in Africa. In the early years of this century the disease made occasional excursions across the Red Sea and along the Nile to Palestine and Syria, e.g. the 1944 enzootic. In 1959 AHS spread eastwards into Iraq, Iran, Afghanistan, India and West Pakistan and in the same year westwards to Cyprus and Turkey. Later, in 1965-6, the disease appeared in Spain. Following the Middle East outbreak in 1960 no clinical cases have been reported from that area in the 15-year period 1963-78.[38]

The mortality rate in susceptible horses is about 90 per cent while mules suffer a lower mortality (50 per cent) and donkeys are even less susceptible. Nevertheless, the disease is a crippling one to mules and donkeys causing gross debility. It has been estimated conservatively that 300,000 equines died during the first phase of the 1960 epizootic in the Near East and south Asia. The spread of AHS has been attributed to the introduction of infected equines into an area where prevailing environmental factors have favoured the establishment of the disease. However, there is other evidence for the spread of the disease by the wind-carriage of infected vectors from enzootic areas into previously disease-free areas.[66]

Evidence for African horsesickness being transmitted by nocturnal biting flies is provided by the fact that horses, accommodated in mosquito-proof stables during the hours of darkness, are protected from infection. This suggests that the vectors are likely to be mosquitoes or biting midges. In 1944 Du Toit[19] incriminated *Culicoides* in the transmission of African horsesickness in South Africa. This finding was questioned, when many years later an attempt was made to repeat this experiment with *Culicoides* and also to extend it to mosquitoes. No transmission occurred with either *Culicoides* or mosquitoes.[80]

One problem with transmission experiments is that there is no small laboratory animal which is susceptible to infection by the bite of an infected vector. Boorman *et al.*[9] overcame this problem, as it had been for bluetongue, by using embryonated hen eggs as infected donors and recipient hosts. Using this technique AHS virus was transmitted from infected eggs to uninfected eggs by the bite of *Culicoides variipennis* seven days after the infective feed. Evidence was also produced that during this period the virus had multiplied in the *Culicoides.*[9]

Mechanical transmission has been suggested but this would appear to be unlikely as tabanids and *Stomoxys* are daytime feeders, against which the stabling of horses at night would be ineffective, and that is known not to be the case. Nine different antigenic serotypes are recognised between which there is no cross-immunity and there are many strains within the serotypes which have antigenic differences.[2] No reservoir host is known for AHS and the only wild equine, the zebra, is highly resistant to infection. Rabbits, sheep and cattle are not susceptible to AHS; dogs are susceptible but only at very high dosages and infection in dogs is a very rare occurrence in nature. The absence of reservoir hosts may be the reason why AHS has apparently disappeared from the Middle East.

Epizootic Haemorrhagic Disease of Deer

Epizootic haemorrhagic disease of deer (EHD) causes epizootics in the Virginian white-tailed deer (*Odocoileus virginianus*) in the United States. This virus does not affect domestic animals but a good deal of work has been done on it because of its similarity to both BT and AHS viruses and it is clearly advisable to use EHD virus for experimental purposes in areas where BT and AHS viruses are absent. As with BT and AHS viruses the vectors are species of *Culicoides*. EHD virus was recovered from *C. variipennis* during an outbreak of the disease in Kentucky in 1971, and two strains of the virus have been transmitted from infected deer to uninfected deer by the bite of the same species.[20, 41] The virus of EHD has been shown to multiply in *Culicoides variipennis* both after oral ingestion and after intrathoracic inoculation, but in the closely related *Culicoides nubeculosus* multiplication of the virus only occurred after intrathoracic inoculation and not after oral ingestion.[8] This suggests that there is a gut barrier to the passage of the virus from the midgut into the haemocoele. This may be one factor in the development of resistance to BTV in strains of *C. variipennis*.

Colorado Tick Fever

Colorado tick fever is endemic in the north-western United States, where it is enzootic in wild rodents, in which it causes no apparent disease. Man is susceptible to infection and encephalitis may occur, particularly in children. The vector is the three-host tick *Dermacentor andersoni* in which transstadial transmission occurs but there is doubt concerning transovarian transmission.[2]

Iridoviridae

Iridovirus particles are icosahedral in shape with a diameter of 125-300 nm, containing one or two molecules of DNA with a molecular weight of $100\text{-}250 \times 10^7$, constituting 12 to 30 per cent of the virus particle by weight.[48] The only member of this family of economic importance is the African swine fever virus.

African Swine Fever[7]

African swine fever (ASF) is a highly fatal, highly contagious disease of pigs which produces no clinical disease in wild pigs. In domestic pigs the morbidity approaches 100 per cent, and infections with a virulent strain are almost always fatal. ASF is enzootic to Africa but in 1957 it appeared in Portugal, in 1960 in Spain, and since then has reached France, Italy and Cuba. It has since been eradicated from the last three countries by extensive slaughter and quarantine programmes.[7]

In Africa the reservoirs of the virus are warthogs, bushpigs and forest hogs, among which it can be transmitted by *Ornithodoros moubata porcinus*, an argasid tick. Transmission is by bite, and virus is also excreted in the coxal fluid.[57] Infected male *O. m. porcinus* are able to transfer virus to clean females during copulation, probably via the seminal fluid, and in one series 88 per cent of females became infected after mating.[57]

References

1. Allmen, S.D. von, Lopez-Correa, R.H., Woodall, J.P., Morens, D.M., Chiriboga, J. and Casta-Velez, A. (1979). Epidemic dengue fever in Puerto Rico 1977: a cost analysis. *American Journal of Tropical Medicine and Hygiene 28*: 1040-4
2. Andrewes, C., Pereira, H.G. and Wildy, P. (1978). *Viruses of Vertebrates*. Baillière Tindall, London
3. Anon. (1911). Quarantine. pp. 709-11, in volume 22, *Encyclopaedia Britannica*, Cambridge University Press, Cambridge
4. _____ (1981). Dengue − Cuba. *Morbidity and Mortality Weekly Report 30*: 317
5. _____ (1982). Yellow fever in 1980. *WHO Chronicle 36*: 120
6. Beaty, B.J., Tesh, R.B. and Aitken, T.H.G. (1980). Transovarial transmission of yellow fever virus in *Stegomyia* mosquitoes. *American Journal of Tropical Medicine and Hygiene 29*: 125-32
7. Blood, D.C., Henderson, J.A. and Radostits, O.M. (1979). *Veterinary Medicine − a Textbook of the Diseases of Cattle, Sheep, Pigs and Horses*. Baillière Tindall, London
8. Boorman, J. and Gibbs, E.P.J. (1973). Multiplication of the virus of epizootic haemorrhagic disease of deer in *Culicoides* species (Diptera, Ceratopogonidae). *Archiv für die Gesamte Virusforschung 41*: 259-63
9. _____ Mellor, P.S., Penn, M. and Jennings, M. (1975). The growth of African horse-sickness virus in embryonated hen eggs and the transmission of virus by *Culicoides variipennis* Coquillett (Diptera, Ceratopogonidae). *Archives of Virology 47*: 343-9
10. Bowne, J.G. and Jones, R.H. (1966). Observations on bluetongue virus in the salivary glands of an insect vector *Culicoides variipennis*. *Virology 30*: 127-33
11. Chambon, L., Wone, I., Brès, P., Cornet, M., Ly, C., Michel, A., Lacan, A., Robin, Y., Henderson, B.E., Williams, K.H., Camain, R., Lambert, D., Rey, M., Diop Mar, I., Oudart, J.L., Causse, G., Bâ, H., Martin, M. and Artus, J.C. (1967). Une epidémie de fièvre jaune au Sénégal en 1965. L'epidémie humaine. *Bulletin of the World Health Organisation 36*: 113-50
12. Coverdale, O.R., Cybinski, D.H. and St George, T.D. (1978). Congenital abnormalities in calves associated with Akabane virus and Aino virus. *Australian Veterinary Journal 54*: 151-2
13. Davies, F.G. (1978). Bluetongue studies with sentinel cattle in Kenya. *Journal of Hygiene 80*: 197-204
14. _____ (1978). A survey of Nairobi sheep disease antibody in sheep and goats, wild ruminants and rodents within Kenya. *Journal of Hygiene 81*: 251-8
15. _____ (1978). Nairobi sheep disease in Kenya. The isolation of virus from sheep and goats, ticks and possible maintenance hosts. *Journal of Hygiene 81*: 259-65
16. _____ and Walker, A.R. (1974). The isolation of ephemeral fever virus from cattle and

Culicoides midges in Kenya. *Veterinary Record,* 20 July, 1974: 63-4

17. Doherty, R.L. (1977). Arthropod-borne viruses in Australia 1973-1976. *Australian Journal of Experimental Biology and Medical Science 55*: 103-30

18. _____ Gorman, B.M., Whitehead, R.H. and Carley, J.G. (1966). Studies of arthropod-borne virus infections in Queensland. V. Survey of antibodies to group A arboviruses in man and in other animals. *Australian Journal of Experimental Biology and Medical Science 44*: 365-78

19. Du Toit, R.M. (1944). The transmission of bluetongue and horse-sickness by *Culicoides. Onderstepoort Journal of Veterinary Science and Animal Industry 19*: 7-16

20. Foster, N.M., Breckon, R.D., Luedke, A.J. and Jones, R.H. (1977). Transmission of two strains of epizootic hemorrhagic disease virus in deer by *Culicoides variipennis. Journal of Wildlife Diseases 13*: 9-16

21. _____ and Jones, R.H. (1979). Multiplication rate of bluetongue virus in the vector *Culicoides variipennis* (Diptera: Ceratopogonidae) infected orally. *Journal of Medical Entomology 15*: 302-3

22. Freitas, R.B., Pinheiro, F.P., Santos, M.A.V., Rosa, A.P.A.T. da, Rosa, J.F.S.T. da and Freitas, E.N. de (1980). Epidemia de virus Oropouche no leste do Estado do Pará, 1979. *Review of Applied Entomology 69*: 3224 (1981)

23. Galindo, P. and Grayson, M.A. (1971). *Culex (Melanoconion) aikenii:* natural vector in Panama of endemic Venezuelan encephalitis. *Science 172*: 594-5

24. _____ Trapido, H., Carpenter, S.J. and Blanton, F.S. (1956). The abundance cycles of arboreal mosquitoes during six years at a sylvan yellow fever locality in Panama. *Annals of the Entomological Society of America 49*: 543-7

25. Gear, J.H.S., Ryan, J., Rossouw, E., Spence, I. and Kirsch, Z. (1977). Haemorrhagic fever with special reference to recent outbreaks in southern Africa. pp. 350-8 in *Medicine in a Tropical Environment,* J.H.S. Gear (ed.), A.A. Balkema, Rotterdam

26. Gorman, B.M., Taylor, J., Finnimore, P.M., Bryant, J.A., Sangar, D.V. and Brown, F. (1982). A comparison of bluetongue viruses isolated in Australia with exotic bluetongue virus serotypes. pp. 101-9 in *Arbovirus Research in Australia,* T.D. St George and B.H. Kay (eds.) CSIRO and QIMR, Brisbane

27. Haddow, A.J. (1965). Yellow fever in Central Uganda, 1964: Part I. Historical introduction. *Transactions of the Royal Society of Tropical Medicine and Hygiene 59*: 436-40

28. Halstead, S.B. (1980). Dengue haemorrhagic fever — a public health problem and a field for research. *Bulletin of the World Health Organization 58*: 1-21

29. _____ (1980). Immunological parameters of *Togavirus* disease syndrome. pp. 107-73 in *The Togaviruses, Biology, Structure, Replication,* R.W. Schlesinger (ed.), Academic Press, New York

30. Hawkins, J.A., Adams, W.V., Wilson, B.H., Issel, C.J. and Roth, E.E. (1976). Transmission of equine infectious anaemia virus by *Tabanus fuscicostatus. Journal of the American Veterinary Medical Association 168*: 63-4

31. Hayes, C.G. and Wallis, R.C. (1977). Ecology of western equine encephalomyelitis in the eastern United States. *Advances in Virus Research 21*: 37-83

32. Hoogstraal, H. (1966). Ticks in relation to human diseases caused by viruses. *Annual Review of Entomology 11*: 261-308

33. _____ (1979). The epidemiology of tick-borne Crimean-Congo hemorrhagic fever in Asia, Europe and Africa. *Journal of Medical Entomology 15*: 307-417

34. _____ (1981). Changing patterns of tickborne diseases in modern society. *Annual Review of Entomology 26*: 75-99

35. _____ Meegan, J.M., Khalil, G.M. and Adham, F.K. (1979). The Rift Valley fever epizootic in Egypt 1977-78. 2. Ecological and entomological studies. *Transactions of the Royal Society of Tropical Medicine and Hygiene 73*: 624-9

36. Hourrigan, J.L. and Klingsporn, A.L. (1975). Epizootiology of bluetongue: the situation in the United States of America. *Australian Veterinary Journal 51*: 203-8

37. Howell, P.G. (1968). African horsesickness. Pp. 73-108 in *Emerging Diseases of Animals,* FAO, Agricultural Studies No. 61, Rome

38. _____ (1979). The epidemiology of bluetongue in South Africa. pp. 3-13 in *Proceedings 2nd Symposium Arbovirus Research in Australia,* T.D. St George and E.L. French (eds.), CSIRO and QIMR, Brisbane

39. Johnson, B.K., Chanas, A.C., Tayeb, E. el, Abdel-Wahab, F.A. and Mohamed, A. el D. (1978). Rift Valley fever in Egypt, 1978. *Lancet 2*: 745
40. Jones, R.H. and Foster, N.M. (1974). Oral infection of *Culicoides variipennis* with bluetongue virus: development of susceptible and resistant lines from a colony population. *Journal of Medical Entomology 11*: 316-23
41. _____ Roughton, R.D., Foster, N.M. and Bando, B.M. (1977). *Culicoides*, the vector of epizootic hemorrhagic disease in white-tailed deer in Kentucky in 1971. *Journal of Wildlife Diseases 13*: 2-8
42. Kalra, N.L., Ghosh, T.K., Pattanayak, S. and Wattal, B.L. (1976). Epidemiological and entomological study of an outbreak of dengue fever in Ajmer, Rajasthan in 1969. *Review of Applied Entomology 65*: 2600 (1977)
43. Karabatsos, N. (ed.) (1978) Supplement to international catalogue of arboviruses including certain other viruses of vertebrates. *American Journal of Tropical Medicine and Hygiene 27*: 372-440
44. Kettle, D.S. and Campbell, M.M. (1980). Bionomics of *Culicoides brevitarsis*. p. 82, *Proceedings 3rd European Multicolloquium of Parasitology*, Cambridge, September 1980
45. Luedke, A.J., Jones, R.H. and Jochim, M.M. (1967). Transmission of bluetongue between sheep and cattle by *Culicoides variipennis*. *American Journal of Veterinary Research 28*: 457-60
46. _____ Jones, R.H. and Walton, T.E. (1977). Overwintering mechanism for bluetongue virus: biological recovery of latent virus from a bovine by bites of *Culicoides variipennis*. *American Journal of Tropical Medicine and Hygiene 26*: 313-25
47. Manson-Bahr, P.E.C. and Apted, F.I.C. (1982). *Manson's Tropical Diseases*. Baillière Tindall, London
48. Matthews, R.E.F. (1979). Classification and nomenclature of viruses. *Intervirology 12*: 129-296
49. McIntosh, B.M., Jupp, P.G. and Dos Santos, I. (1977). Rural epidemic of Chikungunya in South Africa with involvement of *Aedes (Diceromyia) furcifer* (Edwards) and baboons. *South African Journal of Science 73*: 267-9
50. _____ Jupp, P.G., Dos Santos, I. and Meenehan, G.M. (1976). Epidemics of West Nile and Sindbis viruses in South Africa with *Culex (Culex) univittatus* Theobald as vector. *South African Journal of Science 72*: 295-300
51. Metcalf, H.E., Pearson, J.E. and Klingsporn, A.L. (1981). Bluetongue in cattle: a serologic survey of slaughter cattle in the United States. *American Journal of Veterinary Research 42*: 1057-61
52. Murray, M.D. (1970). The spread of ephemeral fever of cattle during the 1967-68 epizootic in Australia. *Australian Veterinary Journal 46*: 77-82
53. Neri, P. (1965). Revue taxonomique aspect écologique et biologique des diptères (Culicidae) présents dans la forêt de Manera (Province du Kaffa) Ethiopie. *Cahiers ORSTOM Entomologie Médicale 3* and *4*: 47-56
54. Parsonson, I.M. (1979). Recent developments on bluetongue (BT) in the United States of America. pp. 13-19 in *Proceedings 2nd Symposium on Arbovirus Research in Australia*, T.D. St George and E.L. French (eds.), CSIRO and QIMR, Brisbane
55. Pinheiro, F.P., Hoch, A.L., Gomes, M.L.C. and Roberts, D.R. (1981). Oropouche virus. IV. Laboratory transmission by *Culicoides paraensis*. *American Journal of Tropical Medicine and Hygiene 30*: 172-6
56. _____ Travassos da Rosa, A.P.A., Travassos da Rosa, J.F.S., Ishak, R., Freitas, R.B., Gomes, M.L.C., LeDuc, J.W. and Oliva, O.F.P. (1981). Oropouche virus. I. A review of clinical, epidemiological and ecological findings. *American Journal of Tropical Medicine and Hygiene 30*: 149-60
57. Plowright, W., Perry, C.T. and Greig, A. (1974). Sexual transmission of African swine fever virus in the tick, *Ornithodoros moubata porcinus* Walton. *Research in Veterinary Science 17*: 106-13
58. Port, G.R. and Wilkes, T.J. (1979). *Aedes (Diceromyia) furcifer/taylori* and a yellow fever outbreak in The Gambia. *Transactions of the Royal Society of Tropical Medicine and Hygiene 73*: 341-4
59. Reeves, W.C. (1982). Gaps in current knowledge of vector biology critical to control or to epidemiological studies of arboviruses. pp. 10-15 in *Proceedings 3rd Symposium*

Arbovirus Research in Australia. T.D. St George and B.H. Kay (eds.), CSIRO and QIMR, Brisbane

60. Roberts, D.R., Hoch, A.L., Dixon, K.E. and Llewellyn, C.H. (1981). Oropouche virus. III. Entomological observations from three epidemics in Pará, Brazil, 1975. *American Journal of Tropical Medicine and Hygiene 30*: 165-71

61. Rosen, L. (1981). The use of *Toxorhynchites* mosquitoes to detect and propogate dengue and other arboviruses. *American Journal of Tropical Medicine and Hygiene 30*: 177-83

62. _____ Gubler, D.J. and Bennett, P.H. (1981). Epidemic polyarthritis (Ross River) virus infection in the Cook Islands. *American Journal of Tropical Medicine and Hygiene 30*: 1294-1302

63. _____ Shroyer, D.A. and Lien, J.C. (1980). Transovarial transmission of Japanese encephalitis virus by *Culex tritaeniorhynchus* mosquitoes. *American Journal of Tropical Medicine and Hygiene 29*: 711-2

64. Rudnick, A. (1978). Ecology of dengue virus. *Asian Journal of Infectious Diseases 2*: 156-60

65. Satti, M.H. and Haseeb, M.A. (1966). An outbreak of yellow fever in the Southern Fung and Upper Nile Province, Republic of the Sudan. *Journal of Tropical Medicine and Hygiene 69*: 36-44

66. Sellers, R.F. (1980). Weather, host and vector — their interplay in the spread of insect-borne animal virus diseases. *Journal of Hygiene 85*: 65-102

67. _____ Pedgley, D.E. and Tucker, M.R. (1978). Possible windborne spread of bluetongue to Portugal, June-July 1956. *Journal of Hygiene 81*: 189-96

68. Sérié, C., Andral, L., Lindrec, A. and Neri, P. (1964). Epidémie de fièvre jaune en Ethiopie (1960-1962). Observations préliminaire. *Bulletin of the World Health Organisation 30*: 299-319

69. Shaplen, R. (1964). *Toward the Well-being of Mankind.* Doubleday, New York

70. Smithburn, K.C., Haddow, A.J. and Gillett, J.D. (1948). Rift Valley fever. Isolation of the virus from wild mosquitoes. *British Journal of Experimental Pathology 29*: 107-21

71. Standfast, H.A., Dyce, A.L., St George, T.D., Cybinski, D.H. and Muller, M.J. (1979). Vectors of bluetongue in Australia. pp. 20-8 in *Proceedings 2nd Symposium Arbovirus Research in Australia*, CSIRO and QIMR, Brisbane

72. _____ St George, T.D., Cybinski, D.H., Dyce, A.L. and McCaughen, C.A. (1978). Experimental infection of *Culicoides* with a bluetongue virus isolated in Australia. *Australian Veterinary Journal 54*: 457-8

73. St George, T.D., Standfast, H.A. and Dyce, A.L. (1976). The isolation of ephemeral fever virus from mosquitoes in Australia. *Australian Veterinary Journal 52*: 242

74. Tesh, R.B. and Chaniotis, B.N. (1975). Transovarial transmission of viruses by phlebotomine sandflies. *Annals of the New York Academy of Sciences 266*: 125-34

75. Theiler, M. and Downs, W.G. (1973). *The Arthropod-borne Viruses of Vertebrates.* Yale University Press, New Haven

76. Tidwell, M.A., Dean, W.D., Tidwell, M.A., Combs, G.P., Anderson, D.W., Cowart, W.O. and Axtell, R.C. (1972). Transmission of hog cholera virus by horseflies (Tabanidae: Diptera). *American Journal of Veterinary Research 33*: 615-22

77. Walker, A.R. (1977). Seasonal fluctuations of *Culicoides* species (Diptera: Ceratopogonidae) in Kenya. *Bulletin of Entomological Research 67*: 217-33

78. Watts, D.M., Pantuwatana, S., Yuill, T.M., DeFoliart, G.R., Thompson, W.H. and Hanson, R.P. (1975). Transovarial transmission of LaCrosse virus in *Aedes triseriatus.* *Annals of the New York Academy of Sciences 266*: 135-43

79. Westaway, E.G. (1980). Replication of flaviviruses. pp. 531-81 in *The Togaviruses*, R.W. Schlesinger (ed.) Academic Press, New York.

80. Wetzel, H., Nevill, E.M. and Erasmus, B.J. (1970). Studies on the transmission of African horsesickness. *Onderstepoort Journal of Veterinary Research 37*: 165-8

81. Woodruff, A.W. (1974). *Medicine in the Tropics.* Churchill Livingstone, Edinburgh

25 TYPHUS AND OTHER RICKETTSIAL DISEASES

This chapter and the next deal with a diverse range of pathogens which, on an evolutionary scale, would be placed above the viruses and below the Protozoa. They are included in the standard reference work, *Bergey's Manual of Determinative Bacteriology.*[5] Three groups of these organisms are relevant to medical entomology: the Rickettsiales, which includes the organisms responsible for typhus and the spotted fevers; Spirochetes of the genus *Borrelia*, which cause relapsing fever in man; and two rod-shaped bacteria, *Yersinia pestis* and *Francisella tularensis*, the causative organisms, respectively, of plague and tularaemia. The Rickettsiales will be dealt with in this chapter and the other two groups in the next chapter.

Rickettsiales[16,31]

Most Rickettsiales are rod-shaped, coccoid and often pleomorphic micro-organisms, which are Gram-negative and multiply inside host cells. All Rickettsiales are regarded as parasitic or mutualistic and are associated with arthropods which may act as vectors or primary hosts.[16] Three families are recognised within the order Rickettsiales: the Rickettsiaceae, the Bartonellaceae and the Anaplasmataceae. The Anaplasmataceae are very small, virus-like particles which occur in the erythrocytes of vertebrates and are transmitted by arthropods. The Bartonellaceae are rod-shaped, bacteria-like parasites, found characteristically in or on the erythrocytes of vertebrates. Transmission by arthropods has been established for some Bartonellaceae and is suspected for others.

The most important family is the Rickettsiaceae which, in vertebrates, are parasites of tissue cells other than erythrocytes and are transmitted by arthropods. Three tribes are recognised within the Rickettsiaceae: the Wolbachieae which are symbionts of arthropods and do not occur in vertebrates; the Ehrlichieae which are pathogenic for certain mammals but not for man; and the Rickettsieae which are capable of infecting suitable vertebrate hosts including man, who may be the primary host but is more often an incidental host.

Symbiotic rickettsias of the Wolbachieae have been described from the common mosquito *Culex pipiens*, from the sheep ked *Melophagus ovinus*, from the bedbug *Cimex lectularius*, and from the *Argas persicus* complex of soft ticks.[16] In addition similar micro-organisms have been described from the human body louse *Pediculus humanus*, and referred to as *Rickettsia pediculi* and *R. rocha-limae*.[7,31] The latter two species are not listed by Moulder.[16] Symbiotic micro-organisms appear to supply essential nutrients to their arthropod hosts (see Chapter 5).

Rickettsiaceae

Within the Rickettsiaceae three genera are recognised; *Rickettsia, Rocha-limaea* and *Coxiella*. *Coxiella* grows preferentially in vacuoles of the host cells and, being highly resistant to physical and chemical conditions in the extracellular environment, can be transmitted in the absence of an arthropod vector. *Rochalimaea* resembles *Rickettsia* but is cultivable on certain bacteriological media and multiplies extracellularly in the arthropod host. Species of *Rickettsia* are not cultivable in the absence of host cells and multiply in the cytoplasm or sometimes in the nucleus of vertebrate cells. They are unstable when separated from host compounds.[16]

Species of *Rickettsia* are the most important disease-causing agents within the Rickettsiales and indeed among all human pathogens. Three groups can be distinguished within the genus: typhus group, spotted fever group and scrub typhus group. The last group contains only one species. J.R. Audy[3] believes that rickettsias were originally associated with soil-dwelling acarines from which they were introduced into rodents by trombiculids. Once established in rodents they were taken up by ticks and blood-sucking fleas and lice. Some rodent fleas will take man as an alternative host and rickettsias were in this way introduced to man, from which they became established in *Pediculus humanus*.

There are varying degrees of adaptation between rickettsias and their arthropod hosts. Their long association with acarines is shown by the ease with which they pass the gut barrier, and disperse in the haemocoele and tissues of the acarine, enabling both transovarian transmission and transmission by bite to occur. In insects the rickettsias are confined to the gut and transmission is via the faeces. Rodent fleas have had longer exposure to rickettsias, in an evolutionary sense, than human lice and are apparently unaffected by infection with *R. mooseri*. The longevity of *P. humanus* is greatly reduced by infection with *R. mooseri* or *R. prowazekii* but greater adaptation has occurred to *Rochalimaea quintana* which is non-pathogenic for *P. humanus*.

Epidemic Typhus *Rickettsia prowazekii*

The aetiological agent of classical epidemic typhus is *Rickettsia prowazekii* named after the American H.T. Ricketts and the Austrian S. von Prowazek, both of whom died from typhus contracted as a result of their researches into the disease. Epidemic typhus is a severe disease with a high mortality (30-60 per cent) in populations weakened by malnutrition.[7] Epidemics of typhus have changed the course of history as Zinsser has documented in his very readable book *Rats, Lice and History*.[32] At the end of the First World War and the period immediately succeeding it

(1917-23) it is believed that 30 million cases of epidemic typhus occurred in Russia and Europe with over three million deaths.[15] Official Soviet statistics maintain that during that period 10 per cent of the population was affected.[31]

A little more than a century earlier typhus had played a major role in the defeat of Napoleon's armies which invaded Russia. Diseases, of which typhus was the major one, rather than military opposition defeated Napoleon.[32] The potato famine in Ireland in the 1840s led to a major movement of the population to America. Of the 75,000 Irish who migrated in 1847, 30,000 (40 per cent) contracted typhus of whom 20,000 (67 per cent) died from the disease, reflecting the debilitated state of the health of the migrants.[3]

The epidemic in Naples in 1943 during the Second World War was the first time an epidemic of typhus had been terminated by human action, and had not exhausted itself. The credit is usually given to the introduction of DDT as an insecticide against the vector *P. humanus*, but there is evidence that other anti-louse preparations had already halted the epidemic before the introduction of DDT.[8]

Although *P. humanus* occurs in all human populations, epidemic typhus is commoner in the temperate regions and in the cooler regions of the tropics above 1,600 m,[15] and is absent from the lowland tropics. Until recently epidemic typhus was present in many parts of the world, including eastern Europe, most parts of the Mediterranean, Ethiopia, South Africa, China, Mexico, Peru, Chile and Argentina.[7, 15, 31] In recent years the incidence of louse-borne typhus has been steadily declining with 10,548 cases in 1975, 8,065 in 1976, and 6,087 in 1977.[1] The mortality during those three years was less than 2 per cent. As in previous years the majority of the cases in 1977 occurred in Africa (96.3 per cent), with most of the remainder occurring in Peru and Ecuador (200/218 = 92 per cent). In 1979 the number of cases increased sharply to 18,359, of which 17,476 (95.2 per cent) were in Ethiopia, but elsewhere the decline continued.[2]

Transmission

The head louse *P. capitis*, and the crab louse *Pthirus pubis*, can transmit *R. prowazekii* experimentally, but epidemics have always occurred in conditions where body lice *P. humanus* were particularly prevalent, and this species is the usual vector.[6] Various species of fleas are susceptible to infection with *R. prowazekii* but they are not known to have a role in transmission.[16]

R. prowazekii multiplies in the epthelial cells of the midgut, and when these burst it is passed out with the faeces of the louse.[7] *R. prowazekii* is pathogenic to the body louse and kills it in about 10 days. Man becomes infected by scratching in response to the feeding of the louse, scarifying the skin, facilitating the entry of *R. prowazekii*. It is possible that *R. prowazekii* can gain entry into the human body by other routes, e.g. by inhalation of louse faeces, or by *R. prowazekii* penetrating the mucosa or the conjunctiva of the eye. Fatalities among early workers arose from their attention being concentrated on the feeding of the louse and not on its faeces. *R. prowazekii* can survive 66 days in dry louse faeces at ambient temperatures. This means that fresh cases of typhus can be contracted for two months after the conclusion of a successful body louse eradication programme.

Survival of R. prowazekii

The question arises as to how *R. prowazekii* survives between epidemics. There is no transovarial transmission; individual lice survive for only about six weeks, less if infected,[7] and *R. prowazekii* survives for only about two months in louse faeces. According to Moulder,[16] 'Man is the primary reservoir. Individuals who recover from typhus probably retain small numbers of organisms, presumably in their lymph nodes for the rest of their lives.'

Brill-Zinsser disease is the recrudescence of epidemic typhus among persons who have recovered from the disease. It occurs in the absence of body lice. In different localities of the USSR recrudescence has been recorded as occurring in 1-16 per cent of recovered patients and may be much higher.[31] Such relapses are considered to be the main reservoir of *R. prowazekii* in eastern Europe.[15] In Peru there is evidence for asymptomatic infections of man with *R. prowazekii*.[31] These could be the reservoirs maintaining endemic areas of infection.

It was shown a long time ago that *R. prowazekii* occurred in domestic animals in Ethiopia, and Reiss-Gutfreund postulated two cycles of transmission.[18,19] The first was the man-louse-man cycle described above, and the other a domestic animal-tick-domestic animal cycle. Strains of *R. prowazekii* have been recovered from domestic animals, and in a survey of 649 sheep, goats and cattle 17 per cent showed serological evidence of previous infection with *R. prowazekii*.[18] In a later survey 69 per cent of 247 animals reacted positively.[19]

Five strains of *R. prowazekii* have been recovered from *Amblyomma variegatum* and *Hyalomma rufipes* by inoculating ground-up ticks into guinea pigs. Larvae and nymphs of both species became infected when fed on rabbits and lambs harbouring *R. prowazekii*, but adult ticks did not.[18] In Ethiopia then there is evidence of a reservoir of *R. prowazekii* in domestic animals which could spread to man through the ticks which are accidental parasites of man.

More recently *R. prowazekii* has been shown to be present as natural infections of flying squirrels in Florida and Virginia in the USA.[25] *R. prowazekii* was recovered from the blood-sucking louse *Neohaematopinus sciuropteri* and the flea *Orchopeas howardii*. The louse is host specific but *O. howardii* has an extensive host range, which includes man. The significance of this finding to the epidemiology of epidemic typhus is not known.

Entomological Aspects of Typhus Epidemics

Epidemics of louse-borne typhus are associated with overcrowded, insanitary conditions. In England, typhus was known as gaol fever. From the sixteenth century until almost recent times epidemic typhus has been prevalent in times of war, occurring among both refugees and fighting men. *P. humanus* is well adapted to spread *R. prowazekii.* It is a permanent ectoparasite of man living on the skin and in the clothing immediately adjoining it. In that situation, on a healthy person the body louse lives in a stable environment. Exposed to a temperature gradient it shows a marked preference for a temperature range of 29-30°C.[30] When the temperature goes above or below this range the louse moves away. This has the effect that lice leave a person in a fever, e.g. suffering from typhus, and also leave a corpse.

When refugees are crowded together for warmth and shelter lice spread rapidly throughout the human population. In experiments in which two volunteers, one infested with 200 lice, shared a large bed, the louse-free individual complained of being bitten in an hour or so if the infested companion had a fever, but if the infested person had a normal body temperature the uninfested individual did not complain for five or six hours.[7]

P. humanus orientates to human odours and the excreta of its own species. Both these responses will keep body lice in the vicinity of their host. Body lice avoid moisture and they will therefore leave a sweating feverish patient, behaviour which will favour the spread of typhus. Body lice prefer rough to smooth surfaces, i.e. woollen stockinette to cotton stockinette and both to silk.[30] This behaviour might explain in part the fashion in earlier times for silk underwear, but although silk would be less favourable to lice it would not prevent infestation.

P. humanus has great powers of reproduction. Buxton[7] has shown that under optimal conditions, a female louse will live for nearly five weeks, during which period she will produce 279 eggs of which 117 will become adults. On these figures a female louse will, in a period of two months, give rise to 15,000 progeny of which 10,500 will be eggs and 4,500 will be larvae and adults. However, under normal conditions an infested human being will take corrective action as the louse population builds up. In practice, 'natural populations of head and body lice commonly consist of about 10 or 20 insects (nymphs and adults) though hundreds are not very rare and populations exceeding 1000 have been recorded'.[7] It is easy to appreciate that, when human society is disrupted by war, famine or natural disaster, personal hygiene practices break down and louse populations flourish. These are the conditions under which louse-borne typhus becomes epidemic.

Rickettsial Pox (Rickettsia akari)

Rickettsia akari is included with the agents of tick typhus in the spotted fever group within the genus *Rickettsia*.[16] Rickettsial pox was first recognised as a new disease of man in the mid 1940s when it was described from Boston and New York in the USA, and a few years later from the USSR. Over a period of three years nearly 500 cases were reported in New York alone.[15] In 1949-50 it occurred in epidemic form in the Ukraine causing approximately 1,000 cases in the Donets basin.[17] The vector is the gamasid mite *Liponyssoides sanguineus*, an ectoparasite of the house mouse, *Mus musculus*. Rickettsial pox has since been identified in South Korea, South Africa and French Equatorial Africa.[17] It is also suspected of occurring in Yugoslavia and Italy (Sicily).[17] In *L. sanguineus R. akari* is transmitted transovarially to the next generation of mites. In the laboratory the tropical rat mite *Ornithonyssus bacoti* can maintain *R. akari* and transmit it transovarially.[17] There is little information on the existence of a cycle of *R. akari* in wild rodents. It has, however, been recovered from a wild rodent in Korea.[16]

Murine Typhus (Rickettsia mooseri)

Rickettsia mooseri (= *R. typhi*) is placed in the typhus group of the genus *Rickettsia* together with *R. prowazekii*.[16] Murine typhus is worldwide in distribution but there are certain areas in which the disease is especially endemic.[15] In the period 1931-46, 42,000 cases of murine typhus occurred in the United States. This may be an underestimate as it is considered that recorded cases may represent only one fifth of the total number of cases. Indeed in an area in the plains of Lahore, Pakistan, more than a third of the resident population gave serological evidence of prior infection with *R. mooseri*.[27] Nevertheless, our understanding of the wider picture of murine typhus is such that Traub *et al.*[27] ended the introduction to their comprehensive review with the statement that 'Murine typhus is unique among the major arthropod-borne diseases, as far as the extent of our ignorance about fundamental information on the ecology of the infection is concerned'.

Although *R. mooseri* causes a milder form of typhus than *R. prowazekii* there can still be a significant death rate, e.g. 5 per cent.[7] Human infections with *R. mooseri* are associated with domestic and peridomestic infestations of commensal rats of the subgenus *Rattus*, especially the black rat *R. rattus* and the brown rat *R. norvegicus*; together with the tropical rat flea *Xenopsylla cheopis*. Although there is this close association between human disease, commensal rats and *X. cheopis* the correlation is not absolute. Commensal rats extend far beyond the known range of murine typhus, and *X. cheopis* may also be abundant outside the range. Traub *et al.*[27] conclude that 'it is by no means clear the coexistence of this rat [*Rattus*] and flea automatically implies occurrence of *R. mooseri* as well'.

Seven species of fleas belonging to six genera have been found infected naturally with *R. mooseri*. Nevertheless, *X. cheopis* is considered to be the major vector as murine typhus has not conclusively been shown to occur in its absence.

In *X. cheopis*, *R. mooseri* multiplies in the cells of the midgut, from which it is released by rupture and exfoliation of midgut cells and is passed in the flea's faeces.[13] The longevity of *X. cheopis* appears to be unaffected by infection with *R. mooseri*. Transmission is via the faeces or by the ectoparasite being crushed on the skin and the infective material scarified into the skin by scratching. *R. mooseri* is not transmitted by the bite of the flea nor is it transmitted transovarially. Although *X. cheopis* is primarily an ectoparasite of rats, it readily feeds on humans in the absence of its main host. In *X. cheopis* feeding and defaecation are closely associated, and infected fleas feeding on people would deposit *R. mooseri* in the human environment.

The transmission cycle involving humans need not be the same as that occurring among the rodent population. Other rodent fleas, e.g. *Leptosylla segnis*, *Echidnophaga gallinaceae*, and rat lice *Polyplax spinulosus* and *Hoplopleura* sp, have been found naturally infected with *R. mooseri*. They almost certainly play a significant role in the maintenance of *R. mooseri* in the rodent population and, although they do not feed on man, it is conceivable that they could cause human infections through the air-borne dispersal of their faeces. It is not known whether cycles of *R. mooseri* exist anywhere in the world in the absence of both commensal *Rattus* and *X. cheopis*.[27]

Once *R. mooseri* has become established in man it could be transmitted among the human population by *Pulex irritans*, acquired by *Pediculus humanus* and become epidemic, but this does not appear to occur. In *P. humanus*, *R. mooseri* becomes intracellular and causes the death of the louse, perhaps even more rapidly than *R. prowazekii* does.[7]

Scrub Typhus (Rickettsia tsutsugamushi)[3]

Rickettsia tsutsugamushi is placed in a separate group of the genus *Rickettsia*. It is the aetiological agent of scrub typhus which is present in a geographical area of the world bounded by West Pakistan, Japan, tropical North Queensland (with rainfall of 1,500 mm or more), and certain islands in the Pacific and Indian Oceans, including Diego Garcia in the Chagos Islands almost midway between Madagascar and the Oriental region.[3] Moulder[16] includes Siberia within the range.

The association between scrub typhus and mites was reported in a sixteenth-century Chinese work on natural history and has been known for at least 200 years by the Japanese who named the disease tsutsugamushi, meaning dangerous mite. The vectors of scrub typhus are trombiculid mites. More than a thousand species of trombiculid mites are known, of which six species in the genus *Leptotrombidium* are vectors of *R. tsutsugamushi* and another 15 species, mostly in the genera *Eutrombicula* and *Schoengastia*, cause scrub itch, an allergic condition. Species of *Leptotrombidium* parasitise mammals whilst those of *Eutrombicula* and *Schoengastia* parasitise birds and reptiles. Although *R. tsutsugamushi* is transmitted to man by species of *Leptotrombidium*, species of *Ascoschoengastia* are involved in its transmission among rodents.

The reservoir hosts of *R. tsutsugamushi* are various species of rats which are abundant in the region with more than 500 named forms being described from the Malaysian subregion alone. Only trombiculid mites which parasitise rodents will have ready access to *R. tsutsugamushi* while species which mainly parasitise birds and reptiles will have little chance of becoming infected. Failure to appreciate the significance of the different feeding habits prevented a clear understanding of the epidemiology of scrub typhus, because the distribution of scrub itch, caused by species normally parasitising birds and reptiles, did not coincide with that of scrub typhus, caused by species parasitising rodents. In addition, when a person is bitten by an infected trombiculid mite an eschar (ulcer) usually develops at the site of infection, and the distribution of eschars on the human body did not coincide with the areas affected by scrub itch.

The main vectors of scrub typhus are *Leptotrombidium akamushi* and *L. deliense* which have a wide geographical distribution, within which they are patchily distributed being abundant in ecologically favourable 'mite islands' and absent from other habitats. In Japan, classical tsutsugamushi was present in limited areas and associated with high mortality. Tsutsugamushi is, in fact, widely distributed throughout Japan but causing a milder disease as in other parts of south-east Asia.

The limited distribution of scrub typhus within a country is well demonstrated by groups undertaking a four-day exercise in Sri Lanka (Ceylon) during the Second World War. At that time *R. tsutsugamushi* was not known to be present in Sri Lanka yet the division engaged in the exercise developed 750 cases of scrub typhus. These were traced to a 'typhus island' at Embilipitiya where slash-and-burn cultivation in virgin forest had produced a mixture of grassy areas and fields of millet. Field rodents established themselves in the grassy areas, fed in the millet fields and built up high populations of their trombiculid parasites.

Scrub typhus is not associated with clearing virgin rainforest or amongst cultivation where weeds are kept to a minimum. However, when such cultivated areas are neglected, scrub typhus is a common infection among the workers who undertake clearance of lapsed cultivation. The environment in which scrub typhus occurs is essentially man-made. In Malaya, Sumatra, New Guinea and tropical Queensland scrub typhus is associated with a coarse, rasping, fire-resistant grass, *Imperata cylindrica*, known as kunai grass in some areas. It provides a suitable habitat for field rodents and its dominance is maintained by the use of fire, which prevents the establishment of shrubs and trees, whose shade would control the grass. Kunai grass represents a pyrophytic subclimax in a succession which should have continued to forest. In areas where the forest is re-established, scrub typhus is either absent or at a negligible level. There is also an ecotone effect with scrub typhus being more likely to occur at the fringes of the grassland habitat.

In the life cycle of a trombiculid mite only the larval stage is parasitic, the active nymph and adult are predators on other arthropods. The larva feeds on only one individual host and therefore has the potential to acquire or to transmit an infection, but it cannot acquire an infection from one host and transmit it to another. This means that trombiculid mites can only be vectors if the pathogen is transmitted transovarially, and *R. tsutsugamushi* is transmitted transovarially in *L. akamushi* and *L. deliense*, so that newly emerged larvae may already be infected.

In the mite the rickettsia passes into the haemocoele from which it establishes itself in the salivary glands and is passed into the host when the mite is feeding, which it does for several days. In the adult female mite the rickettsias invade the ovaries and are passed to the next generation. It is possible to regard trombiculid mites as the main reservoirs of *R. tsutsugamushi* on the grounds that the rickettsia will survive longer by transovarian transmission than in the rodent reservoir in which no transovarian transmission takes place.

Close associations develop between trombiculid species and their vertebrate hosts with each rodent species likely to be host to one or more species of trombiculid. Two types of host may be distinguished. The main host, a rodent, maintains the mite on its home range, creating 'mite islands' while other hosts disperse the mite to new areas. It is considered that *L. deliense* has been introduced into a number of oceanic islands between India and Madagascar, as far west as Diego Garcia, and this is attributed to carriage by birds and possibly flying foxes. Man is an incidental intrusion into a mite-rodent cycle of *R. tsutsugamushi*.

Rodent control may not be the most effective measure to reduce scrub typhus in the short term. The effect of removing many rodent hosts from the ecosystem is to leave large numbers of hungry trombiculid larvae seeking an alternative host. On deserted Jarak island six out of eight scientific investigators who indulged in rodent control contracted scrub typhus, while another group who visited the island later were equally overrun by rats but carried out no control, and none of the ten scientists developed scrub typhus.

Tick-borne Typhus[12]

Spotted fevers or tick-borne typhus are widely spread throughout the world, occurring in every continent and zoogeographical region. They are caused by various species of *Rickettsia* which circulate in a wide range of mammals, and sometimes birds, through the agency of ixodid ticks. The rickettsias are transmitted transstadially and transovarially in the tick vector. They cause benign infections of the non-human host but serious disease in humans, which may be fatal. Hoogstraal[12] cites the following quotation from Dr David B. Lackman: 'Whenever you have ixodid ticks biting man there is the possibility of Rocky Mountain spotted fever.' This remark could be generalised to the effect that wherever ixodid ticks bite man there is the possibility of human infections with spotted fever rickettsias.

Five species of pathogens are involved in tick-borne typhus: *Rickettsia rickettsi, R. sibirica, R. conori, R. australis* and *R. slavaca*. Most detailed information is available on the epidemiology of the first two species and they will be considered at greater length than the others. Hoogstraal's review[12] entitled 'Ticks in relation to human diseases caused by *Rickettsia* species', has the high quality and encyclopaedic coverage of the literature characteristic of his work. The reader is referred to the original article for details as only the major conclusions can be given here.

Rickettsia rickettsi

The disease associated with *R. rickettsi* is usually commonly referred to as Rocky Mountain spotted fever, but the organism is widely distributed outside the Rocky Mountains occurring in the eastern states, particularly Virginia, and in Brazil in South America where the disease is called Sao Paulo fever.

In the USA about 200 cases of this disease are reported annually with some fatalities, but prompt treatment with antibiotics can almost eliminate deaths from *R. rickettsi*. In the eastern United States the vector is *Dermacentor variabilis* which in the immature stages occurs on rodents, and in the adult occurs on larger mammals including man and dog. Infestation of dogs with *D. variabilis* brings infection indoors and disease is also present among women and children. In the western United States, the Rocky Mountain region, the vector is *Dermacentor andersoni*, of which the immature stages are indiscriminate parasites of small mammals, and the adults parasitise hares, larger wild and domestic animals, and also man. In this region Rocky Mountain spotted fever is associated with field workers.

Among wild hosts infections with *R. rickettsi* are transitory, but serological tests have demonstrated antibodies to *R. rickettsi* in 18 species of birds and 31 species of mammals, including 18 species of rodents, five species of leporids and five carnivores. In the laboratory, infected female *D. andersoni* transmit the rickettsia to 100 per cent of their daughters and from them to their progeny. Nevertheless, in the field infections of *D. andersoni* with *R. rickettsi* are much lower, less than 14 per cent. Transstadial and transovarian transmission of the rickettsia does not reduce its virulence. Infection results from the bite of the tick and the faeces of infected *D. andersoni* do not appear to be important in transmission.

Rocky Mountain spotted fever was first recorded in Mexico in 1943 where the vectors were considered to be *Rhipicephalus sanguineus* and *Amblyomma cajennense*. Both these species were associated with an outbreak of Sao Paulo fever in Brazil, and *A. cajennense* has been regarded as the vector in Panama and Columbia. The role of argasid ticks in the transmission of *R. rickettsi* is not clear. In Mexico both *Ornithodoros nicolle* and *Otobius lagophilus* were found infected with *R. rickettsi*. In Brazil *Ornithodoros rostratus* transmitted *R. rickettsi* for less than a month, and while *Ornithodoros turicata* retained rickettsias in its body for more than two years, it was unable to transmit *R. rickettsi* when feeding.

Rickettsia sibirica (spelt *siberica* by Hoogstraal[12])

R. sibirica is closely related to *R. rickettsi*. The two species are geographically distinct with *R. rickettsi* being confined to the western hemisphere, and *R. sibirica* to Asiatic Russia and the central Asian Republics of the USSR. *R. sibirica* is less virulent than *R. rickettsi* and came into prominence during the development of 'The Virgin Lands' of the Soviet Union in the 1930s. Two hundred to 600 cases of Siberian tick typhus are recorded annually at Krasnoyarsk.[12]

Strains of *R. sibirica* have been recovered from at least 18 species of mammals, mostly rodents. Birds are considered to play a secondary role as reservoirs of *R. sibirica*. Nine species of ixodid ticks act as reservoirs and vectors of *R. sibirica*: four species of *Dermacentor*; three of *Haemaphysalis*; *Rhipicephalus sanguineus*; and *Hyalomma asiaticum*. In *Dermacentor marginatus*, naturally or experimentally infected with *R. sibirica*, the rickettsia survives for at least five years or through four generations.

The immature stages of *Dermacentor* occur on small mammals, particularly rodents, hedgehogs, hares and small carnivores, and are rare on birds. This may explain the secondary role of birds as reservoirs of *R. sibirica*. Adult *Dermacentor* parasitise medium to large wild and domestic mammals.

Ticks of the genus *Dermacentor* are common and widely distributed in Eurasia, with species occupying different ecological zones. *Dermacentor marginatus* occurs in lowland and alpine steppes of western Eurasia and further west into central Europe. *D. silvarum* has an eastern distribution, extending from western Siberia to the far eastern coastline of the Soviet Union. It infests the taiga and shrub-wormwood steppes. In the Far East in shrub and fern marshes adjoining taiga, *Haemaphysalis concinna* is the chief vector. It gives way to *Hyalomma asiaticum* in the semi-desert steppe. In central and eastern Siberia *Dermacentor nuttalli* occurs in cisalpine, alpine, forested and desert steppes.

Rickettsia conori

R. conori is widely distributed in the Old World occurring in southern Europe, Africa, India and the Oriental region. The popular names for the disease caused by *R. conori* are often formed from the geographical location plus tick typhus, e.g. Kenya tick typhus, but it is also known as Marseilles fever and *fièvre boutonneuse* (pimply fever). *R. conori* causes acute suffering but few deaths. There have been no extensive epidemiological studies on *R. conori* comparable to those on *R. rickettsi* and *R. sibirica.*

On the South African veld the chief vectors appear to be *Amblyomma hebraeum* and *Rhipicephalus appendiculatus.* The immature stages of both species are common parasites of man. Human infections with *R. conori* in South Africa also occur in urban settings where the vectors are *Haemaphysalis leachi* and *Rhipicephalus sanguineus*, the common dog ticks of tropical and subtropical areas. The normal route of transmission of *R. conori* from tick to man is through the bite of the tick but infection may also result from contamination of eye and nasal mucosa from crushed ticks or tick faeces, particularly when dogs are being de-ticked.[17]

There is lack of agreement as to whether the dog is a reservoir of *R. conori.* In South Africa the dog is not regarded as a reservoir host,[12] but in many countries of southern Europe the dog is suspected of being a major reservoir and in the Crimea the percentage of dogs with antibodies to *R. conori* ranged from 15.1-71.4 per cent.[17] Nevertheless Rehacek[17] concluded his review of *R. conori* in Europe with the statement that the role of the dog as a reservoir host has not yet been proved conclusively. Several species of rodent have been found infected naturally,[16] and antibodies to *R. conori* have been recovered from domestic animals,[17] but their role in the epidemiology of the disease is not fully understood. Although attention in Europe has focused on the dog tick *R. sanguineus*, other species of ixodid ticks may be important locally.

Rickettsia australis, Rickettsia slavaca

Rickettsia australis is the cause of tick typhus in Queensland, Australia. Several species of marsupials, including bandicoots and possums, are considered to be reservoir hosts and, on circumstantial evidence, the probable vector is *Ixodes holocyclus*. *I.holocyclus* is a widely distributed, unusually indiscriminate feeder, attacking almost any bird or mammal.[12]

Rickettsia slavaca, a recently described species, was recovered from *Dermacentor marginatus* from Central Slovakia.[17] It is widely distributed in Slovakia and probably in most parts of Europe. All stages of *D. marginatus* transmit rickettsias by bite and pass rickettsias in the faeces. *R. slavaca* is passed both transstadially and transovarially by *D. marginatus*. Antibodies to *R. slavaca* have been found in wild rodents which are considered to be major reservoir hosts. Nevertheless, the importance of *R. slavaca* in human and animal pathology has not yet been proven, but there is some evidence that this *Rickettsia* can be a human pathogen.[17]

Rochalimaea

Rochalimaea is a monotypic genus of which the sole representative is *R. quintana* which causes trench or five-day fever in man. Epidemics of trench fever occurred on the Western Front in the First World War (1914-18) in which 200,000 cases were recorded in the British Army alone. It was virtually unheard of during the inter-war period but reappeared in Germany in 1941-2 and had become widespread by 1943.[31] The disease is never fatal and nearly half the convalescents recovering from trench fever were carriers of the pathogen, which persisted for months or even years to form a reservoir for further cases. Man is the sole known host for *R. quintana.*

It is spread among human populations by the human louse, *Pediculus humanus.* The louse acquires the pathogen when feeding on the blood of an infected person. *R. quintana* multiplies in the lumen of the midgut in the cuticular margin of the midgut epithelial cells.[15] After six to ten days *R. quintana* appears in the faeces of the louse and infection is caused either by the faeces being scarified into the skin or possibly by inhalation. The longevity of the louse is not affected by being infected with *R. quintana*, and it remains infective for the rest of its life which, in an adult louse, would not exceed five weeks.[7] There is no transovarian transmission so that newly emerged lice are free from infection. However, since transmission of the pathogen is by the faeces of the louse, it is possible for new cases to arise for some time after elimination of the louse population. *R. quintana* remains viable in dry louse faeces for many months and possibly in excess of a year.[31]

Coxiella burneti

Coxiella burneti[16] is the only species at present placed in this genus. It resists drying and relatively elevated temperatures that generally destroy the viability of *Rickettsia.*[16] *C. burneti* was named after Sir McFarlane Burnet, an Australian Nobel Prizewinner in Medicine who first studied this organism. *C. burneti* causes Q-fever, a disease which is now present in most countries of the world, having been introduced into Europe during the Second World War. It causes a moderately severe, but rarely fatal, pneumonia.

C. burneti is enzootic in domestic animals, such as cattle, sheep and goats, and is widely disseminated among other animals, including birds and numerous species of arthropod, especially tick ectoparasites of ungulates, rodents and marsupials.[16] In addition organisms are shed in large numbers by infected animals in their milk, urine, faeces and foetal fluids.[22] *C. burneti* is a highly resistant organism which can remain infective in meat for at least a month and in Wales an outbreak occurred among workers handling infected carcasses. Ixodid ticks play a role in transmitting this disease among wild and domestic animals. In Queensland *C. burneti* is circulated amongst bandicoots by *Ixodes holocyclus*.

The fact that *C. burneti* can be transmitted by an arthropod, by contact with fomites or by being air-borne, favours its wide distribution throughout the world. Liebisch[14] recognises three different epidemiological zones of Q-fever in Germany. In the south-west there is an endemic zone where the ixodid vectors, especially *Dermacentor marginatus*, are present. To the north of the endemic zone there is a zone of sporadic outbreak of Q-fever in man and farm animals. In this zone *C. burneti* is repeatedly introduced by importation of infected farm animals, or by infected raw materials, such as wool. The third zone embraces the more northerly part of Germany, and also includes Belgium, the Netherlands, Denmark and Scandinavia, where Q-fever has never been recorded. Absence of Q-fever from this zone is a reflection of the enforcement of strict quarantine measures.

In the endemic zone of south Germany the main vector is *D. marginatus* which, in the adult stage, occurs on sheep. In this zone more than 20 per cent of sheep and cattle are infected, and the presence of *C. burneti* has been demonstrated in the haemocytes of naturally infected *D. marginatus*. In other countries *Ixodes ricinus* is regarded as a vector of Q-fever. It does not act in that capacity in south Germany but the reason is not known. *C. burneti* is normally regarded as being non-pathogenic for domestic live-stock but there are records of very heavy infections causing abortion in sheep and goats.[9]

Ehrlichieae [16,22,23]

Ehrlichieae are minute rickettsia-like organisms which are pathogenic for certain mammals, but not infectious to man. Most are adapted to existence in ticks but not in insects. *Cowdria ruminantium* and a number of species of *Ehrlichia* and the closely related *Cytoecetes* cause diseases of varying severity in domestic animals. In the vertebrate host *C. ruminantium* is characteristically localised in the vascular endothelial cells, and *Ehrlichia* species in circulating leucocytes.

The known or suspected vectors of the Ehrlichieae of veterinary importance are ixodid ticks in which transstadial transmission occurs.[22,23] At one time it was considered that *E. canis* was transmitted transovarially by

Rhipicephalus sanguineus but this has not been confirmed by more recent work.[11,24] Scott[22] states that transovarial transmission does not occur in *E. bovis, E. canis, E. phagocytophila* and *C. ruminantium.*

Cowdria ruminantium causes heartwater in ruminants in the Afrotropical region. It causes disease in sheep, goats and cattle with mortality rates of 20-95 per cent.[16] This organism also occurs in wild ruminants. After an attack organisms may persist for up to 60 days and be followed by a period of sterile immunity lasting three months to five years.[16]

The most detailed studies have been carried out on *Ehrlichia canis*, a parasite of wild and domestic canidae. The disease in domestic dogs is widely distributed throughout the world occurring from 50°N to 35°S, which is the distribution of the vector *Rhipicephalus sanguineus.* In the 1960s *E. canis* was responsible for a 'highly fatal haemorrhagic disease of U.S. military dogs in south-east Asia'.[16] *E. canis* is able to persist in dogs for at least 13 months after recovery from clinical signs of infection.

Ehrlichia phagocytophila, which causes disease in sheep and cattle in western Europe, has also been recovered from wild deer in Great Britain. In India *Cytoecetes ovis*, which is probably a strain of *E. phagocytophila,* has been described from sheep, and its vector is *Rhipicephalus haemophysaloides.*[22]

E. bovis, which is transmitted by species of *Hyalomma*, causes disease of varying severity, often mild, in cattle in the Middle East, North and Central Africa, and Sri Lanka. A strain of the same organism caused a fatal disease of pigs in Senegal.[22] *E. ovina* causes disease in sheep in North and Central Africa. The vector is considered to be *R. bursa* in North Africa. *E. equi* causes disease in horses in the Sacramento Valley, California, and *Cytoecetes ondiri* causes bovine patechial disease in cattle and sheep in Kenya. The mode of transmission of the last two species is unknown but ixodid ticks are suspected of being the vectors.

Bartonellaceae[16,28]

Members of the Bartonellaceae are rod-shaped micro-organisms which occur in or on erythrocytes and in fixed tissues. They are distinguished from the Anaplasmataceae by cultural and structural characteristics. The Bartonellaceae have cell walls and can be grown on cultural media.

Two genera are included within the Bartonellaceae, *Bartonella* and *Grahamella*. Species of *Grahamella* are worldwide benign parasites of small mammals which are probably transmitted by blood-sucking ectoparasites, particularly fleas. Only one species of *Bartonella* has been described, *B. bacilliformis*, and it is highly pathogenic to man.

Bartonella bacilliformis[21]

B. bacilliformis is restricted to certain high mountain valleys in the western and central Cordilleras of the Andes in South America. *B. bacilliformis* is unusual in that it produces two strikingly different diseases in man, a progressive anaemia with high mortality (40 per cent), referred to as Oroya fever, and a benign cutaneous eruption known as Verruga peruana. These two conditions are referred to jointly as Carrion's disease in memory of Carrion, who in 1885 inoculated himself with the organisms of Verruga peruana, and developed and died from Oroya fever, thus tragically and dramatically proving that the same organism caused both diseases. During the building of the Trans-Andean railway in 1870 Oroya fever was responsible for 7,000 deaths.

Carrion's disease is an anthroponosis. No animal reservoir host is known. Transmission is via the phlebotomine sandfly *Lutzomyia verrucarum*. *B. bacilliformis* is in the circulating blood and is picked up by *L. verrucarum* when it feeds on an infected human. There is no known cycle of development in the sandfly and the pathogen has been found in its gut and on its mouthparts. *L. verrucarum* is nocturnal in habit and the incidence of Carrion's disease among railway workers was greatly reduced by removing them from the high-level valleys before nightfall.[21] The disease is endemic in certain valleys where in some cases it has been known to persist for 300 years. The disease is restricted to mountain valleys between 750 and 2,750 m in altitude. Above that height the night temperatures are too low for *L. verrucarum* to be active and below 750 m the climate is too arid for the survival of *L. verrucarum*. However, that does not explain the absence of *L. verrucarum* and Carrion's disease from well-watered riverine habitats below 750 m.

It is worth noting that the essential features of the epidemiology of Carrion's disease, except for the role of the insect vector, were known by the end of the nineteenth century. It is instructive to read the following paragraph from Weinman and Kreier:[28]

The history of bartonellosis is, in part, a scientific documentation for what seemed one of the most improbable of the New World marvels. The excellent monograph of Odriozola (1898) drew attention to a disease believed to occur only in Western South America. There it was restricted to certain mountain valleys and contracted only at night. This unique disease was said to exist in two forms, clinically distinct and apparently unrelated. One, an anaemia, occurring at times in epidemics, could be fulminant and kill in a few days. The other form was benign and distinguished by a skin eruption, the like of which was unknown outside the Andean valleys. To the surprise of the scientific community all of these facts have proven to be substantially correct.

Anaplasmataceae[4]

The Anaplasmataceae are very small, virus-like particles occurring in the erythrocytes of vertebrates and which are considered to be transmitted by arthropods. They are obligate parasites, which multiply intracellularly by binary fission. They differ from the Bartonellaceae by being in the form of cocci or short rods, by having no cell wall and by not multiplying on culture media. Five genera are included in the family of which two, *Anaplasma* and *Aegyptianella*, are important pathogens of domestic stock but do not infect man.

Anaplasma[20]

Species of *Anaplasma* are restricted to ruminants, especially bovids and cervids. *Anaplasma marginale marginale* is a pathogen of cattle in the tropics and subtropics while *A. m. centrale* occurs in cattle in Africa. *A. m. marginale* is more pathogenic than *A. m. centrale*, which causes a relatively mild disease. Although *A. m. marginale* parasitises a wide range of African bovids, the African buffalo (*Syncerus caffer*) is refractory to infection. Deer can act as reservoirs of anaplasma pathogenic to cattle, and transmission of infection from deer to cattle has been demonstrated.

The severity of the disease is a function of the age of the host. Below two years of age anaplasmosis is rarely fatal in cattle, but the probability of death occurring increases with age, being frequent in cattle over three years. In the early stages of infection *Anaplasma* organisms penetrate erythrocytes and divide to form an inclusion body composed of four to eight organisms. Such inclusion bodies are numerous in the acute stage of the disease.

Anaplasma is transmitted biologically by ticks and mechanically by blood-sucking flies. In ticks the pathogen is said to be transmitted both transstadially and transovarially but Thompson and Roa[26] failed to transmit *A. marginale* transovarially through *Boophilus microplus*. The presence of *Anaplasma* has been demonstrated in the gut and malpighian tubules of infected ixodid ticks. Although more than 20 species of ixodid ticks have been shown to transmit anaplasmosis experimentally, field evidence that ticks are the main vectors of *Anaplasma* is lacking. Experimentally, *Anaplasma* has been transmitted by mosquitoes (*Psorophora*), and by members of the Stomoxinae (*Stomoxys*).

It is considered that horseflies of the genus *Tabanus* are the most important vectors of anaplasmosis. In an area of Tanzania where the cattle tick, *Boophilus decoloratus*, was absent 44 per cent of the cases of anaplasmosis were attributed to *Tabanus taeniola*. Although *T. taeniola* and *T. fraternus* were the most abundant of 12 species of *Tabanus*, cases of anaplasmosis correlated with *T. taeniola* and not with *T. fraternus*.[29] This difference may reflect a difference in behaviour if, for example, *T. fraternus* did not immediately seek another host after having its blood feeding interrupted.

A. ovis causes an inapparent infection in cattle and a mild to severe disease in sheep and goats. It is widely distributed throughout the world.

Aegyptianella pullorum[10]

Until recently (1972) *Aegyptianella pullorum* was included in the Babe-sidae, a family of the class Sporozoa of the Protozoa. It is now included in the Anaplasmataceae on the grounds that, in common with the other members, it has a similar morphology; it has a similar mode of repro-duction, and it affects the same host cell. *A. pullorum* infects a wide range of wild and domestic birds in the warmer parts of the world. It has been recorded from Africa, Asia and southern Europe but its distribution is probably wider.

A. pullorum infects chickens, geese, ducks and quail, and the ostrich has been found infected naturally. There is some uncertainty about the sus-ceptibility of pigeons, turkeys and guinea fowl, which have been recorded as having been found with natural infections[16] and as being refractory to infection (pigeons and turkeys[10]) or of uncertain susceptibility (guinea fowl[10]). A range of wild birds have been infected experimentally but natural infections of wild birds need to be examined more closely before deciding that these are infections with *A. pullorum*.

The effect of infection with *A. pullorum* varies with the age of the bird. Fatalities occur in chickens up to the age of four weeks with mortality declining rapidly over that period. Poultry infected after the age of 12 weeks develop a low persistent parasitaemia. Fowls that have recovered clinically may remain infective to argasid ticks for up to 18 months.

The vectors of *A. pullorum* are ticks of the subgenus *Persicargas* of the genus *Argas*, in particular *A. (P.) persicus* and *A. (P.) walkerae*. Trans-mission in the Argasid is both transstadial and transovarial, although only a small percentage of larvae are infected by the transovarial route which is regarded as being of little epizootological importance.

In *A. (P.) walkerae*, *A. pullorum* develops in the intestinal epithelium, haemocytes and salivary glands. In each of these three separate locations intensive multiplication of the parasite takes place and 30 days are required to complete the cycle. After an infected feed the parasites are to be found in the intestinal epithelium after 24 hours and at the end of 14 days the intestinal cells are heavily parasitised. After two to three weeks the parasites appear in the haemocytes and multiply rapidly until the end of the fourth week, when the parasites appear in the salivary glands. This deve-lopment can take place in all stages of the tick, larva, nymph and adult. Once infected, the tick remains infected for life, with infections even per-sisting for two years in starved nymphs and female ticks. *A. pullorum* is introduced into its bird host with the saliva of the feeding tick.

Eperythrozoon and *Haemobartonella*[10]

Many species of the morphologically very similar *Eperythrozoon* and *Haemobartonella* have been described from a range of vertebrates, both domestic and wild. *Eperythrozoon* has been recorded from mammals and a fish, the pike (*Esox lucius*), and *Haemobartonella* from mammals, several reptiles, frogs and another fish, the tench (*Tinca tinca*). Both genera are worldwide in their distribution occurring on the outside of the erythrocytes of the host and are associated with a mild anaemia, except for *Eperythrozoon suis* which causes icteroanaemia of swine, a disease of some economic importance in the United States. Although little firm data are available on the method of transmission of *Eperythrozoon* and *Haemobartonella*, 'it is widely believed that arthropods including lice, fleas, acarids and biting flies are the vectors'.[10] More is known about the transmission of *Haemobartonella muris* which is spread by the rat louse, *Polyplax spinulosa*, both mechanically and biologically. This organism is also transmitted by the rat flea, *Xenopsylla cheopis*. *Haemobartonella felis* is an exception in that it spreads readily by the oral route and during cat fights.

References

1. Anon. (1978). Louse-borne typhus in 1977: the decline continues. *WHO Chronicle 32*: 401-2
2. _____ (1981). Louse-borne typhus in 1979. *WHO Chronicle 35*: 188-9
3. Audy, J.R. (1968). *Red Mites and Typhus*. Athlone Press, London
4. Blood, D.C., Henderson, J.A. and Radostits, O.M. (1979). *Veterinary Medicine — a Textbook of the Disease of Cattle, Sheep, Pigs and Horses*. Baillière Tindall, London
5. Buchanan, R.E. and Gibbons, N.E. (eds.)(1974). *Bergey's Manual of Determinative Bacteriology*. Williams and Wilkins, Baltimore
6. Busvine, J.R. (1976). *Insects, Hygiene and History*. Athlone Press, London
7. Buxton, P.A. (1950). *The Louse*. Edward Arnold, London
8. Craufurd-Benson, H.J. (1946). Naples typhus epidemic 1943-4. *British Medical Journal 1*: 579-80
9. Crowther, R.W. and Spicer, A.J. (1976). Abortion in sheep and goats in Cyprus caused by *Coxiella burneti*. *Veterinary Record 99*: 29-30
10. Gothe, R. and Kreier, J.P. (1977). *Aegyptianella, Eperythrozoon* and *Haemobartonella*. pp. 251-94 in volume IV, *Parasitic Protozoa*, J.P. Kreier (ed.), Academic Press, New York
11. Groves, M.G., Dennis, G.L., Amyx, H.L. and Huxsoll, D.L. (1975). Transmission of *Ehrlichia canis* to dogs by ticks (*Rhipicephalus sanguineus*). *American Journal of Veterinary Research 36*: 937-40
12. Hoogstraal, H. (1967). Ticks in relation to human diseases caused by *Rickettsia* species. *Annual Review of Entomology 12*: 377-420
13. Ito, S. and Vinson, J.W. (1980). Electron microscopy of rickettsiae in flea tissues. pp. 277-82 in *Fleas*, R. Traub and H. Starcke (eds.), A.A. Balkema, Rotterdam
14. Liebisch, A. (1979). Ecology and distribution of Q-fever rickettsiae in Europe with special reference to Germany. pp. 225-31 in volume II, *Recent Advances in Acarology*, J.G. Rodriguez (ed.), Academic Press, New York
15. Manson-Bahr, P.E.C. and Apted, F.I.C. (1982). *Manson's Tropical Diseases*, Baillière Tindall, London

16. Moulder, J.W. (1974). Order I. Rickettsiales Gieszczkiewicz 1939, 25. pp. 882-914 in *Bergey's Manual of Determinative Bacteriology*, R.E. Buchanan and N.E. Gibbons (eds.), Williams and Wilkins, Baltimore
17. Rehacek, J. (1979). Spotted fever group rickettsiae in Europe. pp. 245-55 in volume II, *Recent Advances in Acarology*, J.G. Rodriguez (ed.), Academic Press, New York
18. Reiss-Gutfreund, R.J. (1956). Un nouveau réservoir de virus pour *Rickettsia prowazeki*: les animaux domestiques et leurs tiques. *Bulletin de la Société de Pathologie Exotique 49*: 946-1021
19. _____ (1961). Nouveaux isolements de *R.prowazeki* a partir d'animaux domestiques et de tiques. *Bulletin de la Société de Pathologie Exotique 54*: 284-97
20. Ristic, M. (1977). Bovine anaplasmosis. pp. 235-49 in volume IV, *Parasitic Protozoa*, J.P. Kreier (ed.), Academic Press, New York
21. Schultz, M.G. (1968). A history of bartonellosis (Carrion's disease). *American Journal of Tropical Medicine and Hygiene 17*: 503-15
22. Scott, G.R. (1978). Tick-borne rickettsial diseases of livestock. pp. 450-73 in *Tick-borne Diseases and their Vectors*, J.K.H. Wilde (ed.), Centre for Tropical Veterinary Medicine, Edinburgh
23. Smith, R.D. and Ristic, M. (1977). Ehrlichieae. pp. 295-328 in volume IV, *Parasitic Protozoa*, J.P. Kreier (ed.), Academic Press, New York
24. _____ Sells, D.M., Stephenson, E.H., Ristic, M. and Huxsoll, D.L. (1976). Development of *Ehrlichia canis*, causative agent of canine ehrlichiosis, in the tick *Rhipicephalus sanguineus* and its differentiation from a symbiotic *Rickettsia*. *American Journal of Veterinary Research 37*: 119-26
25. Sonenshine, D.E., Bozeman, F.M., Williams, M.S., Masiello, S.A., Chadwick, D.P., Stocks, N.I., Lauer, D.M. and Elisberg, B.L. (1978). Epizootiology of epidemic typhus (*Rickettsia prowazekii*) in flying squirrels. *American Journal of Tropical Medicine and Hygiene 27*: 339-49
26. Thompson, K.C. and Roa, J.C. (1978). Transmission (mechanical/biological) of *Anaplasma marginale* by the tropical cattle tick *Boophilus microplus*. pp. 536-9 in *Tick-borne Diseases and their Vectors*, J.K.H. Wilde (ed.), Centre of Tropical Veterinary Medicine, Edinburgh
27. Traub, R., Wisseman, C.L. and Farhang-Azad, A. (1978). The ecology of murine typhus — a critical review. *Tropical Diseases Bulletin 75*: 237-317
28. Weinman, D. and Kreier, J.P. (1977). *Bartonella* and *Grahamella*. pp. 197-233 in volume IV, *Parasitic Protozoa*, J.P. Kreier (ed.), Academic Press, New York
29. Wiesenhütter, E. (1975). Research into the relative importance of Tabanidae (Diptera) in mechanical disease transmission. III. The epidemiology of anaplasmosis in a Dar-es-Salaam dairy farm. *Tropical Animal Health and Production 7*: 15-22
30. Wigglesworth, V.B. (1941). The sensory physiology of the human louse *Pediculus humanus corporis* de Geer (Anoplura). *Parasitology 33*: 67-109
31. Zdrodovskii, P.K. and Golinevich, H.M. (1960). *The Rickettsial Diseases*. Pergamon Press, London
32. Zinsser, H. (1935). *Rats, Lice and History*. Atlantic Monthly Press, Boston

26 RELAPSING FEVERS, BORRELIOSES, PLAGUE AND TULARAEMIA

Relapsing Fevers (*Borrelia spp.*)[24,31]

The Borrelias are loosely helically coiled, Gram-negative, motile, parasitic spirochetes which cause disease in man. Entomologically there are two main groups: *Borrelia recurrentis* which is transmitted by *Pediculus humanus*; and the 18 other species of *Borrelia*, 17 of which are transmitted by ticks, and one species for which the vector is not known. *Borrelia theileri* is transmitted by ixodid ticks and the other 16 species by argasid ticks mostly of the genus *Ornithodoros*. *Borrelia anserina*, the cause of avian spirochetosis, is transmitted by species of the subgenus *Persicargas* of the genus *Argas*.

Epidemic Relapsing Fever (*Borrelia recurrentis*)[18,21,26]

Louse-borne relapsing fever has occurred in epidemic proportions several times in the first half of this century. In 1920 hundreds of thousands of cases occurred in eastern Europe but by 1925 the incidence was almost zero.[21] More than a million cases of epidemic relapsing fever were attributed to the effects of the Second World War and its aftermath.[18] In the 1920s an epidemic of louse-borne relapsing fever raged in northern equatorial Africa. Although the details are not known, millions of people were affected and the death rate was considered to be about 5 per cent.[21] For a variety of reasons mortalities vary from less than 1 per cent to more than 40 per cent.[26]

Epidemic relapsing fever is widely distributed throughout the world, occurring in Europe, Africa, South America and Asia but absent from the Malay Peninsula and Archipelago, and Australia.[21] The disease continues to exist and in the late 1960s nearly 5,000 cases were reported to WHO, of which 95 per cent were recorded from Ethiopia and 2 per cent from the Sudan.[18] The high incidence of the disease in Ethiopia is reminiscent of the survival of the other louse-borne human disease, epidemic typhus, in that country (see p. 477).

Borrelia recurrentis occurs in the circulating blood of a patient during a period of fever. *P. humanus* feeding on a patient at that same time acquires *B. recurrentis* with its blood meal. Most of the spirochetes die in the midgut of the louse but a few survive to penetrate the midgut and reach the haemocoele, in which they multiply. From the sixth day after an infective feed spirochetes become increasingly abundant in the haemolymph of the louse.[21] A few *B. recurrentis* may penetrate the ganglia of the louse but they do not invade other tissues, e.g. salivary glands or ovaries. Their absence from other tissues means that *B. recurrentis* is not transmitted by the bite of the louse and neither is there transovarian transmission.

Few *B. recurrentis* are passed in the faeces of the louse and most, or all, of them are moribund.[21] Transmission via the faeces, therefore, is highly unlikely. Transmission of *B. recurrentis* occurs when a louse is crushed and the infected haemolymph released on to the skin. The borrelias may be scratched into the skin but there is also evidence that *B. recurrentis* can penetrate unbroken skin.[18] This means that transmission involves the death of the louse and an individual louse can only infect one person. Therefore epidemic relapsing fever depends upon high louse populations in the human population. The conditions for this are similar to those associated with epidemic typhus (see p. 479).

No animal reservoir is known for *B. recurrentis.* Man is the only known host for this organism. This raises the problem of the survival of *B. recurrentis* during non-epidemic periods. The life of a louse is less than two months and in the absence of transovarian transmission *B. recurrentis* cannot survive in the louse population. It has been suggested that tick-borne borrelias are introduced into man and become adapted to human lice but the louse-borne relapsing fever appears in many places where tick-borne borrelias are not known to be present.[18] Moreover, *B. recurrentis* does not infect ticks.[37]

Endemic Relapsing Fever (*Borrelia duttoni*)

Borrelia duttoni, named after J.E. Dutton, who died from the disease it causes, is the aetiological agent of endemic relapsing fever found in eastern, central and southern Africa. Endemic relapsing fever differs from the other *Ornithodoros*-borne borrelias in that it is an anthroponosis, with man the only known host. No animal reservoir is, as yet, known.[26] The vector is usually referred to as *Ornithodoros moubata* or one of its subspecies and a note on the *O. moubata* complex is given below.

In the 1940s thousands of cases of endemic relapsing fever occurred in east and central Africa. In 1946 there were 8,200 cases admitted to hospital in East Africa alone and many more thousands of cases remained in the villages and were not reported.[50] Of recent years the number of cases has fallen, partly as a result of the use of synthetic insecticides and improved standards of living, reducing man-tick contact.

When a tick feeds on a person infected with *B. duttoni* it takes in borrelias with the blood into the midgut. The borrelias then penetrate the midgut and enter the haemocoele where they multiply and invade various organs including the central nerve mass, the salivary glands, the coxal glands, and ovaries. Multiplication of *B. duttoni* goes on in both the invaded organs and in the haemolymph. When the tick feeds borrelias are passed into the host through the saliva and, while it is feeding, *O. moubata* excretes infected coxal fluid.[26] Borrelias are able to enter a new host through skin abrasions or by direct penetration of the unbroken skin.

In *O. moubata*, *B. duttoni* is passed both transstadially and transovarially. The distribution of borrelias in the tick changes with age. In nymphs and young adults the salivary glands are the organs involved in transmission, and in old adult ticks the coxal organs play a more important role. *B. duttoni* can be transmitted transovarially through at least five generations, and hence centres of endemic relapsing fever tend to persist for long periods of time.

Transmission of *B. duttoni* to man is associated with populations of *O. moubata*, which are synanthropic and have habits comparable to those of the bedbug. The ticks live and multiply in cracks and crevices of human habitations from which they emerge at night to feed upon the sleeping occupants. Survival of the disease in a location is aided by the long time for which individual ticks may live. Burgdorfer[18] refers to this ability of *Ornithodoros* to survive for long periods and states that he has kept them alive for 15 years without feeding, but the species of *Ornithodoros* was not stated.

Although *B. duttoni* may continue to be transmitted transovarially over several generations, there is a decrease in pathogenicity of the strain concerned unless there is passage through a susceptible host. Some populations of *O. moubata* feed almost exclusively on warthogs (*Phacochoerus*) or chickens but such populations are not infected with *B. duttoni*. The human louse is able to act as a vector of *B. duttoni* but is of secondary importance.[26]

A Note on the *Ornithodoros moubata* Complex[48,50,51]

Walton[50,51] studied *Ornithodoros moubata* in East Africa for many years and concluded that several different forms had been referred to the species *O. moubata*. He recognised four species with two subspecies: *O. compactus*, a parasite of tortoises in Cape Province of South Africa; *O. apertus*, a rare species associated with porcupines in one locality of Kenya; *O. moubata*, a species frequenting huts and the lairs of wild animals in arid conditions, defined as an annual rainfall of 50 mm or less; and a new species, *O. porcinus*, with two subspecies *O. p. porcinus* and *O. p. domesticus*.

O. p. porcinus is described as being exceedingly abundant in lairs of wild animals, particularly warthog (*Phacochoerus*), and occurring on the humid Central African plateau between altitudes of 900 to 1,500 m; *O. p. domesticus* as being completely interfertile with *O. p. porcinus*, but morphologically and physiologically distinct. Later Walton[51] added *O. p. avivora*, a chicken-feeding subspecies present on the East African coast.

Van der Merwe[48] examined a range of material, including some of Walton's, but came to different conclusions. Her studies were entirely morphological and she found difficulty in differentiating between the various forms. She concluded that *O. compactus* was a valid species, but that the other forms were within the single species *O. moubata* in which she recognised three subspecies: *O. m.moubata*, *O. m.apertus* and *O. m. porcinus.* Van der Merwe's[48] *O. m. porcinus* included Walton's *O. porcinus porcinus* and his *O. p. domesticus.* Both workers recognised wild and domestic populations within their taxa: Van der Merwe in her *O. m. moubata* and *O. m. porcinus,* and Walton in his *O. moubata.*

From the medical point of view neither of these two classifications is particularly helpful in that wild and domestic populations are included within the one taxon. Since only domestic populations will play any role in the transmission of *B. duttoni* it would have been preferable, were it taxonomically possible, to have distinguished between wild and domestic populations, i.e. between vectors and non-vectors. Unfortunately that is not possible.

Other *Ornithodoros*-borne relapsing fevers (*Borrelia spp.*)[24]

The quotation regarding tick-borne spotted fevers (see p. 484) can be adapted to cover relapsing fevers carried by *Ornithodoros* spp, to the effect that 'Whenever you have species of *Ornithodoros* biting man there is the possibility of relapsing fever'. Fifteen species of *Ornithodoros* are known to be reservoirs or vectors of *Borrelia* species and they occur in each major zoogeographical region.[31] There are 14 species of *Borrelia* which are transmitted among rodents and other small mammals by *Ornithodoros* ticks. Of these seven are listed as pathogenic to man, two cause mild disease and the other five are not known to infect man.[18,24]

Most foci of *Ornithodoros*-borne borrelias exist in nature in restricted tick biotypes such as burrows, nests or caves. Man becomes exposed to infection when visiting such areas or using caves as shelter. Human infections are accidental and play no role in the population dynamics of the zoonosis among the small mammal population. Two outbreaks of relapsing fever caused by *B. hermsi* in the western United States could be traced to people occupying log cabins infested with rodents and *O. hermsi.* Ten out of 20 boy scouts and scoutmasters who spent at least one night in an infested cabin developed relapsing fever. In 1973, 62 visitors and park service employees contracted relapsing fever caused by *B. hermsi* after spending one or more nights in log cabins in the North Rim Park area of the Grand Canyon in Arizona.[18]

Borrelia hermsi is a zoonosis of chipmunks (*Eutamias* spp) and pine squirrels (*Tamiasciuris* spp). Transmission of rodent borrelias is either via the saliva or the coxal fluid. *Ornithodoros hermsi* secretes too little coxal fluid for it to be the route of infection. Some species of *Ornithodoros* do not secrete coxal fluid until they have left the host and consequently coxal fluid could not be the route of infection. *O. hermsi* and *Ornithodoros turicata* are highly efficient at transmitting borrelias through their saliva, and infections may result from the tick feeding for less than a minute.[18]

Although transovarian transmission of borrelias is common among species of *Ornithodoros* it does not occur in all species, e.g. *O. rudis* does not transmit *B. venezuelensis* transovarially.[18]

Avian borreliosis (*Borrelia anserina*)[24,31]

Borrelia anserina is pathogenic for geese, ducks, turkeys, pheasants, canaries, chickens and grouse. Avian borreliosis occurs in southern Europe, the Middle East, Africa, India, Australia, South America and the western United States. The vectors of *B. anserina* are species of *Argas (Persicargas) persicus* and *A. (P.) arboreus*. *A. (P.) persicus* has been distributed by man along with domestic chickens to many parts of the tropics and subtropics.[32]

The development of *B. anserina* in argasid ticks involves the borrelias penetrating the midgut and appearing in the haemocoele, in which they multiply and invade certain tissues including the central nerve mass, salivary glands and gonads. Heavy infections of *B. anserina* develop in *A. (P.) persicus* and *A. (P.) arboreus*, in which both transstadial and transovarial transmission occur.[23] Two other common Egyptian bird-parasitising argasids, *A. (P.) streptopelia* and *A. (Argas) hermanni*, resist infection. They show only limited transstadial and no transovarial transmission.[54]

Borrelia theileri

Borrelia theileri causes a mild disease in cattle and a febrile disease in horses in South Africa and Australia. *B. theileri* is unusual in that the vectors are species of ixodid ticks, including *Rhipicephalus evertsi* and the cattle ticks *Boophilus decoloratus* and *B. microplus*.[24,31]

Plague (*Yersinia pestis*)[37,47,53]

Plague is a disease of rodents caused by *Yersinia pestis* and to which man is susceptible. *Y. pestis* is a Gram-negative, facultatively anaerobic, non-motile micro-organism, which varies in shape from coccoid to rod-shaped.[38] Three subspecies have been recognised on the basis of their biochemical properties. They are *Yersinia pestis antiqua*, *Y. p. mediaevalis* and *Y. p. orientalis*.[53] At the present day the three subspecies have different distributions throughout the world and each subspecies is regarded as having been responsible for a separate pandemic in the last 1,500 years.[47] A pandemic is an epidemic which is prevalent over a whole country, continent or widespread throughout the world at the same time.

The Pandemics

Plague is considered to have originated in Central Asia from which it has spread virtually throughout the world. It is believed that plague had spread to Asia Minor, Egypt and Africa in pre-Christian times. In the first pandemic plague spread from Arabia in AD 542 into the Byzantine empire of Justinian, throughout Europe and North Africa, and possibly also reached East Africa.[47] The organism responsible is considered to be *Y. p. antiqua*.

The second pandemic, attributed to *Y. p. mediaevalis*, was the 'Black Death' of the Middle Ages which ravaged Europe from the fourteenth to the seventeenth centuries. It originated in Central Asia, probably near Alma Ata, the modern capital of Kazakhstan SSR, and spread eastwards to China, south to India and westwards to the Crimea, which it reached in 1346. From there it spread rapidly throughout Europe reaching France and England in 1348, and in 18 months had spread throughout the whole of England and southern Scotland. In two and a half years the population had been reduced by a third. It took 200 years for the population of Europe to recover numerically from the ravages of the 'Black Death'.

The third pandemic, associated with *Y. p. orientalis*, is currently coming to an end. It originated in Yunnan Province of south-west China in 1892 and two years later reached Canton and Hong Kong, from which it spread rapidly throughout the world through the agency of ocean-going liners. It had spread to Calcutta by 1895, to the Transvaal of South Africa and Santos in Brazil in 1899, and by 1900 plague had reached San Francisco in North America, and Sydney and Brisbane in Australia.[41,47]

The third pandemic continues to produce cases of human plague in many parts of the world. In 1967 there were 6,004 cases reported to the World Health Organisation, and in 1968-71 the number of cases remained steady between 4,000 and 5,000,[28] but since then the incidence has fallen to a low of 505 in 1980.[5] In 1980 there were 283 cases in Asia, including 180 in Vietnam; 142 in South America, mainly in Brazil (98 cases); and 80 in Africa, of which 44 were in Tanzania (Figure 26.1).[5]

Plague took a heavy toll among overcrowded, underfed, poorly housed urban populations of the East. In India, during the period 1898 to 1908,

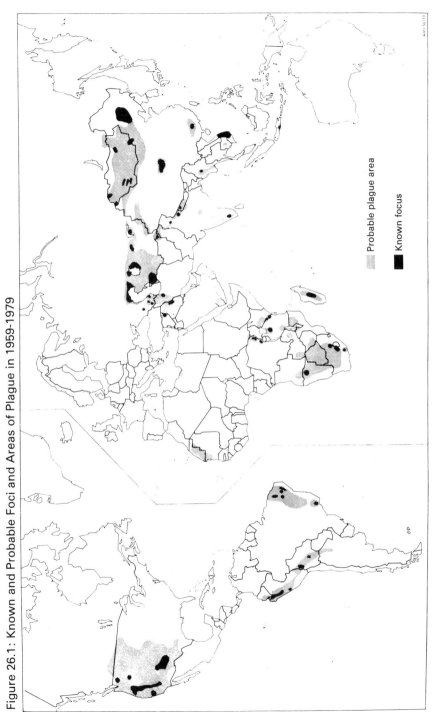

Figure 26.1: Known and Probable Foci and Areas of Plague in 1959-1979

Probable plague area

Known focus

there were more than half a million deaths per annum from plague and in the succeeding decade the annual mortality from it was 420,000.[41] This aroused the compassion of the international community and the British Plague Commission worked for many years combatting this disease. At this time there were five national Plague Commissions in Bombay alone.[20]

In an epidemic the mortality from plague is very high and may reach 60 to 95 per cent of those attacked, with the death rate being inversely proportional to the state of nutrition of those affected. In Hong Kong the death rate from plague among the various social classes varied from 18 per cent among Europeans to 93 per cent among Chinese.[37]

Epidemiology of Plague in India

The Plague Commission (early 1900s). The essential features of the epidemiology of plague were established by the British Plague Commission. In nature plague spread among rats by the agency of rat fleas, and in the absence of fleas there was no epizootic among rats.[3] The first sign of an outbreak of plague was an epizootic among the peridomestic brown rat *Rattus norvegicus*, with numerous deaths. This was followed in about ten days by an epizootic amongst the domestic black rat *Rattus rattus*.[1] After an interval of about two weeks human cases of plague appeared.[3] In the winter of 1905-6 in Bombay peak mortality among *R. norvegicus* was reached on 18 February, peak mortality among *R. rattus* on 17 March, and human deaths reached a maximum on 28 April.[47]

The explanation of these observations was that infected rat fleas left the bodies of dead *R. norvegicus* and some transferred to *R. rattus*, infecting them with plague. The rat flea *Xenopsylla cheopis* readily bites man in the absence of its main host and infected *X. cheopis* would transfer from *R. rattus* to man.[3]

It was shown that epidemics of plague were more likely when the temperature was between 50° and 85°F (10-29°C)[2] and that they declined rapidly at the onset of hot weather. Humidity also played a leading role in the epidemiology of plague. Between 1901 and 1910 there were four winters in which plague was severe and five in which only mild plague occurred. The average temperatures in mild and severe plague years did not differ but the humidities in severe plague years were considerably higher than in the years when plague was less.[27]

The findings of the Plague Commission have been variously quoted as plague being limited by temperatures above 80°F (26.7°C) or 85°F (29.4°C) and humidities above 70 or 80 per cent. These two factors are inter-dependent and Brooks[17] showed that the limiting factor was saturation deficit, which had a critical value of 0.30 inches (10.2 millibars), equal to 70 per cent RH at 80°F; 79 per cent at 90°F; and 60 per cent at 70°F. Epidemic plague ceases when the temperature exceeds 26.7°C and the saturation deficit is more than 10.2 mb; and rapidly wanes when the temperature is below 26.7°C but the saturation deficit exceeds 10.2 mb. Conversely, plague epidemics may commence when the temperature is well above 26.7°C, providing the saturation deficit is less than 10.2 mb.[17]

Rogers[43] extended these findings to take into account the climatic factors of the previous year, in particular temperature and saturation deficit during the hot weather and monsoon seasons. Hot, dry conditions act directly on the transmission of plague by reducing the life expectancy of infected fleas, and indirectly by reducing the flea population by causing higher mortality among larvae, and reducing the fecundity and survival of adult fleas.

More Recent Status of Plague in Calcutta and Bombay. Calcutta and Bombay became free from plague in 1925 and 1935, respectively. Later both cities had epidemics in 1948 and 1949, and Bombay again in 1952. Investigations at this time showed that in the previous 50 years there had been a number of changes in the rodent and flea populations. By 1960 the lesser bandicoot rat (*Bandicota bengalensis*) had become the dominant rodent in both cities, forming 80 per cent of the rodent population in Calcutta and 49 per cent in Bombay. *B. bengalensis* is fairly susceptible to plague but carried fewer *X. cheopis* than *Rattus rattus*, and more *X. astia* which feeds on man less readily. In Calcutta the flea population was 66 per cent *X. astia* and 34 per cent *X. cheopis*. In Bombay, although *X. cheopis* was the dominant flea (76 per cent) on *R. rattus* and *R. norvegicus*, both rats were highly resistant to plague.[45]

Figure 26.2: Development of Blockage in the Alimentary Tract in Fleas. A, fed flea with midgut full of blood containing plague bacilli; B, partially blocked flea; C, D, formation of the plug

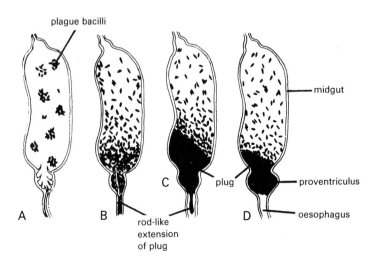

Development of Y. pestis in Fleas

Three forms of plague may be distinguished: bubonic, septicaemic and pneumonic. In bubonic plague the pathogen is largely contained in buboes formed in the lymph glands of the femoral, inguinal and axillary regions. In septicaemic plague, which is regarded as a subset of bubonic plague, *Y. pestis* is abundant in the circulating blood and readily available to blood-sucking fleas. A high level of bacteraemia is required to infect fleas success-fully. Pneumonic plague is highly contagious by the air-borne route and insect vectors play no part in its transmission.

When a flea feeds blood is propelled along the oesophagus to the midgut by the pharyngeal pump, with the proventriculus acting as a valve to pre-vent regurgitation. If the blood is infected *Y. pestis* multiplies in the midgut and in the interstices of the spine-like epithelial cells of the proventriculus (see Chapter 17). The culture of *Y. pestris* in the flea's midgut forms a cohesive, gelatinous body which fills the midgut and proventriculus, effect-ively occluding the lumen of the latter. Such a flea is referred to as 'blocked' (Figure 26.2).

When a blocked flea attempts to feed, the pharyngeal pump is unable to force blood through the proventriculus into the midgut and its pumping distends the oesophagus. When the pharyngeal pump ceases to work, the stretched oesophagus recoils and forces blood, contaminated with frag-ments of the gelatinous bacterial culture, into the host on which the flea has been attempting to feed.[9] Being unable to feed successfully a blocked flea will repeatedly attempt to feed and in so doing has the potential to infect many hosts. Being unable to take in liquid food a blocked flea is susceptible to desiccation and survives only a short time under hot, dry conditions.

Blockage of the gut is not necessarily permanent or fatal to the flea. A passage may be re-established through the plug, giving rise to a partially blocked flea. Such a flea is more dangerous than a fully blocked flea because not only is it able to feed and therefore live longer, but its pro-ventriculus is unable to function as an effective valve, and infective material is regurgitated from the midgut into the flea's host.[8,9]

The process of blockage in the flea is a complicated one and in only a percentage of infected fleas does it develop. Burroughs[19] studied blockage in ten species of fleas and found that the percentage infected varied with the species from zero to 50 per cent, the latter being in *Xenopsylla cheopis.* Bibikova[15] also working with *X. cheopis,* but having a rather larger sample, obtained 33 blocked fleas out of 214 fleas exposed (15 per cent). Many factors influence the development of *Y. pestis* in a flea including: the strain of *Y. pestis*;[15] the temperature at which the flea is held; the frequency and duration of feeding; and the specificity of the host.[29]

From his experimental work Burroughs[19] concluded that: the most important method of transmission of plague was through the blocked flea serving as a biological vector; that mechanical transmission was of considerable importance during an epizootic when mass transmission was occurring; but that a single flea was unlikely to transmit plague mechanically; and transmission by the ingestion of infected fleas, or by crushing such fleas or their faeces, into the skin was a rare occurrence of minor importance.

When a flea feeds it deposits viscous faeces on the hair of its host, and any plague bacilli would be retained in the pellet and not come into contact with the host's skin.[19] Under moderate temperatures *Y. pestis* would remain viable on the mouthparts of a flea for only three hours which, for most species of fleas, is less than the interval between feeds, making mechanical transmission unlikely.[15]

Rat Fleas as Vectors of Plague[10,19,41,42]

Xenopsylla cheopis has a worldwide distribution between 35°S and 35°N where it is a common ectoparasite of rats in cities, ports and rural situations. It is undoubtedly the most important vector of human plague throughout the world. In a comparison of ten species of fleas *X. cheopis* showed: the highest rate of blockage (58 per cent); the highest ratio of transmissions, 35 transmissions from 53 fleas; and the lowest rate of eliminating *Y. pestis* from its body to become plague free.[19,41]

X. brasiliensis is an ectoparasite of *Rattus* spp in rural situations in Africa, South America and India.[10] It is as efficient as *X. cheopis* as a vector of plague and is considered to be the major vector of plague to man in rural situations in Africa and in the hilly, woody tracts of Bombay State in India.[41]

X. astia is a parasite of *Rattus* spp in south-east Asia, where it occurs in fields, villages and ports. It is regarded as a mediocre vector of plague. It was the dominant flea of rats in Madras where in 1931 it formed 94 per cent of the rodent flea population, and Madras was considered to be relatively plague free. The other 6 per cent of fleas on rats were *X. cheopis*. *X. astia* feeds more readily on rats than on man, and will play a greater role in maintaining plague among the *Rattus* population than in transmitting it to man.[47]

The role of the human flea (*Pulex irritans*) is more debatable. It is reluctant to feed on rats, and when it becomes infected the gut rarely blocks.[20] In one series of experiments only one out of 57 *P. irritans* became blocked.[19] *P. irritans* is worldwide in distribution, and it is to be expected that there will be differences between populations in different parts of the world. In Brazil *P. irritans* was implicated in an epidemic of plague when 20 to 70 per cent of *P. irritans* fed on infected *Cercomys* sp, became infected and transmitted *Y. pestis* to healthy *Cercomys*.[34]

Ctenocephalides felis and *Ct. canis*, the dog and cat fleas, are weak vectors of *Y. pestis*. *Nosopsyllus fasciatus* is widely distributed throughout the world in cool, temperate areas and can maintain plague among *Rattus* spp. It is, however, reluctant to feed on man and human cases are rare in epizootics when *N. fasciatus* is the vector.[10] *Leptopsylla segnis* is a cosmopolitan ectoparasite of mice, which also occurs on rats. It is less readily infected with *Y. pestis* than *N. fasciatus* and may play a minor role in plague epizootics but feeds only reluctantly on humans and is considered to play a negligible role in the transmission of plague to man.

The role of *Echidnophaga gallinacea* in the transmission of plague is uncertain. In Burrough's experiments[19] it was a slightly better vector than *N. fasciatus* but considerably less efficient than *X. cheopis*. Although *E. gallinacea* is known as the sticktight flea of poultry it is found on a large range of mammals and birds, and is capable of transmitting *Y. pestis*. Nevertheless, its habit is to attach itself permanently to the head of its host and it does not detach for some time after the host's death. *E. gallinacea* infects the head of its host, and mice and presumably rats clean such fleas off rapidly and devour them, which would reduce the probability of *E. gallinacea* being an effective vector of plague among these rodents.[19]

Strains of the same species of flea may differ in their ability to act as vectors of plague. Divergent results have been obtained with *Diamanus montanus*, a parasite of ground squirrels, which Wheeler and Douglas[52] found to be a better vector of plague than *X. cheopis*, whilst Burroughs[19] found it to be a very poor vector. There was also considerable difference in the vector efficiency of male and female *D. montanus* with females being very much more efficient.[52]

Sylvatic Plague[47] (see Figure 26.2)

A disturbing feature of the third pandemic has been the way in which plague has spread from *Rattus* spp in relatively close association with man to wild rodents in the field. Twigg[47] refers to the first phase when plague is in *Rattus* spp as the murine phase, and the second phase in wild rodents as sylvatic plague, a term in common use. Sylvatic plague is now established in all continents except Australia. Some measure of the complexity of the epidemiology of plague can be given by the numbers of small mammals and their flea parasites which have been found infected. Excluding the cosmopolitan species of rats and commensal mice, 209 taxa (179 species and 30 subspecies) of Rodentia and 16 taxa (15 species and one subspecies) of Lagomorpha have either been found infected in nature or their ectoparasites have been positive for plague.[42] Ninety-nine taxa (95 species and four subspecies) of fleas, associated with these small mammals, have been found infected with *Y. pestis* in nature.[42] In addition in Vietnam and Kampuchea the major carrier of plague is a shrew, *Suncus murinus*, which is parasitised by *X. cheopis*.[47]

USA. Within 40 years of plague being introduced into San Francisco on the west coast of the USA, it had crossed the continental divide and become firmly established east of the Rocky Mountains. This rapid spread was facilitated by the existence of continuous rodent populations. Plague is now enzootic in the USA west of 100°W. On the west coast plague became rapidly established in ground squirrels (*Citellus* spp), which are strongly communal and always infested with fleas. In the interior the primary plague reservoirs were the desert wood rat (*Neotoma desertorum*) and the Zuni prairie dog (*Cynomys gunnisoni zuniensis*), while marmots played a lesser role.

There is a great range in susceptibility to plague among wild rodents. This is conveniently measured using the LD50 value, which is the dosage required to kill 50 per cent of the exposed population. For comparative purposes this can be related to laboratory white mice in which the LD50 was four bacilli. Wild rodents could be put into one of four groups on the basis of their susceptibility to *Y. pestis*. The first group were homogeneously susceptible to infection and *Reinthrodontomys megalotis* had an LD50 of one bacillus, being more sensitive than the laboratory colony of white mice. A second group were those of which the majority died after infection with one to one thousand mouse LD50s. This group included three species of *Peromyscus*. A third group was moderately resistant to infection, tolerating more than one thousand mouse LD50s and this included species of *Citellus* and a vole (*Microtus* sp). The fourth group included two species of kangaroo rat (*Dipodomys*) which were refactory to infection with 1,000,000 mouse LDs. Enzootic plague foci are maintained by rodents of the second and third groups which may have high infection rates. From *Microtus* and *Peromyscus* plague can spread and become epizootic among more susceptible rodents such as prairie dogs.

Southern Africa. In southern Africa plague is now enzootic in wild rodents over a large part of the country where the rainfall is less than 625 mm per annum. The main reservoir of plague is the gerbil, *Tatera brantsi*, which is host to three species of fleas of which *Xenopsylla philoxera* is the most important. Gerbil colonies experiencing an epizootic of plague decline over a period of many months and recovery of the population is even slower, with total recovery being long delayed. There are two routes through which plague may spread from gerbils to man. The first is the more direct route from gerbils to domestic *Rattus rattus* and on to man, and the other involves the peridomestic multimammate mouse *Mastomys natalensis* (= *M. coucha*) as an intermediate host between the gerbil and *R. rattus*. Both *R. rattus* and *M. natalensis* are parasitised by *Xenopsylla brasiliensis*, an extremely efficient vector of plague.[22,47]

Palaearctic Region. Sylvatic plague is unknown in western Europe where plague has not become established in wild rodents. In south-eastern

Europe there are plague foci in the Caspian lowlands at the northern end of the Caspian Sea. Here the main reservoir for plague is the little sisel (*Citellus pygmaeus*), a relative of the ground squirrels of the USA. An extensive campaign, carried out to eradicate plague by controlling the little sisel, has involved the large-scale destruction of colonies of the rodent so that surviving colonies are isolated, and should plague break out in one colony it is unlikely to spread to others. These control measures have been greatly aided by changes in land usage, breaking the originally continuous suitable habitat into isolated small pockets. The campaign has been highly successful and it is confidently anticipated that enzootic plague can be completely eradicated from the area.[25]

In the adjoining region of the Middle East there is the Kurdistan focus which extends for 1,000 km through the mountainous area of southern Turkey and northern Syria, Iraq and Iran. Here a close examination of the gerbil population revealed the existence of two species, *Meriones libycus* and *M. persicus*, which were resistant to plague, and two other species, *M. tristrami* and *M. vinogradovi*, which were very susceptible. The maintenance of plague in Kurdistan results from a balance between resistant and susceptible species.[13]

Plague is transmitted among the gerbils by *Xenopsylla buxtoni*. In this area there are no domestic rats and there is a break in the normal sequence of wild rodent to domestic rat to man. It is considered that epidemics of plague result from rare cases of human plague contracted in the field, infecting *Pulex irritans*, which is abundant in the living quarters of the human population.[13,14] A similar plague focus based on gerbils is present in Transcaucasia, and there are reasons for regarding the Kurdistan and south-eastern European Russian foci as a single unit, the Kurdo-Caspian focus.[14]

There was a plague focus in asiatic Russia, east of Lake Baikal in Transbaikalia, where the reservoir host was the Siberian marmot (*Marmota sibirica*). As a result of control measures between 1939 and 1955 against the marmot no plague has been recorded since 1946. The area is considered to be free from plague but vulnerable to its reintroduction from the adjoining Mongolian People's Republic where foci still exist.[14]

Oriental Region. In the Oriental region sylvatic plague exists in India and in some countries of south-east Asia. In India the main reservoir host is the Indian gerbil (*Tatera indica*), which is not truly sedentary or sufficiently resistant to plague to form permanent pockets of infection.[12] Baltazard and Bahmanyar[12] concluded that the lack of stubborn foci should ensure the disappearance from India of sylvatic plague. This appears to be taking place. In 1951 sylvatic plague was present in foci in northern, central and southern India but by 1969 central India was free, and in southern India only one of three foci was still active.[12,44] Plague continues in the foothills of the Himalayas in Nepal and northern India. In Burma and Vietnam plague has continued to be active since it was introduced 17 years ago.

After a silent period of seven years human plague reappeared in Java in Indonesia,[49] where the situation is unusual, in that the wild reservoir host is another species of *Rattus, R. exulans.* In mobility and susceptibility to plague *R. exulans* is comparable to *T. indica* and unlikely to create permanent foci of infection. The domestic rat in Java is *R. rattus diardi* which is highly susceptible to plague.[11] A similar situation exists in Hawaii where sylvatic plague is maintained in *Rattus hawaiiensis* by its parasite *Xenopsylla hawaiiensis.*[47]

South America. In South America foci of sylvatic plague are present in Brazil, Argentina, Bolivia, Paraguay, Peru and Ecuador.[4]

Survival of Y. pestis[4]

Plague can survive the hot dry season in India by persisting in aestivating Indian gerbils.[12] It can also overwinter in hibernating rodents, and latent infections in rodents can relapse, later become active and initiate an epizootic. It is possible for flea larvae to ingest *Y. pestis* when feeding on the faeces of infected adult fleas. When larvae of *N. fasciatus,* which had been exposed to infected flea faeces, were examined few were positive, and they contained few bacilli showing no signs of multiplication.[7]

The survival of blocked fleas is dependent on external conditions and at 27°C blocked *X. cheopis* survived an average of ten days.[41] Infected fleas, not necessarily blocked, can survive for long periods in the favourable microclimate of a rodent burrow. Davis[22] reported finding infected *X. philoxera* in gerbil burrows which had been deserted for up to four months. There is evidence that infected fleas may live for at least a year, and some species for as long as four years,[4] but the latter claim is refuted by Kir'yakova.[35] In addition plague bacilli can survive, and indeed multiply, in the soil layers of a rodent burrow where microclimatic and other conditions are favourable. Bacilli in soil have infected healthy rodents reoccupying burrows which had been vacant for at least 11 months.[4]

Tularaemia (*Francisella tularensis*)[16,37,40]

Francisella tularensis is a Gram-negative, aerobic micro-organism, which is extremely pleomorphic with rods and cocci occuring in more or less equal numbers. It causes tularaemia in man and many other warm-blooded animals including sheep, horses, pigs, cattle and birds.[16,40,46] In the USSR there were 10,000 cases a year before vaccination was introduced, which reduced the incidence to less than 200 per annum.[39] Tularaemia occurs in Europe, excluding the Iberian peninsula and Great Britain; USSR; Asia Minor; Japan; and north-western USA (Wyoming, Utah, Montana) and adjoining parts of Canada. Recently it has been reported from Virginia, an eastern state, and may therefore be more widely distributed in the USA than had been supposed previously.

In North America the subspecies present is *F. tularensis tularensis*, in the Old World *F. t. palaearctica*, and there is the possibility of a third sub-species *F. t. mediaasiatica* being present in the southern and eastern parts of the species' distribution. The North American subspecies is the most virulent.[39]

F. tularensis can be transmitted from host to host by a variety of routes including blood-sucking arthropods, water, food and inhalation. In addition the organism possesses the potent property of being able to penetrate the unbroken skin, and therefore can be transmitted by contact with infected material.

The natural hosts of *F. tularensis* are mainly rodents, including lemmings in Sweden, jackrabbits in Utah and hares and voles in the USSR.[36,39] Among the rodent population *F. tularensis* is transmitted by fleas and anopluran lice.

The ability of *F. tularensis* to survive away from its vertebrate host favours mechanical transmission by blood-sucking flies, especially tabanids. *Chrysops discalis* is recognised as being a major mechanical vector of *F. tularensis* in the USA. Half (19/39) of the human cases of tularaemia in Utah in the summer of 1971 could be attributed to the biting of *C. discalis* and another quarter (9) were suspected of being due to *C.discalis.*[36] In Sweden, *Aedes cinereus* has been incriminated as a vector of *F. tularensis.*[37]

Ixodid vectors of tularaemia include *Dermacentor andersoni* and *Haemaphysalis leporispalustris* in the USA, and *D. nuttalli* in the USSR.[6,46] Infections of *F. tularensis* in ticks are long-lasting. The organism multiplies in the midgut epithelium and haemolymph of the tick and is transferred when the tick is feeding.[39] Transovarian transmission has been demon-strated in *D. andersoni* and other ixodid ticks in North America.[30]

Hopla[33] has produced evidence for the mechanical transmission of *F. tularensis* among voles by interrupted feeding of fleas. Although tularaemia organisms survive for several weeks in fleas, no transmission occurs when a clean feeding method is used. It is possible for transmission also to occur by contamination with infected flea faeces.

Tularaemia is most severe in sheep in which the morbidity rate in North America may be as high as 40 per cent, with a mortality of 50 per cent.[16] In horses there is fever and foals are more seriously affected than older animals, and in swine tularaemia causes fever in piglets but is latent in adult pigs.[16]

References

1. Anon. (1907). Reports on plague investigations in India. 22. Epidemiological observations made by the Commission in Bombay City. *Journal of Hygiene 7*: 724-98
2. _____ (1908). Reports on plague investigations in India. 31. On the seasonal prevalence of plague in India. *Journal of Hygiene 8*: 266-301
3. _____ (1910). Reports on plague investigations in India. 39. Interim report of the advisory committee for plague investigations in India. *Journal of Hygiene 10*: 566-8
4. _____ (1970). WHO expert committee on plague — fourth report. *WHO Technical Reports Series 447*: 1-25
5. _____ (1981). Human plague in 1980. *WHO Chronicle 35*: 238-9
6. Antisiferov, M.I., Zykina, N.A., Sizykh, L.V., Charnaya, T.G., Zharov, V.R., El'shanskaya, N.I. and Evdokimov, A.V. (1976). Establishment of natural nidality of tularaemia in the Tuva ASSR. *Zhurnal Microbiologii, Epidemiologii i Immunobologii* (2): 75-8
7. Bacot, A.W. (1914). On the survival of bacteria in the alimentary canal of fleas during metamorphosis from larvae to adult. *Journal of Hygiene 13, Plague Supplement III*: 655-64
8. _____ (1915). Further notes on the mechanism of the transmission of plague by fleas. *Journal of Hygiene 13, Plague Supplement IV*: 774-6
9. _____ and Martin, C.J. (1914). Observations on the mechanism of the transmission of plague by fleas. *Journal of Hygiene 13, Plague Supplement III*: 423-39
10. Bahmanyar, M. and Cavanaugh, D.C. (1976). *Plague Manual.* World Health Organisation, Geneva
11. Baltazard, M. and Bahmanyar, M. (1960). Recherches sur la peste à Java, *Bulletin of the World Health Organization 23*: 217-46
12. _____ and Bahmanyar, M. (1960). Recherches sur la peste en Inde. *Bulletin of the World Health Organization 23*: 169-215
13. _____ Bahmanyar, M., Mostachfi, P., Eftekhari, M. and Mofidi, Ch. (1960). Recherches sur la peste en Iran. *Bulletin of the World Health Organization 23*: 141-55
14. _____ and Seydian, B. (1960). Enquête sur les conditions de la peste au Moyen-Orient. *Bulletin of the World Health Organization 23*: 157-67
15. Bibikova, V.A. (1977). Contemporary views on the interrelationships between fleas and the pathogens of human and animal diseases. *Annual Review of Entomology 22*: 23-32
16. Blood, D.C., Henderson, J.A. and Radostits, O.M. (1979). *Veterinary Medicine — a Textbook of the Diseases of Cattle, Sheep, Pigs and Horses.* Baillière Tindall, London
17. Brooks, R. St. J. (1917). The influence of saturation deficiency and of temperature on the course of epidemic plague. *Journal of Hygiene 15, Plague Supplement V*: 881-99
18. Burgdorfer, W. (1976). The epidemiology of the relapsing fevers. pp. 191-200 in *The Biology of Parasitic Spirochetes*, R.C. Johnson (ed.), Academic Press, New York
19. Burroughs, A.L. (1947). Sylvatic plague studies. The vector efficiency of nine species of fleas compared with *Xenopsylla cheopis. Journal of Hygiene 45*: 371-96
20. Busvine, J.R. (1976). *Insects, Hygiene and History.* Athlone Press, London
21. Buxton, P.A. (1950). *The Louse.* Edward Arnold, London
22. Davis, D.H.S. (1953). Plague in South Africa: a study of the epizootic cycle in gerbils (*Tatera brantsi*) in the northern Orange Free State. *Journal of Hygiene 51*: 427-49
23. Diab, F.M. and Soliman, Z.R. (1977). An experimental study of *Borrelia anserina* in four species of Argas ticks. 1. Spirochete localisation and densities. *Zeitschrift für Parasitenkunde 53*: 201-12
24. Felsenfeld, O. (1974). Genus IV. *Borrelia* Swellengrebel 1907, 582. pp. 184-90 in *Bergey's Manual of Determinative Bacteriology*, R.E. Buchanan and N.E. Gibbons (eds.), Williams and Wilkins, Baltimore
25. Fenyuk, B.K. (1960). Experience in the eradication of enzootic plague in the north-west part of Caspian region of the USSR. *Bulletin of the World Health Organisation 23*: 263-73
26. Geigy, R. (1968). Relapsing fevers. pp. 175-216 in volume II, *Infectious Blood Diseases of Man and Animals*, D. Weinman and M. Ristic (eds.), Academic Press, New York

27. Gloster, T.H., White, F.N., Mukhari, A.N., Chaudhuri, J.S.R., Mitra, C.C., Mandal, G.C. and Ram, M. (1917). Epidemiological observations in the United Provinces of Agra and Oudh, 1911-1912. *Journal of Hygiene 15, Plague Supplement V*: 793-880
28. Gratz, N.G. (1980). Problems and developments in the control of flea vectors of disease. pp. 217-40 in *Fleas*, R. Traub and H. Starcke (eds.), A.A. Balkema, Rotterdam
29. Gubareva, N.P., Akiev, A.K., Zemel'man, B.M. and Abdulrakhmanov, G.A. (1976). The effect of some factors on block-formation in the fleas *Ceratophyllus tesquorum* Wagn. 1898 and *Neopsylla setosa setosa* Wagn., 1898. *Parazitologiya 10*: 315-9
30. Guerrant, R.L., Humphries, M.K., Butler, J.E. and Jackson, R.S. (1976). Tickborne oculoglandular tularaemia. *Archives of Internal Medicine 136*: 811-3
31. Hoogstraal, H. (1979). Ticks and spirochetes. *Acta Tropica 36*: 133-6
32. _____ Clifford, C.M., Keirans, J.E. and Wassef, H.Y. (1979). Recent developments in biomedical knowledge of *Argas* ticks (Ixodoidea: Argasidae). pp. 269-78 in volume II, *Recent Advances in Acarology*, J.G. Rodriguez (ed.), Academic Press, New York
33. Hopla, C.E. (1980). Fleas as vectors of tularaemia in Alaska. pp. 287-300 in *Fleas*, R. Traub and H. Starcke (eds.), A.A. Balkema, Rotterdam
34. Karimi, Y., Eftekhari, M. and Almeida, C.R. (1974). Sur l'écologie des puces impliquées dans l'épidémiologie de la peste et le rôle éventuel de certains insectes hématophages dans son processus au nord-est du Brésil. *Bulletin de la Société de Pathologie Exotique 67*: 583-91
35. Kir'yakova, A.N. (1973). On the length of life of fleas in burrows. *Parazitologiya 7*: 261-3
36. Kloch, L.E., Olsen, P.F. and Fukushima, T. (1973). Tularaemia epidemic associated with the deerfly. *Journal of American Medical Association 226*: 149-52
37. Manson-Bahr, P.E.C. and Apted, F.I.C. (1982). *Manson's Tropical Diseases*. Baillière Tindall, London
38. Mollaret, H.H. and Thal, E. (1974). Genus XI. *Yersinia* van Loghen 1944, 15. pp. 330-2 in *Bergey's Manual of Determinative Bacteriology*, R.E. Buchanan and N.E. Gibbons (eds.), Williams and Wilkins, Baltimore
39. Ol'sufyev, N.G. (1978). Personal communication
40. Owen, C.A. (1974). Genus *Francisella* Dorofe'ev 1947, 176. pp. 283-5 in *Bergey's Manual of Determinative Bacteriology*, R.E. Buchanan and N.E. Gibbons (eds.), Williams and Wilkins, Baltimore
41. Pollitzer, R. (1954). *Plague*. WHO, Geneva
42. _____ (1960). Review of recent literature on plague. *Bulletin of the World Health Organization 23*: 313-400
43. Rogers, Sir Leonard (1928). The yearly variations in plague in India in relation to climate: forecasting epidemics. *Proceedings of the Royal Society of London B 103*: 42-72
44. Seal, S.C. (1960). Epidemiological studies of plague in India. 1. The present position. *Bulletin of the World Health Organization 23*: 283-92
45. _____ (1960). Epidemiological studies of plague in India. 2. The changing pattern of rodents and fleas in Calcutta and other cities. *Bulletin of the World Health Organization 23*: 293-300
46. Thorpe, B.D., Sidwell, R.W., Johnson, D.E., Smart, K.L. and Parker, D.D. (1965). Tularaemia in the wildlife and livestock of the Great Salt Lake Desert Region, 1951 through 1964. *American Journal of Tropical Medicine and Hygiene 14*: 622-37
47. Twigg, G.I. (1978). The role of rodents in plague dissemination: a worldwide review. *Mammal Review 8*: 77-110
48. Van der Merwe, S. (1968). Some remarks on the 'tampans' of the *Ornithodoros moubata* complex in southern Africa. *Zoologischer Anzeiger 181*: 280-9
49. Velimirovic, B. (1972). Plague in South-East Asia. *Transactions of the Royal Society of Tropical Medicine and Hygiene 66*: 479-504
50. Walton, G.A. (1962). The *Ornithodoros moubata* superspecies problem in relation to human relapsing fever epidemiology. *Symposia of the Zoological Society of London 6*: 83-156
51. _____ (1979). A taxonomic review of the *Ornithodoros moubata* (Murray) 1877 (sensu Walton, 1962) species group in Africa. pp. 491-500 in volume II, *Recent*

Advances in Acarology, J.G. Rodriguez (ed.), Academic Press, New York
52. Wheeler, C.M. and Douglas, J.R. (1945). Sylvatic plague studies. V. The determination of vector efficiency. *Journal of Infectious Diseases 77*: 1-12
53. Wilson, Sir Graham and Miles, Sir Ashley (1975). *Topley and Wilson's Principles of Bacteriology, Virology and Immunity.* Edward Arnold, London
54. Zaher, M.A., Soliman, Z.R. and Diab, F.M. (1977). An experimental study of *Borrelia anserina* in four species of *Argas* ticks. 2. Transstadial survival and transovarial transmission. *Zeitschrift für Parasitenkunde 53*: 213-23

27 MALARIA (*PLASMODIUM*) AND OTHER HAEMOSPORINA (SPOROZOA)

The sporozoa are parasitic Protozoa which lack cilia and flagella, except in some male gametes; rarely form pseudopodia; and produce either resistant spores or sporozoites. In Baker's classification[3] the Sporozoa are divided into two classes: the Telosporea and the Piroplasmea. The Telosporea have sexual reproduction, and produce sporozoites. The Piroplasmea reproduce asexually by binary fission or schizogony, and there is uncertainty as to whether sexual reproduction occurs. The arthropod-borne members of the Telosporea are placed in the suborder Haemosporina, order Eucoccida, subclass Coccidia. They are characterised by being intracellular parasites which have both asexual and sexual phases of multiplication; undergo schizogony; and, in sexual reproduction, have a motile zygote. Haemosporina have two hosts, with sexual reproduction occurring in a member of the Diptera, and asexual reproduction in the vertebrate host.

Garnham[11] recognises three families within the Haemosporina: the Plasmodiidae, Haemoproteidae and the Leucocytozoidae. The most important of these is the Plasmodiidae, which contains the genus *Plasmodium* and includes the four species responsible for human malaria. In *Plasmodium* schizogony occurs in the blood; gametocytes develop in mature erythrocytes; the end product of the digestion of haemoglobin is a dark pigment, haemazoin; and the vectors are mosquitoes. In the other two families schizogony does not occur in the blood, and the vectors are Diptera other than mosquitoes.

In the Haemoproteidae haemazoin is produced, and the gametocytes develop in mature erythrocytes. In the Leucocytozoidae no haemazoin is produced, and the gametocytes are not found in mature erythrocytes. Two genera of Haemoproteidae, *Haemoproteus* and *Hepatocystis*, and one of Leucocytozoidae, *Leucocytozoon*, are of minor veterinary importance.

The Piroplasmea contains one order, the Piroplasmida, and two families, the Babesiidae and Theileriidae. Species of the type genera for these families, *Babesia* and *Theileria*, cause severe disease in livestock.

The Haemosporina will be dealt with in this chapter and the Piroplasmea in the next.

Malaria

Malaria is the most widespread and persistent disease of mankind. Even today, many tens of millions of the world's population each year suffer

514

from malaria. Malaria is an ancient disease, recognised by Hippocrates about 400 BC, who described the three characteristic stages of an attack — chilly rigor, high fever and profuse sweating.

In the nineteenth century malaria was widely distributed throughout the world and even in 1950, 64 per cent of the world's population (excluding China) was at risk of contracting malaria, which was widespread throughout the Afrotropical, Oriental and Palaearctic regions. It was present in northern Australia, and in western Europe extended as far north as Arkhangelsk (64°N). In the Americas the endemic area embraced South America north of 32°S; Central America; a narrow belt west of the Rocky Mountains extending to Vancouver in Canada; and a broader belt on the eastern coast of North America extending into south-east Canada (Figure 27.1).[42]

Through the strenuous efforts of the World Health Organization the proportion of the world's population (excluding China) exposed to malaria was reduced from 64 per cent to 38 per cent in the period 1950 to 1972. Unfortunately, following a breakdown in control in the Oriental region, half of the world's population was still at risk to malaria in 1981 (Figure 27.2). Before the introduction of control measures the number of cases of malaria in India exceeded 100,000,000 p.a. By 1976 this had been reduced to 7,000,000 cases but with only 37 deaths.[42] Mortality from malaria can be high, and more than a million infants and young children in tropical Africa still die from malaria every year. Even when mortality is low malaria

Figure 27.1: Geographical Distribution of Malaria in the Mid-nineteenth Century. Malarious areas dotted

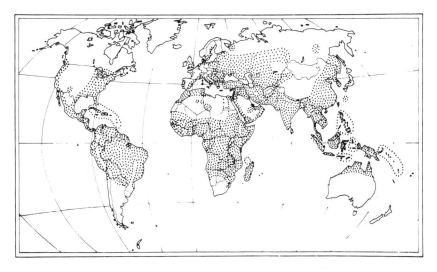

Source: From Wernsdorfer[42]

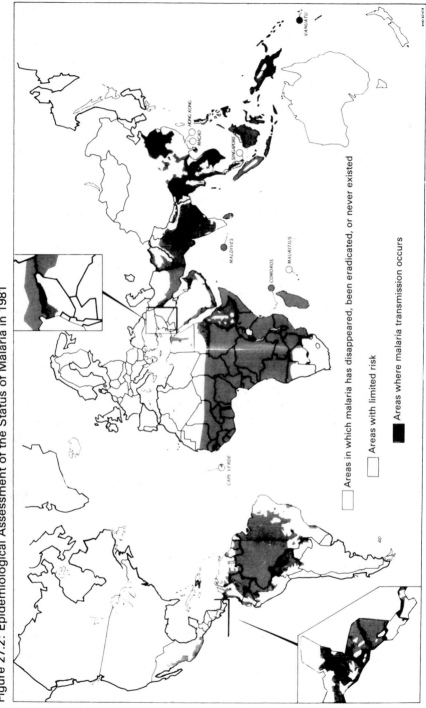

Figure 27.2: Epidemiological Assessment of the Status of Malaria in 1981

Areas in which malaria has disappeared, been eradicated, or never existed

Areas with limited risk

Areas where malaria transmission occurs

Reproduced by permission of the World Health Organization

causes chronic suffering, lowers resistance to other diseases, and reduces life expectancy.[42]

The Malaria Parasites (Plasmodium)

More than a hundred species of *Plasmodium* have been described from vertebrates. Four species occur in man, about 20 species in other primates, a similar number in other mammals, and about 40 each in birds and reptiles.[12,42] The vectors of the mammalian species of *Plasmodium* are invariably species of *Anopheles* mosquitoes while bird plasmodia are transmitted mainly by culicine mosquitoes of the genera *Culex* and *Aedes*.[12]

Before 1940 experimental work on plasmodia was carried out using chickens and various species of bird malaria. This changed with the discovery of plasmodia in rodents in central Africa. These parasites, e.g. *P. berghei*, are readily colonised in laboratory rodents and are transmitted by *Anopheles*, the genus which transmits human malaria. In nature *P. berghei* is transmitted by *An dureni*.[12]

Four species of *Plasmodium* cause malaria in man. Although they produce a similar illness with paroxysms recurring at regular 48 h or 72 h intervals, and are grouped under the one heading 'malaria', there are in fact four different diseases each with its own specific pattern. The species are: *P. falciparum*, which causes malignant tertian malaria; *P. vivax*, which causes benign tertian malaria; *P. malariae*, the cause of quartan malaria; and *P. ovale*. The terms tertian and quartan derive from the Roman way of counting, in which a fever which recurs at 48 h intervals is said to be tertian (third day) because there is fever on day one, normal temperature on day two, and fever again on day three. By the same line of argument *P. malariae* with a 72 h periodicity is said to be quartan (fourth day).

P. falciparum. Malignant tertian malaria is the greatest killer and yet the most easily cured form of malaria. Schizogony occurs in the capillaries and sinuses of the internal organs, interrupting their blood supply. Malignant tertian is said to be the arch simulator of other diseases because the effect it produces will depend upon the organ involved. Cerebral malaria is the most dangerous, producing coma, but malignant tertian can also simulate acute dysentery, heart disease and pulmonary infection. After the initial series of attacks have passed *P. falciparum* commonly causes further clinical disease. These are recrudescences, not relapses. The difference is a technical one. A relapse is 'a renewed manifestation of malarial infection separated from previous manifestations of the same infection by an interval greater than the 48 or 72 hours between the paroxysms,[12] and a recrudescence is 'a renewed manifestation of infection believed due to the survival of erythrocytic forms'.[12]

P. falciparum is associated with two severe reactions: blackwater fever,

Table 27.1: Quantitative Data on the Four Species of *Plasmodium* Which Cause Malaria in Man

| Species | Pre-erythrocytic schizont | | Development in man | | | Persistence in man | | Sporogonic cycle | |
	size	no. of merozoites	prepatent (days)	incubation (days)	periodicity (days)	average (years)	maximum (years)	oocyst size	duration (days)
P. falciparum	60 μm	30,000 40,000	5½	9	2	1	4	60 μm	9
P. vivax	42 μm	10,000	8	12	2	2	8	45 μm	8
P. ovale	n.a.	15,000	9	15	2	1	5	70 μm	12
P. malariae	n.a.	2,000	15	21	3	4	53	45 μm	16

n.a. = not available.

Source: Data extracted from Garnham,[12] Shortt *et al.*[36] and Wernsdorfer[42]

and haemolytic anaemia in children. Blackwater fever was associated with the irregular and inadequate treatment of malignant tertian malaria with quinine. With the replacement of quinine by other drugs blackwater fever is now rarely encountered. The patient passes a urine dark with methaemoglobin. Mortality from blackwater fever could be up to 50 per cent. Haemolytic anaemia is a very rapidly fatal condition of African infants in areas with holoendemic malaria.[12]

P. falciparum has a higher threshold for development than *P. vivax* and is commoner in the warmer areas of the world, being limited by a summer isotherm of 20°C. Some quantitative data on *P. falciparum* are given in Table 27.1.

P. vivax. P. vivax causes a milder disease, but is more persistent than *P. falciparum.* It is widely distributed throughout the world, being limited by the 16°C summer isotherm and is therefore often the only species present in the cooler temperate regions. It can persist up to eight years and cause relapses at two-monthly intervals. It is absent from West Africa because the indigenous people lack the Duffy factor on their erythrocytes, and *P. vivax* fails to penetrate. One subspecies, *P. v. hibernans*, has a prepatent period (period between injection of the parasite and its appearance in the erythrocytes), which varies from 250-350 days.[12]

P. ovale. This is the rarest of the four human malaria parasites, not being described until 1922. It is the least pathogenic, and produces a tertian fever after a longer incubation period than *P. vivax* or *P. falciparum* (Table 27.1).[12] Relapses occur at three-monthly intervals. In West Africa it replaces *P. vivax* among the indigenous people.[12] It is also present in Papua New Guinea and in the area formerly known as Indo-China, i.e. Thailand, Kampuchea and Vietnam.[42]

P. malariae. This is a slow-growing parasite which has a worldwide but patchy distribution. Although widespread it is usually less common than either *P. falciparum* or *P. vivax.* However, it is next to *P. falciparum* in pathogenicity, with death resulting from kidney failure.

P. malariae has remarkable powers of persistence with recrudescences occurring for up to 53 years (Table 27.1).[12] This is highlighted by an incident in Granada in the Caribbean, from which malaria was eradicated in 1962. In 1978 a recrudescence of *P. malariae* occurred in a single individual and produced a number of secondary infections in other people with *An aquasalis* as the vector.[12] *P. malariae* is limited by the 16°C summer isotherm.[42]

Simian Malaria. P. rodhaini, which occurs in chimpanzees, is regarded as identical with the human parasite *P. malariae.* Transmission of *P. malariae* amongst the human population and *P. rodhaini* among chimpanzees take place in two different biological systems with different vectors and present no obstacle to control.[42]

Very rarely, infections with simian parasites occur in human beings. Three cases of human infection with *P. knowlesi* in Malaya and one of *P. simium* in Brazil have been reported.[12] *P. knowlesi* produces a daily paroxysm, i.e. its periodicity is quotidian, and *P. simium* has a tertian periodicity.

Features of Malaria in Man

After the anopheline mosquito has injected sporozoites into a susceptible human there is a prepatent period, defined as 'the minimal time elapsing between the initial sporozoite infection and the first appearance of parasites in the erythrocytes'.[11] There is a further period following the appearance of parasites in the circulating blood before the development of clinical symptoms. This is the incubation period, defined as 'time elapsing between the initial malaria infection in man and the first clinical manifestation'.[12] Values for the prepatent and incubation periods for malaria parasites in man are given in Table 27.1.

Paroxysms occur at the end of schizogony when the merozoites escape from the erythrocytes, releasing a 'toxin'. The paroxysm lasts about six hours, beginning with a short period of shivering, followed by a longer period of fever in which the temperature may reach 41°C, and succeeded by a period of sweating. Paroxysms recur at intervals of 48 h or 72 h with increasing parasitaemia to a maximum after which the parasitaemia declines rapidly. This maximum is reached with *P. falciparum* about 10-14 days after the prepatent period.[11] Further paroxysms from the initial infection may recur after a period of two or three months or even some years. The results of an attack of malaria is anaemia with the possibility of oxygen deprivation to the tissues, and effects of the 'toxin' released when the erythrocytes burst. As part of the immune response the spleen is enlarged.

Passive immunity acquired from the mother lasts for about three months. Certain mutations confer a degree of protection against *P. falciparum* and are prevalent in areas where that parasite is dominant. In the heterozygous state genes for sickle cell anaemia and thalassaemia provide protection against *P. falciparum* but are lethal in the homozygous state.[1,18] There are divided opinions as to the role of the sex-linked gene for glucose-6-phosphate dehydrogenase (G-6-PD) deficiency in protecting against malaria. Luzzatto[18] considers that it does, but Martin *et al.*[22] came 'to the conclusion that clinical evidence of protection against falciparum malaria in G-6-PD-deficient individuals is lacking'.

Life Cycle of *Plasmodium*

History

Laveran was the first person to recognise the malaria parasite within the red blood cells in 1880,[17] and later in the same year he observed the process of exflagellation in fresh preparations. It was the demonstration of exflagellation which convinced Pasteur in 1884 that the object being observed was indeed an independent organism, and not the result of degenerative processes. The significance of exflagellation was shown by MacCullum in 1897 when he observed the formation of microgametes by exflagellation, the fertilization of the macrogamete, and the subsequent development of a motile ookinete in a related genus *Haemoproteus*.[19] MacCullum referred to the anterior tip of the ookinete puncturing erythrocytes with which it made contact. Indeed the pointed end of the ookinete of *Plasmodium* is used to penetrate the cells of the gut of mosquitoes.[11]

At this stage it was not known in what other host exflagellation and formation of the ookinete occurred. In 1897 Ross, working in India, observed oocysts of *P. falciparum* on the midgut of an *Anopheles* mosquito. Ross was then moved to Calcutta but was unable to continue to work on human malaria and turned his attention to bird malaria. In 1898 Ross obtained the complete life cycle of *P. relictum* (= *P. danilevskyi*) in *Culex quinquefasciatus* (= *fatigans*), including the presence of sporozoites in the salivary glands, and transmitted by *P. relictum* from infected to healthy sparrows by the bite of *Cx quinquefasciatus*.[34]

At this stage Ross's work was interrupted and he was not able to extend his findings to human malaria until late 1899 in West Africa. Of this work Ross wrote 'In a few weeks I was able to show that the parasites of quartan, tertian and malignant fever all develop in *Pyretophorus costalis* [now *An gambiae*] or *Myzomyia funesta* [now *An funestus*], precisely as the *Proteosoma* [now *Plasmodium*] of birds develops in *Culex fatigans*'.[34] In the meantime Grassi, Bignami and Bastianelli[14] had followed the development of *P. falciparum* in *An claviger* in 1899. The final seal on their work was the sending of *An maculipennis*, infected with *P. vivax*, from Italy to London where P. Manson fed them on his son, P. T. Manson, who developed malaria.[34]

There remained one problem. Schaudinn had illustrated and described the sporozoites of *Plasmodium* directly invading erythrocytes. If that were so then it should be possible to transmit malaria by blood transfusion soon after the inoculation of sporozoites. This was not the case. Following inoculation of sporozoites there was a period of several days during which it was impossible to transmit infection by blood transfusion. The answer was that the sporozoites did not parasitise red cells but other tissues in the body. In 1936 Raffaele showed that the first cycle of development of the bird parasites, *P. elongatum* and *P. relictum*, was not in the eythrocytes but

Figure 27.3: Life Cycle of Malaria Parasite. 1, sporozoites enter liver cell; 2-5, first pre-erythrocytic schizogony cycle ending with release of merozoites; 6-9, second pre-erythrocytic cycle; 10, an erythrocyte; 11-15, schizogony in erythrocyte; 16-20, repeat of schizogony in erythrocyte; 21-24, development of male and female gametocytes; 25, midgut of mosquito; 26, exflagellation; 27, macrogamete maturing; 28, microgamete; 29, zygote; 30, ookinete; 31-33, developing oocyst; 34, release of sporozoites; 35, sporozoites in salivary gland of mosquito

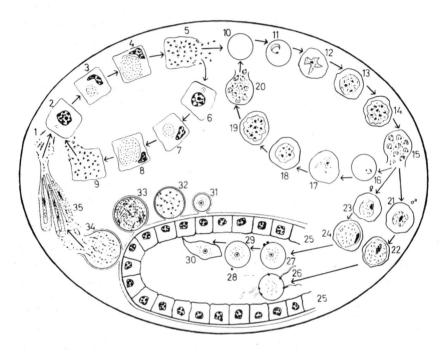

Source: From Garnham[11]

in the cells of the reticulo-endothelial system.[29,30] Later Shortt and Garnham[37] showed that the first cycle of development of *P. vivax*, the exoerythrocytic cycle, occurred in the parenchyma cells of the liver and this was confirmed for *P. falciparum* by Shortt *et al.*[36] The central features of the life cycle of malaria parasites in the vertebrate and invertebrate hosts were now known.

Cycle of Plasmodium in Man and Anopheles (see Figure 27.3)

When an infected *Anopheles* mosquito feeds it injects sporozoites with its saliva. The sporozoites disappear from the circulating blood in 30 min and invade the parenchyma cells of the liver where a cycle of schizogony takes place. This is the exoerythrocytic or pre-erythrocytic cycle of the parasite. A large unpigmented schizont (42 μm)[37] is formed containing several thousand merozoites (Table 27.1). The merozoites are released into the circulation and invade the erythrocytes. Their release coincides more or less with the end of the prepatent period (Table 27.1).

The merozoite attaches to an erythrocyte and is invaginated into the red cell within a parasitophorous vacuole, where it feeds and deposits a pigment, haemazoin. The ingested merozoite becomes a feeding trophozoite and, in the early stages of an infection, the fully grown trophozoite becomes a schizont, producing a small number of new merozoites (6-16).[11] Release of the merozoites from the erythrocytes brings on an attack of malaria, and the interval between attacks is the length of the schizogonic cycle. The released merozoites repeat the cycle and invade other erythrocytes.

After a number of cycles of schizogony some of the trophozoites do not divide but become gametocytes which develop no further in man. Gametocytes are mature in 4 days in *P. vivax* and in 8 days in *P. falciparum*.[42] When a female *Anopheles* takes up blood containing gametocytes they shed the remains of the erythrocyte and are free. Microgametocytes undergo exflagellation producing eight microgametes, the process taking 10-15 min. The microgametes move away to find and enter macrogametes to form zygotes. The zygote is at first immobile and then becomes an active ookinete which enters the midgut epithelium to form an oocyst under the basal laminar.

The oocyst may be recognised by the presence of pigment derived from the gametocyte. As it grows it disrupts the basal laminar and projects into the haemocoele.[38] Considerable nuclear division goes on within the oocyst and sporozoites develop around a number of germinal centres. Mature oocysts measure 45-70 μm (Table 27.1), and in the case of *P. falciparum* contain around 10,000 sporozoites.[28] The time taken to complete sporogony is temperature-dependent and minimum times are given in Table 27.1. Sporogony is not completed at temperatures above 33°C or below 16°C.[33] This is the reason for the association between the distribution of malaria and the summer isotherm of 16°C for *P. vivax* and 20°C for *P. falciparum*.[42] When sporogony is complete the sporozoites escape into the haemocoele and accumulate in the salivary glands. In *P. yoelii nigeriensis* the sporozoites escape from the oocyst through small holes and tears.[38]

The salivary glands of anopheline mosquitoes are paired with each gland consisting of three lobes, two lateral and one median. The central duct in the proximal portion of the lateral lobes is described as being 'a thick chitinised cuticular duct'.[40] Sporozoites that enter cells of the salivary gland in this region have difficulty in penetrating the duct wall. Sporozoites of *P. berghei* in *An stephensi* accumulate in the cells of the distal portion of the lobes where they have easy access into the lumen of the duct.[40] When next the mosquito feeds sporozoites will be passed with the saliva into the host, and if the host is susceptible the cycle is repeated. Once infective, anopheline mosquitoes remain so for up to 12 weeks.[33] For all practical purposes that means that mosquitoes are infected for life.

Epidemiology of Malaria

Malaria is said to be endemic where there is 'a constant measurable incidence of natural transmission over a succession of years'.[42] Four grades are recognised based on the frequency of enlarged spleens in the susceptible two- to nine-year-old age group of children. In holoendemic areas their spleen rate is above 75 per cent and the adult spleen rate low. In hyperendemic areas the adult spleen rate is high and the spleen rate in children above 50 per cent. In hypoendemic and mesoendemic areas the spleen rate is below 10 per cent and between 11 and 49 per cent, respectively.[42] Malaria is said to be epidemic when the 'incidence of cases in an area rises rapidly and markedly above its usual level or when the infection occurs in an area where it was not present previously.[42]

Malaria is also said to be stable or unstable or in an intermediate state. Stable malaria is associated with holoendemic and hyperendemic areas. Characteristically transmission is perennial with little change in the incidence of malaria from season to season; the vector is both strongly anthropophilic, feeding almost exclusively on the human population, and long lived. Stable malaria is associated with the warmer areas of the world, favouring rapid sporogony and with the main parasite being *P. falciparum*. Unstable malaria is associated with sudden, very intense epidemics, a short-lived vector, and a limited transmission period. The vector is not strongly anthropophilic and its importance is derived from it being present in high density. Sporogony is not rapid and the parasite usually involved is *P. vivax*.[42]

About 400 species of *Anopheles* have been described in the world and 67 of these have been found naturally infected with malaria, but only 29 species are significant vectors.[42] Garnham[11] produces rather similar figures with 40 species being infected naturally or experimentally with *P. vivax* and 66 species with *P. falciparum*, but 35 of these species are common to both lists giving a total of 71 different species.

Macdonald[20] attempted a 'tentative classification of some notorious vectors' of malaria, using survival and degree of anthropophily as his criteria. Two problems present themselves in making such a classification. Firstly, data on these aspects of anopheline bionomics are not available for all vector species, and those that are are often unavoidably biased, e.g. anthropophily index being determined on catches made in houses. The second problem arises from the assumption that survival and anthropophily remain constant throughout the species range. Survival will depend on

Table 27.2: *Anopheles* Species Associated With Stable Malaria

Species	Distribution
arabiensis	Afrotropical region
funestus	Afrotropical region
gambiae s.s.	Afrotropical region
melas	West African coast from Senegal to Angola
labranchiae	western Mediterranean
sacharovi	south-east Europe, Near and Middle East
fluviatilis	Oriental region, Arabian Peninsula, Kazakh SSR
minimus	Oriental region

local microclimatic conditions, and the degree of anthropophily on the extent to which a species is an opportunistic feeder, likely to be diverted from man in the presence of abundant domestic animals.

Wernsdorfer[42] has enlarged Macdonald's classification and includes 29 species in place of 20. One interesting feature of the two classifications is that they associate the same eight species with stable malaria (Table 27.2). Macdonald associates five species with intermediate malaria and seven with unstable malaria, while Wernsdorfer has eight and 13, respectively. Only one species, *An pharoensis*, is placed in a different category with Macdonald associating it with intermediate malaria and Wernsdorfer with unstable malaria.

This classification has its uses, providing the dictum attributed to Sir Malcolm Watson, that 'every malaria problem is a local one', is kept in mind. In this connection it must not be assumed that the behaviour of a species will be the same under all conditions. In Italy *An messeae* is zoophilic and not associated with malaria, but in eastern Europe and the Soviet Union after the Second World War *An messeae* was an important vector. Its increased anthropophily was attributed to drastically reduced numbers of domestic stock as a result of the war.

In Malaya *An maculatus* is the principal vector of malaria and would warrant inclusion in the list of vectors of stable malaria. In many other parts of its range, e.g. Borneo, it is not a vector.[31] Part of the explanation for this difference may be found in the fact that even in Malaya *An maculatus* prefers to feed on cattle rather than man, and its survival is greatly reduced by low humidity, declining from an average length of life of 34 days at 80 per cent RH to less than a week at 65 per cent RH.[35]

Eight species are associated with stable malaria (Table 27.2), of which four occur in the Afrotropical region, where three (*An arabiensis, An funestus, An gambiae*) are widespread; two (*An minimus, An fluviatilis*) in the Oriental region; and two (*An labranchiae, An sacharovi*) in the Palaearctic region. Another eight species are associated with intermediate malaria (Table 27.3), including *An quadrimaculatus* and *An darlingi* in the

Table 27.3: *Anopheles* Species Associated With Intermediate Malaria

Species	Distribution
atroparvus	north-western Europe, where it is largely littoral
sergenti	North Africa, Middle East, Pakistan
balabacensis	Oriental region
sinensis	Oriental region and Japan
sundaicus	Oriental region
darlingi	Neotropical region, but not the Antilles
quadrimaculatus	Nearctic region, central and eastern USA, southern Canada and Mexico
farauti	Northern Australia, Moluccas, New Guinea, Bismarck Archipelago and Melanesia

Nearctic and Neotropical regions, respectively; *An farauti* in the Australian region; three species (*An balabacensis, An sinensis, An sundaicus*) in the Oriental region; and two in the Palaearctic region (*An atroparvus, An sergenti*). Thirteen species are associated with unstable (epidemic) malaria, and of these seven are in the Oriental region; two each in the Neotropical and Palaearctic regions; and one in each of the Afrotropical and Australian regions (Table 27.4).

In temperate regions malaria transmission is seasonal and often bimodal with peaks in late spring-early summer and late summer-early autumn with a decline in midsummer. There are two reasons for the midsummer decline. High temperatures, particularly if associated with low humidities, will

Table 27.4: *Anopheles* Species Associated With Unstable Malaria

Species	Distribution
messeae	northern Palaearctic region
superpictus	northern Mediterranean, Middle East, Afghanistan, Pakistan and USSR (Transcaucasia, Middle Asia)
pharoensis	Afrotropical region, Egypt, Israel and Syria
aconitus	Oriental region
annularis	Oriental region
culicifacies	Iraq through India to Vietnam, Sri Lanka
flavirostris	south-east Asia
maculatus	Oriental region
philippinensis	Oriental region
stephensi	Iraq through India to Thailand
albimanus	Florida, Texas, Mexico, Central America, the Antilles, South America to Uruguay
aquasalis	Central America, Lesser Antilles and tropical South America
punctulatus	New Guinea, Bismarck Archipelago, Solomon Islands, Moluccas

markedly reduce the longevity of *Anopheles*, and if high temperatures are maintained they could exceed the threshold (33°C) for sporogony. Infections with *P. vivax* predominate in the spring peak and *P. falciparum* in the autumn peak. The reasons are: higher minimum temperature (20°C) for sporogony of *P. falciparum*; the long periods between infection and production of gametocytes (minimum of 10 days after patency);[37] and the lower parasite reservoir in the population as a result of recoveries during the winter. The probability of recovery from *P. falciparum* is 0.0125 per day, i.e. average duration of infection 80 days.[42]

The main features of the bionomics of *Anopheles* species which determine their importance as vectors of malaria have already been mentioned. They include the frequency with which the species feeds on man, i.e. degree of anthropophily, its longevity and abundance. They will be considered in more detail.

Host Preference

The main factor governing the ability of an *Anopheles* species to act as a vector of malaria is the frequency with which it feeds on man. The vectors associated with stable malaria are those which are strongly anthropophilic, often feeding on man to the exclusion of other hosts. To transmit malaria an individual *Anopheles* has to feed on man at least twice: the first time to acquire an infection and the second to transmit the parasite. This means that the ability of a species to transmit malaria is related to the product of the two probabilities of an individual feeding on man twice and not directly to the proportion feeding on man. This is important in comparing the potential of two species.

If the probability of an *Anopheles* feeding on man (p) is 1.0, i.e. the species feeds exclusively on man, then the probability of it feeding on man twice is p^2, which is also 1.0. If a species takes only half its feeds from man, then $p = 0.5$ and the probability of it feeding twice on man is 0.25. When a species feeds only occasionally on man, e.g. $p = 0.1$, then the probability of that species acting as a vector is 0.01, and when a species feeds infrequently on man, e.g. 1 per cent of feeds, the probability of an individual feeding on man twice is 1 to 10,000. This comparison helps to demonstrate that species with a high rate of anthropophily can transmit malaria when present in low density, while species with low anthropophilic rates only act as vectors when present in high density and include species associated with unstable malaria.

Anopheline mosquitoes show gonotrophic concordancy in which blood feeding and oviposition alternate. A blood meal is required for ovarian development. The gonotrophic cycle begins with a blood meal, and as this is digested the ovaries develop leading to a stage when the meal has been fully digested and the eggs are ready for oviposition. Under optimal conditions this cycle can be completed in two days.

It is possible for a female to oviposit and feed again during the same night, and blood feeding to occur at two-day intervals, but it is more likely that the next blood meal will be taken on the night following oviposition, giving an interval of three days. In the tropics female *Anopheles* collected in the morning can be classified as blood-fed; half gravid; gravid, with fully developed eggs; and empty, which includes newly emerged nullipars and recently oviposited parous females. At lower temperatures both blood digestion and ovarian development will take longer.

In some species, e.g. *An gambiae*, virgin females do not develop eggs after a blood meal. Such females are likely to take another blood meal after mating. The taking of two blood meals early in life will increase the probability of their being infected with *Plasmodium* at an early age.

Longevity

An *Anopheles* mosquito cannot transmit malaria until the sporogonic cycle of the *Plasmodium* has been completed, and this takes a minimum of eight days (Table 27.1), and therefore only those mosquitoes that live at least that time can act as vectors of malaria. A species could be very abundant and feeding mainly on man, but if its mortality was such that few survived long enough to become infective that species would play only a minor role, if any, in transmission. It is important, therefore, to be able to determine the age structure of an *Anopheles* population.

A method of determining the physiological age of an *Anopheles* mosquito, developed by Polovodova,[27] has been applied widely by Detinova.[6,7] The method relies on the fact that in each ovarian cycle each ovariole matures only one egg. When this is deposited the stretched tissues of the ovariole contract to form a dilatation at the position of the former follicle in which the egg developed. A separate dilatation is formed at each ovarian cycle so that the number of dilatations indicates the number of ovarian cycles that have been completed, and the number of blood meals which have been taken. Knowledge of the durations of the gonotrophic and sporogonic cycles under local conditions enables calculation of the proportion of the *Anopheles* population which has lived long enough to be infective.

Gillies and Wilkes[13] used this technique to study the longevity and infectivity of populations of *An gambiae* in Tanzania. At Muheza on the coast survival from one ovarian cycle to the next was 0.62 which, on a three-day ovarian cycle, represented a daily survival of 0.854. Mosquitoes will have to complete a minimum of three ovarian cycles, i.e. be 3-parous, before being infective. The sporozoite rate in 3-parous *An gambiae* was 4.1 per cent and increased to 32 per cent among females which were 7-parous or more. The heavier infection rate in older *An gambiae* was countered by their small numbers. Twenty per cent of the population survived to complete three ovarian cycles or more but only 1 per cent completed seven cycles. The greatest contribution to transmission of *P. falciparum* came from *An gambiae* which has completed four, five and six cycles. These mosquitoes formed only 16 per cent of the population but 73 per cent of those infective.

Gillies and Wilkes[13] made parallel observations on the *An gambiae* population at Gonja, inland from Muheza, where the dry season lasted five months. At Muheza only *An gambiae* s.s. was present, and at Gonja both *An gambiae* s.s. and *An arabiensis*, and this may have had some influence on the findings. At Gonja the daily survival rate of *An gambiae* s.l. was lower than at Muheza (0.791 cf. 0.854). Correspondingly only 14 per cent (cf. 20 per cent) completed three or more ovarian cycles, and only 0.3 per cent (cf. 1 per cent) completed seven cycles. The maximum parity recorded at Gonja was a female that had completed eight cycles and at Muheza 12 cycles. These differences can be attributed to the effect of differences in aridity on survival, and is in agreement with Wernsdorfer[42] who recorded daily survival rates of 0.95, 0.90 and 0.85 at relative humidities of 65 per cent, 55 per cent and 50 per cent, respectively, at mean temperatures of 27-30°C. The survival rate at Muheza corresponds with that found by Wernsdorfer for 50 per cent RH.

Density of Anopheles

Two main factors which influence the abundance of *Anopheles* are temperature and availability of suitable breeding sites. In the tropics the abundance of a species may show very little variation throughout the year. At Muheza the population of *An funestus*, which breeds in permanent bodies of water, shows little change throughout the year and has a stable physiological age structure.[7] *An gambiae* breeds in temporary collections of water and its populations show greater variation throughout the year, being more dependent on rainfall. Nevertheless for much of the year (December-July) the density of *An gambiae* at Muheza was high and the physiological age structure almost constant.[7]

The speed of development of *Anopheles* is temperature-dependent, and its effect can be determined more accurately using non-feeding stages such as eggs or pupae. The length of the egg stage increased from two days at 22-24°C to ten to twelve days at 10-12°C.[16] Muirhead-Thomson[25] found a four-fold increase in the durations of the egg and pupal stages of *An minimus* with a decrease in temperature from 30° to 16°C. Ribbands[32] found that when water temperatures fluctuated from 26.5° to 30.6°C in the summer in Assam the larval stage of *An minimus* was seven days. He considered that under these conditions the complete life cycle from egg to egg would take 14 days — egg to adult eleven days and oviposition of the first egg batch three days. At 16°C the egg to adult cycle can be expected to take about six weeks.

In warmer temperate regions, e.g. North Africa, breeding will continue all the year, but the life cycle be greatly extended during the cooler months. In Egypt the life cycle of *An pharoensis* lasts several months in the winter but adults continue to emerge. In more severe climates breeding ceases and the adult females hibernate. In the Moscow region *An messeae* hibernates for six months (October-March) and there are only two generations in a year: an overwintering generation which feeds and oviposits in the spring and early summer, and a summer generation whose progeny go into hibernation.[7]

Species of *Anopheles* have the potential to increase their populations very rapidly when, under optimal conditions, batches of 100-200 eggs can be laid at intervals of two to three days by females which can complete several cycles in their lifetime. Development from egg to adult may take as little as ten days and it is possible to have an increase of ×50 to ×100 in the *Anopheles* population within two weeks. One limiting factor on this exponential rate of increase is the availability of breeding sites, which are dependent on rainfall. Rainfall increases the humidity of the air and favours greater longevity of the adults, providing further opportunity for population increase.

The effect of rainfall is complex, depending upon the species of *Anopheles* and its particular breeding sites. Heavy rains will flush out water courses and reduce the population of species breeding in pools in river beds. Such autumnal rains in Algeria normally brought the malaria transmission season to an end by flushing out the breeding sites of *An labranchiae*. In 1934 the rains began with steady gentle rain, in place of the more usual violent severe storms, and increased the breeding sites for *An labranchiae*, resulting in a severe late-season epidemic of malaria.

In Ceylon in 1934-5 it was a drought which provided the conditions for a dramatic increase in the population of *An culicifacies*. *An culicifacies* breeds in still water in pools and its breeding sites were greatly increased when the severe drought led to the rivers ceasing to flow, becoming a series of discontinuous pools with no water movement. This was ideal for *An culicifacies* and led to a severe epidemic of malaria. The effect of rainfall will depend upon local conditions, and in northern India *An culicifacies*, which was favoured by drought in Ceylon, has been responsible for severe epidemics in years of excessive rainfall with widespread pool formation.[15]

Sporogony

Sporogony takes place in the female *Anopheles* and is temperature-dependent with an upper threshold of 33°C and a lower one of 16°C for *P. vivax*, and of 20°c for *P. falciparum*. At 30°C sporogony of *P. vivax* is completed in seven to eight days and this time doubles to 15-16 days at 20-21°C.[41] At 16°C sporogony takes 55 days.[42] When an infective *Anopheles* female feeds, only a small percentage of the sporozoites in the salivary gland are injected into its host, with some being deposited directly into capillaries and others into subcutaneous tissues.[41] Although Shortt *et al.*[36] found that relatively few sporozoites of *P. falciparum* developed into schizonts in the liver, yet 'as few as ten sporozoites (of *P. vivax*) is ordinarily sufficient to infect'.[41]

Models of Malaria Transmission

Once the intimate relationship between malaria and the *Anopheles* mosquito was understood efforts were made to express it in quantitative terms. In the first decade of this century Ross[34] was already modelling the transmission of malaria. The development of an efficient model requires that research be concentrated on aspects of the disease on which quantitative information is lacking. Once developed the model can be used to evaluate the likely effects of different strategies, enabling limited facilities (staff, money) to be used in a manner likely to give the best results for the effort expended. The tradition of modelling malaria was continued by Professor G. Macdonald, who appropriately was Director of the Ross Institute of Tropical Hygiene in London. Macdonald's book *The Epidemiology and Control of Malaria,*[20] summarised the existing position in 1957 and gave rise to much field research to test and, where necessary, modify the model proposed.[4,21] A recent book on this subject, received after this chapter had been written, is *The Biomathematics of Malaria.*[2] Various quantitative entomological aspects of malaria transmission are considered below.

Measure of Stability of Malaria

One critical piece of information is the probability of a mosquito surviving long enough for sporogony to be completed. If the daily survival of a female *Anopheles* is p and the sporogonic cycle takes n days, then the probability of an individual mosquito surviving n days is p^n. The life expectancy of the mosquito at emergence is $1/-\log_e p$, and the index of stability is the product of the life expectancy times the average number of humans bitten by one mosquito in one day (a) and is therefore $a/-\log_e p$. Stability of malaria is therefore a function of the longevity of the vector and its degree of anthropophily. Stable malaria is associated with an index exceeding 2.5, unstable malaria with an index less than 0.5 and intermediate malaria with an index of 0.5-2.5.[20,42]

Sporozoite Rate

Macdonald[20] defined the sporozoite rate (s) as: $s = p^n ax/(ax - \log_e p)$ where x is the infectivity of man to the *Anopheles*, i.e. the gametocyte rate. Gillies and Wilkes[13] tested this expression at Muheza for *An gambiae* where daily survival of the mosquito (p) was 0.854; the average number of feeds by a mosquito on man in one day (a) was taken as 0.33, i.e. the gonotrophic cycle was three days; and the duration of the sporogonic cycle (n) was 13 days. The sporozoite rate observed was 2.5 per cent ($s = 0.025$). The unknown variable was the gametocyte rate (x). Substituting the numerical estimates into the formula gave a value for x of 0.1135, i.e. 11.35 per cent of *An gambiae* became infected at each feed, and it would be expected that this would relate to the gametocyte rate in the human population. Ten years earlier the overall gametocyte rate at Muheza had been determined as 7.7 per cent, distinctly lower than the expected 11.35 per cent.

The gametocyte rate is not uniform throughout a population, being low in adults and considerably higher in young children (less than 10 years old) when they are developing immunity. In a holoendemic area such as Muheza gametocyte production would be greatest at two years (35 per cent gametocyte rate) from which it would decline but still exceed 10 per cent in the 12-year olds.[42] The discrepancy between observed and expected gametocyte rates could be accounted for by a change in the rate over ten years or by *An gambiae* feeding preferentially on the younger members of the community, who may be more accessible or more attractive to host-seeking *An gambiae*. I am tempted to change the length of the sporogonic cycle from 13 to 11 days. Gillies and Wilkes[13] found one infective female which had completed only two cycles and would have been seven to ten days old, several which had completed three cycles and would have been ten to 13 days old. When the sporogonic cycle is taken as 11 days the expected gametocyte rate becomes 7.9 per cent, reasonably close to the 7.7 per cent observed.

Basic Reproduction Rate

The reproduction rate (z) is the average number of new infections which will be produced from a single existing infection. The basic reproduction rate (z_0) is the average maximum number of new infections produced by a single infection when an infected individual, possessing no immunity, is introduced into a community where neither the mosquitoes nor the inhabitants are or have been previously infected. The basic reproduction rate is given by the expression:

$$z_0 = ma^2 bp^n / -r \log_e p$$

where b is the proportion of mosquitoes with sporozoites which are actually infective, and in a non-immune population $b = 1$; r is the recovery rate which is taken as 0.0125 for *P. falciparum*;[20,42] and m is the density of *Anopheles* relative to the human population. Note that the reproduction rate is a function of a^2, that is the probability of a mosquito feeding twice on a human being. One important application of this expression is that when the value for z falls below 1.0 the incidence of malaria is declining and if other conditions remain constant the disease will disappear.

Wernsdorfer[42] has calculated various values of z_0 using selected, reasonable values for the other parameters. The values chosen were $m = 10$; $a = 0.4$, i.e. the mosquito is 100 per cent anthropophilic feeding at two- or three-day intervals; $p = 0.90$; $n = 8$; $b = 1.0$ and r $= 0.0125$. When these are substituted in the above expression the calculated value of z_0 is 525.

Any change in m produces a similar proportional change in the value of z_0 while the effect of a change in a produces an effect proportional to the square of the change. Thus when the density of *Anopheles* (m) is reduced by one fifth, from ten to two, the value of z_0 is reduced by the same factor from 525 to 105, but when the *Anopheles* feeds less frequently or there is a change in its degree of anthropophily then the change in z_0 is enhanced. Thus if a changes from 0.4 to 0.16, i.e. feeding at three-day intervals and taking only half of its meals from man, z_0 changes from 525 to 84.

A trebling of the daily mortality, reducing survival (p) from 0.90 to 0.70, has a marked effect on z_0, reducing it from 525 to 21, i.e. to 4 per cent of the initial value. A two-fold increase in the duration of the sporogonic cycle, under the conditions stated above, reduces z_0 to a little less than half (43 per cent) of its previous value. However, changes in n cannot be looked at in isolation because, when dealing with the same species of *Plasmodium* a change in the duration of the sporogonic cycle implies a change in temperature, and there would certainly be changes in the feeding frequency (a) and also in survival(p).

It is possible for anopheline density (m) to vary independently of other factors, but in the same species there will be some correlation between feeding frequency (a) and survival (p). Variations in a independent of p can be obtained using different species. Examination of the effect of different variables on the malarial reproduction rate need not be limited to a particular vector. In field situations the vector could change with the season. The effect of a change in the length of the sporogonic cycle (n) depends on the value of p (survival). When n is doubled from eight to 16 days the basic reproduction rate (z_0) is reduced to a little less than half if $p = 0.9$; but if $p = 0.5$, z_0 is reduced to 0.2 per cent of its original value; and the effect is even greater for smaller values of p.

Under the initial conditions given above the density of *Anopheles* would have to be reduced from ten to 0.019 in order for the basic reproductive rate to fall below 1.0. The basic reproduction rate can also be reduced below unity by reducing the feeding frequency (a) from 0.4 to 0.0174, a very substantial change, or by reducing survival (p) from 0.9 to 0.5. The use of insecticides to control malaria transmission is directed at reducing both the density and longevity of the vector.[42]

Vectorial Capacity

Models need to be continually reassessed against situations actually encountered in the field, and Nájera[26] found that the model he was using in northern Nigeria predicted different results from those found. He attributed these discrepancies to inadequate estimation of the basic variables required for the model, and criticised the preparation not the model. He also blames overestimation of the effects of control measures undertaken by assuming a degree of perfection which was not attainable in the field.

Dietz *et al.*[8] and Molineaux *et al.*[24] produced a revised mathematical model for comparing the effects of alternative control measures against malaria in which the main entomological input was the concept of vectorial capacity, which was defined as:

$$= ma^2 p^n / - \log_e p$$

and is very similar to the basic reproductive rate already considered. The expression for vectorial capacity differs from that of the basic reproduction rate by the omission of terms b (infectivity of sporozoites) and r (recovery rate), but both factors are included elsewhere in the model.

Principles of Control and Current Status of Malaria

There is no single approach to the prevention of malaria because the method or methods to be adopted will depend upon the local situation. In areas where no control measures are in operation the individual must rely on personal protection, using screening of living accommodation, especially bedrooms; sleeping under nets; wearing protective clothing; and using repellents. Such measures can be effective but require a high level of self-discipline. Personal protection may be combined with drug prophylaxis in which the drugs used inhibit the erythrocytic cycle of the parasite and its associated clinical symptoms, but does not prevent the development of exoerythrocytic forms in the liver. Drug prophylaxis does protect groups at high risk, e.g. troops operating in highly malarious areas in wartime.

Any attack on malaria must be a community effort. The attack may be directed against either the parasite or the vector, and in the case of the latter against the immature stages in the breeding sites or against the emerged adults in houses and animal shelters. In practice it is common to include all three approaches but with emphasis on the most vulnerable link in the chain of transmission in the particular locality. Drug treatment would involve curing clinical cases and the detection and treatment of all gametocyte carriers in the community. In theory, if there are no gametocyte carriers then no malaria transmission will take place regardless of the habits and density of the *Anopheles* population. The choice between larval and adult control will depend upon local conditions with larval control being favoured where breeding sites are limited, and adult control where breeding sites are numerous and widespread. Larval control attempts to reduce the *Anopheles* density, that is *m* in the model, while measures against the adult are aimed at decreasing adult longevity, *p* in the model.

Using relatively simple materials considerable success has been achieved against malaria by vector control in many parts of the world. In Central America Gorgas successfully applied measures against mosquitoes to control both yellow fever spread by *Aedes aegypti* and malaria, at first in Cuba and subsequently in the Panama Canal Zone. Larval control measures included modification of the habitat to reduce breeding by such methods as draining swamps and marshes or flooding them, when breeding would be concentrated at the edge of the resultant lake and accessible to chemical control. The use of drainage for mosquito control is particularly associated with the work of Malcolm Watson[43] in Malaya.

Chemical control involved the use of oil and Paris green, a compound containing both copper and arsenic, against *Anopheles* larvae and pyrethrins against adults. Paris green applied as a dust at 1 kg/ha selectively poisoned surface-feeding *Anopheles* larvae, leaving the habitat apparently otherwise undisturbed. Oil was messy and changed the habitat, but was administratively convenient because its application could be easily checked. House spraying with pyrethrins in the evening and early morning was directed at reducing longevity of the vector, and combined with other measures was successful in maintaining communities relatively malaria free in highly malarious areas and used to protect expatriate personnel operating in tropical colonies.

The greatest success achieved by these methods against an *Anopheles* vector was the elimination of *An gambiae* from Brazil, into which it had been introduced from West Africa, and in which it had established itself over a considerable area. Success was only achieved by formulating and implementing a rigorous sustained programme of control which aimed first to contain *An gambiae* in the area already occupied, and then to push the invader steadily back. This splendid achievement of Soper and Wilson[39] was published in 1943 when attention of much of the world was elsewhere and it did not receive full acclaim.

The discovery in the 1940s of the insecticidal properties of DDT and other chlorinated hydrocarbons dramatically changed the approach to malaria control by concentrating the attack against adult *Anopheles*. The outstanding property of DDT and related compounds was their persistence, and deposits applied to resting places of mosquitoes in houses and animal shelters remained insecticidally active for up to six months.[42] Previously adult control measures had to be carried out daily during the transmission season and the extension of this interval to three months opened up the prospect of a more ambitious approach to malaria control. Control, that is the reduction of malaria incidence to a level at which it ceased to a major public health problem, could be extended more widely from the cities into the rural areas, and complete eradication became a distinct possibility.

Considerable success was achieved. In 1950, 143 out of 209 countries in the world were subject to malaria and by 1978, 37 of those countries had been completely freed from malaria (compare Figures 27.1 and 27.2). However, countries from which malaria has been eradicated are of two main classes, being either islands (17 countries) or among the so-called developed countries, including 14 countries in Europe, the USA, Australia and Chile.[42] This success should not disguise the fact that malaria is still firmly established in the tropical areas of the world and although 22 per cent of the world's population originally exposed to malaria have been freed from the disease, one fifth of those still exposed to the disease, largely in tropical Africa, are afforded no protection.[42]

Technical problems have hindered the control of malaria: the development of drug-resistant strains of *Plasmodium*; insecticidal resistance in the vector so that DDT is no longer effective and has had to be replaced by organophosphorous compounds such as malathion, and the carbamates, which have shorter periods of activity, less than one month. Technical problems are solvable but where a government lacks the will to implement control measures no amount of technical expertise can succeed.

In south-east Asia control measures are complicated by the vector, *An balabacensis balabacensis*, being exophilic and therefore not susceptible to control by household spraying. Africa remains the epicentre of malaria in the world and it is the considered opinion of the experts that the best that can be hoped for is long-term malaria control because 'none of the available control tools (singly or in combination) permit the interruption of malaria transmission at a feasible cost'.[42]

Other Haemosporina

Avian Plasmodia

According to Garnham,[12] 'over 30 valid species of malaria parasites have been described from about 500 species of birds'. They are mostly infections of wild birds and where transmissible to domestic poultry cause little disease in local breeds of birds, but cause severe epizootics in introduced poultry. Three species, *P. gallinaceum, P. juxtanucleare* and *P. durae*, are of minor veterinary importance. Species of *Plasmodium* in birds have two preerythrocytic cycles before invading the erythrocytes. The preerythrocytic schizonts are smaller than those in mammals, producing less than 100 merozoites but two successive cycles offer the possibility of releasing more than 1,000 merozoites to invade the erythrocytes.

P. gallinaceum is native to Sri Lanka, India and Malaysia. Its pre-erythrocytic schizonts grow in the cells lining the capillaries and block them causing cerebral damage. Infections develop rapidly in one-day-old chicks but adult birds are only weakly susceptible. *P. juxtanucleare* is more widely distributed in tropical Asia and Japan and has been introduced into Latin America where it has caused more severe epizootics than in its native Asia. Both these species infect jungle fowl, partridges and other wild birds, which form a reservoir of infection.[12] *P. durae* has caused epizootics among domestic turkeys in Kenya and West Africa, and a very similar species, *P. hermani*, has been found in wild turkeys in Florida. *P. durae* causes considerable mortality in domestic turkeys.[12]

Hepatocystis[12]

In *Hepatocystis* the preerythrocytic cycle occurs in the liver of mammals and only gametocytes occur in the erythrocytes. Thirteen species of *Hepatocystis* have been described. They are mostly parasites of arboreal, tropical mammals — lower monkeys, bats and squirrels. There is also one species which occurs in mouse deer (*Tragulus* spp), and another in the hippopotamus. Most work has been done on *H. kochi*, a parasite of monkeys in Africa, for which the vectors are species of *Culicoides*, including *C. adersi* on the East African coast, and *C. fulvithorax*, and probably other species of *Culicoides* in both inland and coastal areas.

The sporogonic cycle in *Culicoides* follows the usual pattern with rapid exflagellation of the microgametocyte with the formation of eight microgametes. In *H. kochi* the ookinete penetrates the basement membrane and enters the haemocoele. Oocysts are free in the haemocoele and accumulate anteriorly in the head, particularly near the eyes and supraoesophageal ganglia. Oocysts measure about 40 μm in diameter, have several germinal centres and produce hundreds of slender sporozoites measuring 11-13 μm. Oocysts mature in five days at 27°C. Sporozoites are rarely seen in the salivary glands and they may invade the mouthparts to be transmitted without being introduced with the saliva.

In the monkey the sporozoites invade the hepatic parenchyma cells and develop into slowly growing schizonts which may take one to two months to reach a size of 2 mm and more. These schizonts are referred to as merocysts. Most of the released merozoites invade erythrocytes to form gametocytes, but some re-invade the liver and repeat schizogony. In the erythrocyte the merozoite produces haemozoin pigment. The presence of free oocysts in *H. kochi* may not be typical of the genus because oocysts of *H. brayi* occur in the usual location on the midgut of *Culicoides (Mono-*

culicoides) nubeculosus and *C. (M.) variipennis*.[23] In some areas infections of *H. kochi* in monkeys can be 100 per cent but its pathogenicity is doubtful. An unusual feature is that parasitaemia increases with the age of the host and there appears to be little or no immunity to *H. kochi.*

Haemoproteus and Parahaemoproteus[9]

More than 80 species of *Haemoproteus* have been named. Schizogony occurs in the tissues and only gametocytes are in the circulating blood. The parasite in the erythrocyte encircles the nucleus of the host cell, in which pigment is deposited. Species of *Haemoproteus* are parasites mainly of birds, but also of lizards and turtles. *H. columbae* is a parasite of pigeons and is transmitted by the hippoboscid *Lynchia maura*. *H. metchnikovi* occurs[5] in turtles and is transmitted by the tabanid *Chrysops callidus*.[5] This is the first record of a tabanid acting as the vector of a species of Haemosporina, and undermines the basis for establishing the genus *Parahaemoproteus* on the grounds that the vectors are not hippoboscids but ceratopogonids. *P. nettionis*, a parasite of ducks, is transmitted by *Culicoides downesi* and other species of *Culicoides*.

The cycle of the parasite in the vector is similar to that of *Leucocytozoon*. The microgamete undergoes exflagellation. The fertilised macrogamete becomes a motile ookinete, about 25 μm long, and forms a oocyst, up to 36 μm in diameter, in which sporozoites are produced from several germinal centres. Sporozoites of *H. columbae* are slender bodies with one end blunt and the other tapered. They are produced in thousands, and those of *H. columbae* are released when the oocyst bursts. The minimum time for the sporogonic cycle in *H. columbae* is ten to twelve days. The sporozoites accumulate in the salivary gland and are passed with the saliva when the vector is feeding.

The cycle of *P. nettionis* in *Culicoides* shows several differences. The oocyst grows very little and there is only a single germinal centre. Fewer sporozoites are produced and they escape gradually from the oocyst. The minimum time for the sporogonic cycle is seven to ten days.

In the vertebrate host schizonts occur in many tissues but are most frequent in the lungs of birds. Those of *H. metchnikovi* occur in the spleens of turtles. Merozoites released from schizonts develop into mature gametocytes in four to six days in birds, and considerably longer (three months) for *H. metchnikovi* in turtles. Infections of *Haemoproteus* are often heavier than those of *Leucocytozoon* but their pathogenicity is uncertain. As with *Leucocytozoon* there is increased parasitaemia in late winter and early spring, favouring infection of the vector and transmission to nestlings.

Leucocytozoon[9,10]

About 70 species of *Leucocytozoon* have been named and they are all parasites of birds. Schizogony occurs in the tissues and only the gametocytes appear in the peripheral circulation. Gametocytes occur in both leucocytes and erythrocytes but no pigment is produced in the latter. Economically important species include *L. simondi*, a parasite of domestic and wild ducks and geese in Europe, North America and south-east Asia; *L. smithi*, a parasite of turkeys in Europe and North America; and probably the most important, *L. caulleryi*, which parasitises chickens in south-east Asia and Africa. *L. caulleryi* is placed in the subgenus *Akiba* which is sometimes raised to generic rank and the species referred to as *Akiba caulleryi*. Species of *Akiba* are characterised by the disappearance of the nucleus of the parasitised cell as the gametocyte matures, and by its transmission by biting midges of the genus *Culicoides*. The vectors of most species of *Leucocytozoon* are species of Simuliidae of various genera, including *Simulium, Prosimulium, Eusimulium* and *Cnephia*.

The life cycle of *Leucocytozoon* will be illustrated using *L. simondi* which has been studied in considerable detail. An infective simuliid injects sporozoites when feeding, and in a susceptible host they develop in the hepatic parenchyma of the liver, growing to a size of 20-40 μm in four to five days. These hepatic schizonts contain several thousand merozoites which invade erythrocytes and erythroblasts to become rounded gametocytes in 48 h. It is not known whether these merozoites are able to invade the liver and produce a second cycle of schizogony. The hepatic schizonts also produce multinucleated syncytia, which are phagocytised by macrophages and grow into megaloschizonts, measuring up to 200 μm, in cells of the reticulo-endothelial system, especially of the spleen and lymph nodes. Megaloschizonts produce a million or more merozoites which either invade the liver to start another cycle of schizogony or enter leucocytes to form elongated gametocytes. Maximum parasitaemia is reached after ten to twelve days after which the infection can remain chronic for two or more years in ducks. The host cell in which a megaloschizont develops becomes hypertrophied.

The density of gametocytes in the peripheral circulation shows a diurnal periodicity with peak numbers being reached in the daytime when simuliids are active and hence favours gametocytes being taken up by feeding simuliids. Both microgametocytes and macrogametocytes escape through a small opening in the pellicle of the host cell. Rounded gametocytes escape more readily than the elongated forms. The microgametocytes undergo exflagellation, producing eight free microgametes. When a microgamete penetrates a macrogamete the two nuclei fuse, and the zygote becomes a motile ookinete measuring 30 μm × 4 μm.

The ookinete penetrates between the cells of the midgut and forms an oocyst beneath the basement membrane. Some ookinetes remain in the midgut for three to four days until the peritrophic membrane disrupts and they are able to reach the midgut epithelium. A mature oocyst is 10-14 μm in diameter and produces about 50 sporozoites from a single germinal centre. The oocyst does not rupture, sporozoites escape gradually from the cyst and move to the salivary glands which they penetrate.

Sporogony occurs at a variable rate even under identical conditions, and in the same vector species sporogony can take 6-18 days at 18-20°C. Exflagellation occurs within one to three minutes of ingestion, with the stimulus being changes in oxygen and carbon dioxide tensions rather than in temperature. It takes 6-12 h for the rounded zygote to become an elongated ookinete, and about 48 h to develop from ookinete to oocyst.

The minimum time from introduction of sporozoites to production of mature gametocytes is six days. Gametocytes will continue to circulate for weeks but their viability declines with time.

L. caulleryi has a similar cycle in *Culicoides arakawae* in which sporozoites are produced in three days at 25°C and six days at 15°C. They remain infective for three to five weeks. The cycle of *L. smithi* in turkeys is slightly different. The primary cycle occurs in the liver, and merozoites released from that cycle either form rounded gametocytes, or invade the liver or kidney producing a second cycle of schizogony; but the schizont and its host cell are not hypertrophied and no megaloschizont is formed.

There is no evidence of a specific relationship between vector and parasite. *L. caulleryi* develops equally well in the major vector *C. arakawae*; in *C. odibilis*, a minor vector which feeds on chickens; and also in *C. schultzei*, which feeds on cattle. Similar observations have been made on other species of *Leucocytozoon*, which parasitise only birds and yet they develop apparently with equal ease in mammal-feeding simuliids. Consequently simuliid-*Leucocytozoon* relationships are more dependent on the simuliid's feeding preferences than on the specificity of the parasite for a particular simuliid.

During winter the parasitaemia in the avian host is low and a small increase occurs in early spring in response to the host's developing reproductive cycle. This ensures that gametocytes will be available in the peripheral blood when the vectors appear in the spring, and when susceptible nestlings will be available for infection. Transmission occurs on the birds' nesting grounds.

Species, such as *L. caulleryi* and *L. simondi*, which include a megaloschizont stage in the reticulo-endothelial system in their cycle are more pathogenic than those, such as *L. smithi*, in which schizogony occurs in the liver and kidneys. Ducks infected with *L. simondi* show some or all of the following symptoms: lethargy, loss of appetite, diarrhoea, convulsions and anaemia. The condition may be fatal. The anaemia cannot be accounted for by simple parasitisation of the erythrocytes but involves intravascular haemolysis. Similar symptoms occur in chickens infected with *L. caulleryi*. There is conflicting evidence as to the pathogenicity of *L. smithi* in turkeys. It may be more important in the presence of other disease. In general *Leucocytozoon* infections are more severe in domestic than wild species, and deaths are commoner in young birds.

References

1. Allison, A.C. (1961). Genetic factors in resistance to malaria. *Annals of the New York Academy of Sciences 91*: 710-29
2. Bailey, N.J.T. (1982). *The Biomathematics of Malaria*. Charles Griffin, London
3. Baker, J.R. (1977). Systematics of parasitic Protozoa. pp. 35-56 in volume I, *Parasitic Protozoa*, J.P. Kreier (ed.), Academic Press, New York
4. Bruce-Chwatt, L.J. (1969). George Macdonald Memorial Lecture. Quantitative epidemiology of tropical diseases. *Transactions of the Royal Society of Tropical Medicine and Hygiene 63*: 131-43
5. DeGiusti, D.L., Sterling, C.R. and Dobrzechowski, D. (1973). Transmission of the chelonian haemoproteid *Haemoproteus metchnikovi* by a tabanid fly *Chrysops callidus*. *Nature, London 242*: 50-1
6. Detinova, T.S. (1962). *Age-grouping Methods in Diptera of Medical Importance*. World Health Organization, Geneva
7. _____ (1968). Age structure of insect populations of medical importance. *Annual Review of Entomology 13*: 427-50
8. Dietz, K., Molineaux, L. and Thomas, A. (1974). A malaria model tested in the African savannah. *Bulletin of the World Health Organization 50*: 347-57
9. Fallis, A.M. and Desser, S.S. (1977). On species of *Leucocytozoon, Haemoproteus* and *Hepatocystis*. pp. 239-66 in volume III, *Parasitic Protozoa*, J.P. Kreier (ed.), Academic Press, New York
10. _____ , Desser, S.S. and Khan, R.A. (1974). On species of *Leucocytozoon. Advances in Parasitology 12*: 1-67
11. Garnham, P.C.C. (1966). *Malaria Parasites and Other Haemosporidia*. Blackwell Scientific Publications, Oxford
12. _____ (1980). Malaria in its various vertebrate hosts. pp. 95-144 in volume I, *Malaria*, J.P. Kreier (ed.), Academic Press, New York
13. Gillies, M.T. and Wilkes, T.J. (1965). A study of the age-composition of populations of *Anopheles gambiae* Giles and *A. funestus* Giles in north-eastern Tanzania. *Bulletin of Entomological Research 56*: 237-62
14. Grassi, B., Bignami, A. and Bastianelli, G. (1899). Ciclo evolutivo delle semilune nell' *Anopheles claviger* ed altri studi sulla malaria dall' ottobre 1898 al maggio 1899. *Atti della Società per gli studi della Malaria 1*: 14-27
15. Hackett, L.W. (1937). *Malaria in Europe*. Oxford University Press, London
16. Kettle, D.S. and Sellick, G. (1947). The duration of the egg stage in the races of *Anopheles maculipennis* Meigen (Diptera, Culicidae). *Journal of Animal Ecology 16*: 38-43
17. Laveran, A. (1880). Note sur un nouveau parasite trouvé dans le sang de plusieurs malades atteints de fièvre palustre. *Bulletin de l'Académie de Médecine Paris Series 2, 9*: 1235-6
18. Luzzatto, L. (1974). Genetic factors in malaria. *Bulletin of the World Health Organization 50*: 195-202
19. MacCullum, W.G. (1897). On the flagellated form of the malarial parasite. *Lancet 2*: 1240-1
20. Macdonald, G. (1957). *The Epidemiology and Control of Malaria*. Oxford University Press, London
21. _____ Cuellar, C.B. and Foll, C.V. (1968). The dynamics of malaria. *Bulletin of the World Health Organization 38*: 743-55

22. Martin, S.K., Miller, L.H., Alling, D., Okoye, V.C., Esan, G.J.F., Osunkoya, B.O. and Deane, M. (1979). Severe malaria and glucose-6-phosphate-dehydrogenase deficiency: a reappraisal of the malaria/G-6-PD hypothesis. *Lancet 1*: 524-6
23. Miltgen, F., Landau, I., Canning, E.U., Boorman, J. and Kremer, M. (1976). *Hepatocystis* de Malaise. III. Développement d'*Hepatocystis brayi* chez *Culicoides nubeculosus et C. variipennis*. *Annales de Parasitologie Humanine et Comparée 51*: 299-302
24. Molineaux, L., Dietz, K. and Thomas, A. (1978). Further evaluation of a malaria model. *Bulletin of the World Health Organization 56*: 565-71
25. Muirhead-Thomson, R.C. (1951). *Mosquito Behaviour in Relation to Malaria Transmission and Control in the Tropics*. Edward Arnold, London
26. Nájera, J.A. (1974). A critical review of the field application of a mathematical model of malaria eradication. *Bulletin of the World Health Organization 50*: 449-57
27. Polovodova, V.P. (1949). Determination of the physiological age of female *Anopheles*. *Meditsinskaya Parazitologiya i Parazitarnye Bolezni 18*: 352-5
28. Pringle, G. (1965). A count of the sporozoites in an oocyst of *Plasmodium falciparum*. *Transactions of the Royal Society of Tropical Medicine and Hygiene 59*: 289-90
29. Raffaele, G. (1936). Il doppio ciclo schizogonico di *Plasmodium elongatum*. *Rivista di Malariologia 15*: 309-17
30. _____ (1936). Presumibili forme iniziali di evoluzione di *Plasmodium relictum*. *Rivista di Malariologia 15*: 318-24
31. Reid, J.A. (1968). *Anopheline Mosquitoes of Malaya and Borneo*. Institute for Medical Research, Kuala Lumpur, Malaysia
32. Ribbands, C.A. (1949). The duration of the aquatic stages of *Anopheles minimus* Theo., determined by a new method. *Bulletin of Entomological Research 40*: 371-7
33. Rieckmann, K.H. and Silverman, P.H. (1977). Plasmodia of man. pp. 493-527 in volume III, *Parasitic Protozoa*, J.P. Kreier (ed.), Academic Press, New York
34. Ross, R. (1911). *The Prevention of Malaria*. John Murray, London
35. Sandoshan, A.A. (1965). *Malariology with Special Reference to Malaya*. Oxford University Press, London
36. Shortt, H.E., Fairley, N.H., Covell, G., Shute, P.G. and Garnham, P.C.C. (1951). The pre-erythrocytic stage of *Plasmodium falciparum*. *Transactions of the Royal Society of Tropical Medicine and Hygiene 44*: 405-19
37. _____ and Garnham, P.C.C. (1948). The pre-erythrocytic development of *Plasmodium cynomolgi* and *Plasmodium vivax*. *Transactions of the Royal Society of Tropical Medicine and Hygiene 41*: 785-95
38. Sinden, R.E. (1975). The sporogonic cycle of *Plasmodium yoellii nigeriensis*: a scanning electron microscope study. *Protistologica 11*: 31-9
39. Soper, F.L. and Wilson, D.B. (1943). *Anopheles gambiae in Brazil 1930 to 1940*. Rockefeller Foundation, New York
40. Sterling, C.R., Aikawa, M. and Vanderberg, J.P. (1973). The passage of *Plasmodium berghei* sporozoites through the salivary glands of *Anopheles stephensi*: an electron microscope study. *Journal of Parasitology 59*: 593-605
41. Vanderbeg, J.P. and Gwadz, R.W. (1980). The transmission by mosquitoes of plasmodia in the laboratory. pp. 153-234 in volume II, *Malaria*, J.P. Kreier (ed), Academic Press, New York
42. Wernsdorfer, W.H. (1980). The importance of malaria in the world. pp. 1-93 in volume I, *Malaria*, J.P. Kreier (ed.), Academic Press, New York
43. Watson, M. (1921). *The Prevention of Malaria in the Federated Malay States*. John Murray, London

28 BABESIOSIS AND THEILERIOSIS

This chapter will deal with babesiosis and theileriosis, clinical diseases produced in domestic animals by species of *Babesia* and *Theileria*, respectively. Two similar terms are used in describing infections with *Babesia*; babesiasis refers to the presence of *Babesia* in the vertebrate host; and babesiosis to clinical disease caused by infection with *Babesia*.[10] The comparable terms for *Theileria* are theileriasis and theileriosis. Both *Babesia* and *Theileria* have an intracellular stage in erythrocytes which is referred to as a piroplasm, a neutral term, non-committal of its role in the life cycle of the parasite. The piroplasms of *Babesia* are larger than those of *Theileria*.

Babesiosis

According to McCosker,[16] 71 species of *Babesia* have been described, of which 18 occur in domestic animals. Their greatest importance is as agents of disease among cattle, to which the greater part of the 1.2×10^9 cattle in the world are exposed.[16] The discovery by Smith and Kilborne[35] of the transmission of *B. bigemina* by the ixodid tick, *Boophilus annulatus*, was the first record of a protozoan being transmitted by an arthropod. As *Bo. annulatus* is a one-host tick the cycle involved transovarian transmission of the *Babesia* by the female tick to the next generation.

Babesia species tend to fall into one of two groups: large or small. Small species have piroplasms measuring 1.0-2.5 μm in length, and include *B. bovis*, the pyriform bodies of which measure 2 × 1.5 μm. Large species measure 2.5-5.0 μm, and include *B. bigemina* which measures 4.5 × 2 μm.[12,22] The parasite multiplies asexually in the erythrocytes by budding. Typically two or four merozoites are formed by schizogony. The division cycle in *B. bigemina* is completed in about 8 h[12] and in a similar time in *B. bovis* which multiplies tenfold in 24 h.[8] The parasite ingests the cytoplasm of the erythrocyte by pinocytosis, and the haemoglobin is completely digested without the production of pigment.[12]

Economic Importance

Mortalities in excess of 50 per cent from babesiosis were often suffered by cattle in the USA and Australia. Babesias cause fever (41-42°C), haemolytic anaemia, haemoglobinuria, and death of infected beasts. Two common terms for the disease are Texas Fever and Red Water. In the USA the disease has been brought under control by the eradication of *Bo.*

annulatus (see Chapter 23). In Australia *B. bovis* (=*B. argentina*)[9] is more important that *B. bigemina*, although both species occur, and both are transmitted by *Boophilus microplus*. The disease is contained by limiting the spread of the vector, and by actions to minimise clinical disease in infected areas.

B. bovis and *B. bigemina* are widely distributed between 32°S and 40°N where they are responsible for serious losses in Latin America and Asia.[16] Losses caused by babesiosis are due to mortality and reduced production; costly maintenance of quarantine and control measures; loss of markets for live grade or pedigree cattle; and 'opportunity losses' by penalising improvement of stock through the introduction of superior but susceptible animals.[16] In the late 1960s it was calculated that annual losses of US$500,000,000 would be suffered by the cattle industry if ticks and babesiosis became established in the endemic areas of the USA.[16] Of this total only 10 per cent was attributed to babesiosis, and 90 per cent to the costs of control and losses in production. These calculations omitted loss of markets and opportunity losses. Losses from babesiosis can be reduced by using Indian Cattle (*Bos indicus*) in place of *Bos taurus*, the former being much more tick resistant and less susceptible to babesiosis.[10]

Immunity to Babesia in Cattle

Two features of infection with *Babesia* influence the severity of the disease produced. They are the destruction of the erythrocytes and the release of pharmacologically active substances.[12] The effect of introducing infective particles of *Babesia* into a mammal is moderated by several factors. Species of *Babesia* show considerable host specificity, and the genetic make-up of the host can limit the severity of the disease. In addition there is the development of immunity among originally susceptible animals. Calves may be protected against reacting severely to infection with *B. bovis* and *B. bigemina* by passive protection acquired via the colostrum from their immune dams, and by a natural immunity. The former lasts for one to two months and the latter for four to seven months.[12]

Cattle that have recovered from infections are immune to developing disease in response to an homologous challenge but may suffer subclinical superinfection. Such animals may develop clinical disease in response to a heterologous challenge. Originally it was considered that acquired immunity was dependent upon retention of a low level of parasitaemia, but there is evidence now that such immunity can continue in the absence of the parasite.[12] Acquired immunity to *B. bovis* and *B. bigemina* persists for more than four years.[12] Protection can be given to susceptible animals by vaccination with an attenuated strain of the parasite which produces a mild disease, but a dead vaccine, which would be ideal, is not yet available.

Species of *Babesia* Parasitising Cattle

Hoyte[9] recognised four species of *Babesia* as parasites of cattle, the two already mentioned, and *B. major* and *B. divergens*. Since then a fifth species, *B. jakimovi*, has been recognised.[20]

Babesia bovis

B. bovis is widely distributed throughout the world occurring in Central and South America, Africa, Asia, Europe and Australia. In tropical and subtropical areas the vectors are species of *Boophilus*, and in southern Europe species of *Rhipicephalus*.[22] Infection is acquired by the female tick, which transmits the parasite transovarially to its larvae which are the infective stage. The larval tick injects infective particles which invade the erythrocytes, and the severity of the reaction is a function of the parasitaemia reached in the host. Maximum parasitaemias of 15,000 parasites per mm^3 (=0.2 per cent parasitaemia) are fatal; non-fatal, severe infections have 5,000 parasites per mm^3; and mild infections less than 1,000 (=0.01 per cent parasitaemia).[22] Infected erythrocytes clump together and block capillaries causing brain damage and anoxia of internal organs.

A beast which has a single infection shows a fluctuating parasitaemia with cycles of three to eight weeks. The fluctuations are due to change in antigenic type of which more than 100 have been recognised. On passage through the tick the strain of *B. bovis* reverts to its basic antigen but this also is variable.[12] In the more natural situation where the infected animal is exposed to repeated infections, i.e. superinfections, the parasitaemia rises smoothly from zero to a maximum in 1-2 years and then declines.[12]

Babesia bigemina

B. bigemina has a similar distribution to that of *B. bovis* and is also found in the southern USSR.[22] One important vector of *B. bigemina* is *Bo. microplus* which acquires the parasite when the adult female is feeding, and transmits the parasite in the succeeding nymphal stage.[8] On introduction into cattle the infective particles appear to invade the erythrocytes. If there is a pre-erythrocytic stage it can only occur in the circulating leucocytes.[8] Clinical disease is produced when the parasitaemia exceeds 1 per cent but there is no clumping of infected red cells and therefore no blockage of capillaries in organs, such as the brain.[12] Because *Bo. microplus* is a vector of several pathogens of cattle the clinical picture can be complicated by synergistic pathogenicity among the various pathogens, such as *B. bigemina*, *B. bovis* and *Anaplasma marginale*.[22] Strains of *B. bigemina* exist, with the African strain being highly pathogenic and the Australian strain considerably less so.[12]

B. divergens

B. divergens is a small parasite which causes disease and death in cattle in northern Europe. It can produce high parasitaemias, exceeding 10 per cent and as high as 24 per cent, but the infected erythrocytes do not clump and therefore there is no cerebral involvement.[22] In western and central Europe the vector is *Ixodes ricinus.*[16] The parasite is acquired by the adult tick and transmitted transovarially to the next generation, of which all stages, but especially the larval, can transmit *B. divergens.* Infection may occasionally continue into the next (F$_2$) generation.[10] There is no such carry over with either *B. bovis* or *B. bigemina.*[28] Since the life cycle of *I. ricinus* extends for three years the parasite may survive up to four years in the tick.[10]

Babesia major

B. major is a large species found in cattle in Europe and the Middle East.[16] The vector is *Haemaphysalis punctata* and although the erythrocytes come together, few fatalities occur in cattle.[22] Infections in American bison, introduced into south-east England, were very severe with 50 per cent mortality before drugs were used to cure the survivors.[22]

Babesia jakimovi

B. jakimovi is a large *Babesia,* whose natural host is the Siberian roe deer (*Capreolus capreolus* – spelt Capreolis in Nikol'skii *et al.*[20]). *B. jakimovi* causes a severe and often fatal disease of cattle. It also infects reindeer and elk. Species of *Ixodes* are vectors in the field, and in the laboratory *I. ricinus* can transmit *B. jakimovi* transovarially. The parasite is acquired by the adult female and transmitted by adults of the succeeding generation.[20]

Species of *Babesia* Parasitising Other Domestic Animals[22]

Sheep

Two species of *Babesia* occur in sheep: a large species, *B. motasi,* and a small one, *B. ovis.* Some strains of *B. motasi* are only infective for sheep, and others for both sheep and goats. *B. motasi* is a significant pathogen on its own but participates in synergistic pathogenicity with *Theileria* and *Ehrlichia. B. motasi* is widely distributed in the Old World where it is transmitted by species of *Haemaphysalis* of which *H. punctata* is a proven vector. Purnell[22] comments that 'there is considerable confusion, then, as to the presence, pathogenicity, and tick vector species of *B. ovis* in sheep and goats in Africa and Asia'. In the USSR the vector is *Rhipicephalus bursa,* in which transovarian transmission has been reported to occur through 44 generations over 20 years.[14]

Horses

Both a large species, *B. caballi,* and a small one, *B. equi,* parasitise equines. *B. equi* used to be referred to the genus *Nuttalia* but this generic name is void. The budding schizont forms four merozoites arranged in the erythrocyte in the form of a Maltese cross. *B. equi* is widely distributed in every continent occurring in all equines, including zebra. Its pathogenicity is variable, and the vectors are species of *Rhipicephalus, Dermacentor* and *Hyalomma.*

B. caballi is less widely distributed than *B. equi* and has not been recorded from zebra. It has the same ixodid vectors as *B. equi,* and in the USA and Central America is transmitted by *D. (Anocentor) nitens,* a one-host tick which infests the ears of equines. In the USA, *B. caballi* caused mortalities of 10 per cent in an outbreak in Florida.

Pigs

Pigs support a large, *B. trautmanni,* and a small, *B. perroncitoi,* species of *Babesia. B. trautmanni* is present in southern Europe, USSR and parts of Africa. It may cause a severe condition with 60-65 per cent of the erythrocytes being parasitised. Infections are commoner in pigs aged four to six months. Wild pigs, warthog and bushpig are likely significant reservoirs of this parasite. *B. perroncitoi* has a very limited distribution in the Sudan, Sardinia and Italy, and may be a significant pathogen of pigs.

Dogs

The large species in dogs is *B. canis,* and the small species *B. gibsoni.* Both parasites are widely distributed but *B. gibsoni* has a more limited distribution. Parasitaemias of 40-45 per cent have been reported in fatal cases where death has been due to anoxia, and parasitaemias of 2 to 14 per cent in non-fatal cases.[12] Foxes and jackals act as reservoirs of *B. gibsoni.* In south-east Asia the vector is *Haemaphysalis longicornis.*

In warmer countries *B. canis* is transmitted by the red dog tick, *Rhipicephalus sanguineus,* and in temperate regions of Europe by *Dermacentor marginatus.* In France infections with *B. canis* have two peaks in the year: a spring-summer peak among domestic dogs with *R. sanguineus* as the vector, and an autumn-winter peak among hunting dogs when *Dermacentor* spp are the vectors.[10] *B. canis* shows synergistic pathogenicity with *Ehrlichia canis,* with *B. canis* destroying the erythrocytes and *E. canis* impeding red cell production. Infected red cells clump together and block capillaries in the brain, leading to death. Young puppies are highly susceptible to *B. canis.*[12] Transovarian transmission of *B. canis* has been observed through five generations.[10]

Cycle of *Babesia* in Tick Vector (see Figure 28.1)

Ixodid ticks acquire infections with *Babesia* by the alimentary route when they feed on an infective host. Infections are also acquired transovarially via the female parent. Strictly speaking transovarian transmission is vertical transmission but it is useful to limit that term to situations where the parasite is passed from generation to generation of the tick without the intake of additional parasites. Such vertical transmission occurs with *B. ovis* in *R. bursa*,[14] while *B. bovis* and *B. bigemina* have only transovarian transmission in *Bo. microplus.*[7] Infections within the tick can be transmitted transstadially, and this is the only mode of transmission for *B. microti* in which infections are acquired by one stage and passed by the same individual in the next stage of its cycle. In this respect *B. microti* resembles *Theileria* in which there is no transovarian transmission.[6] The cycle of the parasite in the tick is still not settled in all details. In particular there is no definite proof of syngamy, i.e. formation of gametes and their fusion. Consequently the terminology to be used is also uncertain.[6]

Figure 28.1: Diagrammatical Representation of the Transmission of a *Babesia* Parasite by a One-host Tick, Accompanied by the Factors Which Determine the Level of Babesial Infection in the Environment

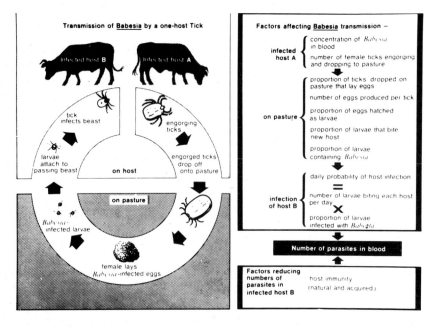

Source: From Mahoney[12]

General Cycle

Friedhoff and Smith[7] have produced a detailed review of the relationships between *Babesia* and its tick vector, and Friedhoff[6] an account of the fine structure of the parasite in the tick. In outline, the cycle involves development within the lumen of the gut; followed by invasion of the epithelial cells lining the gut; release into the haemolymph with multiplication in various organs; and finally penetration of the ovary. Further multiplication takes place in the egg and the tissues of the larva followed by invasion of the salivary glands in which 'sporozoites' (infective particles) are formed and passed when the tick feeds.

Babesia bigemina and *Babesia bovis*

Riek has studied the development of *B. bigemina*[27] and *B. bovis*[28] in *Bo. microplus*. He considers that most of the parasites ingested by the tick are destroyed; and that after 24-36 h club-shaped vermicules, more commonly now referred to as kinetes, appear in the gut and invade the epithelial cells. Multiple fission occurs in these cells and 72 h after detachment of the tick kinetes appear in the haemolymph. The slightly larger kinetes of *B. bovis* (16×3 μm) invade the ovaries, while those of *B. bigemina* (11×2.5 μm) have a second cycle of multiple fission in the malpighian tubules and the cells of the haemolymph, where they form more kinetes which invade the ovary.

A further cycle of multiple fission occurs in the cells of the gut of the developing larva, giving rise to kinetes which appear in the salivary glands of the larva two to three days after attachment. Further multiple fission occurs in the cells of the salivary glands, leading to the production of 'sporozoites' of similar size to the parasites found in the erythrocytes of the vertebrate host, being small in *B. bovis* and large in *B. bigemina*. In the case of *B. bigemina* 'sporozoites' are not formed until eight to ten days after attachment when the tick is in the nymphal stage. It is of interest that heavy parasitaemia in the bovine host (more than 5 per cent) causes mortality among *Bo. microplus*.[28]

Babesia canis, *Babesia ovis* and Other *Babesias*

Infections are usually acquired by the adult female tick, although *R. sanguineus* can transmit *B. canis* in the adult stage having become infected in the preceding nymphal stage.[12] The three-host ticks *I. ricinus*, *H. punctata* and *R. sanguineus* acquire, respectively, *B. divergens*, *B. major* and *B. canis* in the adult stage, and can transmit the parasite in all stages of the next generation, although larvae of *R. sanguineus* only transmit when present in large numbers.[7] Male *R. sanguineus* and *Bo. microplus* can transmit *B. canis* and *B. bigemina*, respectively.[7] *R. bursa* acquires infection with *B. ovis* in the last four hours before detachment, and in this two-host tick transmission is by the adult stage of the succeeding generation.[7]

In *R. bursa*, where both alimentary and vertical infections with *B. ovis* occur, alimentary infections produce higher infection rates and grades of infections than from vertical transmission, but the onset of ovarian infection is retarded compared with vertical transmission.[7] In *Bo. microplus*, where only transovarian transmission occurs, *B. bigemina* does not invade the ovaries until 16-32 h after oviposition has begun. Consequently eggs deposited early in the oviposition cycle, amounting to 13-53 per cent of the egg batch, are uninfected.[7]

In the early stages of alimentary infection of *B. ovis* in *R. bursa*, Friedoff[6] has described five phases of development involving rayed bodies or strahlenkörper. Rayed bodies persist in the gut of the tick up to 120 h after detachment, but some give rise to multiple fission bodies in the epithelial cells of the gut, and developing kinetes become discernible 92 h after detachment.[6] Similar bodies have been described in four species of *Babesia* and three species of *Theileria*.[6]

The development of 'sporozoites' of *B. canis* in *D. reticulatus* has been studied by Schein *et al.*[34] The 'sporozoites' are formed in the salivary glands by binary divisions and not by multiple fission. Development of the 'sporozoites' took two to three days, being competed four to five days after the adult female had attached and transmission occured at engorgement. Development of *B. bigemina* occurs in cells *a* of acinus II and *d* of acinus III, while those of *B. bovis* appeared to be in type *e* cells of acinus III and absent from acini I and II.[2]

Epizootiology

The epizootiology of babesiosis in cattle has been the subject of reviews by Mahoney[12] and Joyner and Donnelly.[10] The treatment of epizootiology is essentially quantitative. Many of the processes involved change steadily with time, e.g. the protection conferred on calves by the colostrum and innate immunity protects them for some months before it wanes. This is not a sudden change but a steady loss of protection with time. It is convenient for the purposes of calculation to subdivide smoothly changing responses into convenient sections but it must be understood that the limits of the sections are arbitrary.

Epizootics occur in three situations: when infected ticks are introduced into a clean area; when susceptible animals are moved into an infected area; and when a temporary reduction in the vector by control or climate leads to animals escaping early infection, and remaining susceptible as adults.[12] In an enzootically stable situation calves become immunised by infection during the period (about nine months) they are protected by colostral and innate immunity, when they suffer minimal clinical disease.[16] In a stable enzootic situation the inoculation rate is high. In an enzootically unstable situation the inoculation rate is too low to infect all the calves before they become adult, leading to the presence of susceptible adult animals, vulnerable to developing severe clinical disease on infection. If the inoculation rate becomes very low there is the possibility of the disease disappearing.[12]

Inoculation Rate

The inoculation rate (h) is an important parameter in the epizootiology of babesiosis. It has been defined as:

$$h = mab$$

when m = bites by vector per day; a = proportion of vectors infected; and b = proportion of infective bites which can infect a host (Figure 28.1). With *Bos taurus* a single larval tick infective with *B. bovis* can cause disease, i.e. $b = 1.0$, but b may have a lower value for resistant cattle, e.g. *Bos indicus*.[12] The inoculation rate is more easily calculated from the proportion of animals infected (I) at age t when

$$I = 1 - e^{-ht}$$

Mahoney[12] has plotted the 'proportion of cattle in a herd that become infective with *B. bovis* within four years after passive immunity wanes for a wide range of inoculation rates' (Figure 28.2). These are the infections which are likely to result in severe clinical disease.

As the inoculation rate increases, the proportion of animals infected rises to a maximum of over 50 per cent and then declines. The critical level for enzootic stability is an inoculation rate of 0.005, which Mahoney[12] equates with 'at least twelve *Boophilus microplus* larvae being required to bite each cow (*Bos taurus*) daily'. Higher rates of infestation with ticks will ensure greater stability and minimal disease, but introduce the complication of other damaging effects of high tick burdens. The zone of maximum risk of babesiosis in this model is when the inoculation rate lies between 0.0005 and 0.005.

Basic Reproduction Rate

Another important parameter is the 'basic reproduction rate which is a hypothetical number representing the number of secondary cases of a

Figure 28.2: Percentage of Animals That Become Infected with *B. bovis* After Passively Acquired Immunity Wanes at Average Inoculation Rates in the Range of 0.0001 to 0.01

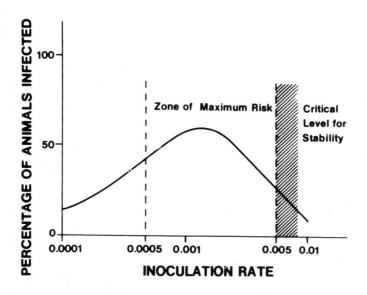

Source: From Mahoney[12]

disease disseminated by a single primary case in a nonimmune individual in an environment in which neither host nor vector populations were previously infected'.[12] The basic reproduction rate is given by the expression:

$$2 \, dna$$

where d = duration of infectivity in days; n = number of female ticks dropped on the pasture per day; and a = the average infection rate in the larval progeny.[12] When the basic reproduction rate is below 1.0 then the parasite will disappear. Mahoney and Ross[13] suggest values of 230-350 days for d for *B. bovis* in *Bos taurus* and 0.04 per cent for a. Using a slightly different expression ($2dn^2a$) they calculated the critical value of n as 1-2 ticks/head/day.[13] This has been repeated by Joyner and Donnelly,[10] who have overlooked the correction given in Mahoney.[12] A higher critical value of about four ticks/head/day is given by the revised expression $2dna$. The actual values are of less importance than the general conclusion that there is a level of transmission below which, other factors remaining constant, the parasite, and therefore the disease, will disappear.

Epizootiology of Babesia divergens

There is no proof of a vertebrate reservoir host for a bovine babesia, although non-bovine hosts may harbour *B. bigemina* for a period, and *B. capreoli* in red deer is very close to and may be identical with, *B. divergens* in cattle.[10] Joyner and Donnelly[10] describe the epizootiology of *B. divergens* and its vector *I. ricinus* in the United Kingdom. Both the vector and the disease have a bimodal seasonal pattern. The autumn rise of *I. ricinus* is composed of new emergences, and the spring rise represents renewed activity of ticks that failed to feed in the autumn. If these are unsuccessful they die off in the late spring. Disease incidence was positively correlated with temperature 14 days earlier, with temperature acting by increasing tick activity. The increase in disease incidence in spring ($\times$ 2.5) compared to autumn was reflected in a similar difference in the inoculation rates, which in spring was $\times$ 2.25 that in autumn by increasing tick activity.

Human Babesiosis

There is no species of *Babesia* which is host specific for man but, under certain conditions, man can become infected with two species with animal hosts. In North America human infections with *B. microti* have been recorded from four islands off the north-east coast of the USA, including Nantucket, Martha's Vineyard and Long Island. One review cites 28 cases on three islands,[36] and a later article 19 cases on four islands.[30] Infection causes a severe anaemia in man with 1-10 per cent of the erythrocytes being parasitised.

B. *microti* is a parasite of deer mice (*Peromyscus leucopus*) and field mice (*Microtus pennsylvanicus*).[36] White-tailed deer (*Odocoileus virginianus*) have increased on the island and with it the deer tick (*Ixodes dammini*), which 'in all instars, attaches to a variety of animals, including man'.[36] (*I. dammini* is the species referred to as *I.* sp. nr. *scapularis* in Spielman and Piesman.[36]) It is considered that the original vector of *B. microti* was *I. muris*, which does not feed on man, and that human infections have resulted from the increase in *I. dammini*.

Cases of babesiosis in man have occurred in splenectomised humans in Europe, where the parasite was *B. divergens*. Five of the seven cases reported ended fatally.[22] Human infections with *Babesia* in intact subjects have been reported from Mexico and Nigeria.[10]

Theileriosis

Three genera, *Theileria, Haematoxenus* and *Cytauxzoon*, have been recognised within the Theileriidae. The economically important parasites of domestic stock, largely cattle, are included in the genus *Theileria*. Species of *Haematoxenus* are non-pathogenic parasites of cattle, sheep and wild bovids, distinguished by some of the piroplasms having a veil on one side.[1] The veil has now been shown to be a crystalline structure and not part of the parasite.[3] *Cytauxzoon* has only been recorded from wild bovids and not from domestic stock. The erythrocytic piroplasms of all three genera are similar, and as some of the grounds for recognising separate genera have been disproved there is a move to drop the generic names *Haematoxenus* and *Cytauxzoon* and recognise only a single genus *Theileria*.[3]

Theileria parva and *T. lawrencei*

The identification of species of *Theileria* is difficult and Barnett[1] refers to species identification as being 'more an art than a science'. Five species of *Theileria* have been recorded from cattle. The two most pathogenic are *T. parva*, which causes east coast fever (ECF), and *T. lawrencei*, the agent of corridor disease. These two forms are closely related and sometimes regarded as subspecies of *T. parva* — *T. p. parva* and *T. p. lawrencei*.[3]

T. parva occurs in eastern tropical Africa from the southern Sudan to Malawi and west to Ruanda and eastern Zaire. *T. parva* is lethal to European (*Bos taurus*) and Indian (*Bos indicus*) cattle, and the water buffalo (*Bubulus bubalis*). It also occurs in the African buffalo (*Synerus caffer*). It is transmitted by the brown ear tick *Rhipicephalus appendiculatus*. Among susceptible stock mortality is high, exceeding 90 per cent, and beasts that recover have a persistent immunity in which piroplasms are not visible.[1] 'The prevailing view is that the majority of recovered animals do not remain long-term carriers of infection',[1] but this view has been challenged by Young *et al.*,[43] who found that in their area of Kenya 'it is possible that the carrier state of *T. parva* in cattle is widespread and extends through all age groups'. There is cross-immunity with *T. lawrencei*.[1]

T. lawrencei is a benign parasite of the African buffalo in which it causes a mild disease, but is lethal to cattle and the water buffalo. Recovered beasts have a good, persistent immunity with piroplasms rarely being visible. *T. lawrencei* occurs in East and Central Africa where the vector is *R. appendiculatus*, and in Angola where *R. appendiculatus* is absent, the vector is probably *R. duttoni*. The absence of *T. parva* and *T. lawrencei* from West Africa is attributed to the absence of their vector *R. appendiculatus*.[1] In Rhodesia there is a related organism which is also considered to be derived from the African buffalo, and which is transmitted by *R. appendiculatus*. It produced a low mortality (15 per cent), and surviving cattle remain infective to ticks for a long period, during which piroplasms are present in the circulating blood.[1]

Development of Theileria parva in Cattle

Infective particles, about 1.5 μm in diameter, are introduced by the tick after it has been feeding for several days. Later they are to be found slightly larger (2 μm), in lymph nodes adjacent to the site of attachment of the tick. They develop into macroschizonts (2-16 μm) containing on average eight medium sized nuclei. The number of macroschizonts increases and in an average infection reaches one macroschizont for every four lymphocytes. Microschizonts, containing 50-120 small nuclei, appear somewhat later. The prefix 'micro' refers to the size of the nuclei and not to the schizont. Micromerozoites, measuring about 1 μm, are released, become piroplasms in the red blood cells, and do not develop further until ingested by the tick.

Fever commences when the density of macroschizonts in the host reaches 7×10^9 and its time of onset is dependent on the number of infective particles injected. 'In three groups of cattle infected with 10, 100 and 1,000 infected ticks, the mean period to day of fever was 13, 11, and 9 days respectively.'[1] The growth rate of the parasite is dependent on the size of the initial inoculation with a tenfold increase occurring in 4.9 days and 1.4 days following inoculations of 2 and 2,000 ticks, respectively. Formation of microschizonts is time dependent, and at all dosages piroplasms appear in erythrocytes in 13 days, i.e. the prepatent period was independent of dosage.[1] Cattle begin to die from the sixteenth day of infection onwards and at death 50 per cent of the erythrocytes may contain piroplasms.[21]

Development of Theileria parva in Rhipicephalus appendiculatus

Until recently very little was known about the early development of *T. parva* in the tick. It has been pointed out that 10^7 to 10^8 piroplasms are ingested when a tick feeds but less than 10 or 100 of these will complete their development in the tick.[21,25] Mehlhorn *et al.*[17] state that in the midgut of *R. appendiculatus* nymphs, the piroplasms escape from the erythrocytes and develop into microgametes or macrogametes. Microgamonts, measuring about 10 μm × 2 μm, produce four slender microgametes (10 μm × 0.2 μm) by a process similar to exflagellation.[17,18] They are considered to fertilise the macrogametes but fertilisation has not actually been observed. Stages that are considered to be zygotes (6-7 μm), appear in the midgut cells 20 days after feeding to repletion, and after the nymph has moulted to the adult. They grow to produce motile kinetes (19 μm × 5.5 μm), which leave the midgut cells and move through the haemocoele to the salivary glands.[19] Within certain cells of the salivary gland the kinetes develop into large sporonts which produce more than 100,000 sporozoites each.[19]

Development of *T. parva* in the salivary glands of a feeding tick has been known for a long time, and it has also been recognised that the parasite is present in the salivary glands of an unfed tick.[1,2] Transmission of

T. parva and other species of *Theileria* is transstadial, but not transovarial. Infections acquired by the larva or nymph are transmitted in the succeeding nymph or adult stage.[1] In adult *R. appendiculatus* which have developed from nymphs fed on a host infective for *T. parva*, the maximum number of parasites are present in the salivary glands three to five days after attachment. They go through a cycle from being small young stages to larger intermediate forms, often known as cytomeres (= sporonts of Mehlhorn *et al.*[17]), to being mature infective particles (= sporozoites[17]). The maximum number of infective particles occurs four to five days after attachment.[24]

There is considerable variation in the proportion of feeding ticks which become infected and in the intensity of infection in individual ticks. One factor that influences this is the parasitaemia of the host. In one series of experiments the overall infection rate among ticks was 35 per cent; but a significantly higher percentage (61 per cent) were infected when the parasitaemia of the host was 41-50 per cent; when the parasitaemia was between 6 and 40 per cent, 33 per cent of the ticks were infected; and when the parasitaemia was below 5 per cent, significantly fewer ticks (27 per cent) became infected.

The mean number of acini per infected tick was 6.0-6.4 at parasitaemias of 1 to 40 per cent, and somewhat higher (8.6) when the host's parasitaemia was 41-50 per cent.[25] There was no close relationship between the intensity of infection in the salivary glands of the tick and the level of parasitaemia in the host animal. It was considered that a random factor, such as juxtaposition of infected gut cells and developing salivary glands during the nymphal moult, was involved.[25] When nymphal and larval *R. appendiculatus* were fed on the same host the infection rate in the resulting adults was higher (45 per cent) than in the nymphs (35 per cent). In addition there were more infected acini in adults than in nymphs, 2.25 compared to 0.7, but infective particles were produced more rapidly in nymphs than in adults, appearing in two days compared to four days in adult *R. appendiculatus*.[23]

In the salivary glands *Theileria* develops preferentially in cells of a particular type. *T. parva*, according to Martins,[15] develops in type *d* cells of type III acini (= alveoli) using the nomenclature of Till.[37] Binnington and Kemp[2] state that *Theileria* develops particularly in cell type *e* using the nomenclature of Coons and Roshdy.[4] Dr. Kemp informs me that both workers are referring to the same cell type and the difference is one solely of nomenclature.

The readiness with which adult ticks feed increases with time since the nymphal moult, and after five weeks 90 per cent of adult females will attach and feed,[11] but if starvation persists for a long time (44 weeks) infectivity with *T. parva* is lost.[1]

Theileria lawrencei

The infection rate among adult *R. appendiculatus* fed in the nymphal stage on infective buffalo is much lower (5.9 per cent) than that obtained with *T. parva* in cattle. Even lower infection rates (2.1 per cent) are obtained when nymphal *R. appendiculatus* feed on infected cattle. The lower infectivity may be related to the presence of fewer piroplasms in erythrocytes. Commonly in cattle less than 0.1 per cent of erythrocytes are infected, and the rate is always below 1 per cent.[44] Buffalo may act as carriers of *T. lawrencei* for more than 26 months but recovered cattle are not carriers.[44] Continued passage of *T. lawrencei* through cattle increases its infectivity to *R. appendiculatus* by increasing the density of piroplasms in the circulating blood and the infection can become indistinguishable from that of *T. parva*.[21,44]

Epizootiology of T. parva and T. lawrencei

The only wild reservoir host for *T. parva* and *T. lawrencei* is the African buffalo (*Synerus caffer*), and the only effective vector of both organisms is *R. appendiculatus*.[1] Seven other species of *Rhipicephalus* and three of *Hyalomma* can transmit *T. parva* experimentally but they are not considered to be able to sustain the parasite in the absence of *R. appendiculatus*.[5] Among susceptible stock morbidity is 100 per cent,[5] and 'with a virulent strain of *T. parva*, single tick infections can kill over 90 per cent of susceptible cattle'.[1] The incubation period in cattle is nine to 24 days, being accompanied by enlargement of the lymph nodes adjacent to the feeding site of the tick; schizonts in lymph nodes, spleen and liver; and a toxic (?) effect on the bone marrow.[1]

In Malawi sporadic cases of east coast fever occur throughout the year with 60-70 per cent of cases occurring in the rainy season (January-March). Local cattle have high resistance and mortality is low (1-5 per cent).[41]

In Sukumaland, north-western Tanzania, Yeoman[42] recognises five zones with varying intensity of ECF and relates these to the density of *R. appendiculatus*. In permanently enzootic areas disease occurs only in calves, of which 40 per cent may die,[5] and infestations of *R. appendiculatus* on cattle exceeed 40 adult ticks per beast. In epizootic areas heavy losses of adult cattle occur and coincide with infestations of one to four adult *R. appendiculatus* per beast. In areas which have passed through the epizootic stage and are classified as 'recent enzootic', mortality shifts from adults to calves and is associated with five to 20 adult *R. appendiculatus* per beast. In areas of sporadic ECF there are localised losses in the presence of 0.3-0.8 adult *R. appendiculatus* per beast; and in ECF-free areas infestations of adult *R. appendiculatus* average one adult for every five or more beasts.[42]

Cattle that recover have immunity to challenge by homologous strains of

ECF but challenge by heterologous strains produces disease and death.[1] There is good, but not perfect, cross-immunity between *T. parva* and *T. lawrencei.*[1] Recovered cattle are not carriers of ECF.

There is no effective multivalent vaccine and control of ticks by dipping is very demanding. Barnett[1] suggests that immune cattle should be kept in a fenced paddock and dipped at seven- or preferably five-day intervals for a period of 15 months to exhaust the pasture of infected ticks. Susceptible stock may now be introduced but dipping should still be carried out weekly, and if there are buffalo in the area, even this regime will not work.

Theileria mutans

T. mutans is widely distributed in the Afrotropical, southern Palaearctic, Oriental and Australian regions.[1,17] It is a parasite of cattle which is rarely pathogenic, but in East Africa there is a pathogenic strain, *T. mutans* (Aitong). In cattle macroschizonts are transient and microschizonts are rare. Piroplasms can be abundant with up to 45 per cent of the erythrocytes being parasitised, and there is marked anaemia with the packed cell volume being reduced to as low as 10-12 per cent.[21,45] *T. mutans* (Aitong) is readily transmissible by blood inoculation, which does not occur in *T. parva* or *T. lawrencei*. It loses its pathogenicity after repeated blood passage but virulence is restored on being cycled in the tick.[45] The vector is *Amblyomma variegatum*, in which transstadial transmission occurs, and *R. appendiculatus* is at the best a very inefficient vector.[39,40,45]

Development of *T. mutans* (Aitong) in *A. variegatum* is similar to that of *T. parva* in *R. appendiculatus* with the following differences. *T. mutans* cannot be seen in the salivary glands of unfed ticks, but appears on the third day of attachment. Development in the salivary glands takes longer, and mature infective particles are not present until day five. The particles are larger than those of *T. parva* and, in appearance, closer to those of *Babesia*. The infection rate of *T. mutans* in *A. variegatum* is lower than that of *T. parva* in *R. appendiculatus* and fewer parasites are produced.[26]

T. mutans (Aitong) may be identical with *T. barnetti*, a similar parasite of the African buffalo. *T. barnetti* is serologically identical with *T. mutans* (Aitong), and has been transmitted from buffaloes to cattle by *A. cohaerens*.[1,21]

More than one species may have been included within *T. mutans*. The South African and East African forms are serologically identical, and different from the Australian and European strains which are serologically closely related. In addition the vectors in Australia and Europe are *Haemaphysalis longicornis*[29] and *H. punctata*,[38] respectively, while the vector of the East African strain is *A. variegatum*, and there are doubts about the vectors in South Africa, which are often cited as *Rhipicephalus evertsi* and *R. appendiculatus*,[1,17] though Uilenberg *et al.*[39] have been unable to find any evidence to support these claims.

Theileria annulata

T. annulata is a parasite of cattle and water buffalo in the southern Palaearctic region, India and northern Sudan. Although less pathogenic than *T. parva*, *T. annulata* may be economically the more important species because of its wider distribution in the world.[1] It is 'moderately lethal for cattle and usually mild in buffalo'.[1] Recovered cattle have a good, persistent immunity of the premunity type in which there is persistent parasitaemia. The vectors are species of *Hyalomma*.

The development of *T. annulata* in *Hyalomma anatolicum excavatum* has been described by Schein *et al.*[32] and Schein and Friedhoff.[33] They described the formation of microgametes and macrogametes, four micro-gametes being formed from each microgamont. These are formed in the first 96 hours, and from day five after repletion zygotes appear in the epithelial cells of the gut and grow steadily to day 12. The zygotes transform into kinetes which at first move within the epithelial cells, and then from day 17 kinetes, measuring about 18 μm, are to be found in the haemolymph.

They reach the salivary glands 18 days after repletion and transform into fission bodies about 10 μm in diameter in type III and less frequently in type II acini. Infected host cells become greatly enlarged, growing from 15 to 110 μm. The parasite divides several times before infective particles ('sporozoites') are formed and released into the saliva. This takes about two days in young ticks; five to seven days in ticks which have been starved for six months; and when ticks have been starved for six to nine months no 'sporozoites' may develop during their feeding period. When ticks feed on hosts with parasitaemias exceeding 40 per cent, they suffer disease and mortality.[33]

The vectors of *T. annulata* are various species of *Hyalomma*, most of which have only one generation a year. Cattle which have recovered from infection with *T. annulata* continue to harbour parasites in the circulating blood and ticks easily become infected with infection rates of up to 64 per cent being recorded for field-collected *H. anatolicum*.[1] *T. annulata* is transmitted by three-host ticks, such as *H. anatolicum anatolicum*, two-host ticks such as *H. detritum*, and even by *H. scupense*, a one-host tick in which the adult remains on the host over the winter period and transmits the disease by moving from one host to another when cattle are in close contact.[1] According to Barnett,[1] *H. anatolicum excavatum* is a two-host tick in which the early stages occur on rodents, and since transmission is transstadial, the tick can not be a vector in the field, although it is readily infected experimentally. In other areas *H. a. excavatum* is described as a three-host tick and a vector of *T. annulata*.[31]

Other *Theileria* in Domestic Stock

T. sergenti is a parasite of cattle in the eastern Palaearctic region where it is transmitted by *Haemaphysalis longicornis*. It is of low pathogenicity but more pathogenic than *T. mutans*. Two species *T. hirci* and *T. ovis* occur in sheep and goats. *T. hirci* has a similar distribution to *T. annulata*, and is highly pathogenic in epizootic areas but of lower pathogenicity in enzootic areas. The vector is *Hyalomma anatolicum*.[1] *T. ovis* is only slightly pathogenic and has a similar distribution to that of *T. hirci* but also occurs in tropical Africa. The vectors are *Rhipicephalus evertsi* in tropical Africa and *R. bursa* in the Palaearctic region.[1]

References

1. Barnett, S. F. (1977). *Theileria*. pp. 77-113 in volume IV, *Parasitic Protozoa*, J.P. Kreier (ed.), Academic Press, New York
2. Binnington, K.C. and Kemp, D.H. (1980). Role of tick salivary glands in feeding and disease transmission. *Advances in Parasitology 18*: 315-39
3. Brocklesby, D.W. (1979). Key note address. *Journal of the South African Veterinary Association 50*: 285-8
4. Coons, L.B. and Roshdy, M.A. (1973). Fine structure of the salivary glands of the unfed *Dermacentor variabilis* (Say) (Ixodoidea: Ixodidae). *Journal of Parasitology 59*: 900-12
5. Cunningham, M.C. (1974). East coast fever — ECF — Cycle in host and vector. pp. 1-2 in *East Coast Fever and Related Tick-Borne Diseases*, Food and Agricultural Organisation, Rome (1980)
6. Friedhoff, K.T. (1981). Morphologic aspects of *Babesia* in the tick. pp. 143-69 in *Babesiosis*, M. Ristic and J.P. Kreier (eds.), Academic Press, New York
7. _____ and Smith, R.D. (1981). Transmission of *Babesia* by tick. pp. 267-321 in *Babesiosis*, M. Ristic and J.P. Kreier (eds.), Academic Press, New York
8. Hoyte, H.M.D. (1961). Initial development of infections with *Babesia bigemina*. *Journal of Protozoology 8*: 462-6
9. _____ (1976). The tick-fever parasites of cattle. *Proceedings of the Royal Society of Queensland 87*: v-xiii
10. Joyner, L.P. and Donnelly, J. (1979). The epidemiology of babesial infections. *Advances in Parasitology 17*: 115-40
11. _____ and Purnell, R.E. (1968). The feeding behaviour on rabbits and *in vitro* of the ixodid tick *Rhipicephalus appendiculatus*, Neumann, 1901. *Parasitology 58*: 715-23
12. Mahoney, D.F. (1977). *Babesia* of domestic animals. pp. 1-52 in volume IV, *Parasitic Protozoa*, J.P. Kreier (ed.), Academic Press, New York
13. _____ and Ross, D.R. (1972). Epizootiological factors in the control of bovine babesiosis. *Australian Veterinary Journal 48*: 292-8
14. Markov, A.A. and Abramov, I.V. (1970). Results of twenty years' observations on repeated life cycles of *Babesia ovis* in 44 generations of *Rhipicephalus bursa*. *Veterinary Bulletin 42*: 1911 (1972)
15. Martins, M.I. (1978). Histochemical studies on the salivary glands of unfed and feeding *Rhipicephalus appendiculatus* during the development of *Theileria parva*. pp. 336-42 in *Tick-borne Diseases and Their Vectors*, J.K.H. Wilde (ed.), Centre of Tropical

Veterinary Medicine, University of Edinburgh

16. McCosker, P.J. (1981). The global importance of babesiosis. pp. 1-24 in *Babesiosis*, M. Ristic and J.P. Kreier (eds.), Academic Press, New York

17. Mehlhorn, H., Heydorn, A.O., Senaud, J. and Schein, E. (1979). La modalités de la transmission des protozoaires parasites des genres *Sarcocystis* et *Theileria* agents de graves malladies. *L'Année Biologique 18*: 97-120

18. _____ and Schein, E. (1976). Elektronenmikroskopische Untersuchungen an Entwicklungsstadien von *Theileria parva* (Theiler, 1904) im Darm der Überträgerzecke *Hyalomma anatolicum excavatum* (Kock, 1844). *Tropenmedizin und Parasitologie 27*: 182-91

19. _____ Schein, E. and Warnecke, M. (1978). Electron microscopic studies on the development of kinetes of *Theileria parva* Theiler, 1904 in the gut of the vector ticks *Rhipicephalus appendiculatus* Neumann, 1901. *Acta Tropica 35*: 123-36

20. Nikol'skii, S.M., Nikiforenko, V.I. and Pozov, S.A. (1977). Epizootiology of piroplasmosis in Siberia. *Veterinariya 4*: 71-5

21. Purnell, R.E. (1977). East coast fever: some recent research in East Africa. *Advances in Parasitology 15*: 83-132

22. _____ (1981). Babesiosis in various hosts. pp. 25-63 in *Babesiosis*, M. Ristic and J.P. Kreier (eds.), Academic Press, New York

23. _____ Boarer, C.D.H. and Peirce, M.A. (1971). *Theileria parva*: comparative infection rates of adult and nymphal *Rhipicephalus appendiculatus*. *Parasitology 62*: 349-53

24. _____ and Joyner, L.P. (1968). The development of *Theileria parva* in the salivary glands of the tick *Rhipicephalus appendiculatus*. *Parasitology 58*: 725-32

25. _____ Ledger, M.A., Omwoyo, P.L., Payne, R.C. and Peirce, M.A. (1974). *Theileria parva*: variation in the infection rate of the vector tick *Rhipicephalus appendiculatus*. *International Journal of Parasitology 4*: 513-7

26. _____ Young, A.S., Payne, R.C. and Mwangi, J.M. (1975). Development of *Theileria mutans* (Aitong) in the tick *Amblyomma variegatum* compared to that of *T. parva* (Muguga) in *Rhipicephalus appendiculatus*. *Journal of Parasitology 61*: 725-9

27. Riek, R.F. (1964). The life cycle of *Babesia bigemina* (Smith and Kilborne, 1893) in the tick vector *Boophilus microplus* (Canestrini). *Australian Journal of Agricultural Research 15*: 802-21

28. _____ (1966). The life cycle of *Babesia argentina* (Lignières, 1903) (Sporozoa: Piroplasmidea) in the tick vector *Boophilus microplus* (Canestrini). *Australian Journal of Agricultural Research 17*: 247-54

29. Roberts, F.H.S. (1970). *Australian Ticks*. CSIRO, Melbourne

30. Ruebush, T.K. (1980). Human babesiosis in North America. *Transactions of the Royal Society of Tropical Medicine and Hygiene 74*: 149-52

31. Samish, M. and Pipano, E. (1978). Transmission of *Theileria annulata* by two and three host ticks of the genus *Hyalomma* (Ixodidae). pp. 371-2 in *Tick-borne Diseases and Their Vectors*, J.K.H. Wilde (ed.), Centre of Tropical Veterinary Medicine, University of Edinburgh

32. Schein, E., Büscher, G and Friedhoff, K.T. (1975). Lichtmikroskopische Untersuchungen über die Entwicklung von *Theileria annulata* (Dschunkowsky und Luhs, 1904) in *Hyalomma anatolicum excavatum* (Koch, 1844). I. Die Entwicklung im Darm vollgesogener Nymphen. *Zeitschrift für Parasitenkunde 48*: 123-36

33. _____ and Friedhoff, K.T. (1978). Lichtmikroscopische Untersuchungen über die Entwicklung von *Theileria annulata* (Dschunkowsky and Luhs, 1904) in *Hyalomma anatolicum excavatum* (Koch, 1844). II. Die Entwicklung in Hämolymphe und Speicheldrüsen. *Zeitschrift für Parasitenkunde 56*: 287-303

34. _____ Mehlhorn, H. and Voigt, W.P. (1979). Electron microscopical studies on the development of *Babesia canis* (Sporozoa) in the salivary glands of the vector tick *Dermacentor reticulatus*. *Acta Tropica 36*: 229-41

35. Smith, T. and Kilborne, F.L. (1893). Investigations into the nature, causation and prevention of Texas or southern cattle fever. *United States Department of Agriculture, Bureau of Animal Industry Bulletin 1*: 1-301

36. Spielman, A. and Piesman, J. (1979). Transmission of human babesiosis on Nantucket. pp. 257-62 in volume II, *Recent Advances in Acarology* J.G. Rodrigues (ed.), Academic Press, New York

37. Till, W.M. (1961). A contribution to the anatomy and histology of the brown ear tick *Rhipicephalus appendiculatus* Neumann. *Memoirs of the Entomological Society of Southern Africa 6*: 1-124

38. Uilenberg, G., McGregor, W., Mpangala, C., Callow, L.L. and Vos, A.J.de (1978). Relationship of some *Theileria* species of cattle. pp. 302-6 in *Tick-borne Diseases and Their Vectors* J.K.H. Wilde (ed.), Centre for Tropical Veterinary Medicine, University of Edinburgh

39. _____ Robson, J. and Pedersen, V. (1974). Some experiments on the transmission of *Theileria mutans* (Theiler, 1906) and *Theileria parva* (Theiler, 1904) by the ticks *Amblyomma variegatum* (Fabricius, 1794) and *Rhipicephalus appendculatus* Neumann, 1901 in Uganda. *Tropenmedizin und Parasitologie 25*: 207-16

40. _____ Schreuder, B.E.C. and Mpangala, C. (1976). Studies on Theileriidae (Sporozoa) in Tanzania. III. Experiments on the transmission of *Theileria mutans* by *Rhipicephalus appendiculatus* and *Amblyomma variegatum* (Acarina, Ixodidae). *Tropenmedizin und Parasitologie 27*: 323-8

41. Wilson, S.G. (1944). Theileriasis in cattle in Northern Province, Nyasaland. *Veterinary Record 56*: 255-8

42. Yeoman, G.H. (1966). Field vector studies of epizootic east coast fever. I. A quantitative relationship between *R. appendiculatus* and the epizooticity of east coast fever. *Bulletin of Epizootic Diseases of Africa 14*: 5-27

43. Young, A.S., Leitch, B.L. and Newson, R.M. (1981). The occurrence of a *Theileria parva* carrier state in cattle from an east coast fever endemic area of Kenya. pp. 60-2 in *Advances in the Control of Theileriosis*, A.D. Irvin, M.P. Cunningham and A.S. Young (eds.), Martinus Nijhoff, The Hague

44. _____ and Purnell, R.E. (1973). Transmission of *Theileria lawrencei* (Serengeti) by the ixodid tick, *Rhipicephalus appendiculatus*. *Tropical Animal Health and Production 5*: 146-52

45. _____ Purnell, R.E., Payne, R.C., Brown, C.G.D. and Kanhai, G.K. (1978). Studies on the transmission and course of infection of a Kenyan strain of *Theileria mutans*. *Parasitology 76*: 99-115

29 TRYPANOSOMIASES AND LEISHMANIASES

The trypanosomiases are diseases of man and livestock, and the leishmaniases largely diseases of man. They are caused by parasitic flagellate Protozoa (superclass Mastigophora) of the order Kinetoplastida. Members of this order are recognised by the possession of a kinetoplast, a DNA-containing particle, close to the flagellar basal bodies, which are inserted on or close to the mitrochondrion.[44] The economically important parasites are in the Trypanosomatidae, the only family in the suborder Trypanosomatina characterised by possession of a single flagellum, which may be free or attached for much or all of its length to the pellicle by the maculae adherentes. Movement of the flagellum lifts up a fold of the pellicle, and this is referred to incorrectly as the undulating membrane.[39]

Species of two genera, *Trypanosoma* and *Leishmania*, are of economic importance, causing, respectively, trypanosomiasis and leishmaniasis. At different stages of the developmental cycle the parasite takes various forms, five of which will be defined briefly. There has been a change in terminology and the older terms will be given in parentheses. In the amastigote (leishmanial form) the flagellar base and kinetoplast are anterior to the nucleus and there is no free flagellum, while in the promastigote (leptomonad) the flagellar base is also anterior to the nucleus and there is a flagellum which emerges from the anterior end of the body. In the opisthomastigote (herpetomonad) the flagellar base is behind the nucleus and there is a long flagellar pocket leading to the anterior end. In the epimastigote (crithidial) the flagellar base is anterior to the nucleus and the flagellum emerges laterally to form an undulating membrane as it runs along the body to the anterior end while in the trypomastigote (trypanosome) the flagellar base is behind the nucleus, the flagellum emerges laterally and there is a long, undulating membrane.[44]

Species of *Trypanosoma* occur as blood parasites in a wide range of vertebrates, from fish to mammals. Trypomastigote and epimastigote stages are common to nearly all trypanosome life cycles. *Leishmania* species are characterised by intracellular amastigotes in the mammalian host and extracellular promastigotes in the gut lumen of phlebotomine sandflies.[44]

In the Mastigophora division is symmetrogenic, equal pairs formed by longitudinal division; there is no sexual reproduction, and recombination of genetic characters is not possible. Lack of recombination leads to the development of strains, which are morphologically identical, but differ in their physiological and biochemical characteristics, and makes the determination of species difficult. Evans and Ellis[8] have produced some evidence suggestive of fusion between organisms with the possibility of genetic interchange.

Trypanosomiases

The economically important and other representative trypanosomes transmitted by insects are listed in Table 29.1. The genus *Trypanosoma* is divided into two sections, the Salivaria and the Stercoraria, which differ in their modes of transmission. Salivarian trypanosomes either undergo cyclic development in the insect before being transmitted with the saliva, or are transmitted mechanically. Stercorarian trypanosomes also undergo development in the insect but the infective forms are deposited in the faeces of the vector. Infection rates of salivarian trypanosomes in the vector are often low, even when the vector has been fed on infective hosts in the laboratory. In contrast vectors of stercorarian trypanosomes fed on an infective host have a very high infection rate, approaching 100 per cent.

In the following account of the trypanosomiases, the salivarian species transmitted by *Glossina* will be considered first, other insect-borne salivarian trypanosomes next, and finally the stercorarian trypanosomes.

Table 29.1: List of Species of *Trypanosoma* Transmitted by Insects

Subgenus Species Subspecies	Vector	Susceptible host
Section Salivaria		
Trypanozoon evansi	tabanids, *Stomoxys*	livestock
Trypanozoon brucei brucei	*Glossina*	livestock (horse)
Trypanozoon brucei gambiense	*Glossina*	man
Trypanozoon brucei rhodesiense	*Glossina*	man
Nannomonas congolense	*Glossina*	livestock
Nannomonas simiae	*Glossina*	pigs
Duttonella vivax	*Glossina*	livestock
Duttonella vivax viennei	tabanids, *Stomoxys*	livestock
Duttonella uniforme	*Glossina*	cattle
Pycnomonas suis	*Glossina*	pigs
Section Stercoraria		
Schizotrypanum cruzi	triatomine bugs	man
Megatrypanum theileri	tabanids	cattle
Megatrypanum melophagium	*Melophagus ovinus*	sheep
Herpetosoma lewisi	rat fleas	rats
Herpetosoma rangeli	triatomine bugs	man, dog
(unresolved) *grayi*[a]	*Glossina palpalis*	crocodile

Note: [a] Dr J.R. Baker informs me that subgenera have only been erected at present for mammalian trypanosomes and hence no subgenus can be given for *T. grayi,* a parasite of crocodiles

Salivarian Trypanosomiases

Salivarian trypanosomes, with two exceptions, are transmitted by species of *Glossina*. The two exceptions are *T. evansi* and *T. vivax viennei*, which are mechanically transmitted by tabanids and *Stomoxys* outside the range of *Glossina*. Various subgenera are recognised within the salivarian species of *Trypanosoma*.[16] Before the establishment of formal subgenera, closely related species were referred to as groups. The main subgenera of economic importance with the group names in parentheses are: *Trypanozoon* (*brucei* group), *Nannomonas* (*congolense* group), *Duttonella* (*vivax* group).

Cycle in Glossina[16]

When a tsetse fly feeds on an infective host it ingests with the blood trypanosomes which are present in the circulating blood in the trypomastigote form. Their further development in *Glossina* depends on the species involved (Figure 29.1).

Duttonella. Individuals of *T. (Duttonella) vivax* and *T. (D.) uniforme* attach to the walls of the food canal in the proboscis where they develop into epimastigotes. If they pass into the midgut of the tsetse fly they develop no further. In the food canal they move to the opening of the salivary duct at the distal end of the hypopharynx. In the salivary duct they undergo further development and multiplication before forming metacyclic trypomastigotes, which are infective to the vertebrate host (epimastigotes are not infective). They are passed into the vertebrate host while *Glossina* is feeding.

Trypanozoon. The development cycle of *T. (Trypanozoon) brucei* is more involved. The trypomastigotes pass with the ingested blood into the midgut where they are contained within the peritrophic membrane, i.e. the endoperitrophic space. They change form in the midgut and appear in the ectoperitrophic space, between the midgut wall and the peritrophic membrane, by movement around its free end. The trypomastigotes move forwards to the proventriculus where the peritrophic membrane is being secreted and is semifluid or soft. They pass through the soft membrane into the foregut, move anteriorly through the oesophagus, and down the food canal to the tip of the proboscis where they enter the opening of the salivary duct. They now swim up the duct for the length of the hypopharynx, and on down the salivary duct in the head to the salivary glands in the thorax. Here epimastigotes are produced before the production of metacyclic trypomastigotes.

When the tsetse feeds the infective metacyclics pass into the host, and, if the individual is susceptible, another infection is started. The probability of

Figure 29.1: Development Patterns of Trypanosomes in *Glossina*. ca,
proventriculus; *cr*, crop; *hg*, hindgut; *hx*, hypopharynx; *l*, labium; *le*, labrum-
epipharynx; *ma*, malpighian tubes; *me*, metacyclic trypanasomes; *mg*,
midgut; *oe*, oesophagus; *ph*, pharynx; *pm*, peritrophic membrane;
r, rectum; *s*, salivary glands (one cut off); *T. grayi* illustrates stercorarian
pattern; others are salivarian. Magnification of trypanosomes about 1300

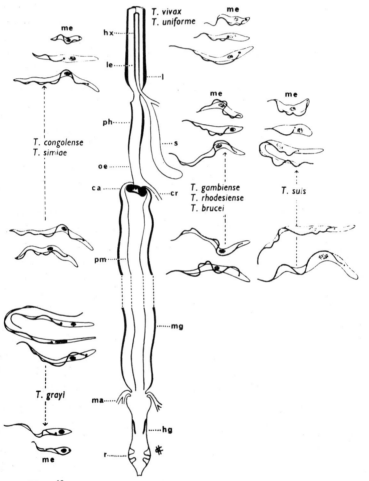

Source: From Hoare[16]

transmission occurring is enhanced by the fact that the first drop of saliva
produced by the feeding fly is the largest and will presumably carry with it
most metacyclics. If feeding is interrupted another large drop of saliva is
produced when the tsetse attempts to feed again.[52] This implies that a
probing fly is almost as likely to transmit as one that feeds to repletion.

The above account follows the classical description of the cycle of *Trypanozoon* in *Glossina*,[16] but recent observations raise doubts about its being the complete story. Trypanosomes have been found in the haemolymph of *Glossina*,[35,38] and penetrating the cells of the midgut.[7] It has been shown that *T. brucei rhodesiense* can penetrate the peritrophic membrane in the central two-thirds of the midgut. Nine days after an infective feed all the trypanosomes were in the endoperitrophic space, but two days later 90 per cent of them were in the ectoperitrophic space.[6] The trypanosomes then actively penetrated the midgut cells and undamaged parasites were seen between the basement membrane of the midgut cells and the haemocoele membrane.[7] The trypanosomes reached the haemocoele and infected the salivary glands, enabling normal transmission to occur when the tsetse fly fed.[8] Penetration of the midgut cells to the haemocoele provides a shorter route to the salivary glands.

Another objection to the classical explanation has been the claim that the pH of the midgut at the open end of the peritrophic membrane was such as to be lethal to trypanosomes.[13] It has also been suggested that trypanosomes and red blood cells pass into the ectotrophic space through the soft anterior part of the peritrophic membrane.[13]

Nannomonas. The development cycles of *T. (Nannomonas) congolense* and *T. (N.) simiae* are intermediate between those of *Duttonella* and *Trypanozoon*. Trypomastigotes pass into the midgut, develop in the manner described for *Trypanozoon*, and finally reach the opening of the salivary duct in the hypopharynx. They do not proceed to the salivary glands, but like *Duttonella* produce epimastigotes and metacyclic trypomastigotes in the salivary duct. When the *Glossina* feeds they pass with the saliva into the host.

More recent observations on the development of infections of *T. congolense* in *Glossina morsitans morsitans* have shown that the trypanosomes penetrate the peritrophic membrane in the central region of the midgut by a similar process to that observed in *T. brucei*. Seven days after an infective feed heavy infections were found in both the endoperitrophic and ectoperitrophic spaces of the midgut; by 21 days epimastigotes were to be found attached to the food canal by their flagella and a week later free forms were found in the hypopharynx.[9] *T. congolense* was found to penetrate the midgut in folds between the midgut cells and not by penetrating the cells.[9] Nantulya *et al.*[36] observed rather faster development of *T. congolense* in *G. m. morsitans*, with 45 per cent of the flies that became infected reaching that stage within 12 days and 76 per cent in 18 days.

T. congolense forms large clusters of organisms on the labrum of *Glossina*, and it has been postulated that they interfere with the sensory receptors of the fly, favouring increased probing and therefore facilitating transmission of the parasite. It has been observed that *Glossina* infected with *T. brucei* or *T. congolense* probe more than uninfected flies.[34]

Implications of Trypanosome Cycle in Glossina

As would be expected from the above descriptions of the developmental cycles of trypanosomes in *Glossina*, the cycle of *T. (D.) vivax* is completed in a much shorter time (5-13 days) than those of *T. (N.) congolense* and *T. (T.) brucei* which takes a minimum of about three weeks. The cycle of *T. (Pycnomonas) suis* in *Glossina* takes a similar time to that of *Trypanozoon*, i.e. about four weeks.[43] This relatively long development time is consistent with the longevity of *Glossina*, which is about six weeks for males and 15 weeks for females. Infections with *Trypanozoon* and *Nannomonas* in *Glossina* last for the life of the fly, while those of *Duttonella* persist in the proboscis for up to eight weeks.[39,43]

In natural populations of *Glossina* there is considerable variation in their infection rates with *Trypanosoma*. In the data tabulated by Jordan,[18] infection rates varied from 0.2 per cent in *G. fuscipes martinii* in Zambia to 76.6 per cent in *G. morsitans submorsitans* in Nigeria. The highest infection rates were of *T. vivax*, and the lowest of *T. brucei*, with infections of *T. congolense* being intermediate in frequency. As a reasonable approximation it can be taken that there is an order of magnitude difference in the percentage infectivity of the three subgenera of *Trypanosoma* in *Glossina*, being of the order of 20 per cent for *Duttonella*, 2 per cent for *Nannomonas*, and 0.2 for *Trypanozoon*.[11,16,18]

Susceptibility to infection with *T. brucei* is a function of age of the vector. Unless a *Glossina* feeds on an infected host very soon after eclosion it is unlikely to become infective. Highest percentages of infection are established in flies that feed on an infected host within 48 h of emergence and preferably within 24 h, that is at the first feed. Even then infectivity is unlikely to exceed 10 per cent. This relationship between early feeding and infectivity gave rise to the observation that flies reared from puparia kept at high temperatures were more readily infected. At eclosion such flies would be deficient in food reserves and feed early.

The dependence of infectivity on age is related to the development of the peritrophic membrane, which is not secreted until after eclosion. Flies that feed early in adult life have shorter membranes, and the trypomastigotes would more easily reach the ectoperitrophic space. When the peritrophic membrane is fully developed the trypomastigotes would have to travel further down the midgut to find the end of the membrane, and this could carry them into the zone where the pH is lethal[13] and account for resistance to infection. The peritrophic membrane is secreted continuously, but particularly after a blood meal.

Three stages (initial, established, mature) can be recognised in the development of an infection of *T. (T.) brucei* in *Glossina*. When *G. morsi-*

tans was fed on infected blood, 50 per cent of the flies developed initial infections in the midgut three days later but only 9 per cent developed established infections in the ectoperitrophic space and foregut. Established infections were detectable five to 30 days after the infective feed. However, the number of mature infections, i.e. flies able to transmit metacyclics, was very low. Only 39 flies out of many hundreds examined successfully transmitted *T. brucei* by bite and in only 15 of those were infections observed in the salivary glands.[5]

Trypanosomes in Vertebrate Host

There is a prepatent period between the injection of metacyclic trypomastigotes and the development of clinical symptoms and/or the presence of trypanosomes in the circulating blood. It is not known if the prepatent period involves a development cycle in an organ. In man, pathogenic trypanosomes produce a chancre (ulcer) at the site of inoculation. This is followed by infection of the vascular system and lymph glands before passing to the second stage involving invasion of the central nervous system, and the development of neurological symptoms which give rise to the common name for the disease: sleeping sickness. Untreated infections are always fatal.

In cattle, *T. vivax* invades the lymph glands and circulating blood, while *T. congolense* remains only in the blood system. The density of parasites in the circulating blood of the vertebrate is cyclical. Numbers of trypanosomes build up to a peak, then decline before increasing again. The explanation is that the surface coat of the trypanosome contains an antigen, a glycoprotein, which can be changed. Trypanosomes with a new antigen multiply rapidly in the blood until the development of an antibody leads to rapid decrease in parasite numbers, the development of a new antigen and further multiplication. One strain of trypanosome is on record as producing 22 different antigens.[39] In *Glossina* the antigenic coat of the trypanosome is lost but reappears in the metacyclic trypomastigote. The antigenic type of the metacyclic is either the same as that ingested or is regarded as having reverted to a basic strain antigen.[19]

Human Trypanosomiasis (Sleeping Sickness)[39]

Two forms of sleeping sickness are recognised in man. Gambian sleeping sickness is caused by *T. (T.) brucei gambiense*, and Rhodesian sleeping sickness by *T. (T.) brucei rhodesiense*. The organisms concerned are morphologically indistinguishable from the animal pathogen *T. (T.) brucei brucei*. These forms will be referred to as *T. gambiense*, *T. rhodesiense* and *T. brucei*.

The only certain way of distinguishing between them is by inoculation into a human volunteer, when *T. brucei* fails to establish but *T. gambiense* and *T. rhodesiense* multiply. Taxonomically there is little justification for differentiating between *T. gambiense* and *T. rhodesiense*, but epidemiologically there is value in making the distinction. They may either be regarded as subspecies of *T. brucei* or as two nosodemes, forms of one subspecies *T. (T.) brucei gambiense* which produce clinically different conditions in man.[39]

At the turn of the century sleeping sickness killed a quarter of a million people around Lake Victoria in East Africa. At the present day about 10,000 new cases are diagnosed in Africa each year.[39] Typically *T. gambiense* sleeping sickness causes a wasting disease which takes several months to several years to prove fatal, whereas *T. rhodesiense* reaches a more rapid climax, killing in a matter of three to nine months. *T. gambiense* occurs in West and Central Africa (see p. 205) and *T. rhodesiense* in East Africa. *T. gambiense* is associated with the *Nemorhina* subgenus of *Glossina*, and its vectors are the riverine and lacustrine tsetse *G. palpalis*, *G. fuscipes* and *G. tachinoides*, whereas the vectors of *T. rhodesiense* are the savanna species of *Glossina* (*Glossina*), *G. morsitans*, *G. pallidipes* and *G. swynnertoni*.

T. gambiense Sleeping Sickness. Until recently *T. gambiense* sleeping sickness had been regarded as an anthroponosis, involving transmission from man to man,[2] but evidence is accumulating that domestic pigs may play an active role as reservoirs of *T. gambiense*.[3,32] In some forest and forest/savanna villages in West Africa where domestic pigs are kept, peridomestic populations of *G. palpalis* and *G. tachinoides* have become established, feeding on pigs and man, and with the pigs acting as hosts of *T. gambiense*, the villages become foci of human trypanosomiasis.[3]

Species of *Glossina* (*Nemorhina*) are opportunist feeders, feeding equally on reptiles, bovids and man and to a lesser extent on suids. Weitz[45] gives percentages of feeds for the respective hosts as 9-34 per cent; 30-38 per cent; 8-40 per cent; and 2-6 per cent. *T. gambiense* sleeping sickness is transmitted when there is close association between tsetse and man and occurs, for example, in the dry season when man and *G. palpalis* concentrate around waterholes.[37] Other hazardous situations occur when palm cutters work in raffia beds (*Raphia sudanica*), the haunt of *G. tachinoides*, or fishermen land on a lake shore frequented by *G. fuscipes*.

T. gambiense sleeping sickness survives in West and western Central Africa in relatively modest-sized foci, more or less separated from each other.[33,39] One problem has been the survival of the disease at low endemic levels. One explanation would be the existence of an animal reservoir, e.g. pigs, as previously mentioned, but there is an alternative explanation. Molyneux *et al*.[33] have presented evidence that tsetse flies can be dispersed by wind over long distances in West Africa. They draw attention to the fact that foci tend to be distributed in south-west to north-east series, an arrangement which could be explained by *Glossina* being carried by winds associated with the Inter Tropical Convergence Zone. The foci would then represent particularly favourable areas for dispersed flies to settle, feed and transmit infection. Wind carriage of insects over long distances in Africa has been well documented for the desert locust (*Schistocerca gregaria*) and *Simulium damnosum* (see pp. 183-4).

T. rhodesiense Sleeping Sickness. This disease is an anthropozoonosis in which the natural cycle is from animal to animal and man is an unimportant, accidental intrusion.[2] *T. rhodesiense* is readily infective to man, laboratory animals and wild and domestic animals. Strains of *T. rhodesiense* retain their infectivity to man, and the strain used in the Tinde experiment has continued to be infective to man over 20 years, during whch it has been cyclically transmitted through antelopes and sheep. Strains pathogenic to man have been isolated from bushbuck,[15] cattle,[17] and some other animals including donkeys. Man becomes infected when his activities as hunter, game warden, entomologist or tourist take him into the habitat of game animals and *Glossina* (*Glossina*) tsetse flies. Man is not their preferred host, 80-90 per cent of the feeds of *G. pallidipes* being made from bushbuck, 65 per cent of those of *G. swynnertoni* on suids, and *G. morsitans* 30-35 per cent on suids and 25-40 per cent on bovids.[45]

Trypanosomiasis of Domestic Animals[43,51]

Virtually all domestic animals suffer from trypanosomiasis caused by one or more species of *Trypanozoon, Nannomonas* or *Duttonella*. Various popular names are given to these diseases in different animals, and those in commonest use are nagana for trypanosomiasis of cattle transmitted by *Glossina*, and surra for the disease in camels and horses caused by *T. (T.) evansi*. The pathogens will be considered briefly starting with those transmitted by *Glossina*.

T. (T.) brucei brucei. T. brucei is a polymorphic species, as are *T. rhodesiense* and *T. gambiense*, in which the parasites in the blood differ in appearance, some being long and slender and others being short and stumpy. Both forms have a free flagellum. *T. brucei* is particularly pathogenic to equines, but like other species it causes disease in a wide range of domestic animals including camels, sheep, goats, cats and dogs. It produces only a benign infection in cattle. Indeed cattle and game animals are the main reservoirs of *T. brucei*. Its pathogenicity to horses has led Ford[11] to write '*T. brucei* more than any other trypanosome has protected African people from invasion and African wildlife from destruction' (p.64). *T. brucei* is transmitted by the subgenus *Glossina* and other species.

T. (N.) congolense. T. congolense is a sluggish, monomorphic trypanosome which lacks a free flagellum, and is a major cause of trypanosomiasis in cattle. It is particularly liable to produce chronic infections in cattle, sheep, goats, camels and horses, and is transmitted by members of the subgenus *Glossina* and *G. (A.) brevipalpis* and *G. (A.) longipennis.*

T. (N.) simiae. T. simiae occurs naturally in warthogs in East and Central Africa, where it is highly pathogenic to domestic pigs. In view of the high feeding rates of *Glossina* species on suids, this trypanosome is transmitted by five species of *Austenina*, four *Glossina* and two *Nemorhina*. Cattle are resistant.

T. (D.) vivax. T. vivax is very motile, monomorphic trypanosome with a free flagellum. It is a main cause of trypanosomiasis in domestic animals, especially cattle, to which it maintains high virulence, particularly in West Africa. It is also pathogenic to sheep, goats, horses and camels but not to cats or dogs. The main vectors are species of the subgenus *Glossina.*

T. (D.) uniforme. T. uniforme produces a mild disease in cattle in East Africa, where it is transmitted by *G. palpalis* and *G. fuscipes.*

T (Pycnomonas) suis. T. suis is an uncommon, stumpy, monomorphic trypanosome with a free flagellum. It has only been recorded from Tanzania and the Congo, where its natural host is the warthog. It is pathogenic to domestic pigs, and transmitted by *G. (A.) brevipalpis* and *G. (A.) vanhoofi.*

T. (T.) evansi.[27,51] *T. evansi* is a monomorphic trypanosome with a free flagellum. It causes severe disease in camels, horses, dogs and the Indian elephant, but produces only benign infections in cattle, water buffaloes, pigs, sheep, goats and donkeys, which can act as reservoir hosts. In horses the disease can be rapidly fatal, and in general a high mortality rate can be expected in untreated camels. In dogs the disease is more severe in imported dogs. *T. evansi* is widespread in the tropics and subtropics, being found in South and Central America, North Africa, India, the Middle East and south-east Asia. It has no cycle in the vector, but is transmitted mechanically by tabanids, biting muscids, e.g. *Stomoxys*, and vampire bats. The relationship between *T. evansi* and vampire bats is most unusual in that the bats act both as vectors and hosts, with *T. evansi* multiplying in the bats. Infection in bats lasts about a month, during which time the bat may die from the infection.

Tabanids are the most capable vectors of *T. evansi* in most areas of the world, and in the Sudan there is a definite correlation between outbreaks of *T. evansi* infections and the increase in number of tabanids in the rainy season.[27]

T. (D.) vivax viennei. T. v. viennei is a form of *T. vivax* which has developed in Guadeloupe, Martinique and the countries of Central and

South America bordering the Caribbean. *T. viennei* is transmitted mechanically by tabanids and biting muscids and is no longer competent to develop in *Glossina.*[51] However, the possibility of cyclical development in an unknown vector cannot be excluded.[47] *T. v. viennei* is pathogenic to cattle and sheep, and it is not known whether a reservoir has been established in the indigenous wildlife.

Trypanosomiasis in African Wildlife[11]

The response of wildlife to infection with trypanosomes differs from species to species. Some such as baboons are totally resistant to infection. Others such as the suids and buffalo develop a scanty parasitaemia and are tolerant of infection. This suggests a long relationship between parasite, *Glossina* and host, as suggested when considering the evolution of *Glossina* (p. 216). Some bovidae are tolerant of infection but develop high parasitaemias which could make them important reservoir hosts. This group includes eland, reedbuck, bushbuck and impala, all of which are browsers on vegetation at the forest edge, and in thickets where close contact would be made with *Glossina*. High parasitaemias suggest that their association with *Glossina* and *Trypanosoma* is, in evolutionary terms, of recent origin. Other bovids and families of mammals are intolerant of infection and develop fatal parasitaemias. These include the plains-dwelling gazelles which would rarely have contact with *Glossina* in nature, and hyrax on which tsetse do not commonly feed.

Surveys of infection rates of game animals with *T. vivax*, *T. congolense* and *T. brucei* give overall values of 6 per cent, 10 per cent and 4 per cent, respectively, which are quite different from those found in *Glossina* where the infection rates are closer to 20 per cent, 2 per cent and 0.2 per cent. This difference highlights the effect of selective feeding by *Glossina* and its varying susceptibility to infection.

Some data concerning trypanosome infections in wildlife are presented in Table 29.2. Infection rates in buffalo, zebra and suids are low. (Zebra are plains animals with little contact with tsetse.) There is considerable difference between the specific infections found in different mammals. High infection rates occur in the Reduncinae, Tragelaphinae of the Bovidae, and in the Giraffidae. Infections with *T. vivax* were common in giraffe, waterbuck and reedbuck. *T. congolense* infections were particularly abundant in the Tragelaphinae, reedbuck and giraffe. Infections with *T. brucei* were 5 per cent or more in hartebeeste, waterbuck, reedbuck, eland and bushbuck. The last named is particularly important because an isolation of *T. b. rhodesiense* has been made from it,[15] and it is a major host of tsetse (Table 12.2).

General Observation on Glossina-borne Trypanosomiases

It should be clear that transmission of salivarian trypanosomes to man and

Table 29.2: Infections in Game Animals, Expressed as Percentages of Animals Examined

Family	Subfamily	Genus	Common name	n	Percentage infected			
					T.v.	T.c.	T.b.	All
Suidae	Suinae	*Phacochoerus*	warthog	154	1	6	2	10
		Potamochoerus	bushpig	26	12	0	0	12
				180	2	5	2	10
Giraffidae		*Giraffa*	giraffe	68	16	28	1	37
Bovidae	Alcelophinae	*Alcelophus*	hartebeeste	76	1	3	9	13
		Connochaetes	wildebeeste	38	0	0	0	0
		Damaliscus	topi	30	3	3	3	13*
				144	1	2	6	10
	Reduncinae	*Adenota*	cob	70	3	0	1	4
		Kobus	waterbuck	110	33	9	24	52*
		Redunca	reedbuck	39	25	15	8	43
				219	22	7	14	35
	Aepycerotinae	*Aepyceros*	impala	151	1	9	1	11
	Antilopinae	*Gazella*	gazelles	20	0	0	0	0
	Tragelaphinae	*Strepsiceros*	kudu	40	3	45	0	45
		Taurotragus	eland	63	5	21	5	29
		Tragelaphus	bushbuck	55	2	25	5	31
				158	3	28	4	34

Bovinae	Syncerus	buffalo	87	0	3	3	7
Equidae	Equus	zebra	109	2	3	0	6*

* One unidentified infection included in total.

T.v., *T.c.* and *T.b.* indicate, respectively, *T. vivax*, *T. congolense* and *T. brucei*.

Source: From Lumsden.[26]

livestock is very complex, depending on the distribution of the reservoir host and the species of *Glossina* involved. Even when reservoir host and tsetse coincide in the same habitat their interaction will be influenced by the feeding preferences of the fly, and susceptibility of both host and fly to the strain of trypanosome. In general, species of *Glossina* (*Nemorhina*) are relatively poor vectors of *Trypanosoma* (*Nannomonas*) species.[18] Finally, the onset of fresh cases of trypanosomiasis will depend on contact being established between susceptible hosts and infective *Glossina*.

Stercorarian Trypanosomiasis

The only stercorarian trypanosome of economic importance is *Trypanosoma (Schizotrypanum) cruzi*, the causative organism of Chagas' disease, a widespread and dangerous disease of man in the Neotropical region, where ten million people are affected.[30]

Chagas' Disease (*Trypanosoma (Schizotrypanum) cruzi*)[10,53]

Chagas' disease is of greatest importance in Argentina, Brazil and Venezuela. The parasite is present in its animal host from 46°S to 40°N, as far north as Maryland, but in the USA cases are very rare, in spite of the coexistence of reservoir host and vector, because the vectors rarely become domestic.[30] The vectors of *T. cruzi* are species of haematophagous triatomine bugs (Reduviidae, Hemiptera; see Chapter 19).

Cycle of T. cruzi

T. cruzi is a monomorphic trypanosome which is present in the circulating blood of its vertebrate host. When a triatomine bug feeds on an infected host the trypanosomes are ingested and taken into the midgut where the trypomastigotes multiply and develop into epimastigotes. They move slowly down the gut of the insect, and in the rectum metacyclic trypomastigotes are formed and passed out with the faeces. The cycle in the bug takes two to four weeks. If metacyclic forms are deposited on the skin of a susceptible host they enter either through abrasions or through the intact mucous membrane. In the vertebrate host amastigotes are formed intracellularly in muscle cells where they multiply and release trypomastigotes into the blood in which they become available to a vector.

Triatomine Vectors of T. cruzi

Various species of triatomine bugs are vectors of *T. cruzi* and they differ in their ecological requirements and geographical distributions. *Triatoma dimidiata* is found in dry areas where the climate is not too warm, and occurs in Mexico, Central America, Colombia and Ecuador. *Triatoma infestans* occurs in warmer but equally dry habitats in Argentina, Paraguay, Bolivia, Chile, and parts of Peru and Brazil. It is the most domestic of the triatomines and extends widely, being found at 3,682 m in Argentina and as far south as 45°S. *Panstrongylus megistus* occurs in the moister areas of Brazil and Peru. It requires a high humidity for breeding (above 60 per cent RH), and is found as wild, peridomestic and domestic populations in rural situations, and even as urban populations in the city of Salvador.[53] By contrast *Triatoma braziliensis* flourishes under dry conditions in north-east Brazil where *P. megistus* cannot survive.

Rhodnius prolixus occurs north of the equator in the mainland countries bordering the Caribbean, i.e. Mexico, Central America (except Panama and Costa Rica), Colombia, Venezuela and the Guianas. It is an ancient pest of man, well adapted to poor households. In Venezuela it occurs as high as 1,500 m and in Colombia it has been found at 2,600 m.[53] In El Salvador *R. prolixus* is replaced by *T. dimidiata* above 340 m. Below 340 m *R. prolixus* is dominant (91.5 per cent); between 340 and 600 m it forms only 18.3 per cent of the triatomine population, and above 600 m a mere 3 per cent.[50]

Epidemiology and Epizootiology of Chagas' Disease

T. cruzi occurs in a wide range of wild and domestic animals. The main wild hosts are opossums, marsupials of the genus *Didelphys*, which are widely distributed from Argentina to the USA. They are parasitised by triatomine bugs, and have a high incidence of infection with *T. cruzi.* In a sylvatic situation the disease is enzootic, but opossums become established near houses where they infect peridomiciliary triatomines. Human infections result when these triatomines enter houses and infect the residents directly, or by infecting dogs and cats which become sources of infection for resident domiciliary triatomines, which in turn will feed on the human occupants of the house and infect them.

T. cruzi is spread by faecal contamination of the host by the bug. Since bugs only visit hosts to feed it follows that they will only be potential vectors if they defaecate while feeding. Some bugs, e.g. *Triatoma infestans*, do so and are vectors, while *Triatoma protracta* defaecates off the host and is not a vector.

In infected houses in Bahia, Brazil, Minter[30] found that the infection rate of *T. cruzi* in *P. megistus* increased steadily with age. In 1st instar nymphs the infection rate was 6.5 per cent, and in adults of both sexes 70 per cent. In laboratory experiments Miles *et al.*[29] found that both *P. megistus* and *T. infestans* were more readily infected than *R. prolixus*, and this applied to both the percentage of the bugs which became infected and the degree of infection established, but there was no correlation between the size of the blood meal and the development of infection. In El Salvador Wilton and

Cedillos[50] found that 17 per cent of *T. dimidiata* examined were infected with *T. cruzi* compared to 1 per cent in *R. prolixus*. The reverse occurred with *Trypanosoma rangeli* with no infections being found in *T. dimidiata* compared to 23 per cent in *R. prolixus*. The authors state that these findings require confirmation.

The infection rate in bugs will depend upon available hosts, even in the case of domestic triatomine populations. Minter[30] found 529 *P. megistus* in one house, of which 225 were in the living room and 304 in the bedroom. The infection rate with *T. cruzi* in the bedroom bugs was 56 per cent, compared to 10 per cent in those from the living room. Similar differences were apparent in the sources of their blood meals, with 82 per cent of the bedroom bugs having fed on humans, while the living room bugs had fed almost exclusively (97 per cent) on chickens which roosted along the walls in which the bugs were found.

Other Stercorarian Trypanosomes[28]

None of the other stercorarian trypanosomes are of economic importance but some are of interest for other reasons.

Trypanosoma (Herpetosoma) rangeli.[4] *T. rangeli* resembles *T. cruzi* in being transmitted by triatomine bugs, particularly *R. prolixus*. It occurs in Central and South America in a range of mammals including man and dogs, and must be differentiated from infection with *T. cruzi*. *T. rangeli* is not pathogenic to vertebrates, but is pathogenic to the triatomine vector. In the midgut of the vector the ingested trypomastigotes transform into epimastigotes which multiply extracellularly throughout the midgut. They eventually migrate to the hindgut and ultimately typical metacyclic trypomastigotes develop in the hindgut and can infect new mammalian hosts by the contaminative route.[28] D'Alessandro[4] regards transmission by the contaminative route as controversial, and claims that transmission is mainly, if not exclusively, by the salivarian route.

After infections have been established for at least three weeks, *T. rangeli* invades the haemolymph and subsequently the salivary glands. *R. prolixus* has been recorded as being capable of transmitting *T. rangeli* by bite for up to nine months.[4] In experimentally infected bugs salivary gland infections occurred in 30 per cent of *R. prolixus* and 63 per cent of *R. neglectus*, and in two-thirds of these bugs infections were limited to the glands.[4]

Trypanosoma (Herpetosoma) lewisi. *T. lewisi* has a worldwide distribution as a benign parasite of rats (*Rattus* spp), and is much used in laboratory studies of trypanosomes. It is transmitted by the rat fleas *Nosopsyllus fasciatus* in temperate regions and *Xenopsylla cheopis* in the warmer parts of the world.

Trypanosoma (Megatrypanum) theileri.[46] *T. theileri* is a large trypanosome which occurs in low density in cattle causing benign infections. Most of the evidence regarding transmission incriminates tabanid flies, especially those of the genera *Tabanus* and *Haematopota*, as the main vectors, but the possibility of vectors other than tabanids cannot be ruled out. The developmental cycle of *T. theileri* in its vector has not been adequately worked out but the assumption is that metacyclic trypomastigotes are passed with the faeces.

Trypanosoma (Megatrypanum) melophagium.[46] *T. melophagium* is another large, non-pathogenic trypanosome which occurs in sheep and completes its cycle in the sheep ked (*Melophagus ovinus*), a hippoboscid fly. It is most probable that sheep become infected when they ingest keds.

Trypanosoma grayi. T. grayi is a parasite of crocodiles and is transmitted by *Glossina palpalis* by faecal contamination of the mucosa of the reptiles' mouth while the tsetse is feeding. Epimastigotes and metacyclic trypomastigotes occur in the hindgut of infected *Glossina.*[44]

Leishmaniasis

Leishmaniasis is a disease of man and dogs caused by infection with *Leishmania*. In these hosts the parasites are intracellular in macrophages. They are transmitted from host to host by the bites of phlebotomine sandflies in which the parasites are motile and extracellular. In man infections take three principal forms – cutaneous, visceral and mucocutaneous. The cutaneous form may be self-curing; the visceral form is usually fatal unless treated; and the outcome of the mucocutaneous form is variable. It may remain localised in the skin or, sometimes long after the primary skin lesion has healed, it may attack the nasopharyngeal tissue with fatal results. Man is the main, if not the only, host of some leishmanias but most cause infections in wild mammals with man being an accidental introduction into a natural cycle.

Taxonomy and Vectors of Leishmania[25,54]

Leishmanias occur in a wide range of hosts, including eutherian mammals, marsupials and reptiles. The species of *Leishmania* infective for man are morphologically identical and are traditionally classified on the clinical syndromes they produce. The validity of this classification has been confirmed and extended by modern taxonomic techniques involving serological, immunological and biochemical studies.[49] The mammalian species can be arranged in four groups (Table 29.3). *Leishmania donovani* and *L. tropica* complexes occur predominantly in Europe, Africa and Asia, while the *L. mexicana* and *L. brasiliensis* complexes are restricted to Central and South America.

Leishmania donovani Complex. The three species in this group cause visceral leishmaniasis, known sometimes as kala azar, in man. *L. donovani*, which occurs in the Oriental region and Africa, has no known animal host, i.e. the disease is an anthroponosis. Vectors of *L. donovani* include *Phlebotomus argentipes* in India, *P. chinensis* in north-east China, and *P. martini* in Kenya. In the Palaearctic region visceral leishmaniasis, caused by *L. infantum*, is a zoonosis of canines and porcupines (*Hystrix*), which principally affects children. The vectors include *P. ariasis* in France and *P. major* in Turkestan. In the Neotropical region a similar visceral leishmaniasis is caused by *L. chagasi*, and it also is a zoonosis involving dogs and foxes with the vector being *Lutzomyia longipalps*. (*Lutzomyia* will be abbreviated to *Lu.* to avoid confusion with *Leishmania*.)

Leishmania tropica Complex. These three species cause cutaneous leishmaniasis (oriental sore). *L. tropica* is associated with dry cutaneous leishmaniasis, an anthroponosis of urban areas, while *L. major* is associated with wet cutaneous leishmaniasis, a zoonosis of rural areas. Vectors of *L. tropica* include *P. papatasi* in Asia and *P. perfiliewi* in Europe. *L. major* parasitises ground-dwelling rodents, particularly the giant gerbil *Rhombomys opimus*. The main vector of *L. major* among gerbils is *P. caucasicus*, which is strongly zoophilic, while the disease is spread to man by *P. papatasi*, which is markedly but not exclusively anthropophilic. Control of *L. major* has been achieved in Central Asia by applying insecticides and rodenticides to gerbil burrows to control both the reservoir hosts and the vectors.

   L. aethiopica is a parasite of rock hyraxes (*Procavia habessinica* and *Heterohyrax brucei*), of which the vectors are *P. longipes* and *P. pedifer*.[1] These sandflies feed equally easily on hyraxes and cattle, and man is bitten and becomes infected when he associates closely with the sandflies' main hosts. It has been calculated that in compounds where human disease was present the average biting rate was as low as 21 bites/man/month.[12]

Leishmania mexicana Complex. The species in this complex produce mild cutaneous lesions in man. They are parasites of rodents and opossums, and are transmitted by species of the *Lu. intermedia* group in which they develop in the midgut. *L. mexicana mexicana* infects the log cutters and collectors of chicle (chewing gum latex) who work in the forest for periods of about six months during the rainy season. The main host is the rodent *Ototylomys phyllotis*, and the vector *Lu. olmeca olmeca*, which is not especially attracted to man, except when its daytime resting places in the leaf litter on the forest floor are disturbed. It is particularly liable to bite if

Table 29.3: List of Species and Subspecies of *Leishmania* Which Infect Man, Together with Their Distributions, Reservoir Hosts, Vectors and the Type of Disease Caused in Man

Leishmania	Geographical distribution	Reservoir host	Vector	Disease in man
donovani complex				
L. donovani	Oriental region Afrotropical region North-east China	none	*P. argentipes* *P. martini* *P. chinensis*	visceral (kala azar)
L. infantum	Mediterranean littoral Palaearctic region	dog, fox	*P. ariasi* *P. major*	visceral in children
L. chagasi	Neotropical region	dog, fox	*Lu. longipalpis*	visceral
tropica complex				
L. tropica	Palaearctic Region Afghanistan, India	dog?	*P. papatasi* *P. perfiliewi*	cutaneous
L. major	Deserts of Asia and Sahara	*Rhombomys opimus* desert rodents	*P. caucasicus* *P. papatasi*	cutaneous
L. aethiopica	Highlands of East Africa	*Procavia habessinica,* *Heterohyrax brucei*	*P. longipes*	cutaneous
mexicana complex				
L. m. mexicana	Mexico, Central America	forest rodents *Ototylomys phyllotis*	*Lu. olmeca olmeca*	cutaneous
L. m. amazonensis	Amazon, Trinidad, Mato Grosso	forest rodents and marsupials	*Lu. flaviscutellata*	cutaneous (rare)
L. m. pifanoi	Amazon, Venezuela, Mato Grosso	forest rodents	?	very rare
braziliensis complex				
L. b. braziliensis	Tropical South America	forest rodents	*Lu. intermedia* *Lu. wellcomei*	mucocutaneous (espundia)
L. b. guyanensis	Guyanas, N. Brazil	?	*Lu. anduzei* *Lu. trapidoi*	cutaneous
L. b. panamensis	Panama	rodents, sloths procyonids	*Lu. panamensis*	cutaneous
L. peruviana	Peruvian Andes	dog	*Lu. verrucarum* *Lu. peruensis*	cutaneous (uta)

Source: Based on information available in Zuckerman and Lainson.[54]

disturbed in the hour or so after dawn.[48] By contrast *L. m. amazonensis* rarely causes infections in man because the vector *Lu. flaviscutellata* is zoophilic, and rarely feeds on man.[42]

Leishmania brasiliensis Complex. The most important member of this group is *L. brasiliensis brasiliensis*, a slow-growing parasite which causes espundia in man, when the parasite invades and destroys tissue in the nasopharyngeal region. The primary skin lesions, although few in number, are long lasting, extensive and disfiguring. The vectors are members of the *Lu. intermedia* group and *Lu. (Psychodopygus) wellcomei*, in which the parasites multiply in the hindgut before moving anteriorly. The reservoir hosts are poorly known, but include forest rodents.

Leishmania peruviana. The taxonomic position of *L. peruviana* is uncertain, but it is close to the *L. brasiliensis* complex because in the laboratory, *L. peruviana* develops in the hindgut of *Lu. longipalpis*.[25] It causes self-healing skin lesions in man in the high Peruvian Andes, a condition known as 'uta'. It is possible that dogs may be the only reservoir of infection for man, although the existence of other hosts cannot be excluded. The disease was effectively controlled when houses were sprayed with DDT against Carrion's disease (see Chapter 26), indicating that peridomestic sandflies were the most likely vectors. *Lu. verrucarum* was highly suspected as being the main vector with *Lu. peruensis* as a less important vector.[25]

Cycle of Leishmania in Phlebotomine Vectors

When a phlebotomine sandlfy feeds the ingested blood passes to the midgut where it is enclosed in the peritrophic membrane formed by the cells lining the posterior midgut. In infected blood some of the ingested macrophages will contain amastigote leishmanias, i.e. non-motile forms. They become free and develop into slender flagellate promastigotes (nectomonads) with terminal or subterminal kinetoplasts. They multiply rapidly and are abundant by the third day after feeding when the blood meal is almost digested and the peritrophic membrane disintegrating.

Broader promastigotes (haptomonads) then appear and move anteriorly in the cardiac portion of the midgut, and attach to the cuticle of the oesophageal valve.[23] The two forms of promastigotes differ in their abilities to attach. Nectomonads insert their flagella into villi projecting from midgut cells, whereas haptomonads attach to the cuticle by hemi-desmosomes in the flagellum, i.e. definite junctional complexes are formed.[23]

L. brasiliensis brasiliensis develops largely in the anterior, broader portion (pylorus) of the hindgut. Few promastigotes are to be seen in the midgut or in the long, narrower distal portion of the hindgut (ileum), and none in the rectum.[24]

The role of the peritrophic membrane, and particularly its duration, is of paramount importance in the successful development of *Leishmania*. In *P. mongolensis* the blood meal is surrounded by a permanent peritrophic membrane in which leishmanias multiply at first but later die. Finally the membrane containing the remains of the blood meal and the surviving parasites is excreted with the faeces. This action prevents the establishment of *Leishmania* in *P. mongolensis*, which is not a vector.[31]

Transmission of Leishmania by Vectors

It has been comparatively easy to obtain development of *Leishmania* in the midgut of phlebotomines but difficult to obtain transmission of the parasite by allowing infected phlebotomines to feed on susceptible hosts. Williams and Coelho consider that human infections commonly occur when infected flies are crushed when biting and the body contents scarified into the skin.[49] It has also been proposed that promastigotes form a plug at the junction of the oesophagus and midgut, preventing the ingestion of blood. When the sandly attempts to feed, blood is pumped into the oesophagus but is unable to reach the midgut, and when the fly relaxes some of the ingested blood flows back into the host together with promastigotes detached from the plug.[31] Killick-Kendrick[20] considers this most unlikely as transmission requires the deposition of morphologically characteristic forms into the skin when the sandfly feeds.

In the oesophagus, pharynx and cibarium of the sandfly small rounded sessile flagellates (paramastigotes), which are not easily seen in fresh preparations, are produced.[21] Paramastigotes have their flagella modified for attachment to cuticle by means of hemidesmosomes. They are considered to give rise to promastigotes with unmodified flagella, and which invade the proboscis. These proboscis promastigotes are the infective forms.[22] It is believed that the midgut forms give rise to a steady supply of paramastigotes to the foregut, in which they do not divide but give rise to the proboscis promastigotes. Both the paramastigotes and the succeeding promastigotes have a short life and the infectivity of the fly depends on there being a steady supply from the midgut.

The conditions under which the parasite invades the foregut and proboscis of the sandfly are still imperfectly known. *L. donovani* has been successfully transmitted by the bite of experimentally infected *P. argentipes* when the sandflies were allowed to feed on raisins, and Killick-Kendrick[21,22] considers that plant sugars may (a) influence the anterior migration of the parasites to the proboscis, (b) be an important source of nutrients to the foregut forms, and (c) affect the production of proboscis promastigotes.

Infected phlebotomines take small blood meals, if any, and it has been postulated that this may be due to parasites blocking the cibarial sensilla, which are few in number. There are no pharyngeal sensilla, and the absence of sensory information from the cibarium would restrict or inhibit ingestion, but not affect probing. Increased probing would be beneficial to the parasites in ensuring that some were deposited in sites suitable for development.[22]

Epidemiology

Killick-Kendrick[20] has tabulated 52 species and subspecies of *Phlebotomus* and *Lutzomyia* which are known or suspected of being vectors of leishmaniasis. In *Phlebotomus* there is a specific association between vector and parasite with complete development, involving the invasion of the head and proboscis, occurring in the vector. In *Lutzomyia* there appears to be no such specific association with parasites developing equally successfully in vectors and non-vectors.[20,49] Development of the parasite is rapid and in most species of *Leishmania* is complete in one gonotrophic cycle and the sandfly is potentially capable of transmitting the parasite at the first blood meal after the infecting meal. In *L. donovani* development is slower and transmission is not possible until the second blood meal after the infecting feed.[20]

Three weeks after feeding on a dog infected with *L. infantum*, *P. ariasi* transmitted the parasite to a healthy dog.[41] In the Cevennes region of southern France the greatest risk of infection with *L. infantum* is in the late summer from mid-August to mid-September when the proportion of parous females in the *P. ariasi* population is high.[14] In the same area the parasite is dispersed by movement of infected dogs and by dispersal of *P. ariasi* which has been found to disperse 750 m.[40]

Infection rates in wild-caught phlebotomines have varied from zero to 15.4 per cent, the latter being found in *Lu. trapidoi*.[49] These infections will include both pathogenic and non-pathogenic leishmanias. Dissection of substantial numbers of *P. orientalis* in the Sudan and *P. longipes* in Ethiopia gave infection rates of 2.4 and 3.1 per cent, respectively.[49] Infection rates in *P. papatasi* have ranged from 0.2 to 8.7 per cent, and in *P. caucasicus* from 2.6 to 10.5 per cent.[49] In 11 out of 17 species of *Lutzomyia* infection rates were low, mostly below 1 per cent, while in the other six species they were much higher.[49]

References

1.　Ashford, R.W., Bray, M.A., Hutchinson, M.P. and Bray, R.S. (1973). The epidemiology of cutaneous leishmaniasis in Ethiopia. *Transactions of the Royal Society of Tropical Medicine and Hygiene 67*: 568-601

2.　Baker, J.R. (1974). Epidemiology of African sleeping sickness. pp. 29-50 in *Trypanosomiasis and Leishmaniasis with Special Reference to Chagas' Disease*, Ciba Foundation Symposium 20, Elsevier, Amsterdam

3.　Baldry, D.A.T. (1980). Local distribution and ecology of *Glossina palpalis* and *G. tachinoides* in forest foci of West African human trypanosomiasis, with special reference to associations between peri-domestic tsetse and their hosts. *Insect Science and Its Application 1*: 85-93

4. D'Alessandro, A. (1976). Biology of *Trypanosoma (Herpetosoma) rangeli* Tajera, 1920. pp. 327-403 in volume I, *Biology of the Kinetoplastida*, W.H.R. Lumsden and D.A. Evans (eds.), Academic Press, New York

5. Dipeolu, O.O. and Adam, K.M.G. (1974). On the use of membrane feeding to study the development of *Trypanosoma brucei* in *Glossina*. *Acta Tropica 31*: 185-201

6. Ellis, D.S. and Evans, D.A. (1977). Passage of *Trypanosoma brucei rhodesiense* through the peritrophic membrane of *Glossina morsitans morsitans*. *Nature, London 267*: 834-5

7. Evans, D.A. and Ellis, D.S. (1975). Penetration of mid-gut cells of *Glossina morsitans morsitans* by *Trypanosoma brucei rhodesiense*. *Nature, London 258*: 231-3

8. _____ and Ellis, D.S. (1979). Development of *Trypanosoma brucei* and *T. congolense* in *Glossina*. *Transactions of the Royal Society of Tropical Medicine and Hygiene 73*: 126

9. _____ Ellis, D.S. and Stamford, S. (1979). Ultrastructure studies of certain aspects of the development of *Trypanosoma congolense* in *Glossina morsitans morsitans*. *Journal of Protozoology 26*: 557-63

10. Fife, E.H. (1977). *Trypanosoma (Schizotrypanum) cruzi*. pp. 135-73 in volume I, *Parasitic Protozoa*, J.P. Kreier (ed.), Academic Press, New York

11. Ford, J. (1971). *The Role of the Trypanosomiases in African Ecology*. Clarendon Press, Oxford

12. Foster, W.A., Boreham, P.F.L. and Tempelis, C.H. (1972). Studies on leishmaniasis in Ethiopia. IV. Feeding behaviour of *Phlebotomus longipes* (Diptera: Psychodidae). *Annals of Tropical Medicine and Parasitology 66*: 433-43

13. Freeman J.C. (1973). The penetration of the peritrophic membrane of the tsetse flies by trypanosomes. *Acta Tropica 30*: 347-55

14. Guilvard, E., Wilkes, T.J., Killick-Kendrick, R. and Rioux, J.A. (1980). Ecologie des leishmanioses dans le sud de la France. 15. Déroulement des cycles gonotrophiques chez *Phlebotomus ariasi* Tonnoir, 1921 et *Phlebotomus mascittii* Grassi, 1908 en Cévennes. Corollaire épidémiologique. *Annales de Parasitologie Humaine et Comparée 55*: 659-64

15. Heisch, R.B., McMahon, J.P. and Manson-Bahr, P.E.C. (1958). The isolation of *Trypanosoma rhodesiense* from a bushbuck. *British Medical Journal 2*: 1203-4

16. Hoare, C.A. (1972). *The Trypanosomes of Mammals*. Blackwell Scientific Publications, Oxford

17. Hoeve, K. van, Onyango, R.J., Harley, J.M.B. and Raadt, P. de (1967). The epidemiology of *Trypanosoma rhodesiense* sleeping sickness in Alego Location, Central Nyanza, Kenya. II. The cyclical transmission of *Trypanosoma rhodesiense* isolated from cattle to a man, a cow and to sheep. *Transactions of the Royal Society of Tropical Medicine and Hygiene 61*: 684-7

18. Jordan, A.M. (1974). Recent developments in the ecology and methods of control of tsetse flies (*Glossina* spp) (Dipt., Glossinidae) — a review. *Bulletin of Entomological Research 63*: 361-99

19. _____ (1976). Tsetseflies as vectors of trypanosomes. *Veterinary Parasitology 2*: 143-52

20. Killick-Kendrick, R. (1978). Recent advaces and outstanding problems in the biology of phlebotomine sandflies. *Acta Tropica 35*: 297-313

21. _____ (1979). Biology of *Leishmania* in phlebotomine sandflies. pp. 395-460 in volume II, *Biology of the Kinetoplastida*, W.H.R. Lumsden and D.A. Evans (eds.), Academic Press, New York

22. _____ Leaney, A.J., Ready, P.D. and Molyneux, D.H. (1977). *Leishmania* in phlebotomid sandflies. IV. The transmission of *Leishmania mexicana amazonensis* to hamsters by the bite of experimentally infected *Lutzomyia longipalpis*. *Proceedings of the Royal Society of London B 196*: 105-15

23. _____ Molyneux, D.H. and Ashford, R.W. (1974). *Leishmania* in phlebotomid sandflies. I. Modifications of the flagellum associated with attachment to the mid-gut and oesophageal valve of the sandfly. *Proceedings of the Royal Society of London B 187*: 409-19

24. _____ Molyneux, D.H., Hommel, M., Leaney, A.J. and Robertson, E.S. (1977). *Leishmania* in phlebotomid sandflies. V. The nature and significance of infections of the

pylorus and ileum of the sandfly by leishmaniae of the *braziliensis* complex. *Proceedings of the Royal Society of London B 198*: 191-9

25. Lainson, R. and Shaw, J.J. (1979). The role of animals in the epidemiology of South American leishmaniasis. pp. 1-116 in volume II *Biology of the Kinetoplastida*, W.H.R. Lumsden and D.A. Evans (eds.), Academic Press, New York.

26. Lumsden, W.H.R. (1962). Trypanosomiasis in African Wildlife. pp. 66-95, *Proceedings of the First International Conference on Wildlife Diseases, New York*

27. Mahmoud, M.M. and Gray, A.R, (1980). Trypanosomiasis due to *Trypanosoma evansi* (Steel, 1885) Balbiani, 1888. A review of recent research. *Tropical Animal Health and Production 12*: 35-47

28. Mansfield, J.M. (1977). Nonpathogenic trypanosomes of mammals. pp. 297-327 in volume I. *Parasitic Protozoa*, J.P. Kreier (ed.), Academic Press, New York

29. Miles, M.A., Patterson, J.W., Marsden, P.D. and Minter, D.M. (1975). A comparison of *Rhodnius prolixus, Triatoma infestans* and *Panstrongylus megistus* in the xenodiagnosis of a chronic *Trypanosoma (Schizotrypanum) cruzi* infection in a rhesus monkey (*Macaca mullatta*). *Transactions of the Royal Society of Tropical Medicine and Hygiene 69*: 377-82

30. Minter, D.M. (1978). Triatomine bugs and the household ecology of Chagas's disease. pp. 85-93 in *Medical Entomology Centenary Symposium Proceedings*, S. Willmott (ed.), Royal Society of Tropical Medicine and Hygiene, London

31. Molyneux, D.H. (1977). Vector relationships in the Trypanosomatidae. *Advances in Parasitology 15*: 1-82

32. _____ (1980). Animal reservoirs and residual 'foci' of *Trypanosoma brucei gambiense* sleeping sickness in West Africa. *Insect Science and Its Application 1*: 59-63

33. _____ Baldry, D.A.T. and Fairhurst, C. (1979). Tsetse movement in wind fields: possible epidemiological and entomological implications for trypanosomiasis and its control. *Acta Tropica 36*: 53-65

34. _____ Lavin, D.R. and Elce, B. (1979). A possible relationship between salivarian trypanosomes and *Glossina* labrum mechano-receptors. *Annals of Tropical Medicine and Parasitology 73*: 287-90

35. Mshelbwala, A.S. (1972). *Trypanosoma brucei* infection in the haemocoele of tsetse flies. *Transactions of the Royal Society of Tropical Medicine and Hygiene 66*: 637-43

36. Nantulya, V.M., Doyle, J.J. and Jenni, L. (1978). Studies on *Trypanosoma (Nannomonas) congolense*. II. Observations on the cyclical transmission of three field isolates by *Glossina morsitans morsitans*. *Acta Tropica 35*: 339-44

37. Nash, T.A.M. (1978). A review of mainly entomological research which has aided the understanding of human trypanosomiasis and its control. pp. 39-47 in *Medical Entomology Centenary Symposium Proceedings*, S. Willmott (ed.), Royal Society of Tropical Medicine and Hygiene, London

38. Otieno, L.H. (1973). *Trypanosoma (Trypanozoon) brucei* in the haemolymph of experimentally infected young *Glossina morsitans*. *Transactions of the Royal Society of Medicine and Hygiene 67*: 886-7

39. Raadt, P. de and Seed, J.R. (1977). Trypanosomes causing disease in man in Africa. pp. 175-237 in volume I, *Parasitic Protozoa*, J.P. Kreier (ed.), Academic Press, New York

40. Rioux, J.A., Killick-Kendrick, R., Leaney, A.J., Turner, D.P., Bailly, M. and Young, C.J. (1979). Ecologie des leishmanioses dans le sud de la France. 2. Dispersion horizontale de *Phlebotomus ariasi* Tonnoir, 1921. Expériences préliminaires. *Annales de Parasitologie Humaine et Comparée 54*: 673-82

41. _____ Killick-Kendrick, R., Leaney, A.J., Young, C.J., Turner, D.P., Lanotte, G. and Bailly, M. (1979). Ecologie des leishmanioses dans le sud de la France. 11. La leishmaniose viscerale canine: succès de la transmission expérimentale 'chien — phelbotome — chien' par la piqûre de *Phlebotomus ariasi* Tonnoir, 1921. *Annales de Parasitologie Humaine et Comparée 54*: 401-7

42. Shaw, J.J., Lainson, R. and Ward, R.D. (1972). Leishmaniasis in Brazil. VII. Further observations on the feeding habitats of *Lutzomyia flaviscutellata* (Mangabeira) with particular reference to the biting habits at different heights. *Transactions of the Royal Society of Tropical Medicine and Hygiene 66*: 718-23

43. Soltys, M.A. and Woo, P.T.K. (1977). Trypanosomes producing disease in livestock in

Africa. pp. 239-68 in volume I, *Parasitic Protozoa*, J.P. Kreier (ed.), Academic Press, New York

44. Vickerman, K. (1976). The diversity of the kinetoplastid flagellates. pp. 1-34 in volume I, *Biology of the Kinetoplastida*, W.H.R. Lumsden and D.A. Evans (eds.), Academic Press, New York

45. Weitz, B.G.F. (1970). Hosts of *Glossina*. pp. 317-26 in *The African Trypanosomiases*, H.W. Mulligan (ed.), Wiley, New York

46. Wells, E.A. (1976). Subgenus *Megatrypanum*, pp. 257-84 in volume I, *Biology of the Kinetoplastida*, W.H.R. Lumsden and D.A. Evans (eds.), Academic Press, New York

47. _____ Betancourth, A. and Page, W.A. (1970). The epidemiology of bovine trypanosomiasis in Colombia. *Tropical Animal Health and Production 2*: 111-25

48. Williams, P. (1970). Phlebotomine sandflies and leishmaniasis in British Honduras (Belize). *Transactions of the Royal Society of Tropical Medicine and Hygiene 64*: 317-64

49 _____ and Coelho, M. de V. (1978). Taxonomy and transmission of *Leishmania*. *Advances in Parasitology 16*: 1-42

50. Wilton, D.P. and Cedillos, R.A. (1978). Domestic triatomines (Reduviidae) and insect trypanosome infections in El Salvador, C.A. *Bulletin of the Pan American Health Organization 12*: 116-23

51. Woo, P.T.K. (1977). Salivarian trypanosomes producing disease in livestock outside of sub-saharan Africa. pp. 269-96 in volume I, *Parasitic Protozoa*, J.P. Kreier (ed.), Academic Press, New York

52. Youdeowei, A. (1975). Salivary secretion in three species of tsetse flies (Glossinidae). *Acta Tropica 32*: 166-71

53. Zeledón, R. and Rabinovich, J.E. (1981). Chagas' Disease: an ecological appraisal with special emphasis on its insect vectors. *Annual Review of Entomology 26*: 101-33

54. Zuckerman, A. and Lainson, R. (1977). *Leishmania*. pp. 57-133 in volume I, *Parasitic Protozoa*, J.P. Kreier (ed.), Academic Press, New York

LYMPHATIC FILARIASIS (*WUCHERERIA BANCROFTI,*
BRUGIA MALAYI)

The most important group of Helminths, transmitted by insects, belongs to the superfamily Filarioidea, order Spirurida, class Nematoda. The classification used here is that given in the *CIH Keys to the Nematode Parasites of Vertebrates*.[1] Members of this superfamily, often referred to as filarial worms, are responsible for serious, widespread diseases of man and comparatively minor conditions in domestic animals. The vectors of the economically important filarial worms are various species of blood-sucking Diptera, mostly Nematocera, particularly mosquitoes. Other Spirurida have a wide range of intermediate hosts, including insects of many different orders, and some species are of minor veterinary importance (*Habronema, Thelazia*). A few species of tape-worms (Cestoda) use insects as their intermediate hosts and are of minor veterinary importance.

In the vertebrate host the Filarioidea are parasites of the blood or lymphatic system, muscles or connective tissue or of the serous cavities of their host. The Filarioidea contains two families, the Onchocercidae and the Filariidae. All the medically important species are in the Onchocercidae, including *Wuchereria bancrofti* and *Brugia malayi,* the causative organisms of bancroftian and brugian filariasis; *Onchocerca volvulus,* the cause of onchocerciasis or river blindnes; *Loa loa, Dipetalonema perstans, D. streptocerca* and *Mansonella ozzardi,* which cause relatively benign filariasis in man.

Parasites of veterinary importance in the Onchocercidae include species of *Onchocerca; Dirofilaria immitis,* the heartworm of dogs; and species of *Setaria* and *Elaeophora.* In the Filariidae species of *Parafilaria* and *Stephanofilaria* are of minor veterinary importance.

The diseases caused by these parasites, with emphasis on the role played by the insect vectors, will be dealt with in this and the following two chapters. Bancroftian and brugian lymphatic filariasis will be dealt with in this chapter, onchocerciasis in the next, and other helminths transmitted by insects in Chapter 32.

Bancroftian and Brugian Filariasis

The World Health Organization estimated that in 1974 there were more than 250,000,000 cases of bancroftian or brugian filariasis.[9] Infections with *Wuchereria bancrofti* and *Brugia malayi* produce a chronic debilitating condition, which may culminate in disfiguring elephantiasis, in which areas of the body are excessively swollen. The disease is becoming more prevalent but less severe, with the grosser manifestations becoming more rare.[21] Filariasis has been controlled in many countries, including China, Japan, Sri Lanka, west Malaysia and many Pacific islands, yet in some other areas 40 per cent of the male population may suffer from hydrocoele, and 1-2 per cent of the adult population from elephantiasis.[21,38] The greatest concentration of lymphatic filariasis is in India and Africa where the disease is spreading in urban areas as a result of increased populations of the vector, *Cx quinquefasciatus* (= *Cx pipiens fatigans*).[21]

Nature of the Disease

The adult worms live in the lymphatic system and obstruct the flow of lymph, causing local inflammation of the lymphatic vessels (lymphangitis), swelling of the lymphatic glands (lymphadenitis), and oedema of the affected area, frequently the legs.[18] Chronic obstruction of the lymphatic system leads to permanent oedema and the development of fibrous tissue resulting in permanent elephantiasis. Elephantiasis particularly affects the legs either below the knees or the whole limb, the arms, breasts, labia and scrotum. In males hydrocoele is a common complication but both it and lymph scrotum are amenable to surgical treatment.[18] Obstructed abdominal lymphatic vessels may rupture leading to the excretion of lymph in the urine, a condition known as chyluria.[18]

Discovery of Transmission of W. bancrofti

The discovery of the insect vector of *W. bancrofti* is of particular significance to medical entomologists because it is considered to be the birth of medical entomology, and the centenary of this event was celebrated by a symposium in London in 1977.[27] It was the first time that an insect had been incriminated as the vector of an agent of any human or animal disease. Microfilariae of the parasite were found by Wucherer in the urine of a patient suffering from chyluria in Bahia, Brazil, in 1866. (Nelson[22] states that they were seen earlier in 1863 by Demarquay.) Interest in filariasis was worldwide. Microfilariae were seen in the blood of patients in India by Lewis in 1872 and by Manson and Bancroft in China and Australia, respectively, in 1876. In the same year Bancroft found the adult worms and sent them to Cobbold in England, who named the worm after Bancroft as *Filaria bancrofti* in 1877.[27]

The existence of microfilariae in the blood suggested the possibility that a blood-sucking insect might be involved in transmission. In 1877, at Amoy in China, Manson was able to follow the development stage of the microfilariae in *Cx quinquefasciatus* to the infective third stage. At the time it was thought that mosquitoes only fed once and therefore Manson considered that transmission occurred through drinking water infected with worms which had escaped from mosquitoes, trapped in the surface film.

This view persisted until Bancroft in 1899 showed that transmission occurred during the feeding of an infective mosquito.[27]

Geographical Distribution of Parasites

W. bancrofti is widespread throughout the tropics and subtropics while *B. malayi* has a more limited distribution, occurring in the Oriental region, particularly south-east Asia.[9] Populations of both species show variations in the abundance of microfilariae in the circulating blood at different times of the day. These variations are adaptations to the feeding habits of the local vector. Manson recognised a marked nocturnal periodicity in China in 1877,[27] and Thorpe in 1896 found that microfilariae were more abundant in the circulating blood during the day than at night in Fiji and Tonga.[21] These two populations are now referred to as the nocturnal periodic and the diurnal subperiodic forms of *W. bancrofti*, and geographically they are separated in the Pacific islands at the 170° east longitude. Malaria and periodic filariasis occur to the west of this line of demarcation and islands to the east have the diurnal subperiodic form of *W. bancrofti* and no malaria.[21] Nocturnal periodic and nocturnal subperiodic forms of *B. malayi* occur.[25] Recently a second species of *Brugia* infecting man, *B. timori*, has been described from Timor and nearby islands.[23]

Life Cycle of Parasite

The female worm is viviparous, liberating embryos into the lymphatic system in large numbers. The embryos or microfilariae are enclosed in a membrane and are said to be sheathed. They ultimately escape from the lymphatics and appear in the peripheral blood.[18] The microfilariae of *W. bancrofti* are long and slender, measuring 260 μm and those of *B. malayi* are somewhat shorter measuring 210 × 6 μm.[9,25] The microfilariae are taken up with the blood ingested by the vector. In the midgut they shed their sheaths and penetrate the midgut epithelium to reach the haemocoele through which they migrate to the thoracic flight muscles. Here the microfilariae develop into thicker, shorter 'sausage' forms, which undergo two moults before developing into elongate, snake-like mature infective larvae measuring about 1.5 × 0.02 mm. Mature third-stage larvae leave the thoracic musculature and enter the haemocoele in which they move around actively and accumulate in the head.[33] They escape when the mosquito is feeding, by entering the labium and rupturing the labella. They are deposited in a drop of haemolymph, and enter the host through the puncture made by the feeding mosquito.[20,25]

The number of adult worms in a host cannot exceed the number of infective larvae introduced. A year after a leaf monkey (*Presbytis melalophos*) had been subcutaneously inoculated with 471 infective larvae of *W. bancrofti*, it died, and 77 adult worms were recovered.[28] The sexes are separate and the female has to pair before producing microfilariae. In the experimentally infected leaf monkey microfilariae first appeared 287 days after inoculation.[28] In man development of the worm is considered to take three to six months or a year or longer before becoming mature.[18,25]

The development of disease is a slow process with the later stages being associated with youth or early adult life.[18] Microfilariae of *W. bancrofti* are seldom found in children less than three years of age, but in areas where there is a high level of transmission of *B. malayi* microfilariae can be found in the blood at an earlier age. In East Pahang, Malaysia, microfilariae were present in 8 per cent of children under one year, and in 60 per cent of children aged five to nine years.[10]

The adult worms are long and slender with male and female *W. bancrofti* measuring 40 × 0.1 mm and 90 × 0.7 mm, respectively, and being about twice the size of adult *B. malayi*.[9,25] It is not known how long adult worms live, but Webber[31] produced evidence that the reproductive expectancy of *W. bancrofti* in the Solomon Islands was about eight years.

Forms of W. bancrofti and B. malayi

Quite early in the history of filariasis the term 'periodic' was coined for forms of *W. bancrofti* which were abundant in the peripheral blood at night and virtually absent by day, and 'subperiodic' for forms in which the contrast between densities by day and by night were less strongly marked. This distinction reflects the adaptation of the parasite to its mosquito vector and it should be expected that in different ecosystems populations of parasites will have arisen which are adapted to the biting habits of the local vector. Hawking[14] points out the need to indicate at what time in the 24 h cycle the peak is reached, diurnal or nocturnal, and to give quantitative expression to the fluctuations throughout the 24 h period. For the latter he uses a periodicity index which is the standard deviation expressed as a percentage of the mean, and therefore the same as the statistical coefficient of variation. Hawking[14] recognises four forms of *W. bancrofti* (Table 30.1). In addition there are differences in vector susceptibility to urban and rural forms of nocturnal periodic *W. bancrofti*.[35]

During the time when microfilariae are absent from the peripheral blood they accumulate in the lungs in the terminal arterioles before the

Table 30.1: Forms of *W. bancrofti*

Form of *W. bancrofti*	Peak time	Periodicity index %
Nocturnal periodic	23.00–03.00	90–110
Nocturnal subperiodic	22.00–24.00	20–30
West Thailand form	21.00	50
Diurnal subperiodic	14.00–17.00	20–25

capillaries.[14] In the nocturnal periodic *W. bancrofti* and *B. malayi* this accumulation is in response to a greater difference in oxygen tension between the alveolar and arterial blood by day than by night (55 mm Hg cf. 45 mm).[14] There is no simple explanation for the accumulation of microfilariae of the diurnal subperiodic form in the lungs at night.

The nocturnal periodic *B. malayi* has a similar periodicity to the comparable form of *W. bancrofti* with a peak at 23.00-03.00 h and a periodicity index of 90-110 per cent, and it is controlled by the difference in oxygen tension.[14] There are two other forms of *B. malayi*, a nocturnal subperiodic form associated with dense swamp forest in south-east Asia and a more localised, sympatric, diurnally subperiodic form in west Malaysia.[9,14] The latter has a periodicity similar to that of the diurnal subperiodic *W. bancrofti*.[14]

Microfilariae of nocturnal subperiodic *B. malayi* show a peak in the peripheral blood in the early evening,[18] and a periodicity index of 30 per cent.[25] This form of *B. malayi* is common in wild monkeys and domestic and wild carnivores (dogs and cats). The closely related *B. pahangi* is sympatric with nocturnal subperiodic *B. malayi* and occurs in a similar range of hosts but rarely, if ever, occurs in man; and the two have been shown by hybridisation to be good species.[9,36]

Some Factors Affecting Infectivity of Mosquito

Nelson[21] states that a temperature of 25-30°C and a relative humidity greater than 70 per cent are required for development of the worm in the mosquito, and that no development occurs if the relative humidity is below 50 per cent. The number of microfilariae taken up by feeding mosquitoes is greater than would be expected from the size of the blood meal. For example, although *Ma dives* takes up the number of microfilariae found in 5 mm^3 of blood, it ingests only 3 mm^3 of blood.[33] An even greater discrepancy is found with *Cx quinquefasciatus* which ingests 4 mm^3 of blood and the number of microfilariae found in three times that volume.[35] Both mosquitoes excrete a clear fluid either while feeding or shortly afterwards, so that the blood volume could be underestimated, but it is possible that microfilariae respond to the feeding mosquito, e.g. its saliva, and accumulate at the site of feeding. This would be more likely with pool feeding rather than capillary feeding.

Wharton[33] found that microfilariae of *B. malayi* reached the thorax of *Ma dives* in 12 hours, and that half of these were mature after 11 days. The number of larvae matured was directly related to the density of microfilariae in the blood of the host, and to the numbers taken up. However, when large numbers of microfilariae were ingested (50 or more) there was a high mortality among the infected mosquitoes after seven days. When the density of microfilariae in the blood exceeded two per mm^3 there was 100 per cent infection in *Ma dives*.[34] Wharton[33] proposed an index of experimental infection based on survival of the mosquitoes, proportion infected, density of the infection which was equivalent to:

$$\frac{\text{Total no. of mature larvae}}{\text{No. of mosquitoes fed}}$$

When this expression was applied to *B. malayi* and *Ma dives* the index increased to a peak between three to eleven microfilariae per mm³, and then decreased due to the lethal effects of developing larvae.[34]

Bryan and Southgate[5] reported that *Ae polynesiensis* ingested more microfilariae of diurnal subperiodic *W. bancrofti* than expected from their concentration in the circulating blood. They found no effect of parasite load on mosquito survival but they were working with very low infections (less than 0.01 microfilariae/mm³). Rosen,[24] working with much heavier human infections (8-10 microfilariae/mm³), found that the longevity of *Ae polynesiensis* was adversely affected by large numbers of maturing larvae. Such deaths occurred at the time of parasite maturation, i.e. 13 days after an infective feed.

Fate of Deposited Infective Larvae. Infective larvae of the related filarioid worm *Dirofilaria immitis* escape from the tip of the labella of *Ae aegypti* in a drop of haemolymph which, under laboratory conditions, evaporated in 4 min.[20] Larvae that fail to enter via the mosquito's puncture in that time will perish on the surface of the skin. This finding is in accord with observations on the fate of larvae of *B. pahangi* deposited from *Ae togoi*, of which 62-90 per cent die on the skin surface.[11,15] Conflicting results have been obtained with larvae of *B. pahangi* deposited from *Ae aegypti* on to cats in which it was found that 90 per cent of the deposited larvae penetrated and that penetration was independent of humidity (20 per cent or 80 per cent RH). The only difference was that at the lower humidity fewer larvae escaped on to the skin.[9]

Larvae escape rapidly from the labium, the main stimulus being the bending of the labium.[20] The nature of the host on which the mosquito is feeding also plays a role. When *Ae togoi* probed a cat, 57 per cent of the infective larvae of *B. pahangi* escaped in the first five seconds; at the end of a minute this value had risen to 77 per cent; and to 91 per cent on engorgement. The corresponding figures when infected *Ae togoi* fed on a mouse were 28 per cent in five seconds, 44 per cent in one minute, and 74 per cent at engorgement.[16]

Cibarial and Pharyngeal Armatures. Wharton[34] found that there was no appreciable loss of larvae of *B. malayi* in *Ma dives* (= *Ma longipalpis*), and Bryan and Southgate[5] that *Ae polynesiensis* was easily infected with *W. bancrofti* even when its microfilariae were present in low density. The ease of development of microfilariae is in part due to the absence of cibarial armature in these mosquitoes. Denham and McGreevy[9] state that none of the vectors of *B. malayi* has cibarial armature, and the effect of their pharyngeal armatures is unknown.

In some *Anopheles* vectors of *W. bancrofti*, e.g. *An gambiae* s.s., *An arabiensis* (= *An gambiae* B) and *An farauti* No 1, the cibarial armature is well developed and damages microfilariae during feeding.[19] *An gambiae* s.s. damaged 49 per cent of ingested microfilariae of *W. bancrofti*, rendered 36 per cent amotile, and inflicted even greater damage on *B. pahangi*, of which 96 per cent were damaged, and 61 per cent rendered amotile.[19]

Cibarial armatures were absent in four species of *Anopheles* (*Anopheles*) and five species of *Aedes*, including *Ae polynesiensis*, *Ae togoi* and *Ae aegypti*, and only weakly developed in *Cx quinquefasciatus*.[19] *Cx quinquefasciatus* damaged and rendered amotile only 6 per cent of ingested microfilariae of *W. bancrofti*, while the corresponding results for ingested microfilariae of *B. pahangi* were 9 per cent damaged and 6 per cent amotile in *Ae aegypti* and 22 per cent and 11 per cent, respectively, in *Ae togoi*.[19] Clearly an efficient cibarial armature can play a substantial role in reducing infections in the mosquito host.

Facilitation and Limitation. When Brengues and Bain[4] fed *An gambiae* s.s. on a heavily infected (1.25 microfilariae/mm^3) volunteer, 97 per cent of them ingested microfilariae. The average number ingested was 26.5, but the distribution was not normal. More than half the females ingested less than 20 microfilariae, and a small number (2 per cent) ingested more than 100. Passage of microfilariae through the midgut epithelium was rapid with more than 60 per cent of the mosquitoes having microfilariae in the haemocoele two hours after engorging, but the numbers of microfilariae entering the haemocoele became proportionately larger the greater the number of microfilariae ingested. Thus where one to ten microfilariae were ingested only 20 per cent had entered the haemocoele 12-18 h after engorging compared with 52 per cent when more than 50 microfilariae had been ingested. This increasing proportion with numbers ingested has been called facilitation.[4]

When *Ae aegypti* was fed on the same carrier of *W. bancrofti* it ingested, on the average, rather more microfilariae (36.8) but the opposite response occurred. When a few microfilariae were ingested (1-10), 58 per cent successfully penetrated the gut epithelium and were free in the haemolymph; but as the number of microfilariae ingested increased, the percentage reaching the haemocoele decreased; and where more than 70 microfilariae were taken in, only 8 per cent successfully reached the haemocoele. This response was called limitation.[4] A similar limiting response was found when *Ae aegypti* was infected with *Dipetalonema dessetae*, when in light infestations six out of 14 microfilariae reached the haemocoele in six hours, and in heavy infestations none out of 20 had reached the haemocoele in seven hours.[2]

Limitation and facilitation are features of the host rather than the parasite. Brengues and Bain[4] and Bain and Chabaud[2] associate the different responses with changes in the midgut epithelium. Microfilariae escape from the midgut of *An gambiae* s.s. by penetrating the columnar cells at the anterior and posterior ends of the midgut. Following penetration of the first microfilariae the neighbouring cells enlarge and protrude into the midgut, facilitating subsequent penetration by other microfilariae.[2] The reaction of the midgut cells of *Ae aegypti* is quite different and they undergo severe lysis, which impedes passage of microfilariae.[2]

Other Factors. Escape of microfilariae from the blood meal into the haemocoele of the mosquito is likely to be affected by the formation of the peritrophic membrane, and by the speed with which the blood clots. Blood rapidly coagulates in the midgut of *Ae aegypti*, and only 30 per cent of ingested *Dirofilaria immitis* microfilariae reached the haemocoele, but this proportion increased to 80 per cent when an anticoagulant was added to the ingested blood.[9] Most microfilariae have escaped from the midgut before formation of the peritrophic membrane, and there is no evidence on whether microfilariae can penetrate the membrane, once it has been formed.[9]

Conclusions. Denham and McGreevy[9] concluded that 'facilitation and limitation in the various filaria-vector combinations is the summation of microfilarial interactions with the pharyngeal and cibarial armatures, the blood clot, digestive enzymes, putative antifilarial toxins, peritrophic membrane and the gut epithelium.'

Genetics of Susceptibility of Mosquitoes to Infection

Although *Ae aegypti* is not a vector of filariasis in the field it is a convenient species to work with in the laboratory. Susceptibility of this species to *B. malayi* was increased from 17 to 90 per cent in one generation, and subsequently retained for 15 generations. Susceptibility to *B. malayi*, *B. pahangi* and *W. bancrofti* is controlled by a sex-linked, recessive gene designated f^m.[17,30] This gene has no effect on susceptibility to *Dirofilaria immitis* and *D. repens*, which is controlled by another sex-linked, recessive gene, f^t. It is considered that these genes act through the tissues in which the worms develop. Development of *Dirofilaria* takes place in the malpighian tubes and of *Brugia* and *W. bancrofti* in the thoracic musculature.[17,30]

Even in a susceptible strain of *Ae aegypti*, 75-80 per cent of *B. malayi* die in the course of development with the peak number of deaths occurring two to three days after the infecting meal, and this agrees with observations on *B. pahangi.* In the same strain of *Ae aegypti, B. pahangi* suffers 25 per cent mortality in the course of development in the thoracic muscles. This probably occurs early in development because third-stage larvae intro- duced into the thorax survive equally well in susceptible and refractory hosts.[3,30]

Ae polynesiensis and *Ae pseudoscutellaris* are both vectors of diurnal subperiodic *W. bancrofti* and they are also susceptible to infection with urban nocturnal periodic *W. bancrofti* and *B.pahangi.*[17] *Ae malayensis* is not considered to be a vector of subperiodic *W. bancrofti* in the field and in the laboratory is refractory to both urban periodic *W. bancrofti* and *B. pahangi.*[17] Cross-mating of *Ae polynesiensis* and *Ae malayensis* and testing the progeny for susceptibility to *B. pahangi,* shows that susceptibility is a recessive character because the hybrids are refractory.[17]

All populations of *Cx quinquefasciatus* tested were very susceptible to urban periodic *W. bancrofti* but had only a low susceptibility to rural periodic *W. bancrofti* (5 per cent infective cf. 87 per cent);[35] and were refractory or with low susceptibility to *B. pahangi.*[17] Susceptibility to *B. pahangi* is a sex-liked recessive gene, which has no effect on susceptibility to *W. bancrofti.*[17]

Mosquito Vectors of Bancroftian and Brugian Filariasis

The most widespread cause of lymphatic filariasis is the nocturnal periodic form of *W. bancrofti* which is widely distributed throughout the tropical and subtropical regions of the world. In urban areas the main vector is *Cx quinquefasciatus,* a highly anthropophilic species which feeds readily both indoors and out of doors and has its peak biting period between midnight and 03.00 h, coinciding with the peak microfilarial abundance in the peripheral blood.[6] In rural areas the vectors are species of *Anopheles* of which Nelson[21] lists 26 species. Eighteen species are vectors of *W. ban- crofti,* three of *B. malayi,* and five species transmit both parasites. Many of these species are also vectors of malaria, and 11 are included in Werns- dorfer's[32] list of vectors of malaria. Four species (*An gambiae* s.s., *An funestus, An melas* and *An minimus*) are associated with stable malaria in tropical Africa and the Oriental region, three with intermediate malaria and four with unstable malaria.

The main vector of diurnal subperiodic *W. bancrofti* of the eastern zone of the South Pacific is the day-biting, exophilic *Ae polynesiensis* which breeds in a wide range of small water containers, including coconut shells, tins, tyres, drums, tree holes, crab holes, canoes and the axils of *Pandanus.*[6] *Ae polynesiensis* has a minor peak of feeding at 08.00 h and a major one just before sunset at 17.00-18.00 h, which more or less corresponds with the time of microfilarial maximum abundance at 16.00 h.[6,14]

Chow[6] lists 13 species of *Aedes* as vectors of diurnal subperiodic *W. bancrofti,* of which six are important vectors and include *Ae vigilax,* an exophilic, day-biting species which breeds mainly in brackish water, but also occurs in freshwater pools in New Caledonia where it is the main vector. In west Thailand the vector of nocturnal subperiodic *W. bancrofti* is *Ae niveus*.[25] In the Philippines an important vector of nocturnal periodic *W. bancrofti* is *Ae poecilus* which breeds in the axils of the Abaca (*Musa textilis*) and banana. It is an exophilic species which bites man indoors, mostly before midnight.[6]

The vector of nocturnal periodic *W. bancrofti* in a focus on the Pahang River in Malaysia was *An whartoni* (= *An letifer* auct.), which had a low infection in the wild, but when fed on a carrier nearly 40 per cent became infective while *Cx quinquefasciatus* was a comparatively poor vector with only 5 per cent becoming infective.[35] *An whartoni* is exophilic, exophagic, and active all night with maximum activity in the two hours after sunset.[35] This species breeds in shaded swamp forest, open grass swamp and clear seepage pools.[35]

Nearer the coast of west Malaysia the main vectors of nocturnal sub-periodic *B. malayi* are four species of *Mansonia* (*Mansonioides*), including *Ma dives*, *Ma bonneae* and *Ma uniformis*.[36] The first two species breed in dense swamp forest where the larvae attach to the pneumatophores of trees. The adults are exophilic and exophagic and largely zoophilic. At ground level in swamp forest biting occurred all day and night with a peak after sunset. In more open areas around houses there was a sharp peak in biting after sunset, and within houses the peak of biting occurred after midnight. These species act as vectors because of their large numbers and the catholicity of their responses. Although they are largely zoophilic and exophagic, they will enter houses and feed on man, when available. Around houses 10 per cent of *Ma dives* and *Ma bonneae* were found to have fed on man.[36] They fed preferentially on the lower limbs and conse-quently elephantiasis was almost confined to them.[29,36]

On the coastal rice-plains in west Malaysia nocturnal periodic *B. malayi* is largely transmitted by three species of *Anopheles*, including *An campestris* and other members of the *An barbirostris* group. These species are poor hosts for nocturnal subperiodic *B. malayi*. The reverse response is shown by the *Mansonia* vectors of nocturnal subperiodic *B. malayi* in which no larvae of the periodic form develop in *Ma bonneae* and few in *Ma dives*.[36] *An campestris* is an anthropophilic, endophilic and endophagic species which breeds in ditches, wells and 'burrow-pits' under semi-shade.[6]

Ae togoi is a vector of nocturnally periodic *B. malayi* in China, Japan and South Korea where it breeds in brackish water in rock holes and also rain-filled artificial containers. The adults are endophilic with the peak biting rate occurring after sunset.[6,25] *Ae togoi* is readily colonised in the laboratory and has proved to be an excellent experimental intermediate host of many filarial species.[25]

Epidemiology

W. bancrofti is a parasite of man and bancroftian filariasis is spread by the vector from man to man.[25] *B. malayi* is found in man and domestic and wild animals but the periodic form is seldom found in animals in nature and is generally considered not to be a zoonosis. The nocturnal subperiodic form is common in wild monkeys and is limited to foci in swamp forests in south-east Asia where man and his domestic animals are surrounded by virgin forest with wild animals and mosquitoes.[9] The relative importance of domestic and wild animals is not known but it is likely that transmission to man would occur with greater frequency from domestic animals.[9] Wharton[36] summarised the situation with the subperiodic form as being the result of 'the catholic feeding habits of *Mansonia* combined with their occurrence in large numbers in houses, kampong (village) and forest, and their ability to transmit both *B. malayi* and *B. pahangi*, are sufficient explanation for the high infection rates in man, particularly in children, and the maintenance of the animal reservoir of *B. malayi* and *B. pahangi*, which extends through a bewildering array of domestic and wild animals.' Wharton also states that '*B. pahangi* is rarely if ever found in man'.

Transmission requires the presence of microfilariae for the vector to take up when it feeds. In *W. bancrofti* and periodic *B. malayi* the proportion of the population with microfilariae increases with age whereas with subperiodic *B. malayi* the highest infection rates are found in children below the age of five years and there is a decrease in infection with age.[37] Abundant microfilariae are produced during the inflammatory and early obstructive stage while in advanced cases of elephantiasis microfilariae are rarely present and the patients are non-infective.[9,18] Nevertheless, infected individuals remain infective for a long time, the reproductive life of *W. bancrofti* being about eight years.[31] In addition some mosquitoes, e.g. *Ae polynesiensis*, can acquire infections when the density of microfilariae in the host is very low.[5]

Limiting Factors involving the Vector. When microfilariae are ingested by a susceptible host they undergo a cycle of development which is temperature-dependent and in western Samoa infective larvae of *W. bancrofti* were present in the proboscis of *Ae polynesiensis* in 12 days.[5] A short time of nine days was reported for *B. malayi* in a susceptible strain of *Ae aegypti*,[3] and Sasa (p. 77)[25] cites the results of Feng (1936) who found that *B. malayi* completed its development in *An sinensis* in 6-6½ days at 29-32°C. To become infective the mosquito must survive long enough for the worm to complete its development. Daily survival rates of 0.80-0.85 have been obtained in Malaysia for *Ma dives* and *Ma bonneae*,[36] and a survival rate of 0.80 per day for *Cx quinquefasciatus* throughout the year in

Rangoon.[7] A survival rate of 0.80 gives 26 per cent survival after six days and 7 per cent after 12 days.

De Meillon *et al.*[7] found that the infection rate of *Cx quinquefasciatus* with *W. bancrofti* in Rangoon was more or less constant throughout the year with 4.8 per cent of the mosquito population infected and 0.36 per cent infective. In west Malaysia infection rates of *B. malayi/ B. pahangi* in *Ma dives* and *Ma bonneae* around houses were 1.1-1.4 per cent infected and 0.5-0.6 infective. Two miles away in swamp forest the rates were somewhat lower, 0.7 per cent infected and 0.4 per cent infective. Unlike malaria where an infected *Anopheles* mosquito remains infective for the rest of her life, filarial infections are limited and can be exhausted. Infected *Ma dives* and *Ma bonneae* contained an average of five mature larvae and a similar number of immature larvae, but the distribution was skewed with 60 per cent of the infective mosquitoes containing one to four larvae and a similar distribution occurred with the immature stages.[36]

Transmission Rate. The transmission rate depends not only on the proportion of the vectors that are infective but also on vector density. In Rangoon the infection rate of *Cx quinquefasciatus* with *W. bancrofti* remained unchanged throughout the year, but the risk of infection was markedly seasonal, being lowest in the monsoon season when the breeding sites of *Cx quinquefasciatus* were flushed away and highest at the end of the dry season.[7] In addition the risk of infection was greater late in the evening, towards midnight, than in the period following sunset and also greater outdoors than indoors.[7] In the west Malaysian *Brugia/Mansonia* system the intensity of transmission was highest in the swamp forest on account of the larger number of vectors, lower around houses and lowest at night within houses where the rate was 31 infective bites per annum.[36]

Three comparable investigations of the transmission of nocturnal periodic *W. bancrofti* by *Cx quinquefasciatus* have been carried out in Rangoon,[13] Calcutta[12] and Jakarta.[26] The findings with regard to the mosquito populations and their infectivity are summarised in Table 30.2. The average annual biting rate per person was of the order of 100,000, of which 0.3 to 1.6 per cent of the mosquitoes were infective, carrying 3.0 to 4.5. infective larvae per infective mosquito. De Meillon *et al.*[8] calculated that during blood-feeding 41.4 per cent of the infective larvae were deposited on the skin. Using this correction the average number of infective larvae deposited on a person each year in the three cities ranged from 560 in Rangoon to nearly 2,500 indoors in Calcutta.

Bryan and Southgate[5] calculated the input of infective larvae into a population from the expression:

$$y = M \, map^n ib$$

Table 30.2: Selective Data on the Transmission of Nocturnal Periodic *W. bancrofti* by *Cx quinquefasciatus* in Rangoon, Calcutta and Jakarta. Figures, where not otherwise defined, indicate rate per person, per annum

	Rangoon Hairston & De Meillon[13]	Calcutta Gubler & Bhattacharya[12]		Jakarta Self et al.[26]
		Indoors	Outdoors	
(a) annual biting rate	83,000	115,000	117,000	223,000
(b) number of infective bites (% mosquitoes infective)	298 (0.36)	1,850 (1.61)	1,352 (1.16)	647 (0.29)
(c) number of infective larvae (mean/infective mosquito)	1,353 (4.5)	5,904 (3.2)	4,056 (3.0)	1,941 (3.0)
(d) number of infective larvae deposited during feeding = 0.414 × line c	560	2,444	1,679	804

Source for correction factor in (d): From De Meillon et al.[8]

where *m*, *a*, *p*, *n* refer to mean density of vector in relation to man, average number of humans bitten by vector in one day, daily survival rate and duration of the extrinsic cycle, respectively, as in similar expressions concerned with the transmission of malaria. The new factors are: *M*, the number of carriers in the population; *i*, the proportion of vectors infective; and *b* the number of infective larvae per infected mosquito. Applying this to *W. bancrofti* and *Ae polynesiensis*, the human population was being exposed to an annual injection of 1.37 million larvae per annum. The above expression is a contribution towards the mathematical model, which Nelson[22] considers to have priority in future research.

Comparison with Malaria. Unlike malaria, where a single inoculation of sporozoites will produce clinical malaria, filariasis requires repeated infection.[18] Webber[31] made a comparison between the transmission of *Plasmodium falciparum* and *W. bancrofti* by *An farauti* in the Solomon Islands and found that the critical density of mosquitoes to maintain transmission was of the order of ten times greater for filariasis than for malaria. In other words malaria transmission would continue after transmission of filariasis had ceased, but this comparison is dependent upon accurate knowledge of the recovery rates from malaria and filariasis, and the number of bites required to produce a case of malaria or filariasis. In Rangoon it was calculated that 15,500 infective bites were needed to produce microfilaraemia, and at a rate of 300 infective bites per annum, on average 50 years would be required to achieve that level.[13]

Principles of Control

The worms are long lived and produce microfilariae over a period of years, even up to ten years,[31] so that control measures against filariasis must be maintained at an appropriate level over many years. Measures can be directed against the parasite or against the vector or to minimising the man-vector contact. Chemotherapy, using diethylcarbamazine (DEC) has been successful in west Malaysia,[38] Japan, and some Pacific islands, and is the approach favoured by Sasa,[25] but mass treatment has not been successful in India.[21] DEC acts against microfilariae and, except in very large dosages, has little action on the adult worm, and repeated therapy is required at intervals of about a year.[18] A control programme should preferably include several different lines of attack with effort being concentrated on the approach which offers the maximum benefit for effort in the particular situation.

Prospects for successful control are highest against nocturnal periodic filariasis transmitted by endophilic vectors, such as *Cx quinquefasciatus* and *Anopheles* spp, against which residual insecticides and personal protection will be most effective. The use of mosquito nets and rendering houses, especially bedrooms, mosquito-proof can produce significant reduction in biting intensity.[9] In addition, raising living standards, in particular by the introduction of piped water supply with accompanying drainage and sewerage, removes breeding sites of *Cx quinquefasciatus*, and has given control of filariasis in the southern USA, Puerto Rico and the Mediterranean.[21] Development of insecticide resistance in vectors of filariasis has complicated chemical control of the vector, and here possible elimination of breeding sites is preferable.[22]

When the vector is exophilic and diurnal, control is more difficult. Mosquito-proofing of houses offers little protection, neither do mosquito nets. This is the situation with the *Ae scutellaris* group which are vectors of the diurnal subperiodic *W. bancrofti* in the Pacific. They breed in a wide range of small containers, which are too numerous to locate and deal with individually so that larval control is not practical.[17] In that situation mass chemotherapy offers the best prospect of control.

Control of subperiodic *B. malayi* transmitted by *Mansonia* species is a formidable task. Although residual insecticides had little effect on the overall vector population, house-spraying with dieldrin halved the transmission rate.[36] Wilson[38] has shown that supervised administration of DEC to a high proportion of the human population can bring about a long-lasting reduction in infection rates of both periodic and subperiodic *B. malayi*. Another possible approach to the control of subperiodic *B. malayi* involves eliminating the reservoir in domestic animals. This might make a significant contribution to the reduction of human filariasis.[9]

References

1. Anderson, R.C., Chabaud, A.G. and Willmott, S. (eds.) (1974) *CIH Keys to the Nematode Parasites of Vertebrates*, Commonwealth Agricultural Bureaux, Slough
2. Bain, O. and Chabaud, A.G. (1975). Le mécanisme assurant la régulation de la traversée de la paroi stomacale du vecteur par les microfilaires (*Dipetalonema dessetae — Aedes aegypti*). *Comptes Rendus Hebdomadaire des Séances de l'Académie Scientifique, Paris, Série D 281:* 1199-202
3. Beckett, E.W. and Macdonald, W.W. (1971). The survival and development of subperiodic *Brugia malayi* and *B. pahangi* larvae in a selected strain of *Aedes aegypti*. *Transactions of the Royal Society of Tropical Medicine and Hygiene 65:* 339-46
4. Brengues, J. and Bain, O. (1972). Passage des microfilaires de l'estomac vers l'hémocèle du vecteur, dans les couples *Wuchereria bancrofti-Anopheles gambiae A, W. bancrofti-Aedes aegypti* et *Setaria labiatopapillosa-Aedes aegypti. Cahiers ORSTOM, Entomologie Médicale et Parasitologie 10:* 235-49
5. Bryan, J.H. and Southgate, B.A. (1976). Some observations on filariasis in Western Samoa after mass administration of diethylcarbamazine. *Transactions of the Royal Society of Tropical Medicine and Hygiene 70:* 39-48
6. Chow, C.Y. (1973). Filariasis vectors in the Western Pacific Region. *Zeitschrift für Tropenmedizin und Parasitologie 24:* 404-18
7. De Meillon, B., Grab, B. and Sebastian, A. (1967). Evaluation of *Wuchereria bancrofti* infection in *Culex pipiens fatigans* in Rangoon, Burma. *Bulletin of the World Health Organization 36:* 91-100
8. _____ Hayashi, S. and Sebastian, A. (1967). Infection and reinfection of *Culex pipiens*

fatigans with *Wuchereria bancrofti* and the loss of mature larvae in blood-feeding. *Bulletin of the World Health Organization 36*: 81-90

9. Denham, D.A. and McGreevy, P.B. (1977). Brugian filariasis: epidemiological and experimental studies. *Advances in Parasitology 15*: 243-309
10. Edeson, J.F.B. and Wilson, T. (1964). The epidemiology of filariasis due to *Wuchereria bancrofti* and *Brugia malayi. Annual Review of Entomology 9*: 245-68
11. Ewert, A. and Ho, B.C. (1967). The fate of *Brugia pahangi* larvae immediately after feeding by infective vector mosquitoes. *Transactions of the Royal Society of Tropical Medicine and Hygiene 61*: 659-62
12. Gubler, D.J. and Bhattacharya, N.C. (1974). A quantitative approach to the study of bancroftian filariasis. *American Journal of Tropical Medicine and Hygiene 23*: 1027-36
13. Hairston, N.G. and De Meillon, B. (1968). On the inefficiency of transmission of *Wuchereria bancrofti* from mosquito to human host. *Bulletin of the World Health Organization 38*: 935-41
14. Hawking, F. (1975). Circadian and other rhythms of parasites. *Advances in Parasitology 13*: 123-82
15. Ho, B.C. and Ewert, A. (1967). Experimental transmission of filarial larvae in relation to feeding behaviour of the mosquito vectors. *Transactions of the Royal Society of Tropical Medicine and Hygiene 61*: 663-6
16. _____ and Lavoipierre, M.M.J. (1975). Studies on filariasis. IV. The rate of escape of the third-stage larvae of *Brugia pahangi* from the mouthparts of *Aedes togoi* during the blood meal. *Journal of Helminthology 49*: 65-72
17. Macdonald, W.W. (1976). Mosquito genetics in relation to filarial infections. *Symposia of the British Society of Parasitology 14*: 1-24
18. Maegraith, B. (1980). *Adams and Maegraith: Clinical Tropical Diseases.* Blackwell Scientific Publications, Oxford
19. McGreevy, P.B., Bryan, J.H., Oothuman, P. and Kolstrup, N. (1978). The lethal effects of cibarial and pharyngeal armatures of mosquitoes on microfilariae. *Transactions of the Royal Society of Tropical Medicine and Hygiene 72*: 361-8
20. _____ Theis, J.H., Lavoipierre, M.M.J. and Clark, J. (1974). Studies on filariasis. III. *Dirofilaria immitis*: emergence of infective larvae from the mouthparts of *Aedes aegypti. Journal of Helminthology 48*: 221-8
21. Nelson, G.S. (1978). Mosquito-borne filariasis. pp. 15-25 in *Medical Entomology Centenary Symposium Proceedings*, S.Willmott (ed.), Royal Society of Tropical Medicine and Hygiene, London
22. _____ (1981). Issues in filariasis — a century of enquiry and a century of failure. *Acta Tropica 38*: 197-204
23. Partono, F., Purnomo, Dennis, D.T., Atmosoedjono, S., Oemijati, S. and Cross, J.H. (1977). *Brugia timori* sp.n. (Nematoda: Filariodea) from Flores Island, Indonesia. *Journal of Parasitology 63*: 540-6
24. Rosen, L. (1955). Observations on the epidemiology of human filariasis in French Oceania. *American Journal of Hygiene 61*: 219-48
25. Sasa, M. (1976). *Human Filariasis.* University of Tokyo Press, Tokyo
26. Self, L.S., Usman, S., Sajidiman, H., Partono, F., Nelson, M.J. Pant, C.P., Suzuki, T. and Mechfudin, H. (1978). A multidisciplinary study on bancroftian filariasis in Jakarta. *Transactions of the Royal Society of Tropical Medicine and Hygiene 72*: 581-7
27. Service, M.W. (1978). Patrick Manson and the story of bancroftian filariasis. pp. 11-14 in *Medical Entomology Centenary Symposium Proceedings*, S. Willmott (ed.), Royal Society of Tropical Medicine and Hygiene, London
28. Sucharit, S., Harinasuta, C. and Choochote, W. (1982). Experimental transmission of subperiodic *Wuchereria bancrofti* to the leaf monkey (*Presbytis melalophos*), and its periodicity. *American Journal of Tropical Medicine and Hygiene 31*: 599-601
29. Turner, L.H. (1959). Studies on filariasis in Malaya: the clinical features of filariasis due to *Wuchereria malayi. Transactions of the Royal Society of Tropical Medicine and Hygiene 53*: 154-69
30. Wakelin, D. (1978). Genetic control of susceptibility and resistance to parasitic infections. *Advances in Parasitology 16*: 219-308
31. Webber, R.H. (1977). The natural decline of *Wuchereria bancrofti* infection in a vector

control situation in the Solomon Islands. *Transactions of the Royal Society of Tropical Medicine and Hygiene 71*: 396-400

32. Wernsdorfer, W.H. (1980). The importance of malaria in the world. pp. 1-93 in volume I, *Malaria*, J.P. Kreier (ed.), Academic Press, New York

33. Wharton, R.H. (1957). Studies in filariasis in Malaya: observations on the development of *Wuchereria malayi* in *Mansonia (Mansonioides) longipalpis. Annals of Tropical Medicine and Parasitology 51*: 278-96

34. _____ (1957). Studies in filariasis in Malaya: the efficiency of *Mansonia longipalpis* as an experimental vector of *Wuchereria malayi. Annals of Tropical Medicine and Parasitology 51*: 422-39

35. _____ (1960). Studies on filariasis in Malaya: field and laboratory investigations of the vectors of a rural strain of *Wuchereria bancrofti. Annals of Tropical Medicine and Parasitology 54*: 78-91

36. _____ (1962). *The Biology of Mansonia Mosquitoes in Relation to the Transmission of Filariasis in Malaya.* Bulletin No. 11, Institute for Medical Research, Federation of Malaya

37. _____ (1963). Adaptation of *Wuchereria* and *Brugia* to mosquitoes and vertebrate hosts in relation to the distribution of filarial parasites. *Zoonoses Research 2*: 1-12

38. Wilson, T. (1969). An example of filariasis control from west Malaysia. *Bulletin of the World Health Organization 41*: 324-6

31 HUMAN ONCHOCERCIASIS (*ONCHOCERCA VOLVULUS*)

Human onchocerciasis is an economically important disease of man, which is not directly fatal but causes untold misery in certain tropical areas of Africa and Central America. It is caused by infection with *Onchocerca volvulus* and transmitted by blackflies of the genus *Simulium*. It has been estimated that there are 30,000,000 people suffering from onchocerciasis in Africa where it occurs between latitudes 15°S-15°N but causes its most severe effects in the savanna region between 8°-12°N.[21,27] It places an intolerable burden on whole communities, and denies vast fertile areas to human settlement and agricultural development. Thus, although the valleys of the White Volta and Red Volta in Upper Volta have the most fertile and best irrigated soils in the Republic, they are devoid of humans.[21,27]

The disease results in an unsightly and irritating dermatitis, and eye lesions which result in blindness. On the West African savanna 30 per cent of the population are estimated to have impaired vision, and blindness often exceeds 10 per cent of the population.[27] In certain areas of Mexico and Guatemala 20 per cent of infected individuals develop eye lesions, and a proportion of these become totally blind.[23] In Central America onchocerciasis is present in Mexico, Guatemala, Venezuela, Colombia and Brazil.[27,35] Infections with *O. volvulus* are cryptic, and new foci are found by chance, e.g. the one in the Yemen which was not discovered until the mid-1950s, and Nelson[27] considers that onchocerciasis 'should be looked for in all parts of the world where simuliids bite man'.

The long, slender, long-lived adult worms are to be found free in the subcutaneous tissue or in nodules which may be up to 60 mm in diameter.[23] The female worm is considerably longer than the male, measuring 335-500 × 0.27-0.40 mm compared to 18-32 × 0.13-0.21 mm for the male.[35] The adults are of secondary importance and the severe clinical manifestations of the disease are due to the microfilariae, which occur in the skin where their density is greatest in the vicinity of adult worms. The distribution of nodules and microfilariae differs with the strain of parasite, being most abundant on the lower part of the body in West Africa; mainly around the buttocks and upper thigh in East Africa; and on the torso in Central America.[27] This distribution is correlated with, but not necessarily determined by, the biting habits of the vectors, of which *S. ochraceum* in Central America attacks the upper part of the body and *S. damnosum* in West Africa the lower parts of the body.

The presence of large numbers of active microfilariae in the skin causes intense itching and scratching leading to loss of pigment in patches in the

605

affected area. These contrast strikingly with the normal dark skin and are an obvious sign of infection with *O. volvulus*. In the later stages there is thickening of the skin and a loss of elasticity, giving the sufferer a prematurely aged appearance, and in rare cases a condition known as 'hanging groin'.[27]

Onchocerciasis develops slowly, with nodules being rare in children less than three years of age[23] and eye lesions commonest in adult males over 40 years of age. Living microfilariae invade the conjunctiva and cornea of the eye, causing little reaction, but opacities develop around dead microfilariae resulting in loss of vision. Microfilariae invade the anterior chamber of the eye, where dead ones accumulate, and in some cases posterior lesions may occur, leading to optic atrophy and complete loss of vision.[23] According to Maegraith,[23] 'Microfilariae have not been identified in the living retina'. One puzzle is the lower incidence of blindness in the forest zone of West Africa compared to the savanna zone (less than 1 per cent cf. 10 per cent), in spite of the higher transmission rate of *O. volvulus* in the forest.[27]

Onchocerciasis is diagnosed by a skin snip in which a small piece of skin is removed and examined for the presence of living microfilariae. Surgical removal of nodules is traditional treatment in Central America where it is claimed to reduce the number of microfilariae in the skin, but similar results have not been obtained in Africa.[27] Three drugs are available for chemotherapy but none are suitable for mass treatment as diethylcarbamazine (DEC) has to be used at a higher dosage than for mass treatment of bancroftian filariasis.[23] DEC kills microfilariae but not adult worms, and can produce severe reactions; while suramin kills both microfilariae and adults worms, but is much more toxic. Both should be given under close medical supervision. Melarsan W kills adult worms, but has no effect on microfilariae, and can produce serious complications.[27]

Simuliid Vectors of *Onchocerca volvulus*

The vectors of Onchocerciasis will be considered under three headings: the *S. damnosum* group of species, the *S. neavei* group, and the vectors in Central America.

Simulium damnosum Complex

For many years *S. damnosum* was considered to be a single species widely distributed throughout the Afrotropical region except for: the coastal area of eastern Africa, the Red Sea coast, and the arid lands of the Kalahari and Namib deserts of south-western Africa.[5] Examination of the polytene chromosomes of different populations led to the recognition of four different forms in 1966, which had increased to nine by 1969, and stood at 26 in 1981.[16] At that stage eight of the species had been formally named, and another 18 designated by locality only. Only two species, *S. damnosum* s.s. and *S. sirbanum*, occur in both East and West Africa; eight species are found only in West Africa; and 16 only in East Africa. In agreement with the greater level of onchocerciasis in West Africa six of its species are anthropophilic, of which *S. damnosum* s.s., *S. sirbanum* and *S. squamosum* are the most important, and *S. sanctipauli, S. soubrense* and *S. yahense* of lesser importance.[16] The East African species are mainly zoophilic and only two, *S. damnosum* s.s. and *S. sirbanum*, are recognised vectors, and another two species are considered possible vectors.[16]

Unravelling the different ecologies of these closely-related forms is a challenging prospect requiring many years of patient study by workers in many parts of the continent. Cytotaxonomic methods can only be applied to larvae, and a lot of work has been devoted to developing sound methods of separating the different forms in the adult stage, when the females can act as vectors of onchocerciasis. Attention has been concentrated on the six important West African species. Peterson and Dang[30] have tabulated comparisons between these species for 31 characters, from which they have derived a simplified pictorial key.[7] Additional detailed information on the length of the antennae, the breadth of the antennal segments, and the number of teeth on the maxillae has been given by Quillévéré *et al.*[33] Another approach has been used by Meredith and Townson[26] who studied 44 enzyme systems and found only two to be taxonomically useful; but they enable *S. squamosum* and *S. yahense* to be separated from each other, and from the other four West African anthropophilic species.

The distribution of the anthropophilic species in West Africa is given in map form by Crosskey,[5] and in greater detail by Vajime and Quillévéré,[36] who summarised their distributions in terms of ecological zones. With increasing distance from the coast, zones of increasing aridity can be recognised. The moist forest zone occupies, except for the Dahomey Gap, a coastal belt of varying width. Moving inland this is succeeded by the forest-savanna mosaic zone; an undifferentiated, relatively moist Guinea or woodland savanna; a relatively dry Sudan or woodland savanna; the Sahel savanna; subdesert; and finally desert.[14] Onchocerciasis extends into the Sudan savanna but not further inland.

S. sirbanum is predominant in the Sudan savanna, spreads into the Guinea savanna and is almost absent from the forest zone. *S. damnosum* s.s. is abundant in the Guinea savanna, well represented in the Sudan savanna and present in smaller numbers in the forest. *S. squamosum* is mainly a forest species being present in heavily shaded or forested areas in the Guinea savanna but almost absent from the Sudan savanna. The other three species are mainly found in the forest zone although *S. soubrense* also occurs in the Guinea savanna.

Dunbar and Vajime[16] comment that in general West African species prefer 'long rivers running through gently rolling country', and East

African species 'usually prefer mountain streams'. There are exceptions to these statements and '*S. squamosum* and *S. yahense* prefer rivers coming from upland areas'. Distribution of species along a stream is associated with its trace chemical composition of which pH is the best single indicator.[16]

Simulium neavei Group

Six species of the *S. neavei* group occur in East Africa and another two in Angola.[22] *S. neavei* is the main vector in East Africa,[25] but at Amani in the Usambara mountains of northern Tanzania *S. woodi* is the vector.[34] The larvae and pupae of species of the *S. neavei* group have a phoretic association with crabs, with those of *S. neavei* occurring on the carapace of *Potamonautes* (*Potamon*) *niloticus*, which lives in the rockier parts of rivers near cascades.[25,37] The eggs of *S. neavei* are deposited on vegetation in clusters near cascades.[9]

S. woodi has a bimodal cycle of biting activity with morning and afternoon peaks in which nulliparous flies are commoner in the morning and parous flies in the afternoon.[34] When *S. woodi* feeds on man it attacks, almost exclusively, the legs where the greatest concentration of microfilariae is to be found. In one survey 17 per cent of the parous flies were infected and 3 per cent were infective.[34]

Central American Vectors

Dalmat[6] made a detailed study of the taxonomy, biology and ecology of the blackflies of Guatemala. The majority of the species were zoophilic with only six species readily attacking man, and only three — *S. ochraceum*, *S. metallicum* and *S. callidum* — were present in the onchocerciasis region. Dalmat[6] considered that *S. ochraceum* was the most important vector because its distribution coincided with that of the disease, being present only in small numbers outside the onchocerciasis region.

S. ochraceum is a predominantly anthropophilic species occurring between 900-1500 m above sea level, where it breeds in trickles and streams less than 1.5 m in width and 2-12 cm deep, classified by Dalmat[6] as infant and young streams. *S. ochraceum* is diurnal with peak activity occurring between 08.00-10.00 h. It attacks selectively the upper region of the body where the microfilariae of *O. volvulus* are most abundant. High biting rates were associated with high humidities and sunny skies, conditions found in the coffee-growing regions where onchocerciasis is rife.

S. metallicum is widely distributed both inside and outside the onchocerciasis zone, breeding in a wide range of streams including those classified by Dalmat[6] as adolescent and mature, which are larger water courses with a greater volume flow. Although *S. metallicum* feeds more readily on equines, it is the commonest species biting man, attacking the lower parts of the body where the density of microfilariae is lower. It is considered to be a good secondary vector of onchocerciasis[6] and the main vector in Venezuela.[27]

S. callidum has a sporadic distribution throughout the onchocerciasis zone and is the least common of the three species. Like *S. metallicum* it is strongly zoophilic, feeding more readily on equines than man and showing a more marked preference for feeding on the lower parts of the body; all of which operate against *S. callidum* being an important vector of onchocerciasis.

In Colombia the only man-biting Simuliid is *S. exigum* and it is considered to be the vector of onchocerciasis in that country.[35]

Development of O. volvulus in Simulium

Blacklock, working in Sierra Leone, showed that *O. volvulus* was ingested by *S. damnosum* when it fed on a host with microfilariae in the skin, and that these developed in the thoracic muscles, giving rise to infective larvae which escaped from the labium of the fly during feeding.[2,3] The worm undergoes a very similar cycle of development to that of *W. bancrofti* in its mosquito vector. The simuliid takes up microfilariae as it scrapes its way through the skin, and hence the uptake of microfilariae is more likely to be related to the distribution of microfilariae in the skin and the time taken to penetrate the skin than to the size of the blood meal. Wegesa (quoted by Nelson[27]) and Philippon[31] relate the number of microfilariae ingested to the duration of feeding, which may reflect the time spent penetrating the skin.

There is a great deal of variation in the uptake of microfilariae by flies feeding on the same host and it is preferable to work with geometric rather than arithmetic means. Duke[10] showed that the intake of microfilariae varied with their concentration in the skin up to a maximum of 150 microfilariae per mg of skin. The intake of microfilariae by flies fed on the same host, ranged from 0-171 with 55 per cent of *S. damnosum* ingesting ten or fewer microfilariae, and 15 per cent ingesting more than 50.[19] In this series the arithmetic mean was 26.2 and the modified geometric mean (William's mean, Mw) was 10.1.

Microfilariae must penetrate the midgut quickly to avoid being trapped within the peritrophic membrane, which is secreted around the blood meal. In two series of experiments the proportions of microfilariae which avoided such imprisonment were 0.44[13] and 0.75,[19] but in individual flies the proportion varied from none to all microfilariae.[13,19] There was no correlation between the proportion of microfilariae which escaped into the haemocoele and the number ingested, i.e. there was no evidence of facilitation or limitation as observed with *Wuchereria bancrofti* and different mosquito hosts.[13]

In the simuliid the first microfilaria reached the thorax in 20 min and invaded the flight muscles in two hours. The numbers of microfilariae in the thorax increased steadily from 30 min to six hours after feeding, when

62 per cent of the ingested microfilariae had reached the thorax.[19]

Once microfilariae have escaped from the midgut, a high proportion (0.91) completed development to become infective larvae.[13] The success rate for ingested microfilariae developing into infective forms was around 35-40 per cent and took seven to eight days.[10,13] A similar time (6-7 days) was found for the development of *O. volvulus* in *S. neavei* in Uganda at 21°C and 75 per cent RH.[27] Wegesa found the threshold for development of *O. volvulus* in *S. woodi* to be 18°C, and the optimum temperature 24°C. In *S. ochraceum* development of *O. volvulus* is at least eight days at 25°C, and four days at 30°C.[29]

Between oviposition and the next blood meal female *S. damnosum* s.l. take a meal of nectar during which some infective larvae of *O. volvulus* are lost.[40] This proportion may be as high as one third of the infective larvae.[31] Further loss of infective potential occurs when not all the infective larvae (about 80 per cent) escape while the female is taking a blood meal.[40]

Development of *O. volvulus* does not damage the simuliid host as much as one might expect. Blackflies invading the Onchocerciasis Control Programme in West Africa are considered to have come from localities several hundred kilometres away, and yet they have a high infection rate. Female *S. metallicum*, which have fed on heavily infected carriers of *O. volvulus*, suffer high mortality as a result of physical damage. *S. ochraceum* does not suffer this damage because a high proportion of the microfilariae ingested are damaged by its buccopharyngeal armature, recalling similar destruction wrought on microfilariae of *Wuchereria bancrofti* by the comparable armature of *An gambiae.*[29]

Strains of Onchocerca volvulus

The strains of *Onchocerca volvulus* in Central America and Africa behave quite differently, partly in adaptation to the vectors. In Central America microfilariae are seven to ten times as abundant in the face, neck and arms than in the legs, making them more accessible to the vector, *S. ochraceum,* which preferentially feeds on the upper parts of the body. In contrast, in Africa microfilariae are more abundant in the legs and lower parts of the body where 98 per cent of the biting of *S. damnosum* occurs.[8]

When fed on carriers with comparable densities of microfilariae in the skin *S. ochraceum* ingests 20-25 times more of the Guatemalan strain of *O. volvulus* than of either the forest or Sudan savanna strains from West Africa.[8] When either forest or Sudan savanna *S. damnosum* are fed on a host containing the Guatemalan strain of *O. volvulus* there is no concentration of microfilariae. Indeed forest *S. damnosum* ingested two to 4.5 times as many microfilariae of the forest strain of *O. volvulus* than of the Guatemalan strain, and both the forest and Sudan savanna forms of *S. damnosum* rapidly eliminated microfilariae of the Guatemalan strain.[15] The success rate of microfilariae of the forest strain *O. volvulus* in *S. dam-*

nosum was 47 per cent compared with 2 per cent for microfilariae of the same strain in *S. ochraceum*, although slightly more microfilariae were ingested by *S. ochraceum*.[8]

Duke *et al*.[14] recognised two parasite-vector complexes, one existing in the forest and Guinea savanna and the other in the Sudan savanna. They pointed out that microfilariae of *O. volvulus* from the forest area of Cameroon developed well in *S. damnosum* of the forest and Guinea savanna zones, but not in *S. damnosum* from the Sudan savanna; and, conversely, that microfilariae of *O. volvulus* from the Sudan savanna developed well in *S. damnosum* of the same zone but achieved little or no development in *S. damnosum* from the forest or Guinea savanna.[14]

When *S. damnosum* from the Sudan savanna ingested microfilariae of the forest *O. volvulus* it eliminated nearly all the parasites as microfilariae. A similar response occurred when forest *S. damnosum* ingested microfilariae of *O. volvulus* from the Sudan savanna zone, but in this case there were further eliminations of parasites during development in the thorax with heavily infected flies dying early.[11]

The differences between vectors can be related to sibling species of the *S. damnosum* complex. No comparable separation is available for the recognition of forms of *O. volvulus* but there is evidence for the existence of two strains of *O. volvulus* in West Africa differing in their pathogenicities, biochemical structure and vectors.[32] The savanna strain is associated with *S. damnosum* s.s. and *S. sirbanum*, and causes severe disease involving serious eye lesions and blindness, urinary excretion of microfilariae, and depressed immunity in the host. The forest strain of *O. volvulus* has low pathogenicity to man; is poorly transmitted by *S. damnosum* and *S. sirbanum*, but is well adapted to local vectors; and shows certain characteristic biochemical features.[32]

Epidemiology of Onchocerciasis

Onchocerciasis is not a zoonosis, although natural infections have been found in a spider monkey (*Ageles geoffroyi*) in Guatemala and a gorilla in the Congo; and chimpanzees can be infected in the laboratory.[27] The disease is passed from man to man by the bites of *Simulium* and can only rarely be passed before the third blood meal providing the simuliid becomes infected at its first blood meal. The gonotrophic cycle of *S. damnosum* s.s. and *S. sirbanum* is normally three to four days, made up of a period of less than 24 h between oviposition and feeding; ovarian development of 48 h; and a variable time (less than 12 h) between the eggs being fully mature and oviposition.[1]

One hypothesis which was put forward to explain the difference in severity of onchocerciasis between the Sudan savanna and the forest and

Guinea savanna, was that in the Sudan savanna the flies were long lived, and had more limited dispersal so that a higher rate of transmission existed. In contrast it was postulated that in the forest the life expectancy of the vector was shorter, and it dispersed more widely spreading infection more evenly over a greater area.[20]

Observation showed that indeed *S. damnosum* was longer lived in the Sudan savanna with 61 per cent of the population being parous compared with 40 per cent in the Guinea savanna and forest. This higher parity rate resulted in a higher proportion of the infected flies being infective, with this proportion reaching nearly 50 per cent in the Sudan savanna, compared to 20-36 per cent in the Guinea savanna and forest.[12] However, these calculations do not take into account the different sizes of the man-biting population of *S. damnosum* in the different regions, and the density of microfilariae in the human population available to the vectors. Simuliid populations in the Sudan savanna were only 12 per cent of those in the Guinea savanna, and less than 10 per cent of those in the forest.[12]

Using the number of infective larvae per infective fly as an estimate of the microfilarial reservoir in the human population, that in the Sudan savanna was 40 per cent of that in the forest. Putting all these factors together Duke[12] calculated that the infective biting density (the number of infective bites per man per day) was five in the Sudan savanna, 14 in the Guinea savanna, and depending upon the season, ranged from 18-83 in the forest. The transmission potential (number of infective larvae per man per day) was 12 in the Sudan savanna, 42 in the Guinea savanna, and 99-556 in the forest. These figures confound the hypothesis. The severity of onchocerciasis in the Sudan savanna is not related to the transmission rate which is actually lower than in the forest.[12]

Principles of Control

The problems of controlling onchocerciasis are formidable on account of the longevity of *O. volvulus*, and the habits of the vector which bites by day, and both bites and rests out of doors. This pattern of behaviour renders ineffective most methods of personal protection, e.g. screening of houses, use of nets, and the application of residual insecticides to houses. Some degree of personal protection can be achieved with repellents, and the wearing of long trousers offers some protection against *S. damnosum* which feeds preferentially on the lower parts of the body. Adult simuliids disperse widely, and the population is most concentrated in the immature stages which occur in running water. Control measures have therefore been directed against the immature stages with success.

East African Control Schemes

Control can be achieved by modifying the habitat so that it is no longer suitable for the vector, or by chemical control. It is possible to combine simuliid control with engineering works being carried out for an entirely different purpose. The Ripon Falls at Jinja in Uganda marked the source of the River Nile as it flowed from Lake Victoria. They were a prolific breeding ground for *S. damnosum,* and the onchocerciasis rate in the riverside dwellers was around 99 per cent.[25] Construction of the Owen Falls hydroelectric power station involved the building of a dam which raised the level of the Nile, and completely submerged the Ripon Falls, eliminating breeding of *S. damnosum.*

Advantage was taken of the controlled water outlet from the dam to introduce DDT into the released water and this controlled breeding of *S. damnosum* for 80 km below the dam, freed 4,000 sq km from *S. damnosum* making it available for more intensive settlement and agriculture without the fear of onchocerciasis.[27] However, it is important that engineering works reduce breeding sites and not increase them. Spillways which are often incorporated in a dam to allow a steady release of excess water can become highly productive breeding sites of *S. damnosum.*[4] Clearly engineers should seek the advice of public health authorities and medical entomologists lest their constructions for the benefit of the local population have the reverse effect.

In the Nyanza province of Kenya, which forms part of the north-eastern shore of Lake Victoria, the vector of *O. volvulus* in the inland hilly region was *S. neavei.* Four foci were discovered with onchocerciasis rates varying from 21-72 per cent, and eye lesions from 1.6-10.5 per cent.[25] An area of 12,000 sq km was freed from onchocerciasis by eradicating *S. neavei* from 323 rivers in which it was present by dosing them with DDT.[25] DDT was applied at a dosage which killed the larvae of *S. neavei,* but had no effect on fish or on the crabs with which *S. neavei* has a phoretic association. As there was no residual effect because the insecticide was carried away by the flow of water, treatments were repeated at ten-day intervals which was less than a minimum period for larval development. Adult *S. neavei* live for up to two months and so control was maintained for nine cycles of ten days, and eradication of the vector was achieved.[25] Nelson[27] listed a number of features of this particular situation which contributed to its success. Firstly, *S. neavei* had a limited flight range of 16 km along the course of bush-covered rivers but would not cross open country. Secondly, breeding was restricted to perennial streams at altitudes of 1,000-2,100 m, and the infected area was geographically isolated.

The eradication of *S. neavei* provided the opportunity to obtain information on the longevity of infections. Eleven years after the successful campaign no new infections had occurred, but 60 per cent of the older people were still infected and, worse still, those that had mild eye lesions earlier were now completely blind. The maximum life of *O. volvulus* is probably 16 years with microfilariae persisting in the skin for 30 months.[27] The fact that the worm is so long lived means that where eradication is not practical, control measures must be maintained at a high level of efficiency for a very long time, if transmission is to be prevented.

Onchocerciasis Control Programme in West Africa

Control of *S. damnosum* is more formidable because the adults have a flight range exceeding 100 km, and the ability to survive the dry season when many breeding sites dry up. In face of this long flight range, control measures must be carried out over a very large area to be successful. The Onchocerciasis Control Programme (OCP) began in 1975 with the aim of attaining and maintaining a zero incidence of serious and irreversible ocular lesions among those who were not infected at the start of the programme.[39] It is being financed by the World Bank for Development at a cost of $250,000,000 over a period of 20 years.[28]

The selected area of Sudan and Guinea savanna covered 654,000 sq km and extended across seven countries where 1,000,000 people suffered from onchocerciasis, and 70,000 were blind or had seriously impaired vision.[39] It was based on the Volta river system, extending west to the north-east flowing Niger, and east to the south-east flowing Niger. (The Niger flows from west to east in a vast northerly directed arc before flowing southwards into the Gulf of Guinea.)

Since the aim of the programme was not eradication it was necessary to define the desired level of control consistent with 'a tolerable level of onchocerciasis infection'.[39] Two criteria were adopted, an annual biting rate (ABR) of less than 1,000 per individual per year, and an annual transmission rate (ATP) of less than 100 infective larvae per year. At the start of the programme the ABR in most of the Volta river basin exceeded 8,000, and at over 90 per cent of the assessment points within the programme area the ABR exceeded 4,000.[39] By 1978 the effect of the control programme had been to reduce the ABR in the majority of localities to less than 500.[39] There was some variation in the relationship of ATP to ABR, and at Naboulgou the ATP was only 64 in spite of the ABR being 4,017.[39] The opposite was recorded at Nangodi bridge where an ATP of 102 coincided with an ABR of 587.[38]

Mounting a control programme over such a large area was a major administrative and logistic exercise, bristling with difficulties. It is a great credit to the organisers that the programme has been established, is working well, and appears to be attaining its aim. During its first 30 months of operations the OCP was treating 14,500 km of river length in the wet season, and this was increased to 18,000 km in 1978 with the inclusion of an extra 100,000 sq km in the Ivory Coast. Even at the height of the dry season 6,000 km of river length required weekly treatment. In 1980 consideration was given to adding a further 111,000 sq km to the southeast, involving parts of Ghana, Togo and Benin, which would require treatment of a further 4,000 km of river.[38]

Under the favourable temperatures (22-32°C) of West Africa, *S. damnosum* can develop from egg to pupa in eight days, therefore weekly treatment of all breeding sites, actual and potential, was made with temephos (= Abate®), an organophosphorus insecticide. The insecticide was applied from the air, using helicopters in narrow situations and aircraft on broader rivers. In the dry season the reduction in river flow necessitated a change in the method of insecticide application.[38] The programme has succeeded so well that treatment of some rivers has been discontinued. An interesting observation has been made that in areas where *S. damnosum* has been eliminated from the river system, other species such as *S. adersi* and *S. griseicolle* have survived, which may reflect different larval feeding habits.[38]

Two particular problems merit mention. *S. sanctipauli* and *S. soubrense* have developed resistance to temephos so that increasing the dosage by a factor of four or eight proved ineffective. Resistance to temephos by *S. sanctipauli* has increased over 30 times.[18] An alternative insecticide has been used and the problem overcome, for the present.

From the start of the control programme it was noticed that there was an increase in the density of *Simulium* during the rainy season and this was attributed to the wind-carriage of adults along the track of the monsoon winds during the northwards movement of the Inter Tropical Convergence Zone (ITCZ). This invasion takes place along a SW-NE track bringing flies 300 km or more, even up to 500 km.[17] The flies concerned are mainly older parous *S. damnosum* s.s. and *S. sirbanum*, many of which are infective (15 per cent). Clearly, infection with *O. volvulus* does not reduce the ability of flies to be dispersed by wind.

It is believed that the flies feed before migrating, arrive gravid, and move to the rivers to oviposit, after which they stay close to the rivers and do not disperse into the surrounding countryside in the same way as a population of younger flies.[17] Magor and Rosenberg[24] have analysed data relating to flies invading the control area, and consider that both nulliparous and parous flies participate in the migration. South of the ITCZ the flies are carried in a NE direction, the main route of migration, but in addition there is some carriage north of the ITCZ in a SW direction. To prevent this invasion, south-westerly expansion into the Ivory Coast was undertaken in 1978.

It is appropriate here to mention that the Royal Entomological Society of London recognised the outstanding contribution of Dr René Le Berre to the planning and execution of OCP by awarding him the Society's new medal for Major Achievement in Applied Entomology on 24 November 1981.

References

1. Bellec, C. and Hébrard, G. (1980). La durée du cycle gonotrophique des femelles du complexe *Simulium damnosum* en zone préforestière de Côte d'Ivoire. *Cahiers ORSTOM Entomologie Médicale et Parasitologie 18*: 347-58
2. Blacklock, D.B. (1926). The development of *Onchocerca volvulus* in *Simulium damnosum*. *Annals of Tropical Medicine and Parasitology 20*: 1-48
3. _____ (1926). The further development of *Onchocerca volvulus* Leukart in *Simulium damnosum* Theob. *Annals of Tropical Medicine and Parasitology 20*: 203-18
4. Burton, G.J. and McRae, T.M. (1965). Dam-spillway breeding of *Simulium damnosum* Theobald in northern Ghana. *Annals of Tropical Medicine and Parasitology 59*: 405-12
5. Crosskey, R.W. (1981). Geographical distribution of Simuliidae. pp. 57-68 in *Blackflies*, Marshall Laird (ed.), Academic Press, New York
6. Dalmat, H.T. (1955). The blackflies (Diptera, Simuliidae) of Guatemala and their role as vectors of onchocerciasis. *Smithsonian Miscellaneous Collection 125*: 1-425
7. Dang, P.T. and Peterson, B.V. (1980). Pictorial keys to the main species and species groups within the *Simulium damnosum* Theobald complex occurring in West Africa (Diptera: Simuliidae). *Tropenmedizin und Parasitologie 31*: 117-20
8. De Leon, J.R. and Duke, B.O.L. (1966). Experimental studies on the transmission of Guatemalan and West African strains of *Onchocerca volvulus* by *Simulium ochraceum*, *S. metallicum* and *S. callidum*. *Transactions of the Royal Society of Tropical Medicine and Hygiene 60*: 735-52
9. De Meillon, B. (1957). The bionomics of the vectors of onchocerciasis in the Ethiopian geographical region. *Bulletin of the World Health Organization 16*: 509-22
10. Duke, B.O.L. (1962). Studies on factors influencing the transmission of onchocerciasis. II. The intake of *Onchocerca volvulus* microfilariae by *Simulium damnosum* and the survival of the parasite in the fly under laboratory conditions. *Annals of Tropical Medicine and Parasitology 56*: 255-63
11. _____ (1966). *Onchocerca-Simulium* complexes. III. The survival of *Simulium damnosum* after high intake of microfilariae of incompatible strains of *Onchocerca volvulus*, and the survival of parasites in the fly. *Annals of Tropical Medicine and Parasitology 60*: 495-500
12. _____ (1968). Studies on factors influencing the transmission of onchocerciasis. VI. The infective biting potential of *Simulium damnosum* in different bioclimatic zones and its influence on the transmission potential. *Annals of Tropical Medicine and Parasitology 62*: 164-70
13. _____ and Lewis, D.J. (1964). Studies on factors influencing the transmission of onchocerciasis. III. Observations on the effect of the peritrophic membrane in limiting the development of *Onchocerca volvulus* microfilariae in *Simulium damnosum*. *Annals of Tropical Medicine and Parasitology 58*: 83-8
14. _____ Lewis, D.J. and Moore, P.J. (1966). *Onchocerca-Simulium* complexes. I. Transmission of forest and Sudan-savanna strains of *Onchocerca volvulus*, from Cameroon, by *Simulium damnosum* from various West African bioclimatic zones. *Annals of Tropical Medicine and Parasitology 60*: 318-36
15. _____ Moore, P.J. and De Leon, J.R. (1967). *Onchocerca-Simulium* complexes. V. The intake and subsequent fate of microfilariae of a Guatemalan strain of *Onchocerca volvulus* in forest and Sudan-savanna forms of West African *Simulium damnosum*. *Annals of Tropical Medicine and Parasitology 61*: 332-7
16. Dunbar, R.W. and Vajime, Ch. G. (1981). Cytotaxonomy of the *Simulium damnosum* complex. pp. 31-43 in *Blackflies*, Marshall Laird (ed.), Academic Press, New York
17. Garms, R., Walsh, J.F. and Davies, J.B. (1979). Studies on the reinvasion of the Onchocerciasis Control Programme in the Volta River basin by *Simulium damnosum* s.l.

with emphasis on the south-western areas. *Tropenmedizin und Parasitologie 30*: 345-62

18. Guillet, P., Escaffre, H., Ouedraogo, M. and Quillévéré, D. (1980), Mise en évidence d'une résistance au téméphos dans la complexe *Simulium damnosum* (*S. sanctipauli et S. soubrense*) en Côte d'Ivoire (zone du programme de lutte contre l'onchocercose dans la région du Bassin de la Volta). *Cahiers ORSTOM Entomologie Médicale et Parasitologie 18*: 291-9

19. Laurence, B.R. (1966). Intake and migration of the microfilariae of *Onchocerca volvulus* (Leuckart) in *Simulium damnosum* Theobald. *Journal of Helminthology 40*: 337-42

20. Le Berre, R., Balay, G. Brengues, J. and Coz, J. (1964). Biologie et ecologie de la femelle de *Simulium damnosum* Theobald, 1903, en fonction des zones bioclimatiques d'Afrique occidentale. *Bulletin of the World Health Organization 31*: 843-55

21. _____ Walsh, J.F., Davies, J.B., Philippon, B. and Garms, R. (1978). Control of onchocerciasis: medical entomology — a necessary pre-requisite to socio-economic development. pp. 70-75 in *Medical Entomology Centenary Symposium Proceedings*, S. Willmott (ed.), Royal Society of Tropical Medicine and Hygiene, London

22. Lewis, D.J. and Hanney, P.W. (1965). On the *Simulium neavei* complex (Diptera: Simuliidae). *Proceedings of the Royal Entomological Society of London (B) 34*: 12-16

23. Maegraith, B. (1980). *Adams and Maegraith: Clinical Tropical Diseases*. Blackwell Scientific Publications, Oxford

24. Magor, J.I. and Rosenberg, L.J. (1980). Studies of winds and weather during migrations of *Simulium damnosum* Theobald (Diptera: Simuliidae), the vector of onchocerciasis in West Africa. *Bulletin of Entomological Research 70*: 693-716

25. McMahon, J.P., Highton, R.B. and Goiny, H. (1958). The eradication of *Simulium neavei* from Kenya. *Bulletin of the World Health Organization 19*: 75-107

26. Meredith, S.E.O. and Townson, H. (1981). Enzymes for species identification in the *Simulium damnosum* complex from West Africa. *Tropenmedizin und Parasitologie 32*: 123-9

27. Nelson, G.S. (1970). Onchocerciasis. *Advances in Parasitology 8*: 173-224

28. _____ (1981). Issue in filariasis — a century of enquiry and a century of failure. *Acta Tropica 38*: 197-204

29. Ogata, K. (1981). Preliminary report of Japan-Guatemala onchocerciasis control pilot project. pp. 105-15 in *Blackflies*, Marshall Laird (ed.), Academic Press, New York

30. Peterson, B.V. and Dang, P.T. (1981). Morphological means of separating siblings of the *Simulium damnosum* complex (Diptera: Simuliidae). pp. 45-56 in *Blackflies*, Marshall Laird (ed.), Academic Press, New York

31. Philippon, B. (1977). Etude de la transmission d'*Onchocerca volvulus* (Leuckart, 1893) (Nematoda, Onchocercidae) par *Simulium damnosum* Theobald, 1903 (Diptera, Simuliidae) en Afrique tropicale. *Travaux et Documents de l'ORSTOM 63*: 1-308

32. Prost, A., Rougemont, A. and Omar, M.S. (1980). Caracteres épidémiologiques cliniques et biologiques des onchocercoses de savane et de forêt en Afrique occidentale, Revue critique et éléments nouveaux. *Annales de Parasitologie Humaine et Comparée 55*: 347-55

33. Quillévéré, D., Sechan, Y. and Pendriez, B. (1977). Etude du complexe *Simulium damnosum* en Afrique de l'Ouest. V. Identification morphologiques des femelles en Cote d'Ivoire. *Tropenmedizin und Parasitologie 28*: 244-53

34. Raybould, J.N. (1967). A study of anthropophilic female Simuliidae (Diptera) at Amani, Tanzania: the feeding behaviour of *Simulium woodi* and the transmission of onchocerciasis. *Annals of Tropical Medicine and Parasitology 61*: 76-88

35. Sasa, M. (1976). *Human Filariasis*. University of Tokyo Press, Tokyo

36. Vajime, C. and Quillévéré, D. (1978). The distribution of *Simulium damnosum* complex in West Africa with particular reference to the Onchocerciasis Control Programme area. *Tropenmedizin und Parasitologie 29*: 473-82

37. Van Someren, V.D. and McMahon, J. (1950). Phoretic association between *Afronurus* and *Simulium* species, and the discovery of the early stages of *Simulium neavei* on freshwater crabs. *Nature, London 166*: 350-1

38. Walsh, J.F., Davies, J.B. and Cliff, B. (1981). World Health Organization Onchocerciasis Control Programme in the Volta River basin. pp. 85-103 in *Blackflies*,

Marshall Laird (ed.), Academic Press, New York
39. _____ Davies, J.B. and Le Berre, R. (1979). Entomological aspects of the first five years of the Onchocerciasis Control Programme in the Volta River basin. *Tropenmedizin und Parasitologie 30*: 328-44
40. Wenk, P. (1981). Bionomics of adult blackflies. pp. 259-79 in *Blackflies,* Marshall Laird (ed.), Academic Press, New York

32 OTHER HELMINTHS TRANSMITTED BY INSECTS

This chapter will deal with a miscellaneous collection of helminths transmitted by insects to man and domestic animals. The human parasites will include *Loa Loa* and three species of benign filarioid worms: *Dipetalonema perstans*, *D. streptocerca* and *Mansonella ozzardi*. Animal parasites dealt with will include species of *Onchocerca* and other filarioid parasites of domestic animals; *Habronema*, *Thelazia*; and two cestodes, *Dipylidium* and *Hymenolepis*.

Loiasis

Loiasis, a filarial disease of man caused by infection with *Loa Loa*, occurs in the rainforest areas of tropical Africa, extending roughly from 10°N to 5°S, including countries in West Africa, Central Africa and eastwards to the Great Lakes.[39] Sasa[57] gives a rather wider distribution adding 5° to the northern distribution and 10° to the southern distribution to include Zambia and Malawi. It was estimated that in the 1940s about 13,000,000 people suffered from loiasis, the effects of which range from trivial to severe and painful, often complicated by a psychological factor.[39] The disease is marked by temporary oedematous swellings the size of a hen's egg, the so-called Calabar or fugitive swellings, which may occur anywhere on the body but are particularly found on the arms, legs and orbit.[39,57] Swellings last several days before subsiding, and usually only one is present at a time but occasionally two or three may occur together.[39]

The adult worms live a nomadic life moving through loose connective tissue, and at times can be seen moving under the skin causing minimal local reaction. The most disquieting demonstration of their mobility is when they move across the eye under the conjunctiva at a speed of 1 cm per minute. No permanent damage is done to the eye which becomes oedematous, and is said to feel like having been 'kicked in the eye'.[39] As in other filarial infections there is a pronounced eosinophilia with the eosinophil count being, at times, as high as 60-90 per cent of the white blood cells.[57] The microfilariae occur in the circulating blood. Loiasis can be treated with diethylcarbamazine (DEC) which as 'considerable effect on the microfilariae and less on the adults'.[39]

Loa loa in the Vertebrate Host

Two subspecies of *L. loa* are recognised; *L. loa loa* occurs in man, its microfilariae have a diurnal periodicity in the circulating blood, and it is transmitted by day-biting *Chrysops*; *L. loa papionis* is a larger worm which parasites monkeys, its microfilariae show a nocturnal periodicity, and it is transmitted by crepuscular or nocturnal biting *Chrysops*.[47] Male *L. loa loa* measure 30-34 × 0.35-0.43 mm, and females 50-70 × 0.5 mm.[57]

In monkeys the worms become mature and microfilariae appear in the circulating blood four to five months after the introduction of infective larvae,[22] while in man maturation of the worm is considered to take somewhat longer, six to twelve months.[39] The sheathed microfilariae of *Loa loa* are similar to those of *Wuchereria bancrofti* which also occur in the circulating blood. In monkeys, and probably also in man, the female passes microfilariae into the connective tissue, from which they enter the vascular system and accumulate in the pulmonary blood before entering the peripheral circulation about three weeks after being released.[22]

Development of Loa loa in Chrysops

Connal and Connal[12] were the first to demonstrate the development of *L. loa* in two species of tabanid flies, *Chrysops silacea* and *C. dimidiata*. Later Williams[68] carried out a detailed study of the development of *L. loa* in *C. silacea* and found that the worm developed in the fat-body of the fly where it underwent two moults before reaching the infective stage. At 28-30°C and 92 per cent RH microfilariae developed to the infective stage in seven days, and in the process increased in length from 275 μm to more than 2 mm. Most microfilariae developed in the fat-body of the abdomen, and a smaller number in the fat-body of the thorax and head. In the initial stages of development the parasite is intracellular but later it becomes free.[38] Infective larvae move to the head where they accumulate in the subcibarial haemocoelic space and escape, when the fly is feeding, by rupturing the delicate labio-hypopharyngeal membrane.[38]

When *C. silacea* and *C. dimidiata* feed they take in about twice their bodyweight of blood with the heavier species, *C. silacea*, taking in about 20-25 per cent more blood.[36] *C. silacea* ingests only about half the number of microfilariae that would be expected from the density of microfilariae in the circulating blood and the size of the blood meal. After ingestion there is little mortality of microfilariae during development.[36] Duke[22] found in the field that the number of *L. loa* in *C. silacea* and *C. dimidiata* were almost identical, 79 and 81 respectively, and, in view of the smaller blood meal taken by *C. dimidiata*, this suggests that *C. dimidiata* takes in proportionally more microfilariae than *C. silacea.*

The number of infective larvae developing from one intake of microfilariae is limited, and flies that have infective larvae after ten to twelve days are considered to become free of infective forms five to seven days later, i.e. after one or two blood meals.[39] However, Williams[68] has pointed out that development of the worm in *C. silacea* may be delayed or arrested, in which case the fly would not be infective until much later.

Ecology of the Vector and Epidemiology of Loiasis

L. l. loa and *L. l. papionis* are good biological entities which form hybrids on cross-mating, that have a characteristic periodicity, differing markedly from that of either parent, or from a 50:50 mixture of the two periodicities.[22] Connal and Connal[12] incriminated *C. silacea* and *C. dimidiata* as vectors of *L. loa,* and Woodman and Bokhari[72] and Woodman[71] showed that *L. loa* would develop in *C. distinctipennis* and *C. longicornis* in the southern Sudan. Duke[14] considers 'that all members of the genus *Chrysops* are potential vectors of the parasite'. He considers that *C. silacea* is the most important vector, and that *C. dimidiata* is an equally efficient, but usually less numerous, vector. He also considers that *C. distinctipennis* and *C. zahrai* are less effective local or subsidiary vectors, and that *C. langi* and *C. centurionis* are zoophilic and responsible for the transmission of *L. l. papionis.* Duke[22] concluded that transmission of *L. loa* from man to monkey could occur rarely but that the reverse transmission from monkey to man was most unlikely.

   C. silacea, which at this time included a taxon later designated *C. dimidiata* (Bombe form), was most abundant in the canopy of the rainforest, and in the open area just below the canopy. About 7 per cent occurred above the canopy, and 17 per cent were taken at ground level.[15] The biting cycle of these two species in the canopy was bimodal with morning and afternoon peaks in which nulliparous females were more numerous in the morning and parous females in the afternoon.[21] *C. langi* and *C. centurionis* were crepuscular, biting from about 17.00 h to 21.00 h.[18] It is unlikely that *C. silacea* and *C. dimidiata* (Bombe form) would acquire infections by feeding on monkeys, because during the daytime monkeys are active and would quickly catch biting tabanids. Even if some fed successfully, there would be virtually no microfilariae in the monkeys' peripheral blood at that time. At night *C. langi* and *C. centurionis* would find it easier to feed on sleeping monkeys at a time when the microfilarial density in their circulating blood would be high, favouring infection.

   In the daytime *C. silacea* and *C. dimidiata* (Bombe form) descend to the forest floor where they are likely to find human hosts. They become more numerous in the presence of a wood fire, increasing man-fly contact. In the absence of a wood fire *C. dimidiata* (Bombe form) is more efficient than *C. silacea* at finding a stationary human bait.[20]

   In a mixed farmland-forest region tabanid larvae and pupae were more numerous in 'small patches of mud in deep valleys in deep forest', and diminished with reduction of the forest to reach their lowest level in mud in open ground.[69] The distribution of immature *Chrysops* followed that of the biting densities of *C. silacea* and *C. dimidiata* (Bombe form), which formed 60-70 per cent of all *Chrysops* bred to the adult. This suggests that these species do not readily cross open ground.[69] If this applies to hungry as well as gravid females, then the risk of infection with *L. loa* should decrease with distance from forest. Certainly the biting intensity decreases with distance from forest with the rate of decline depending on the degree of cover available. Thus where there are only saplings 0.5 m high in the clearing the biting density was reduced to one tenth of its original value at 90 m from the forest, but where the saplings were taller (3-3.5 m) the same reduction was not reached until 500 m.[16] Even in the tropical rainforest the biting densities of *C. silacea* and *C. dimidiata* (Bombe form) is not constant throughout the year but shows a seasonal cycle, with *C. silacea* being abundant from April to December and *C. dimidiata* (Bombe form) having two peaks of abundance, November to January and March to May.[20]

Other Filarial Infections of Man

Three other species of filarial worms infect man, to whom they are usually no more than mildly pathogenic. They produce unsheathed microfilariae which, in the case of *Dipetalonema perstans* and *Mansonella ozzardi*, occur in the circulating blood, and in the case of *Dipetalonema streptocerca* in the skin. The latter need to be differentiated from the sheathed microfilariae of *Onchocerca volvulus* which also occur in the skin in the same part of the world. The three species will be considered separately.

Dipetalonema perstans

Dipetalonema perstans, sometimes referred to as *Acanthocheilonema perstans*, is the most widespread of the three species, occurring in West, Central and East Africa, Brazil, northern Argentina, Trinidad, Guyana and Surinam.[39,57] The adult worms occur free in the body cavities of man, and the microfilariae, which are present in the circulating blood, show no periodicity. Usually no clinical symptoms are associated with infection with *D. perstans*, but there are some accounts of *D. perstans* causing clinical disease and they have been reviewed by Sasa.[57] Treatment with diethylcarbamazine is effective against the microfilariae, and may also act against the adult worms.[57]

The vectors of *D. perstans* are species of *Culicoides*, among which there is some confusion concerning the status of certain species. *C. austeni* and *C. milnei* were treated originally as separate species; then *C. austeni* was regarded as a synonym of *C. milnei*; and later it was re-established as a separate species. For that reason, in this account the specific names used by the original authors will be retained.

Sharp[59] followed the development of *D. perstans* in *C. austeni*, observing that microfilariae escaped from the midgut into the haemocoele in six hours and in 20-30 h had reached the thorax. Infective larvae were present in the head after seven days, and emerged from the membranous end of the labium eight to ten days after the infected blood meal. The role of *C. austeni* as a vector of *D. perstans* was confirmed by finding that 7 per cent of wild-caught flies were infected.[59] These observations were confirmed by Hopkins and Nicholas[33] who found that 40 per cent of *C. austeni* became infected after feeding on a carrier of *D. perstans*. Nicholas and Kershaw[51] showed that *C. austeni* took up more microfilariae (about × 2) than expected from their concentration in the circulating blood. Allowing for difficulties in measuring the size of a blood meal of a *Culicoides*, it is clear that there is no barrier to the uptake of microfilariae of *D. perstans* by *C. austeni.*

The role of *C. grahamii* is less clear cut. Sharp[59] considered it to be a possible vector but Chardome and Peel[10] and Henrard and Peel[29] in Zaire found that *C. grahamii* did not ingest microfilariae of *D. perstans*. Nicholas *et al.*[50] and Nicholas and Kershaw[51] showed that *C. grahamii* did take up microfilariae of *D. perstans* at a rate comparable with their density in the circulating blood. It is possible that the workers in Zaire and Cameroon were working with different, but related, species of *Culicoides*.

Hopkins and Nicholas[33] found that, after feeding on a carrier of *D. perstans*, only two out of 418 *C. grahamii* became infective, and they considered that *C. grahamii* was a poor host for *D. perstans*, as did Nicholas and Kershaw.[51] Using more accurate measurements of the size of the blood meal, Duke[17] found that when *C. grahamii* and *C. inornatipennis* fed on the same carrier, similar proportions, 77 and 76 per cent, respectively, took up microfilariae, but six to nine days later few *C. grahamii* (6 per cent) were infected compared to 41 per cent of *C. inornatipennis*.

Dipetalonema streptocerca

Dipetalonema streptocerca, also referred to as *Acanthocheilonema streptocerca*, is geographically limited to the rainforest areas of West and Central Africa from Ivory Coast to Zaire, and including Upper Volta.[39,57] The adult worms are subcutaneous in the upper parts of the body, and microfilariae occur on the upper trunk and upper arms.[13] No clinical disease is associated with *D. streptocerca* other than an itchy skin, which responds to treatment with diethylcarbamazine.[39] Chardome and Peel[10] and Henrard and Peel[29] described the development of *D. streptocerca* in *C. grahamii* with infective larvae being produced in seven to eight days and 1.2 per cent wild-caught *C. grahamii* being naturally infected.

Duke[13,19] showed that *C. grahamii* readily took up microfilariae of *D. streptocerca* with 15 per cent and 39 per cent *C. grahamii* taking up microfilariae in two separate experiments. During development there was some loss of infection, and seven to nine days after feeding on a carrier the percentage of infected flies had fallen from 39 to 19, and the number of larvae per infected *C. grahamii* from 2.1 to 1.4.[13] *C. milnei* (= *C. austeni*) takes in very few microfilariae of *D. streptocerca*, less than one tenth of that taken in by *C. grahamii*, and must be considered to be no more than a poor vector of *D. streptocerca*.[19]

Mansonella ozzardi

Mansonella ozzardi is found only in the Neotropical region where it occurs in Central America, certain Caribbean Islands, the north coast of South America, Brazil, Bolivia and the northern province of Argentina.[39,57] No particular symptoms are associated with *M. ozzardi*, against which diethyl-carbamazine is considered to be ineffective.[39,57] Adult worms have been found in fat tissue beneath the peritoneum and in other body cavities.[39] Microfilariae usually occur in the circulating blood, in which they show no periodicity, but in a survey in Brazil microfilariae were found with almost equal frequency in bloodless skin snips (295/701) and in blood (350/701).[43]

Buckley[8] followed the development of *M. ozzardi* in *Culicoides furens* at Calliaqua, St. Vincent, where a high proportion of the human population (37.5 per cent) was infected with *M. ozzardi*. When *C. furens* fed on a carrier, microfilariae reached the thorax in 24 h and infective larvae were present in the head after seven to eight days. These laboratory observations were supported by finding 5 per cent of *C. furens* infected naturally.

Buckley[8] referred to the possibility that *C. paraensis* might act as a vector, and this has been confirmed in northern Argentina by Romaña and Wygodzinsky, cited in Wirth.[70] Cerqueira, cited by Sasa,[57] incriminated *Simulium amazonicum* as the vector of *M. ozzardi* in Amazonas, Brazil. It is of interest that this is the same area in which Moraes[43] found micro-filariae of *M. ozzardi* in the skin, and raises the question as to whether there are two forms of *M. ozzardi* or two separate species, one with micro-filariae in the blood and transmitted by *Culicoides*, and another with microfilariae in the skin and transmitted by *Simulium*.

On the island of Trinidad, Nathan[44] found that *Culicoides phlebotomus* was the vector of *M. ozzardi*. The proportion of *C. phlebotomus* females infected was very low, being 0.8 per cent and 1.3 per cent in two large samples. The proportion infective was even lower being 0.07 per cent and 0.13 per cent of all females, but nearly 4 per cent of parous females, i.e. those which had had the opportunity to become infected. Transmission of *M. ozzardi* is assured by the large numbers of *C. phlebotomus* biting man, which can easily exceed 100 per hour in the early morning. Indeed, using simple assumptions, Nathan[44] calculated that a person spending one hour per day on the beach in the early morning would receive 38 infective bites in the course of a year.

Filarioid Parasites of Domestic Animals Transmitted by Insects

Onchocerca Species

Bain *et al.*[4] list 21 species of *Onchocerca* in addition to *O. volvulus*. Nine of these have been recorded from cattle and water buffalo, four from equines, six from wild cervids, and a single species each from camels (*O. fasciata*) and from a wild boar in Malaysia (*O. dewittei*). The species of *Onchocerca* are not easy to identify, and the cattle parasites *O. guttturosa* and *O. linealis* have only been separated with confidence comparatively recently.[3,55] Although species of *Onchocerca* are referred to as parasites of cattle or of equines, Ottley and Moorhouse[54] have shown that species are not necessarily host specific. In a group of 20 horses, 11 were infected with *O. cervicalis* (regarded as an equine parasite), and 12 with the cattle parasite, *O. gutturosa*. Ottley and Moorhouse[54] have also found the cattle parasite *O. gibsoni* in sheep.

Economic Importance and Vectors

Onchocerciasis of cattle, water buffaloes and horses occurs widely throughout the world wherever these domestic animals have been introduced and there are suitable vectors. Steward[61] associated infection of horses with *O. cervicalis* with fistulous withers and poll evil, but as Nelson[46] has pointed out high infection rates with *O. cervicalis* occur in areas where fistulous withers is very rarely seen. Eichler and Nelson[25] regarded *O. linealis* (*O. gutturosa* auct.) as an unobtrusive parasite which produced no marked pathological changes or evidence of clinical disease. Losses in the beef industry arise because 'free worms cause aesthetically displeasing blemishes' to the carcase, and encapsulated adult worms in nodules have to be trimmed from the carcase.[53] Microfilariae occur in the skin and subcutaneous lymph, with the exception of those of *O. armillata* which occur in the blood.[46] Microfilariae are ingested by blood-sucking flies and develop in various species of *Simulium*, *Culicoides* and *Lasiohelea*.[56,61,62]

Onchocerca Species in Domestic Bovines

Adult *O. linealis* occur in the gastroplenic ligament and its microfilariae are concentrated in the region of the umbilicus, while adults of *O. gutturosa* are found in the cervical ligament and microfilariae in the skin of the head, neck and back.[3] Bain and Beveridge[1] classify the nodule-forming onchocercas in terms of their geographical distribution and the location of the adults in the bovine host. In Africa, adults of *O. dukei* are subcutaneous, and those of *O. ochengi* are dermal parasites, which cause a dermatitis resembling mange or pox.[7] In Asia, adults of *O. gibsoni* and possibly those of *O. indica* occur in the subcutaneous tissues, while *O. cebei* and possibly *O. sweetae* are dermal parasites.[1] Nodules of *O. gibsoni* are most prevalent on the brisket.[53] Also in Asia, *O. armillata* causes striking lesions in the wall of the thoracic aorta.[46]

Transmission of Bovine Onchocercas. Steward[62] showed that microfilariae of a bovine onchocerca could develop in *Simulium ornatum*. It is not clear which species he was working with since adult worms were present in both the cervical and gastroplenic ligaments, and he could have been dealing with a mixed infection of *O. linealis* and *O. gutturosa*. Microfilariae occurred at a depth of about 1 mm from the skin surface, and 42 per cent of *S. ornatum* ingested microfilariae when feeding. Development was relatively slow with the 'sausage' stage, measuring 200×20 µm, being reached in ten days, and infective forms being present in the head 19 days after the infective feed. No development was observed in two other species of *Simulium*, and none in *Culicoides nubeculosus*, which is a vector of *O. cervicalis* to horses.

S. *ornatum* is well adapted to transmitting *O. linealis* (*O. gutturosa* auct.) because it feeds preferentially in the umbilical regions where the microfilariae of *O. linealis* are concentrated.[25] The number of microfilariae ingested is a function of the period of time spent feeding, and not of the volume of blood (about 3 mg) taken in. On average, about 15 microfilariae were ingested in three minutes and 30 in six minutes, and few were lost when *S. ornatum* discharged blood from the anus during feeding.[23] Within one hour 25 per cent of the microfilariae had reached the haemocoele and most were in the thorax in six hours, some even entering the thoracic musculature within one hour of feeding. The ingested blood is quickly surrounded by a peritrophic membrane which becomes progressively thicker with time, and is probably a factor in preventing escape of microfilariae from the midgut.[24]

Buckley,[9] working in Malaysia, found that *Culicoides pungens* ingested microfilariae of *O. gibsoni* when feeding on infected cattle. Microfilariae of *O. gibsoni* have their maximum concentration at a depth of 50-200 µm from the surface of the skin. The infection rate in *C. pungens* was less than 1 per cent, but this is compensated for by the very large numbers biting cattle. Some other species of *Culicoides* were also considered to be able to act as vectors.

Ottley and Moorhouse[56] showed that *Lasiohelea townsvillensis* could transmit *O. gibsoni*, the microfilariae of which completed their development in the midge in six days at 30°C and 85 per cent RH. *Culicoides marksi* and *C. actoni* ingested microfilariae of *O. gibsoni* when feeding on infected cattle.[6,56] Although microfilariae of *O. gutturosa* occur mainly on the dorsal surface of cattle, particularly in the withers, *C. brevitarsis*, which attacks preferentially the dorsal surface of cattle, did not ingest any microfilariae.[56]

Microfilariae of *O. ochengi* are located in the umbilical area and legs of cattle. They developed normally in females of the *Simulium damnosum* complex, probably *S. sanctipauli,*[52] with infective larvae of *O. ochengi* being present six days after an infective feed. Although microfilariae of *O. gutturosa* and *O. dukei* were also ingested by *S. damnosum* s.l., they did not develop.[52] Microfilariae of the water buffalo parasite *O. sweetae* were ingested only by *Culicoides* sp 'M' in which they developed.[60] Of interest was the fact that *C. schultzei* and *C. peregrinus* fed on areas of skin known to contain microfilariae of *O. sweetae* but did not ingest them.[60]

Equine Onchocercas

Three species of *Onchocerca* have been recorded from horses and a fourth species from donkeys. Adult *O. reticulata* occur in the suspensory ligament of the fetlock of horses; *O. cervicalis* in the cervical ligament of horses; *O. bohmi,* originally placed in the genus *Elaeophora,* is found in the walls of arteries and veins in the limbs of horses; and *O. raillieti* has recently been described from domestic donkeys in Africa.[2]

Steward[61] followed the development of *O. cervicalis* in *Culicoides nubeculosus* in which infective larvae were produced in 24-25 days. Development also occurred in *C. obsoletus* and *C. parroti,* but not in *C. pulicaris* or in *Simulium.* Mellor[42] confirmed the development of *O. cervicalis* in *C. nubeculosus,* and showed that development also occured in *C. variipennis.* At 23°C development was faster than that obtained by Steward[61] with infective forms being produced in 14-15 days. When *C. nubeculosus* fed on an infected horse, 17 per cent of the flies ingested microfilariae with an average intake of 1.9 microfilariae per infected fly. Rather lower infection rates were obtained with *C. variipennis* with 7 per cent ingesting an average of 1.3 microfilariae per infected fly. As with other skin-dwelling microfilariae the number ingested was a function of the duration of feeding and not of the volume of the blood meal.[42]

Microfilariae of *O. cervicalis* escape from the midgut of *C. nubeculosus* within five minutes of the fly finishing feeding, and 60 per cent of the microfilariae reached the haemocoele within one hour. About 40 per cent of the microfilariae fail to escape from the midgut. Most of those which enter the haemocoele have reached the thorax in 16-36 h. *C. variipennis* is a less efficient vector with about two thirds of the microfilariae being retained within the midgut. Early death of the midge can occur when large numbers of microfilariae penetrate the gut wall.[42]

Microfilariae of *O. cervicalis* are predominantly (95 per cent) present in the skin along the abdominal midline of the host which brings them into close contact with *C. nubeculosus,* 85 per cent of which land and feed on the ventral midline of the horse from the front legs to the mammae or sheath.[41] While the numbers of microfilariae in the whole skin remain unchanged over the year, during the active season of *C. nubeculosus* (June to September) microfilariae were most abundant just under the epidermis, favouring their ingestion by blood-sucking insects.[28] During the cooler months of the year, October to February, the microfilariae were deeper (1-2 mm) in the skin. A similar seasonal movement of microfilariae of *O. gutturosa* in the skin of cattle has been shown to coincide with the period of activity of the vector *S. ornatum*.[28]

Other Filarioid Parasites of Domestic Animals

Dirofilaria immitis in the Dog

Dirofilaria immitis, the heartworm of dogs, occurs mainly in the tropics and subtropics where it infests dogs, other canids, and rarely cats or humans.[30] Adult worms, measuring 12-20 cm in the male and 25-31 cm in the female, are found in the right ventricle of the heart and in the pulmonary artery. They restrict the circulation, leading to a loss of exercise tolerance, chronic cardiac insufficiency and heart failure.[5,30] Wharton[67] found that *D. immitis* was common in domestic and forest carnivores in Malaya. *D. immitis* appears to be spreading into more temperate regions along the east coast of Australia and in the USA, where infection rates of 5 to 50 per cent have been recorded.[5,30]

The unsheathed microfilariae of *D. immitis* show a nocturnal periodicity in the circulating blood. When they are ingested by mosquitoes the micro-filariae escape from the midgut into the haemocoele and develop in the malpighian tubes, in which development is completed in 15-16 days in temperate regions, and in eight to ten days in tropical regions. Infective larvae move into the head and enter the labium from which they escape when the mosquito is feeding. Mature worms reach the heart in three to four months, and microfilariae are produced in six to eight months.[30] More than 70 species of mosquitoes can act as vectors of *D. immitis*.[5]

Intermill[34] found that 96 per cent of *Ae triseriatus* ingested microfilariae of *D. immitis*, but in only a little over 50 per cent of the mosquitoes did microfilariae produce infective larvae. On average 24 microfilariae were ingested, of which 40 per cent developed further, and 11 per cent reached the infective stage. At 21-27°C and 70-80 per cent RH infective larvae reached the labium in 13 days.

The relationship between *D. immitis* and its mosquito vectors is complex. The microfilariae have a nocturnal periodicity which coincides with the feeding cycle of the vector and in northern temperate regions there is a seasonal cycle with a five- to ten-fold increase in microfilariae in the circulating blood in August and September, when mosquitoes are most abundant.[28] Nayar and Sauerman[45] found that when the mosquito's saliva contained an anticoagulant, as in *Ae sollicitans* and *Ae taeniorhynchus*, ingested microfilariae readily escaped into the haemocoele, but in the absence of an anticoagulant, as in *Cx quinquefasciatus* and *Ae aegypti*, the rapidly clotting blood trapped microfilariae in the midgut.

In some *Ae sollicitans* and *Ae aegypti* substantial numbers of micro-filariae that reach the malpighian tubes do not complete development. In *Ae aegypti* the gene f^t controls susceptibility to infection with *D. immitis.* It is considered to act via the site of development of the parasite, i.e. the malpighian tubes, because the development of *D. immitis* is not affected by the gene f^m which controls susceptibility to infection with *Brugia malayi,* which develops in the thoracic musculature.[66]

Elaeophora schneideri in Sheep

Infections of sheep with *Elaeophora schneideri* have been recorded in North America and Italy,[7] and the history of the investigation into the transmission of this worm in North America has been summarised by Krinksky.[37] *E. schneideri* is a benign parasite of the mule deer *Odocoileus hemionus.* which causes clinical disease in abnormal hosts such as sheep, elk (*Cervus canadensis*) and moose (*Alces alces*).[32] The worm inhabits the carotid arteries, and in mule deer moves to larger arteries as it grows, but in abnormal hosts, e.g. domestic sheep, the worm does not migrate and restricts blood circulation, causing blindness, deafness, and circling. Frequently animals become comatose and die.[32] Sheep that survive the establishment of the worm show a severe dermatitis on the head and feet.[7] Infections occur in sheep which are grazed at high altitudes (1,800 m) in the summer months, and has an incidence of about 1 per cent.[7]

In Gila National Park, New Mexico, the vector of *E. schneideri* is a tabanid *Hybomitra laticornis,* of which in one survey 16 per cent were infected with an average of 25 developing worms.[11] Ingested microfilariae escape from the midgut into the haemocoele and enter the fat-body for the initial stage of development. Later developing larvae leave the fat-body, develop in the abdomen into infective larvae, measuring 4.5 mm by 50 μm, before moving to the head and mouthparts from which they escape when the fly is feeding.[32]

Stephanofilariasis in Cattle

Stephanofilaria stilesi. S. stilesi is found in cattle in North America, Hawaii and the Soviet Union, and may occur more widely in the world.[31] It causes lesions in the skin along the midventral line between the brisket and navel, which remain raw and bloody for several years. The adult worms and the sheathed, very small microfilariae (52 × 3 μm) occur in the lesions from which they are ingested by feeding flies. In New Mexico the vector is the blood-sucking muscid, *Haematobia irritans.*[31] An infection rate of 12 per cent was found in field-collected female flies and a similar infection rate was obtained when laboratory-reared females were fed on infected lesions, but infections in male flies, both field-collected and laboratory-reared, were very low (less than 0.5 per cent). The infection rate in cattle is variable, and was 98 per cent in beef cattle but lower (25 per cent) in drylots where the manure was removed or scattered, reducing the populations of *H. irritans.* Infection rates in *H. irritans* were highest in spring and autumn when the maximum temperature was 21-27°C, and low in July and August when the temperature was 32-38°C.[31]

Stephanofilaria assamensis. S. assamensis is a parasite mainly of cattle but occurs in other ungulates, infesting the subcutaneous layer and skin of the ears and back.[35] In Bangladesh the vector is *Musca conducens,* which has well developed prestomal teeth and interdental armature on its proboscis, which enable it to scratch and rasp the skin.[31] *S. assamensis* produces eggs which are ingested by the fly and hatch in the midgut. Second-stage larvae occur in the abdomen and thorax, while third-stage larvae migrate to the proboscis, and are deposited on to the skin of cattle when the fly feeds.[58]

The overall infection rate in cattle was 30 per cent but it varied according to locality being as high as 95 per cent in swampy areas. Transmission occurred all the year round but had a marked maximum in July and August. Natural infection rates of *M. conducens* were low (2 per cent) with infected flies containing one to seven larvae.[58] In Uzbekistan the vector is *Haematobia thirouxi titillans* (*Lyperosia titillans* auct.), in which the natural infection rate was 0.7 per cent, and the infection rate in cattle only 1 per cent. At 26-32°C development of *S. assamensis* in *H. t. titillans* took 21-24 days.[25]

Parafilariasis in Cattle and Equines

Parafilaria bovicola. P. bovicola has been recorded from cattle in Europe, North Africa, South Africa, India and the Philippines.[48] The adult worm causes slimy, bruise-like, subcutaneous lesions which reduce the value of carcases. The ovipositing female worm perforates the skin and deposits egg and/or microfilariae into the blood which trickles down over the surface of the skin. These blood spots occur in the hottest part of the day and attract muscid flies. Nine species of *Musca* were collected off cattle, and infective third-stage larvae were found in three species belonging to the subgenus *Eumusca, M. lusoria, M. xanthomelas* and an undescribed species.[48]

Infection rates in the field were usually less than 1 per cent, but in the laboratory rates of 40-45 per cent were obtained.[48] Infective larvae escape from the mouthparts when the fly feeds on warm (38-40°C) citrated ox blood, but not when it feeds on blood at 22°C, or warm saline or 15 per cent sucrose solution.[49] The stimulus to emergence of infective larvae would appear to be a high temperature and the presence of blood proteins. *P. bovicola* was successfully transmitted when infected *M. lusoria* fed at a skin incision. Cattle were also infected when infective larvae were instilled inside the eyelids.[49]

Parafilaria multipapillosa. P. multipapillosa is a parasite of equines in Europe and Asia.[7] In the USSR the vector is a blood-sucking muscid (*Haematobia atripalpis*), in which infective larvae develop only in female flies.[26]

Setaria Species in Domestic Animals

Several species of *Setaria* occur in the peritoneal cavity of cattle, horses and pigs.[7] The adult worms are 5-10 cm long and of little pathological significance in their normal host, but can cause severe infections in unnatural hosts, in which the worm migrates abnormally invading the central nervous system and causing cerebrospinal nematodiasis. Outbreaks of *Setaria*, reaching epizootic proportions, have caused the deaths of horses, sheep and goats in Israel and Asia.[7]

S. digitata occurs in the Oriental and eastern Palaearctic regions, and *S. cervi* is worldwide in distribution.[63] One survey in India found just under 50 per cent of *Bos indicus* and *Bos bubalis* infected with *Setaria*, but the infection of *B. indicus* was predominantly (97 per cent) *S. digitata*, and in *B. bubalis* 89 per cent *S. cervi*.[63]

Sheathed microfilariae in the circulating blood are ingested by mosquitoes in which they have the usual filarioid cycle in the thoracic musculature. Third-stage, infective larvae, measuring 2-2.5 mm × 40-50 µm, reach the proboscis in 11 to 13 days at laboratory temperature.[63] Vectors of *S. digitata* include *An sinensis*, *Armigeres obturbans*, *Ae vittatus* and *Ae togoi.*[63]

Other Helminths

Habronemiasis in Horses

Habronema muscae, H. microstoma and *H. megastoma*, are the cause of gastric habronemiasis in horses. The adult worms measure 1-2.5 cm, and those of *H. megastoma* occur in gastric 'tumours', which may cause pyloric obstruction.[7] The other two species can cause inflammation and ulceration but not tumours. When larvae of *Habronema* are deposited in wounds they give rise to cutaneous habronemiasis causing a condition known as summer sores or swamp cancer. Similar lesions may develop on the nictitating membrane, causing conjunctival habronemiasis.[7] Habronemiasis has a worldwide distribution being commoner in warmer, wetter areas, and also in adult horses.[7]

Greenberg[27] has reviewed early work on the transmission of *Habronema*. Larvae are passed out in the faeces of the horse and ingested by muscid larvae, in which they penetrate into the haemocoele where *H. megastoma* develops in the malpighian tubes and *H. muscae* in the fatbody. The infective stage of the worm is reached in the pupal stage of the fly so that newly emerged adults are capable of transmitting the worm.

Horses become infected when they ingest parasitised flies or deposited larvae. Larvae emerge from the fly's proboscis when it is feeding on the lips, nostrils or wounds. Larvae of *H. muscae* readily escape when flies are feeding on horse blood, but not on horse saliva or other media.

H. muscae and *H. megastoma* develop in larvae of *Musca domestica* and those of *H. microstoma* in *Stomoxys calcitrans*. Other species of muscid flies may be involved in transmission, but the suggestion that *M. vetustissima* is a vector is unlikely because this species breeds in cow dung, and its larvae would have no contact with *Habronema*. The behaviour of infected *S. calcitrans* is modified and it feeds on the moist surfaces of the horse and no longer pierces the skin to feed on blood. This behaviour favours deposition of larvae of *H. microstoma* on the skin of the horse where they can develop further.

Thelaziasis

Species of *Thelazia* (*Thelazia*), the eyeworms of mammals, have a worldwide distribution.[7] Greenberg[27] lists five species which inhabit the conjunctival sac and lachrymal ducts of animals, and occasionally occur in man. Infections, which are commoner in cattle than horses, can result in blindness due to opacity of the cornea from abrasion by the rough cuticle of migrating worms. *T. rhodesi* occurs in cattle, sheep and goats in Europe, Asia, Africa and the USA.

T. rhodesi produces larvae in summer (June-September) when muscid vectors are abundant. Larvae, ingested by an adult fly when it feeds at the eye, penetrate to the haemocoele and enter the ovary where they develop to the infective form which moves to the proboscis. Infective larvae escape from the labella when the female fly is feeding on eye secretions. The worm develops in *Musca autumnalis*, *M. larvipara* and other muscids. It is not know to what extent there is any specific association between the species of *Thelazia* and species of muscid. As the vectors are exophilic, infection with *Thelazia* only occurs outdoors. Natural infections of 3 per cent have been found in the vector, and up to 90 per cent of cattle may be infected.[27]

Cestodes with Insect Intermediate Hosts

Dipylidium caninum. *D. caninum* is the commonest parasite of dogs and cats with 72 per cent of racing greyhounds being found infected on post mortem examination.[5] It has a worldwide distribution, occurs in some wild carnivores, and is rarely found in man.[64] *D. caninum* occurs in the small intestine causing anal irritation, digestive disturbances and a subtle nutritional deficiency, but occasionally, heavy infestations produce more severe symptoms with vomiting, convulsions and chronic enteritis.[5,64]

Proglottids of the tapeworm either crawl out of the anus of the host or are passed with the faeces. They move about vigorously expelling egg capsules containing eight to 15 eggs each. These are ingested by the intermediate host, usually larvae of dog or cat fleas, *Ctenocephalides canis* and *Ct. felis.* In the midgut of the flea the eggs give rise to oncospheres with three pairs of hooks, which penetrate to the haemocoele and develop to the infective cysticercoid stage. Further development occurs when the infected flea is swallowed by a suitable host. Development can also occur in the human flea, *Pulex irritans*, and the dog louse, *Trichodectes canis.*[64]

Development of the tapeworm is related to the growth and metamorphosis of the flea. Little growth occurs in the larval flea, but there is a rapid growth in the pupa, and differentiation of the cysticercoid in the adult flea. *D. caninum* causes no mortality of flea larvae but significant mortality of infected flea pupae when the parasite is growing most rapidly.[40]

Hymenolepis nana and H. diminuata. Both *H. nana* and *H. diminuata* have worldwide distributions, occurring predominantly in rodents but also in some monkeys and man. *H. nana* occurs in man, particularly in the tropics and subtropics, and is more pathogenic than *H. diminuata*, the effects of which are mild or inapparent.[64] Intermediate hosts of these cestodes are fleas and flour beetles such as *Tribolium confusum*, but eggs of *H. nana* can also develop in another definitive vertebrate host.[64]

Eggs of *Hymenolepis* ingested by *T. confusum* hatch in the midgut releasing oncospheres which penetrate into the haemocoele where they develop to the infective cysticercoid stage. At 30°C development of *H. nana* is complete in five days and of *H. diminuata* in eight days.[65] When *Hymenolepis* developed in *Ct. felis* there was no correlation between growth of the cestode, and growth and metamorphosis of the flea. Mature cysticercoids were present in both active larvae, and pharate adults in cocoons.[40] Infection occurs when the definitive host ingests an infected intermediate host.

References

1. Bain, O. and Beveridge, I. (1979). Redescription d'*Onchocerca gibsoni* C. et J., 1910. *Annales de Parasitologie Humaine et Comparée 54*: 69-80
2. _____ Muller, R.L., Khamis, Y., Guilhon, J. and Schillhorn van Veen, T. (1976). *Onchocerca raillieti* n.sp. (Filarioidea) chez l'ane domestique en Afrique. *Journal of Helminthology 50*: 287-93
3. _____ Petit, G. and Poulain, B. (1978). Validité des deix espèces *Onchocerca linealis* et *O. gutturosa*, chez les bovins. *Annales de Parasitologie Humaine et Comparée 53*: 421-30
4. _____ Ramachandran, C.P., Petter, F. and Mak, J.W. (1977). Description d'*Onchocerca dewittei* n.sp. (Filariodea) chez *Sus scrofa* en Malaisie. *Annals de Parasitologie Humaine et Comparée 52*: 471-9
5. Beresford-Jones, W.P. and Jacobs, D.E. (1979). Endoparasites. pp. 362-78 in *Canine Medicine and Therapeutics*, Blackwell Scientific Publications, Oxford
6. Beveridge, I., Kummerow, E.L. Wilkinson, P. and Copeman, D.B. (1981). An investigation of biting midges in relation to their potential as vectors of bovine onchocerciasis in north Queensland. *Journal of the Australian Entomological Society 20*: 39-45

7. Blood, D.C., Henderson, J.A. and Radostits, O.M. (1979). *Veterinary Medicine — a Textbook of the Diseases of Cattle, Sheep, Pigs and Horses.* Baillière Tindall, London
8. Buckley, J.J.C. (1934). On the development, in *Culicoides furens* Poey, of *Filaria* (= *Mansonella*) *ozzardi*, Manson, 1897. *Journal of Helminthology 12*: 99-118
9. _____ (1938). On *Culicoides* as a vector of *Onchocerca gibsoni* (Cleland and Johnston, 1910). *Journal of Helminthology 16*: 121-58
10. Chardome, M. and Peel, E. (1949). La répartition des filaires dans la région de Coquilhatville et la transmission de *Dipetalonema streptocerca* par *Culicoides grahamii.* *Annales de la Société Belge Médecine Tropicale 29*: 99-119
11. Clark, G.C. and Hibler, C.P. (1973). Horse flies and *Elaeophora schneideri* in the Gila National Forest, New Mexico. *Journal of Wildlife Diseases 9*: 21-5
12. Connal, A. and Connal, S.L.M. (1922). The development of *Loa loa* (Guyot) in *Chrysops silacea* (Austen) and in *Chrysops dimidiata* (van der Wulp). *Transactions of the Royal Society of Tropical Medicine and Hygiene 16*: 64-89
13. Duke, B.O.L. (1954). The uptake of the microfilariae of *Acanthocheilonema streptocerca* by *Culicoides grahamii* and their subsequent development. *Annals of Tropical Medicine and Parasitology 48*: 416-20
14. _____ (1955). IV. The development of *Loa* in flies of the genus *Chrysops* and the probable significance of the different species in the transmission of loiasis. *Transactions of the Royal Society of Tropical Medicine and Hygiene 49*: 115-21
15. _____ (1955). Studies on the biting habits of *Chrysops.* I. The biting cycle of *Chrysops silacea* at various heights above the ground in the rain-forest at Kumba, British Cameroons. *Annals of Tropical Medicine and Parasitology 49*: 193-202
16. _____ (1955). Studies on the biting habits of *Chrysops.* IV. The dispersal of *Chrysops silacea* over cleared areas from the rain-forest at Kumba, British Cameroons. *Annals of Tropical Medicine and Parasitology 49*: 368-75
17. _____ (1956). The intake of microfilariae of *Acanthocheilonema perstans* by *Culicoides grahamii* and *C. inornatipennis* and their subsequent development. *Annals of Tropical Medicine and Parasitology 50*: 32-8
18. _____ (1958). Studies of the biting habits of *Chrysops.* V. The biting-cycles and infection rates of *C. silacea, C. dimidiata, C. langi* and *C. centurionis* at canopy level in the rain-forest at Bombe, British Cameroons. *Annals of Tropical Medicine and Parasitology 52*: 24-35
19. _____ (1958). The intake of the microfilaria of *Acanthocheilonema streptocerca* by *Culicoides milnei* with some observations on the potentialities of the fly as a vector. *Annals of Tropical Medicine and Parasitology 52*: 123-8
20. _____ (1959). Studies on the biting habits of *Chrysops.* VI. A comparison of the biting habits, monthly biting densities and infection rates of *C. silacea* and *C. dimidiata* (Bombe form) in the rain-forest at Kumba, Southern Cameroons, U.U.K.A. *Annals of Tropical Medicine and Parasitology 53*: 203-14
21. _____ (1960). Studies on the biting habits of *Chrysops.* VII. The biting-cycles of nulliparous and parous *C. silacea* and *C. dimidiata* (Bombe form). *Annals of Tropical Medicine and Parasitology 54*: 147-55
22. _____ (1972). Behavioural aspects of life cycle of *Loa.* pp. 97-107 in *Behavioural Aspects of Parasite Transmission,* E.U. Canning and C.A. Wright (eds.), Academic Press, London
23. Eichler, D.A. (1971). Studies of *Onchocerca gutturosa* (Neumann, 1910) and its development in *Simulium ornatum* (Meigen, 1818). II. Behaviour of *S. ornatum* in relation to the transmission of *O. gutturosa. Journal of Helminthology 45*: 259-70
24. _____ (1973). Studies on *Onchocerca gutturosa* (Neumann, 1910) and its development in *Simulium* (Meigen, 1818). 3. Factors affecting the development of the parasite in its vector. *Journal of Helminthology 47*: 73-88
25. _____ and Nelson, G.S. (1971). Studies on *Onchocerca gutturosa* (Neumann, 1910) and its development in *Simulium ornatum* (Meigen, 1818). I. Observations on *O. gutturosa* in cattle in south-east England. *Journal of Helminthology 45*: 245-58
26. Gnedina, M. and Osipov, A. (1960). Contribution to the biology of *Parafilaria multipapillosa* (Condamine and Drouilly, 1878) parasitic in the horse. *Helminthologia 2*: 13-16

27. Greenberg, B. (1973). *Flies and Disease. II. Biology and Disease Transmission.* Princeton University Press, Princeton
28. Hawking, F. (1975). Circadian and other rhythms in parasites. *Advances in Parasitology 13*: 123-82
29. Henrard, C. and Peel, E. (1949). *Culicoides grahami* Austen. Vecteur de *Dipetalonema streptocerca* et non de *Acanthocheilonema perstans. Annales de la Société Belge Médecine Tropicale 29*: 127-43
30. Heyneman, D. (1973). Nematodes. pp. 203-320 in *Parasites of Laboratory Animals,* R.J. Flynn (ed.), Iowa State University Press, Ames
31. Hibler, C.P. (1966). Development of *Stephanofilaria stilesi* in the horn fly. *Journal of Parasitology 52*: 890-8
32. _____ and Metzger, C.J. (1974). Morphology of the larval stages of *Elaephora schneideri* in the intermediate and definitive hosts with some observations on their pathogenesis in abnormal definitive hosts. *Journal of Wildlife Diseases 10*: 361-9
33. Hopkins, C.A. and Nicholas, W.L. (1952). *Culicoides austeni,* the vector of *Acanthocheilonema perstans. Annals of Tropical Medicine and Parasitology 46*: 276-83
34. Intermill, R.W. (1973). Development of *Dirofilaria immitis* in *Aedes triseriatus* Say. *Mosquito News 33*: 176-81
35. Kabilov, T.K. (1980). New data on biology of *Stephanofilaria assamensis* (Nematoda, Filariata). *Helminthologia 17*: 191-6
36. Kershaw, W.E., Deegan, T., Moore, P.J. and Williams, P. (1956). Studies on the intake of microfilariae by their insect vectors, their survival and their effect on the survival of their vectors. VIII. The size and pattern of the blood-meals taken in by groups of *Chrysops silacea* and *C. dimidiata* when feeding to repletion in natural conditions on a rubber estate in the Niger Delta. *Annals of Tropical Medicine and Parasitology 50*: 95-9
37. Krinsky, W.L. (1976). Animal disease agents transmitted by horse flies and deer flies (Diptera: Tabanidae). *Journal of Medical Entomology 13*: 225-75
38. Lavoipierre, M.M.J. (1958). Studies on the host-parasite relationships of filarial nematodes and their arthropod hosts. 1. The sites of development and the migration of *Loa loa* in *Chrysops silacea,* the escape of the infective forms from the head of the fly, and the effect of the worm on its insect host. *Annals of Tropical Medicine and Parasitology 52*: 103-21
39. Maegraith, B. (1980). *Adams and Maegraith: Clinical Tropical Diseases.* Blackwell Scientific Publications, Oxford
40. Marshall, A.G. (1967). The cat flea, *Ctenocephalides felis felis* (Bouché, 1835) as an intermediate host for cestodes. *Parasitology 57*: 419-30
41. Mellor, P.S. (1974). Studies on *Onchocerca cervicalis* Railliet and Henry 1910: IV. Behaviour of the vector *Culicoides nubeculosus* in relation to the transmission of *Onchocerca cervicalis. Journal of Helminthology 48*: 283-8
42. _____ (1975). Studies on *Onchocerca cervicalis* Railliet and Henry 1910: V. The development of *Onchocerca cervicalis* larvae in the vectors. *Journal of Helminthology 49*: 33-42
43. Moraes, M.A.P. (1976). *Mansonella ozzardi* microfilariae in skin snips. *Transactions of the Royal Society of Tropical Medicine and Hygiene 70*: 16
44. Nathan, M.B. (1981). Transmission of the human filarial parasite *Mansonella ozzardi* by *Culicoides phlebotomus* (Williston) (Diptera: Ceratopogonidae) in coastal north Trinidad. *Bulletin of Entomological Research 71*: 97-105
45. Nayar, J.K. and Sauerman, D.M. (1975). Physiological basis of host susceptibility of Florida mosquitoes to *Dirofilaria immitis. Journal of Insect Physiology 21*: 1965-75
46. Nelson, G.S. (1970). Onchocerciasis. *Advances in Parasitology 8*: 173-224
47. _____ (1978). Mosquito-borne filariasis. pp. 15-25 in *Medical Entomology Centenary Symposium Proceedings,* by S. Willmott (ed.), Royal Society of Tropical Medicine and Hygiene, London
48. Nevill, E.M. (1975). Preliminary report on the transmission of *Parafilaria bovicola* in South Africa. *Onderstepoort Journal of Veterinary Research 42*: 41-8
49. _____ (1979). The experimental transmission of *Parafilaria bovicola* to cattle in South Africa using *Musca* species (subgenus *Eumusca*) as intermediate hosts. *Onderstepoort Journal of Veterinary Research 46*: 51-7

50. Nicholas, W.L., Gordon, R.M. and Kershaw, W.E. (1952). The taking up of microfilariae in the blood by *Culicoides* spp. *Transactions of the Royal Society of Tropical Medicine and Hygiene 46*: 377-8

51. _____ and Kershaw, W.E. (1954). Studies on the intake of microfilariae by their insect vectors, their survival and their effect on the survival of their vectors. III. The intake of microfilariae of *Acanthocheilonema perstans* by *Culicoides austeni* and *C. grahamii*. *Annals of Tropical Medicine and Parasitology 48*: 201-6

52. Omar, M.S., Denke, A.M. and Raybould, J.N. (1979). The development of *Onchocerca ochengi* (Nematoda: Filarioidea) to the infective stage in *Simulium damnosum* s.l. with a note on the histochemical staining of the parasite. *Tropenmedizin und Parasitologie 30*: 157-62

53. Ottley, M.L. and Moorhouse, D.E. (1978). Bovine onchocerciasis: aspects of carcase infection. *Australian Veterinary Journal 54*: 528-30

54. _____ and Moorhouse D.E. (1978). Equine onchocerciasis. *Australian Veterinary Journal 54*: 545

55. _____ and Moorhouse, D.E. (1979). *Onchocerca* (Nematoda: Filarioidea) from Queensland cattle: a redescription of *Onchocerca gibsoni* (Cleland and Johnston) and *O. lienalis* (Stiles). *Zoologischer Anzeiger 203*: 369-77

56. _____ and Moorhouse, D.E. (1980). Laboratory transmission of *Onchocerca gibsoni* by *Forcipomyia (Lasiohelea) townsvillensis*. *Australian Veterinary Journal 56*: 559-60

57. Sasa, M. (1976). *Human Filariasis*. University of Tokyo Press, Tokyo

58. Shamsul, A.V.M. (1971). Biology of *Stephanofilaria assamansis* and the epizootiology of stephanofilariasis of zebu cattle. *Veterinariya 3*: 112-3

59. Sharp, N.A.D. (1928). *Filaria perstans*: its development in *Culicoides austeni*. *Transactions of the Royal Society of Tropical Medicine and Hygiene 21*: 371-96

60. Spratt, D.M. Dyce, A.L. and Standfast, H.A. (1978). *Onchocerca sweetae* (Nematoda: Filarioidea): Notes on the intermediate host. *Journal of Helminthology 52*: 75-81

61. Steward, J.S. (1933). *Onchocerca cervicalis* (Railliet and Henry 1910) and its development in *Culicoides nubeculosus* Mg. *Review of Applied Entomology B 22*: 58-9 (1934)

62. _____ (1937). The occurrence of *Onchocerca gutturosa* Neumann in cattle in England, with an account of its life history and development in *Simulium ornatum* Mg. *Parasitology 29*: 212-9

63. Varma, A.K., Sahai, B.N., Singh, S.P., Lakra, P. and Shrivastava, V.K. (1971). On *Setaria digitata* ; its specific characters, incidence and development in *Aedes vittatus* and *Armigeres obturbans* in India with a note on its ectopic occurrence. *Zeitschrift für Parasitenkunde 36*: 62-72

64. Voge, M. (1973) Cestodes. pp. 155-202 in *Parasites of Laboratory Animals*, R.J. Flynn (ed.), Iowa State University Press, Ames

65. _____ and Heyneman, D. (1957). Development of *Hymenolepis nana* and *Hymenolepis diminuata* (Cestoda: Hymenolepididae) in the intermediate host *Tribolium confusum*. *University of California Publications in Zoology 59*: 549-80

66. Wakelin, D. (1978). Genetic control of susceptibility and resistance to parasitic infections. *Advances in Parasitology 16*: 219-308

67. Wharton, R.H. (1963). Adaptations of *Wuchereria* and *Brugia* to mosquitoes and vertebrate hosts in relation to the distribution of filarial parasites. *Zoonoses Research 2*: 1-12

68. Williams, P. (1981). Studies on Ethiopian *Chrysops* as possible vectors of loiasis. II. *Chrysops silacea* Austen and human loiasis. *Annals of Tropical Medicine and Parasitology 55*: 1-17

69. _____ (1962). The bionomics of the tabanid fauna of streams in the rain-forest of the Southern Cameroons. III. The distribution of immature tabanids at Kumba. *Annals of Tropical Medicine and Parasitology 56*: 149-60

70   Wirth, W.W. (1977). A review of the pathogens and parasites of the biting midges (Diptera: Ceratopogonidae). *Journal of the Washington Acadamy of Science 67*: 60-75

71. Woodman, H.M. (1949). *Filaria* in the Anglo-Egyptian Sudan. *Transactions of the Royal Society of Tropical Medicine and Hygiene 42*: 543-58

72. _____ and Bokhari, A. (1941). Studies on *Loa loa* and the first report of *Wuchereria bancrofti* in the Sudan. *Transactions of the Royal Society of Tropical Medicine and Hygiene 35*: 77-92

SUBJECT INDEX

Note: numbers in italic type represent pages on which illustrations appear.